Color Atlas of Urologic Surgery

Color Atlas of Urologic Surgery

Abraham T.K. Cockett, M.D.

Professor of Urology, Department of Urology, Univerity of Rochester Medical Center, Rochester, NY

Ken Koshiba, M.D.

Professor and Chairman, Department of Urology, Kitasato University School of Medicine, Sagamihara, Japan
Director, Kitasato Institute Medical Center Hospital, Kitamoto, Japan

SANS TACHE

Williams & Wilkins
A WAVERLY COMPANY

BALTIMORE • PHILADELPHIA • LONDON • PARIS • BANGKOK
BUENOS AIRES • HONG KONG • MUNICH • SYDNEY • TOKYO • WROCLAW

Executive Editor: Carroll C. Cann
Managing Editor: Susan Hunsberger
Production Coordinator: Peter J. Carley
Book Project: Jennifer D. Weir
Designer: Arlene Putterman
Illustration Planner: Peter J. Carley
Cover Designer: Arlene Putterman
Typesetter: Maryland Composition
Printer: Walsworth Publishing
Digitized Illustrations: Maryland Composition
Binder: Walsworth Publishing

351 West Camden Street
Baltimore, Maryland 21201-2436 USA

Rose Tree Corporate Center
1400 North Providence Road
Building II, Suite 5025
Media, Pennsylvania 19063-2043 USA

Accurate indications, adverse reactions, and dosage schedules for drugs are provided in this book, but it is possible that they may change. The reader is urged to review the package information data of the manufacturers of the medications mentioned.

Printed in the United States of America

First Edition,

Library of Congress Cataloging-in-Publication Data

Cockett, Abraham T. K., 1928-
Color atlas of urologic surgery / Abraham T. K. Cockett, Ken Koshiba.
p. cm.
Rev. ed. of: Manual of urologic surgery / Abraham T. K. Cockett, Ken Koshiba.c1979.
Includes bibliographical references and index.
ISBN 0-683-02045-5
1. Genitourinary organs—Surgery—Atlases. I. Koshiba, Ken, 1932- . II. Cockett, Abraham T. K., 1928- Manual of urologic surgery. III. Title.
[DNLM: 1. Urogenital System—surgery—atlases 2. Urogenital Diseases—surgery—atlases. WJ 17 C666c 1996]
RD571.C63 1996
617.4′6—dc20
DNLM/DLC
for Library of Congress 96-13528
CIP

The publishers have made every effort to trace the copyright holders for borrowed material. If they have inadvertently overlooked any, they will be pleased to make the necessary arrangements at the first opportunity.

To purchase additional copies of this book, call our customer service department at **(800) 638-0672** or fax orders to **(800) 447-8438.** For other book services, including chapter reprints and large quantity sales, ask for the Special Sales department.

Canadian customers shall call **(800) 268-4178,** or fax **(905) 470-6780.** For all other calls originating outside the United States, please call **(410) 528-4223** or fax us at **(410) 528-8550.**

Visit Williams & Wilkins on the Internet: **http://www.wwilkins.com** or contact our customer service department at **custserv@wwilkins.com**. Williams & Wilkins customer service representatives are available from 8:30 am to 6:00 pm, EST, Monday through Friday, for telephone access.

96 97 98 99
1 2 3 4 5 6 7 8 9 10

This color Atlas is dedicated to ***Elmer Belt, MD,***
an excellent surgeon and humanitarian,
and to ***Willard E. Goodwin, MD,***
our Professor and teacher who provided the environment
and the support in the early years of our residency at UCLA.

We also dedicate the manual to our wives, ***Willia Cockett*** *and* ***Kiyo Koshiba,***
who assisted materially and editorially in the preparation of this atlas.
They provided encouragement and editorial assistance
as we labored diligently for 15 years, frequently exchanging
color photographs, sketches, illustrations,
and comments across a distance of 9000 miles.

Foreword

The color photographs and illustrations appearing in select monographs over the past decade represent a significant advance in surgical communication. Previously, black and white renderings were standard because color printing had not been perfected and its cost was prohibitive. We believe the gradual change from black and white etchings and reproductions to detailed color illustrations represents a tremendous twentieth century achievement.

In our own urologic practices it became evident that the use of black and white sketches for teaching operative urology, while helpful, left too much to the surgeon's imagination. Even the dimension of depth, produced by varying the intensity of shading, often was inadequate in demonstrating subtle surgical details in a fossa or bed.

Since color photography recently has been used to demonstrate operative techniques, we climbed on the bandwagon and photographed in color many of the major operative procedures. However, the reflection of light caused by normal tissue fluid significantly reduces the clarity of photographs. Not infrequently, the crucial operative step is obscured by light reflected on a trickle of blood. Even when meticulous care is taken to irrigate and clean the surgical field, the tissue sheen obscures portions of the field. Color paintings by a gifted artist are not only unique, but can be extraordinary; the vividness with which subtleties can thus be portrayed cannot be matched by photography, black and white or color.

We have carefully selected the new procedures in this text. Laparoscopy, percutaneous lithotripsy, and the new surgical procedures such as the Walsh technique for preservation of the neurovascular bundles at the time of radical retropubic prostatectomy are included.

The illustrations and the descriptions in writing should materially assist the urologic resident in training. We learned from the Surgical Operating Supervisors at UCLA and the Peter Bent Brigham Hospitals that the first edition of our manual needed to be chained outside the urologic operating room. The color illustrations and descriptions provided a quick review for the urologic surgeon performing the major urological procedures.

A.T.K. Cockett
K. Koshiba

Preface

Since the publication of our first "Manual of Urologic Surgery" in 1979, a significant number of advances have occurred in Urology. During this interval we have seen renal transplantation programs in Urology expand in number. The addition of cyclosporine to the standard regimen of azathioprine and corticosteroids has improved the survival rates of renal allografts in the recipient population. We include several vascular modifications when harvesting kidneys. Incorporating the donor's vena cava to extend renal vein length, particularly when the right renal allograft is used, is an important advance first described by John Barry.

The prostate gland. BPH and prostate cancer have generated significant research and clinical studies warranting a revision of our first text. Today prostate cancer—Gleason grade 5 to 7—is the indication for radical retropubic prostatectomy. When moderate undifferentiated cancer is located within the capsule, 12 to 15 year surgical cure rates are possible. The neurovascular bundles are clearly demonstrated in the retropubic surgical approach, which we describe in detail. Preservation of potency is important.

BPH has attracted the attention of Urologists worldwide. The American Urological Association Symptom Score, which was tested, retested, and validated by Mike Barry and other urologists, including this author (ATKC), has provided a framework for clinical studies. The added question for "bothersomeness" is also important and an impact index is now validated. The classical operation—TURP—is still a very effective procedure. We have avoided illustrating new, non-FDA approved procedures focusing on devices or new technologies. Even the prostatic vaporizing procedure, while promising, does not leave any prostatic tissue available for histology in older men. Clinical research studies have demonstrated the efficacy of two medications. Until the effectiveness of new devices to treat BPH are proven by randomized studies using TURP as the standard, the FDA will not sanction approval of these experimental devices, since 1 year of follow-up data are required in both groups. At present, the new devices are undergoing clinical studies. Finasteride, a 5 alpha-reductase blocker of dihydrotestosterone (DHT), reduces prostate size by 20% after 1 year of treatment due to a marked reduction of this potent androgen. Five mg of finasteride daily reduces epithelial cell hyperplasia. Since PSA is intimately associated with the epithelial cells and the neuroendocrine cells nearby, the PSA is reduced by 50% after 1 year of therapy. The Symptom Score improves and urinary flow rates increase by 2.1–2.5 mL/sec.

Professor Koshiba and coworkers have had excellent experience with VLAP for prostatic ablation in men with BPH. Local anesthesia is employed and VLAP can be performed in an office setting.

Alpha blockers are also effective in relaxing the smooth muscles in the stroma of the prostate gland. The alpha blockers, terazosin and doxazosin, have demonstrated greater efficacy then prazosin and several studies have demonstrated an improvement in urinary flow of nearly 2.0–3.0 cc per second.

Many of the classical surgical procedures focusing on the kidney, ureter, and bladder have been retained. In many countries worldwide, nephrectomies, ureteral reconstructive surgery, and bladder surgery are still important when the clinical indications are demonstrated by CT scans, biopsies, or by other noninvasive radiologic or ultrasonic tests.

A new section on laparoscopy is included. The basic approaches to the kidney for percutaneous nephrostomy, dilatation, and stone extraction or nephroscopic lithotripsy are also included.

Following cystectomy for infiltrative bladder carcinoma, we now have quite an array of procedures for continent urinary diversion. The major continent diversions available are included in this text. The reader will appreciate the color illustrations and the step-by-step techniques.

Urethra and bladder. Urethral reconstructive procedures in the female for urinary incontinence are expanded. Even while collagen injections into the bladder neck are being performed and evaluated in some women with stress incontinence, our color atlas focuses on the newer surgical procedures to correct urinary incontinence.

We have retained the classical procedures for urethroplasty in the male. In our travels around the world, we noted that in Egypt and China, traumatic injuries or strictures secondary to specific infections still occur. This color atlas will materially assist the neophyte urologist in reconstructive surgery, particularly overseas.

Endourology. Percutaneous nephrolithotripsy is described in great detail. The anatomic approach is carefully described. The intrarenal arterial blood supply is illustrated. The use of ultrasonic devices to fragment stones in the upper calyces is also described. The rocket wire technique for retrograde nephrostomy is described for percutaneous removal of calculi in the calyces.

Laparoscopy. Laparoscopic surgery is still one of the most difficult of all the procedures to master, particularly for the urologist who uses the technique infrequently. Today, with proper skills, laparoscopic surgery can replace open surgery for selected procedures. We describe several procedures including laparoscopy for an undescended testicle in this Atlas. Varicocelectomy for male infertility is also illustrated.

We believe that you will appreciate the new procedures and advances that have occurred over the past 15 years in this color atlas. Residents in training will also benefit from the illustrations in this color atlas.

Acknowledgments

The authors wish to thank Lora Tiede for her excellent assistance in the preparation of this text. The editorial assistance of Willia Cockett is again acknowledged.

The authors also thank Isao Takamoto for his beautiful color anatomic renditions. The color renditions clearly illustrate the surgical steps in the major urological operations.

Contents

The Kidney

1

Surgical Anatomy

LOCALIZATION AND FASCIAL RELATIONSHIPS

The kidneys are located in the retroperitoneal space at the level of the upper lumbar region and lie on each side of the spinal column (Fig. 1). The upper half of each kidney lies within the bony thorax. The right kidney is normally at a slightly lower level than the left because of the right hepatic lobe.

The area surrounding the left kidney is quadrilateral in shape, bounded by the 12th rib, iliac crest, vertebral column, and an imaginary vertical line extending upward from the anterior superior iliac spine.

The superficial fascia is arranged between two layers, and the muscles in this region are in three groups:

1. Superficial—the latissimus dorsi and external abdominis oblique;
2. Middle—the posterior inferior serratus, sacrospinalis, and internal abdominis oblique; and
3. Deep—the quadratus lumborum muscle of the loins, the psoas major, and the transverse abdominis muscle.

The latissimus dorsi muscle originates from the lower six thoracic vertebrae, all lumbar and upper sacral spinal processes, and also from the supraspinous ligament as it merges with the posterior layer of the lumbodorsal fascia. It derives from fleshy fibers at the outer lip of the iliac crest posteriorly, the last four ribs, and, at times, the inferior angle of the scapula. It inserts as a tendon into the floor of the intertubercular sulcus on the humerus.

The anatomic details of the external oblique muscle are discussed in the Operative Techniques section later in this chapter.

The posterior inferior serratus muscle merges with the lumbar fascia and, thus, attaches to upper lumbar and lower thoracic spinal processes. It is beneath the latissimus dorsi and passes upward and transversely to ribs 9–12. This muscle depresses these four ribs. Its lowest fibers lie superficial to the posterior lumbocostal ligament that overlies the lowermost pleural border. Incisions in this area can lead to a pneumothorax as a result of entry into the pleura.

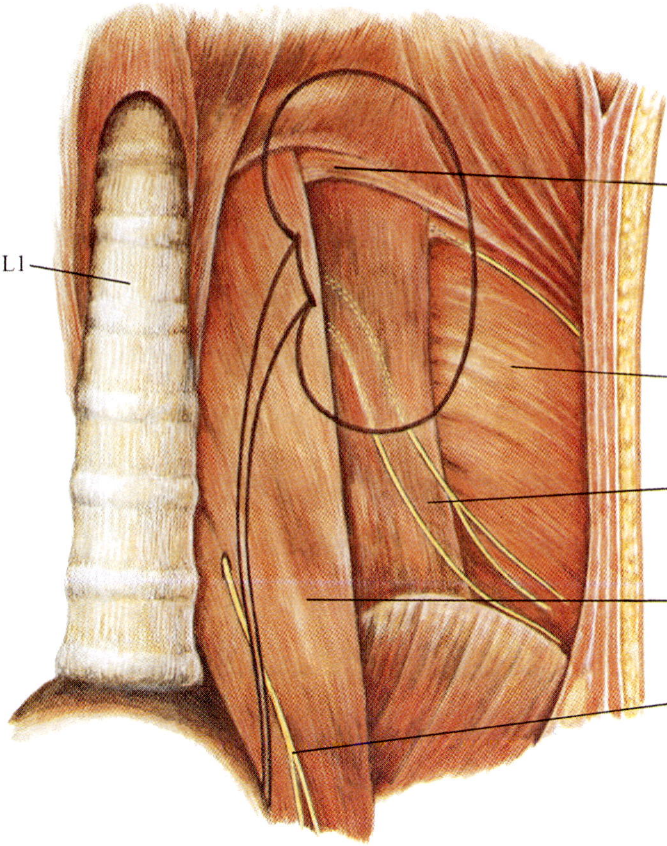

FIG. 1.
Normal anatomic relationships of the kidney.

The sacrospinalis muscles are elongated and comprise a group extending from the dorsal sacrum and posterior iliac crest. The group is surrounded by the aponeurotic sheath formed by the posterior and middle layers of lumbodorsal fascia. It has three subdivisions: the iliocostal, the most lateral; the longissimus, the widest and bulkiest; and the spinalis muscle, the most medial and shortest.

The internal oblique muscle arises from the iliac crest and inferior part of the lumbodorsal fascia. It forms the floor of Petit's triangle. Its origin and insertion in relation to exposure of the left kidney are discussed in the Operative Techniques section.

The quadratus muscle of the loins is a flat muscle lying lateral to the psoas. It arises from the fifth lumbar transverse process to the posterior part of the iliac crest and the iliolumbar ligament. It inserts into the lower border of the 12th rib. The anterior and middle layers of the lumbodorsal fascia surround this muscle. The anterior layer of the lumbodorsal fascia separates the muscle from the transversalis fascia.

The psoas major is considered an upward migration of the iliac muscle. It occupies the trough between the transverse processes and the bodies of the lumbar vertebrae.

Figure 5 describes the transversus abdominis muscle.

The right kidney's anterior surface is related to: the liver superiorly, the descending part of the duodenum near the kidney hilus, and the hepatic flexure of the colon inferiorly (Fig. 2). The left kidney is adjacent to the stomach superiorly, to the spleen laterally, to the tail of the pancreas near the kidney hilus, and to the splenic flexure of colon inferiorly. Both kidneys are capped by adrenal glands. The gastric and splenic surfaces are covered by peritoneum, as is the hepatic surface, except for a bare fibrotic area attaching to the posterior wall.

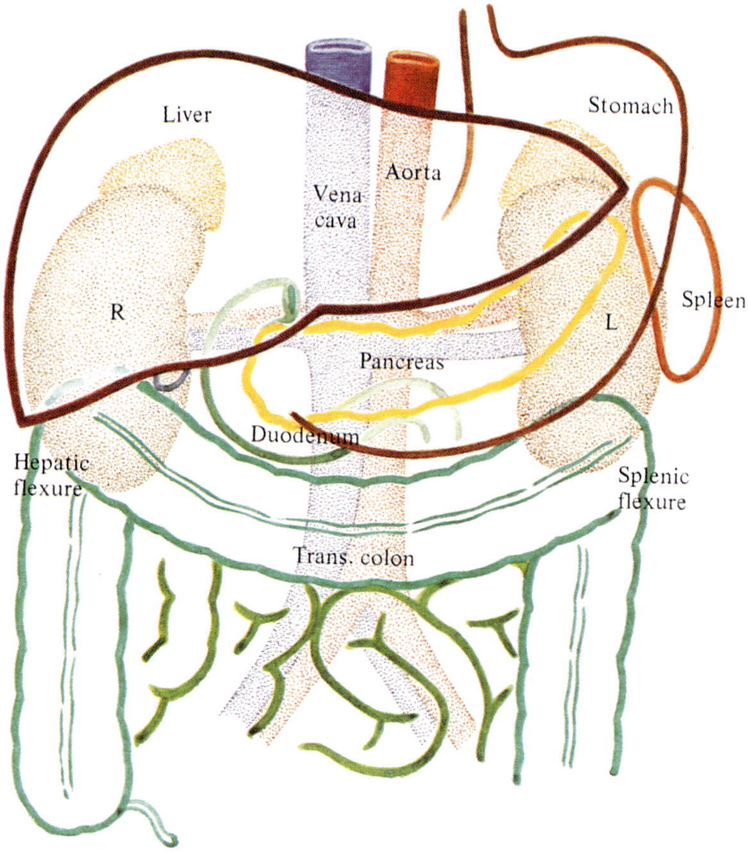

FIG. 2.
The kidney's anterior surface.

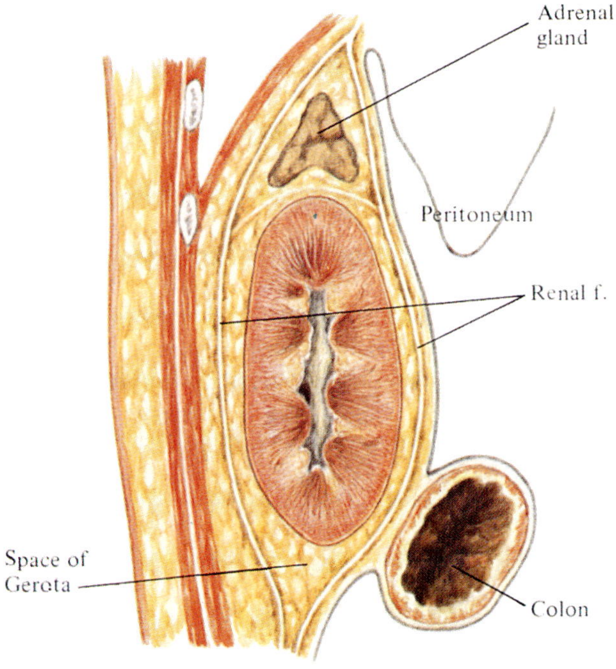

FIG. 3.
Capsule of Gerota, enclosing the kidney, adrenal gland, renal vessels, ureter, and perirenal fat.

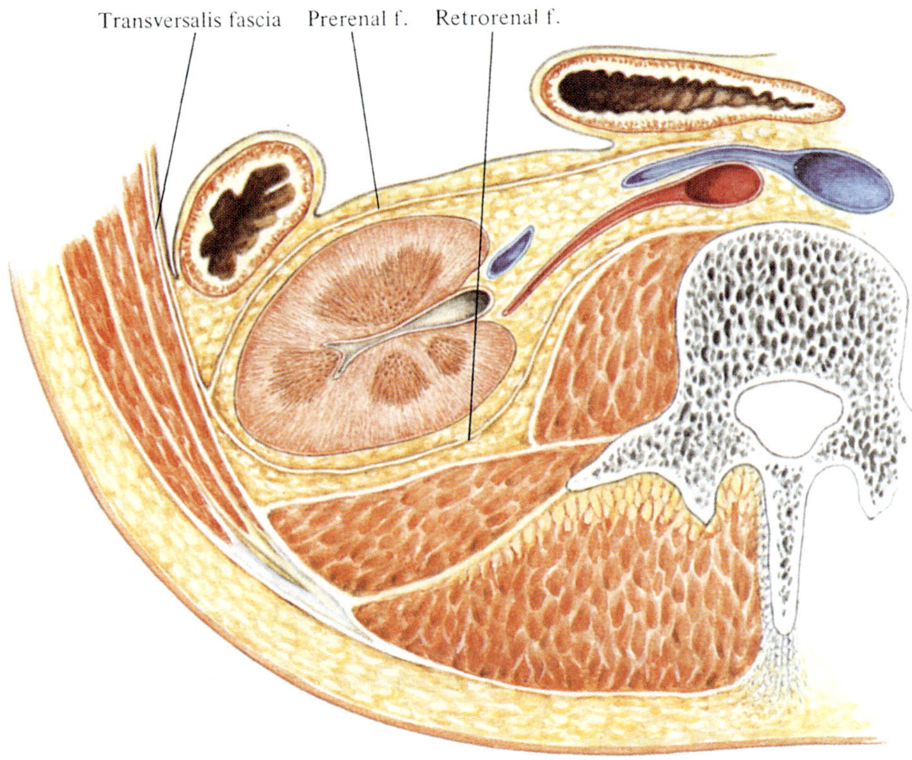

FIG. 4.
A cross section of the mid-left kidney, revealing anatomic relationships.

The transversalis fascia splits into anterior prerenal and posterior retrorenal fascial layers, forming the capsule of Gerota that encloses the kidney, adrenal gland, renal vessels, ureter, and perirenal fat (Fig. 3). These two layers of fascia fuse at the upper pole of the kidney and adrenal gland, but remain open inferiorly and medially. Within this fascial space, the kidney is slightly movable in a thin person.

The lumbodorsal fascia has three layers: anterior, middle, and posterior. The posterior and middle layers are dense and strong. The posterior layer arises from tips of the lumbar, sacral, and thoracic vertebrae. The middle layer arises from the transverse processes of the lumbar vertebrae. The anterior layer arises from the anterior surfaces of the lumbar transverse processes near their roots. The psoas fascia begins from this layer.

As the three layers continue laterally, they fuse near the outer border of the quadratus lumborum. This merger forms a dense tendinous structure—the aponeurosis (origin) of the transversus abdominis muscle. The aponeurosis gives rise, in part, to the internal oblique muscle. Between the posterior and middle layers of lumbodorsal fascia is the sacrospinal muscle group. The quadratus muscle of the loins is between the middle and anterior layer. A cross section of the mid-left kidney (Fig. 4) reveals the full anatomic relationships.

THREE MUSCLE LAYERS

The external abdominal oblique muscle arises from the lower eight ribs (Fig. 5A)(5–12). It inserts on the anterior half of the iliac crest. *Fascia covering this muscle extends* from the anterior border of Petit's triangle *between the 12th rib and the iliac crest.* The external oblique aponeurosis forms the inguinal and Cooper's ligaments. The free posterior border is located at the midpoint of the iliac crest.

The internal oblique muscle is a fan-shaped muscle with a narrow origin and a

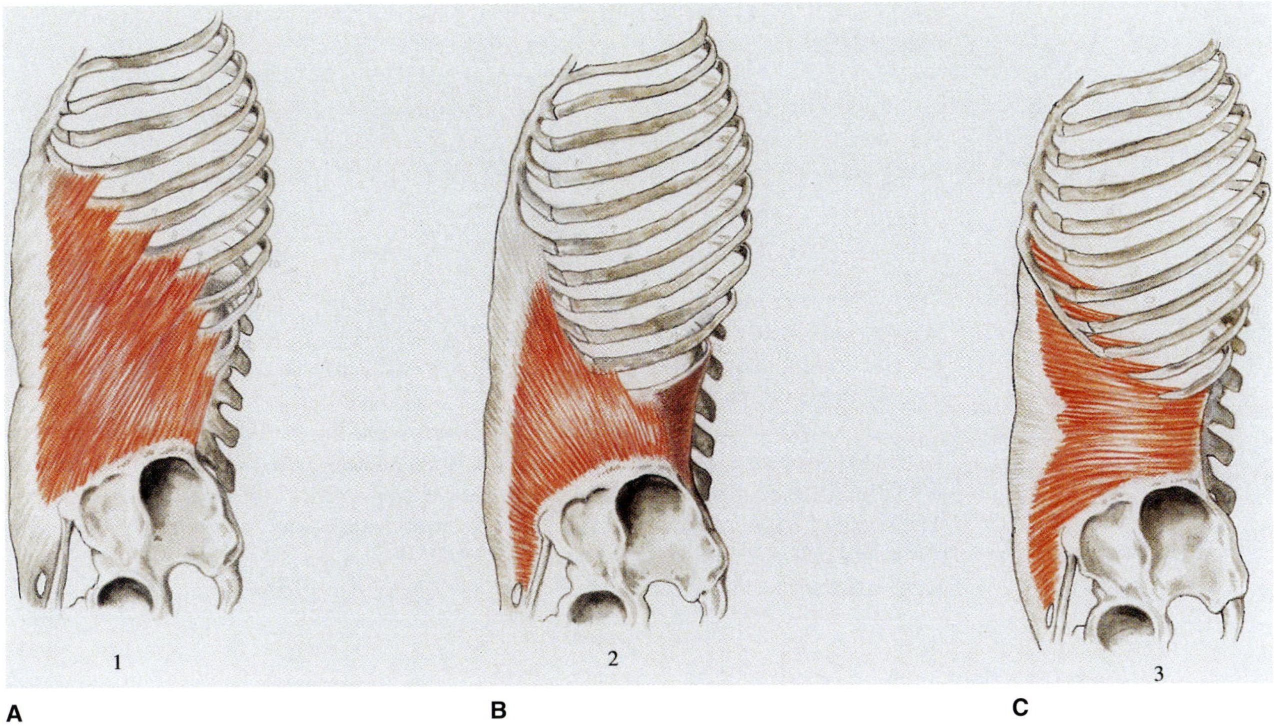

FIG. 5.
Three muscle layers.

broad insertion (Fig. 5B). It lies between the external oblique and transversus abdominis muscles, and it originates from the outer half of the inguinal ligament, the intermediate line on the iliac crest, and the posterior lamella of the lumbodorsal fascia.

This muscle has no free posterior border. The uppermost fibers run vertically upward into the lower four ribs and other cartilages. The intermediate fibers form an aponeurosis at the line of Douglas. Above the semicircular line it divides into two lamellae at the lateral wall of the rectus muscles. The anterior wall of the rectus sheath consists of the aponeurosis of the external oblique and the anterior layer of the internal oblique aponeurosis. The posterior rectus sheath or wall is made up of the posterior layer of the internal oblique aponeurosis, the aponeurosis of the transversus abdominal muscle, and the transversalis fascia. Below the line of Douglas, the combined aponeuroses of all three lateral abdominal muscles fuse and pass in front of the rectus muscle as the anterior rectus sheath. Its fibers in the flank region run at right angles to the more superficial external oblique muscle.

The internal oblique muscle is now incised, exposing the transversus abdominis muscle and lumbodorsal fascia (Fig. 5C).

The transversus abdominis muscle is the deepest of the three lateral abdominal muscles. It originates from the outer third of the inguinal ligament, from the inner lip of the iliac crest, from the middle layer of the lumbodorsal fascia, and from the inner surface of the lower six costal cartilages. Insertion is to the linea alba and through the conjoined tendon into the pubic crest. Its fibers, in the main, are directed horizontally. The aponeurosis passes behind the rectus muscle to the level of the line of Douglas. Below this level it passes in front of the rectus.

Transversalis fascia (endoabdominal fascia) covers the entire internal surface of the abdomen. The fascia covers certain muscles and assumes its name from that muscle. Below the inferior margins of the internal oblique and transversus abdominis muscles, the fascia is well developed. It forms the floor of Hesselbach's triangle; weakness leads to a direct inguinal hernia. It lies between transversus abdominis muscle and the properitoneal fat layer. In lean patients, it adheres to the parietal peritoneum as one layer.

Care should be taken to preserve the 12th thoracic and first lumbar nerves coursing between the internal oblique and the transversus abdominis muscles. A window is made in the lumbodorsal fascia to facilitate blunt separation of the transversus abdominis.

GROSS STRUCTURE

The kidney is bean-shaped, reddish-brown in color, slightly soft in consistency, and covered by the capsule, a fibrous membrane that strips easily from the normal kidney (Fig. 6). The adult kidney is 9- to 12-cm long, 4.5- to 6.5-cm wide, and 3- to 4-cm thick. It weighs about 110 to 140 g.

The kidney parenchyma consists of the cortex and the medulla. The cortex is thinner than the medulla, about 4- to 5-mm thick, and contains the glomeruli and convoluted tubules. The medulla is composed of 8 to 15 striated, conical masses called pyramids. The bases of the pyramids are continuous with the cortex, and their apexes project into the minor calices of the renal pelvis. The tips of the apexes are called the papillae and have openings for the papillary ducts forming the cribriform plate.

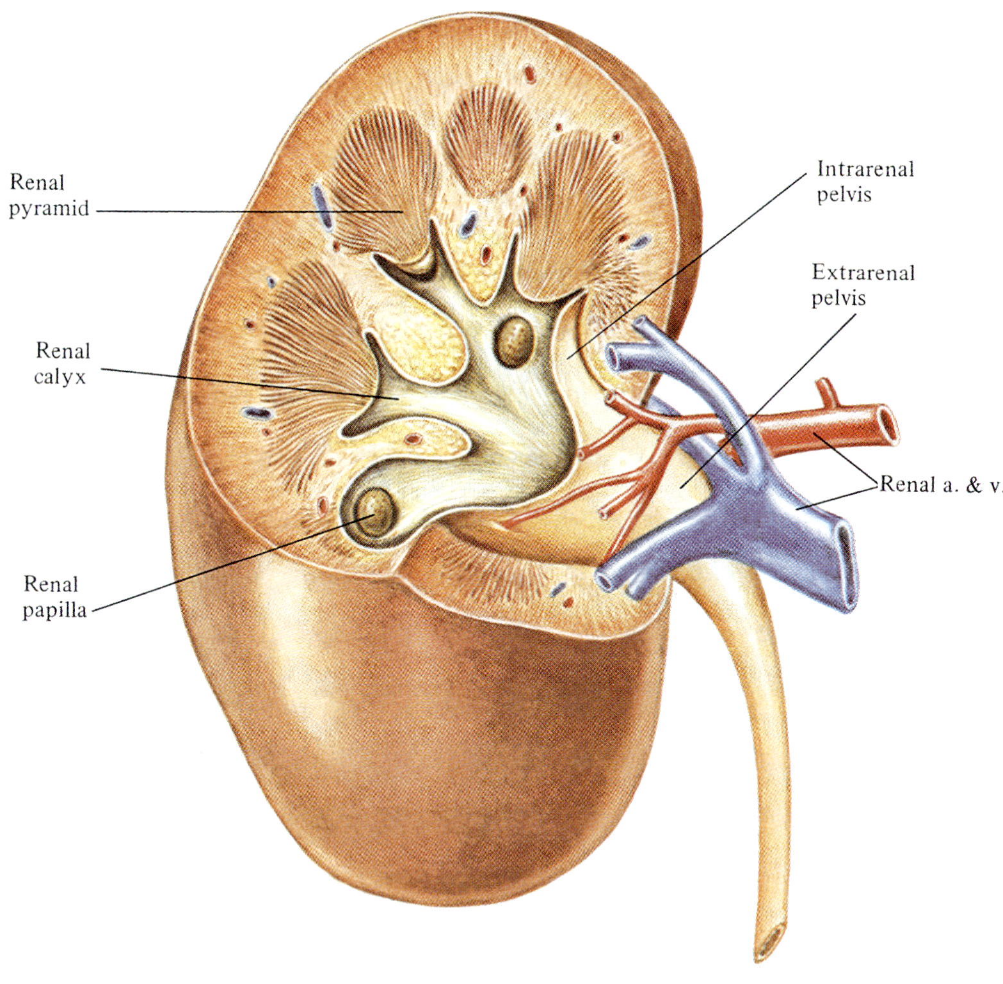

FIG. 6.
Gross structure of kidney.

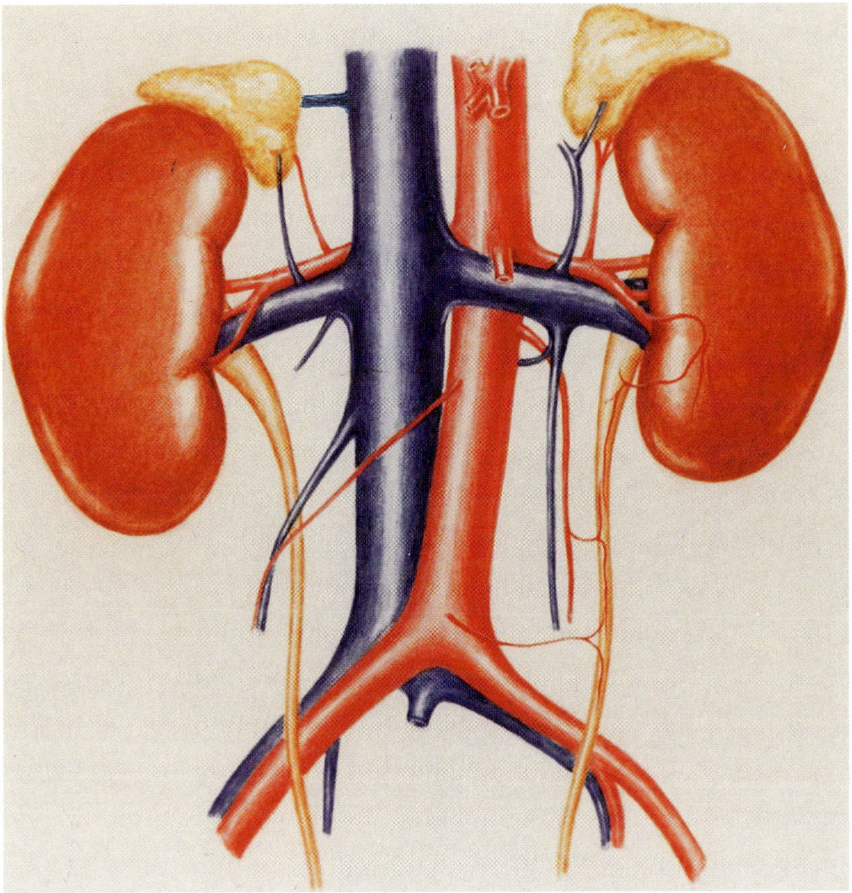

FIG. 7.
Vascular supply to the kidney.

Minor calices join to form two or three major calices and open into a single cavity called the intrarenal pelvis. The extrarenal pelvis is funnel-shaped, situated at the hilus of the kidney, and joins the ureter at the ureteropelvic junction.

VASCULAR SUPPLY

The renal arteries arise laterally from the abdominal aorta just below the superior mesenteric artery and pass laterally to each kidney (Fig. 7). The right renal artery courses behind the inferior vena cava and is longer than the left artery. The renal artery may divide into major branches before entering the kidney hilus. It also sends some branches to the adrenal gland and ureter. Accessory renal arteries may branch from the aorta and enter the kidney near the upper or lower pole. Occasionally, the inferior accessory artery passes behind the ureter and interferes with urinary drainage from the kidney. These accessory branches may cause troublesome bleeding if unrecognized during surgery.

The renal veins lie anterior to the accompanying arteries and anastomose freely. The left renal vein courses anterior to the aorta, and is longer than the right vein. The left ovarian or spermatic vein joins the left renal vein, whereas the right empties directly into the inferior vena cava. Duplication of the left renal vein is rare; however, the right renal vein may be single, double, or triple, and is shorter than the left vein. The vena cava lies in close proximity to the right kidney and can be injured if it is unrecognized and traumatized when the kidney is mobilized during surgery. Accessory renal veins are infrequent. Accessory renal arteries are not usually accompanied by veins.

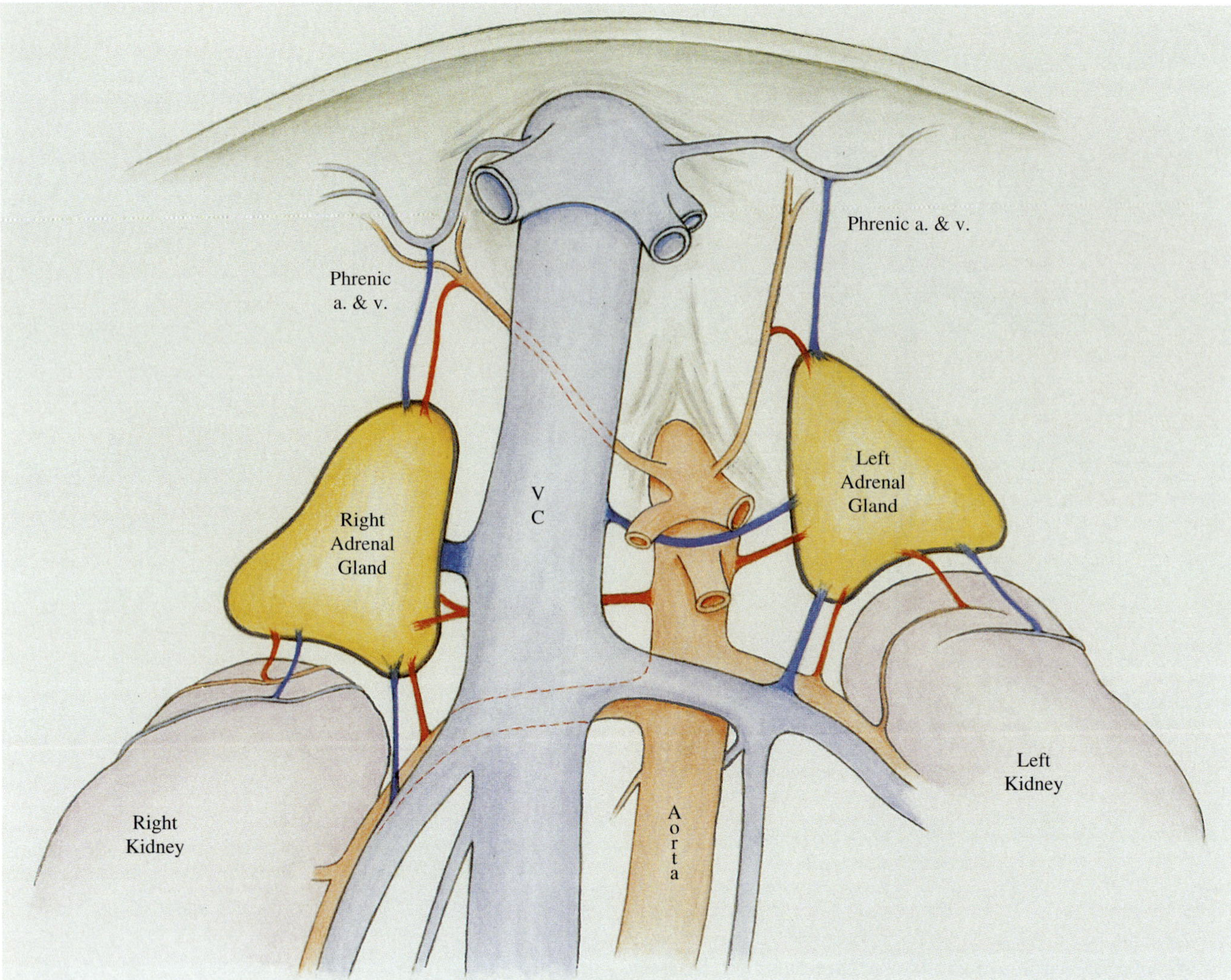

FIG. 8.
The definitive blood supply derived from the renal vessels, aorta, vena cava, and the superior branches from the phrenic vessels, and from superficial renal vessels.

BLOOD SUPPLY TO THE ADRENAL GLANDS

Figure 8 illustrates the blood supply to both adrenal glands. From a surgical standpoint, a right adrenalectomy as part of a radical nephrectomy is a concern to the surgeon since there is a significant venous connection between the medial aspect of the right adrenal gland and the vena cava lying superior to the renal veins. This significant communication with the vena cava, if unrecognized, can cause significant bleeding. At the time of a right radical nephrectomy for cancer, the possibility exists that the connection between the vena cava and the right adrenal gland can be severed or traumatically disrupted. The surgeon should keep in mind that exposure is often difficult in this region and the surgeon should carefully dissect and look for this adrenal vein connection as demonstrated. Careful ligation of this vein without disruption of the adjacent structures can help to maintain a bloodless field.

On the left side, the adrenal gland does not have such a major connection and the left radical nephrectomy, including adrenalectomy, can proceed with dispatch. The venous connections on the left side are shown. One can usually find an artery and vein running together, as the illustration depicts. There is a venous communication from the

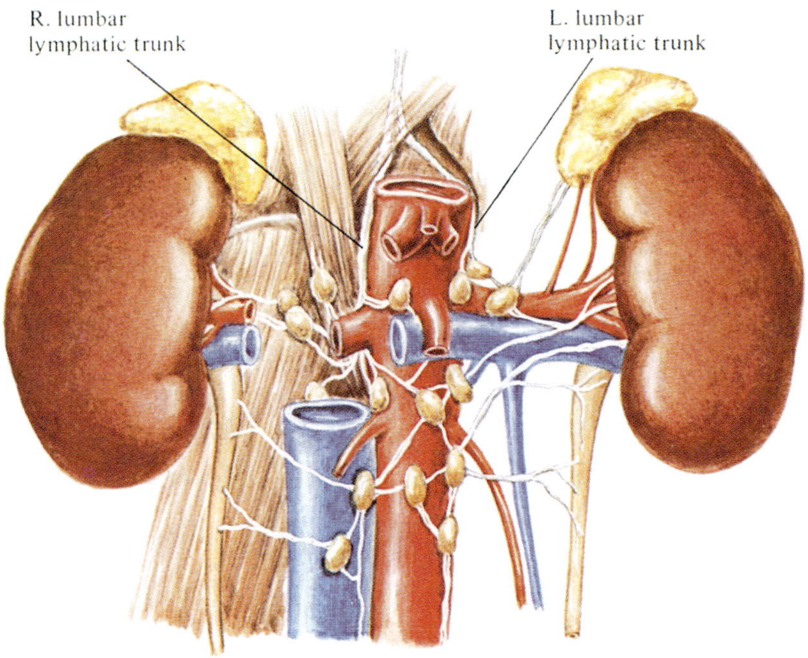

FIG. 9.
Lymphatic network of the kidney.

adrenal vein to the left renal vein. A second connection to the vena cava and, at times, a phrenic or diaphragmatic connection may be encountered. This venous connection to the diaphragm may be bilateral.

LYMPHATIC NETWORK

The intrarenal lymphatics within the renal parenchyma consist of a cortical and a medullary network and drain into lymph nodes surrounding the renal pedicle (Fig. 9). The lymphatics emerge from the hilus via larger trunks. From there they drain into retrocaval trunks in the region of the inferior vena cava and aorta. The extrarenal lymphatic network of the kidney communicates freely with the adrenal gland lymphatics and periureteral sheath.

Cortical lymphatics at the outer renal cortex communicate with the lymphatics of the renal capsule. The lymphatics at the inner cortex and corticomedullary junction course through the medulla to the hilar network.

NERVE SUPPLY

The kidneys are supplied with sympathetic and parasympathetic nerves (Fig. 10). Sympathetic fibers are derived from the greater and lesser splanchnic nerves and pass to the renal plexus via the celiac and superior mesenteric ganglia. Parasympathetic fibers also course to the kidney. The majority of nerve fibers run along the renal artery to the kidney, along the upper, lower, and posterior aspects of the artery. They are adherent to the distal portion of the renal artery. A few nerve fibers are received directly from the solar plexus and course as splanchnic nerves to the kidney and its capsule.

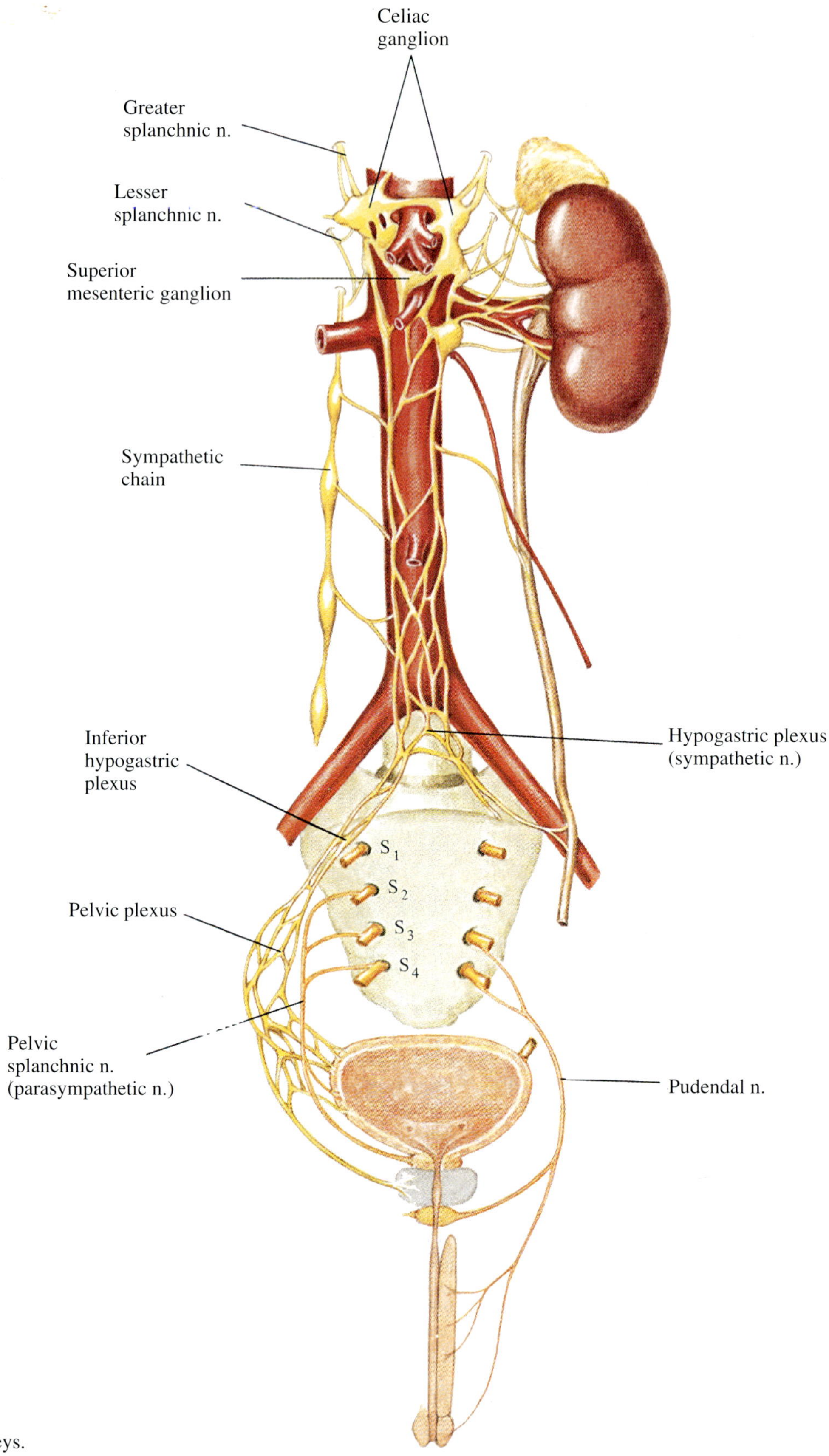

FIG. 10.
Autonomic nerve supply to kidneys.

Operative Techniques

1. Lumbar-Flank Approach

1-1. After the induction of anesthesia and insertion of an endotracheal tube, *the patient is positioned on his or her side* with the appropriate kidney exposed. The surgical table is flexed to place tension at the incision site. Adhesive tape (3-inch) can be placed at the hip and shoulder to secure the position. The arm is elevated on a horizontal plane. The knees should be protected.

1-2. The *line of incision can be made below the 12th rib* or over the distal half of the 12th rib. It is carried through the skin and subcutaneous fat, exposing the external oblique muscle. If rib resection is required, the incision is extended over the body of the 12th rib.

1-3. *A lumbar incision, left anterior oblique approach, can be used* as an alternative to the approach seen in 1–1. Ribs 10, 11, and 12 are depicted for orientation.

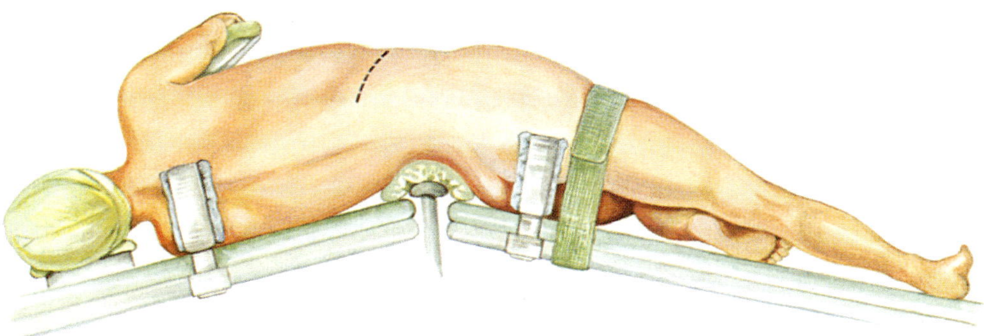

1-1

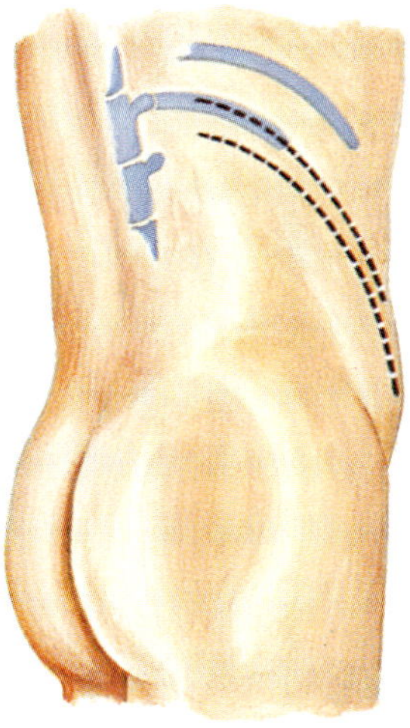

1-2

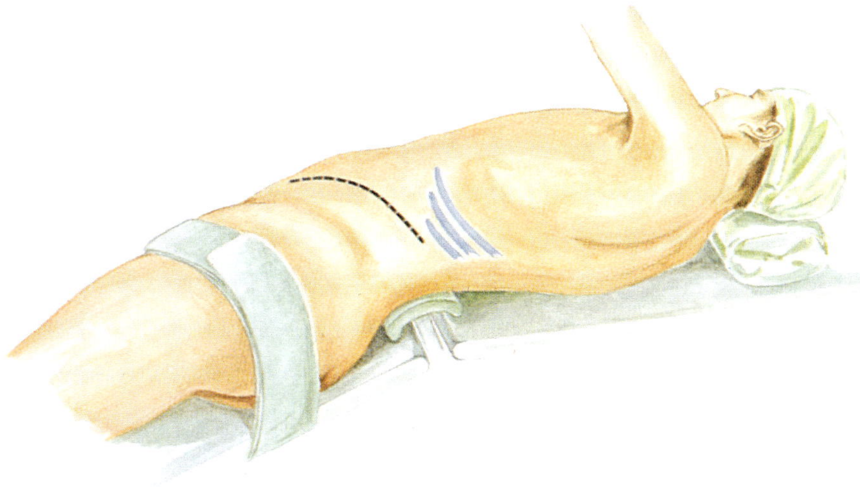

1-3

Exposure of Left Kidney

1-4. Skin and subcutaneous bleeders are secured. *The incision is carried* in depth *to obtain exposure of the external oblique muscle.* The external abdominal oblique muscle arises from the lower eight ribs. It inserts on the anterior half of the iliac crest. *Fascia covering this muscle extends* from the anterior border of Petit's triangle *between the 12th rib and the iliac crest.* The external oblique aponeurosis forms the inguinal and Cooper's ligaments. The free posterior border is located at the midpoint of the iliac crest.

1-5. *The internal oblique muscle is a fan-shaped muscle* with a narrow origin and a broad insertion. It lies between the external oblique and transversus abdominis muscle and originates from the outer half of the inguinal ligament, the intermediate line on the iliac crest, and the posterior lamella of the lumbodorsal fascia.

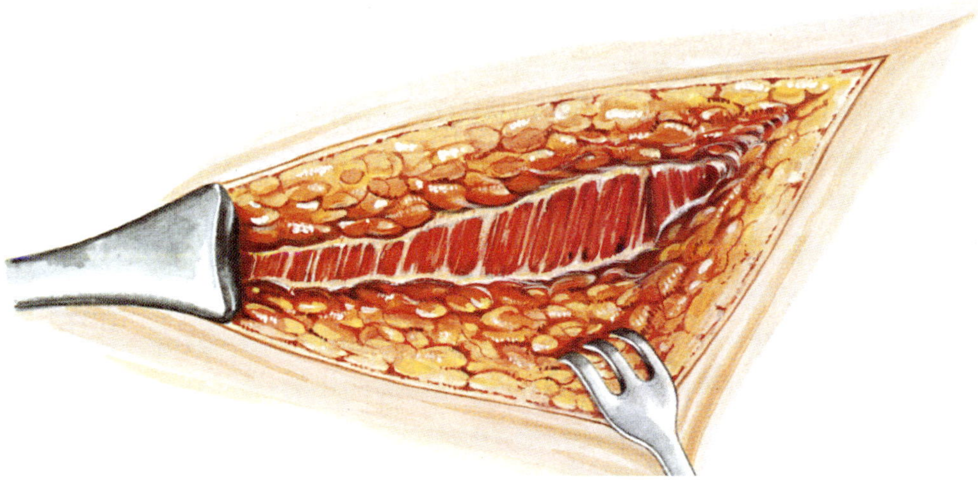

1-4

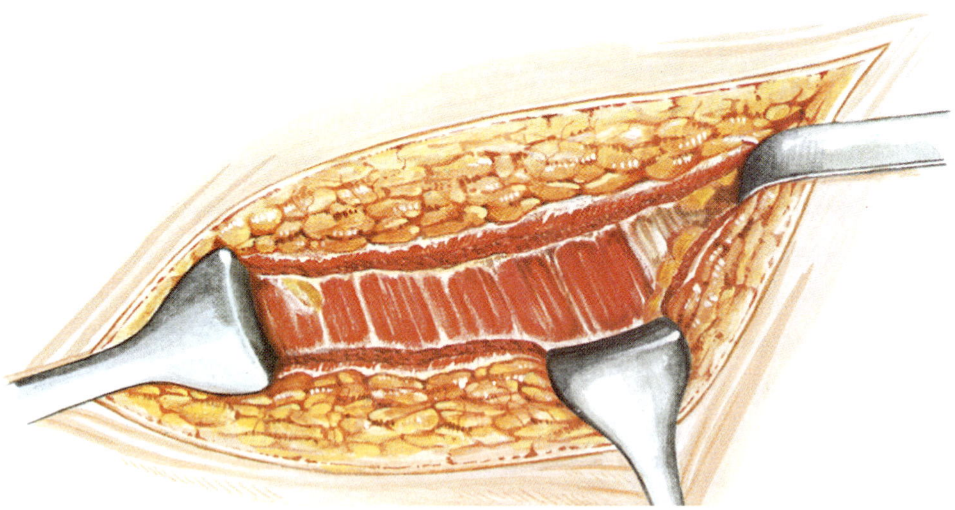

1-5

This muscle has no free posterior border. The uppermost fibers run vertically upward into the lower four ribs and their cartilages. The intermediate fibers form an aponeurosis at the line of Douglas. Above the semicircular line it divides into two lamellae at the lateral wall of the rectus muscles. The anterior wall of the rectus sheath consists of the aponeurosis of the external oblique and the anterior layer of the internal oblique aponeurosis. The posterior rectus sheath or wall is made up of the posterior layer of the internal oblique aponeurosis, the aponeurosis of the transversus abdominis muscle, and transversalis fascia. Below the line of Douglas, the combined aponeuroses of all three lateral abdominal muscles fuse and pass in front of the rectus sheath as the anterior rectus sheath. Its fibers in the flank region run at right angles to the more superficial external oblique muscle.

1-6. The internal oblique muscle is now incised, exposing the transversus abdominis muscle and lumbodorsal fascia.

The transversus abdominis muscle is the deepest of the three lateral abdominal muscles. It originates from the outer third of the inguinal ligament, from the inner lip of the iliac crest, from the middle layer of the lumbodorsal fascia, and from the inner surface of the lower six costal cartilages. Insertion is into the linea alba and through the conjoined tendon into the pubic crest. Its fibers, in the main, are directed horizontally. The aponeurosis passes behind the rectus muscle to the level of the line of Douglas. Below this level it passes in front of the rectus.

Transversalis fascia (endoabdominal fascia) covers the entire internal surface of abdomen. The fascia covers certain muscles and assumes its name from that muscle. Below the inferior margins of the internal oblique and transversus abdominis muscles, the fascia is well developed. It forms the floor of Hesselbach's triangle; weakness leads to a direct inguinal hernia. It lies between transversus abdominis muscle and the properitoneal fat layer. In lean patients it adheres to the parietal peritoneum as one layer.

Care should be taken to preserve the 12th thoracic and first lumbar nerves coursing between the internal oblique and the transversus abdominis muscles. A window is made in the lumbodorsal fascia to facilitate blunt separation of the transversus abdominis.

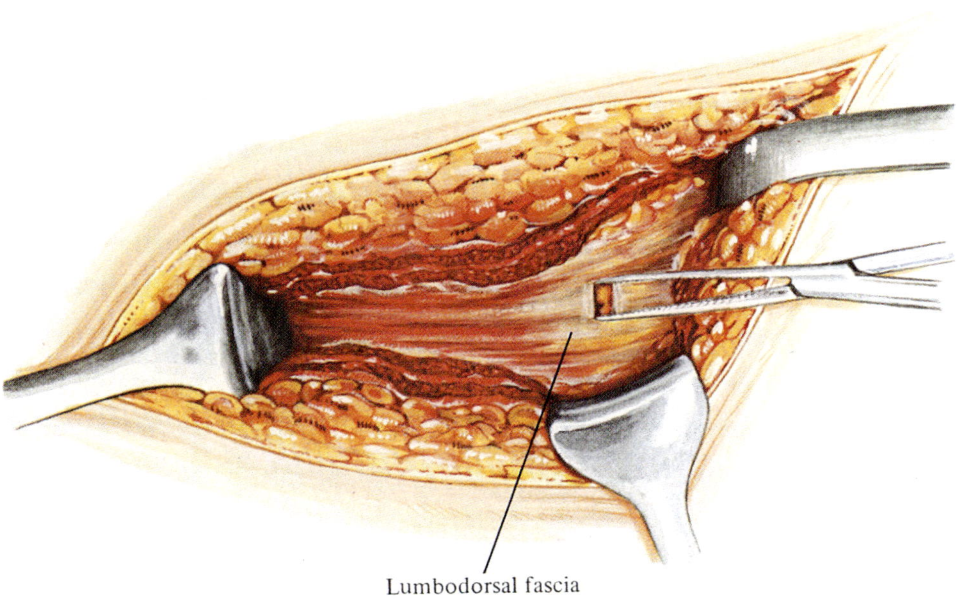

1-6

1-7. *Gerota's fascia, which encloses the kidney, has been opened,* allowing exposure of the perirenal fat.

1-8. *The ureter is identified and carefully exposed* by lifting the lower pole of the kidney and moving it medially. This maneuver is done to avoid possible damage to the ureter.

Once the kidney has been exposed in this fashion, a number of operative procedures can be undertaken. See the sequence of illustrations for pyelolithotomy. On occasion, when the lumbar flank approach is being used and greater exposure is needed, the technique of rib resection can facilitate the operative procedure. (Technique of 12th rib resection, right side.)

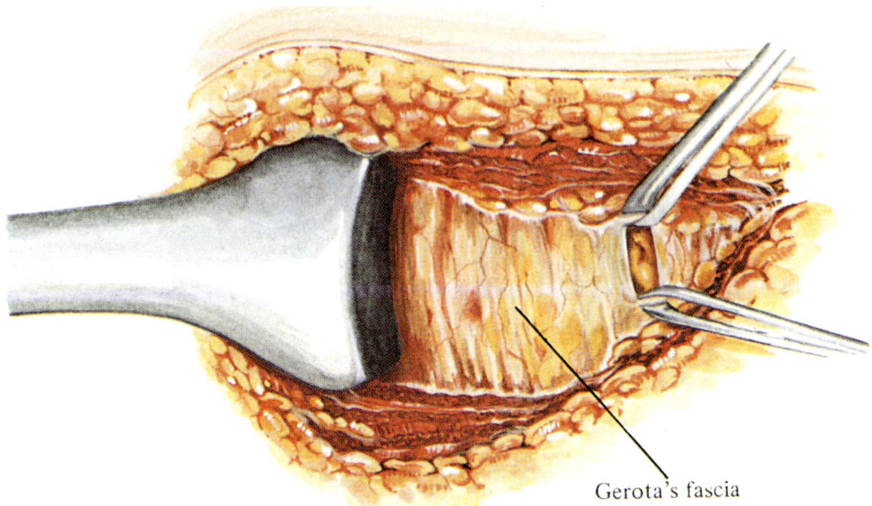

1-7

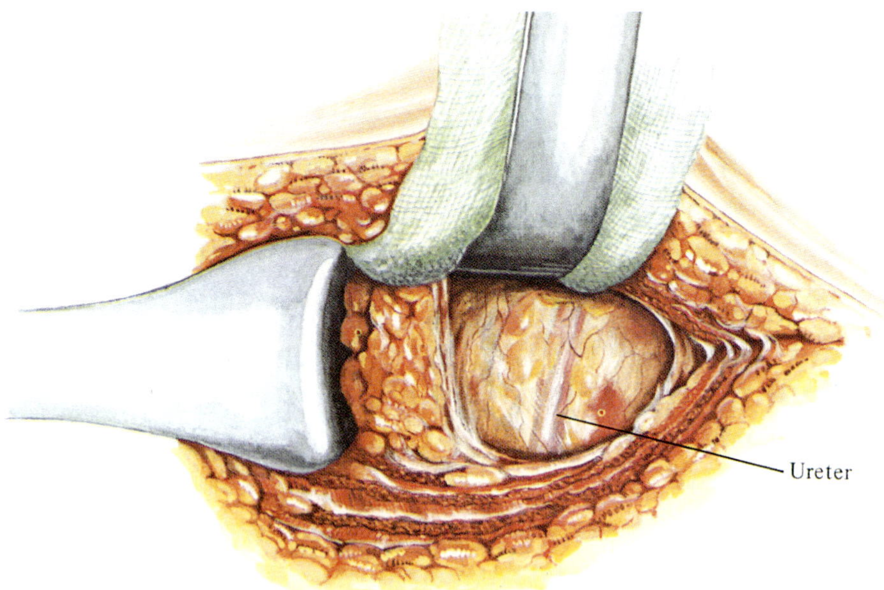

1-8

1-9. After the incision is made, exposing the external oblique muscle (see Figs. 1 and 3), *the incision is extended over the body of the 12th rib.* In sequence, the appropriate slips of the external oblique, internal oblique, and latissimus dorsi muscles are transected to expose the body of the rib. Care is taken to avoid exposing the inferior concave end of the rib because of the intercostal blood vessels and nerve.

1-10. The *periosteum is incised along the body of the rib,* and a periosteal elevator is used to develop the subperiosteal plane. Dissection of the periosteum at the lateral rib borders is facilitated by use of the Alexander periosteotome. If the surgeon wishes to expose the 11th rib, care is necessary to avoid tearing the underlying pleura. If the pleural space is opened inadvertently, a catheter (16–17 French) is left in place during closure and removed after residual air is expressed by hyperinflation of the lungs before the skin closure is completed.

1-11. *The Doyen instrument (left or right) is used to develop the subperiosteal space* behind the rib and free it for the next surgical maneuver. If bleeding is encountered from the intercostal vessels, hemostasis is established. If the procedure for exposing the external oblique muscle has been followed, then clamping and dividing the intercostal vessels are obviated, thus preserving the subcostal nerve which parallels the vessels.

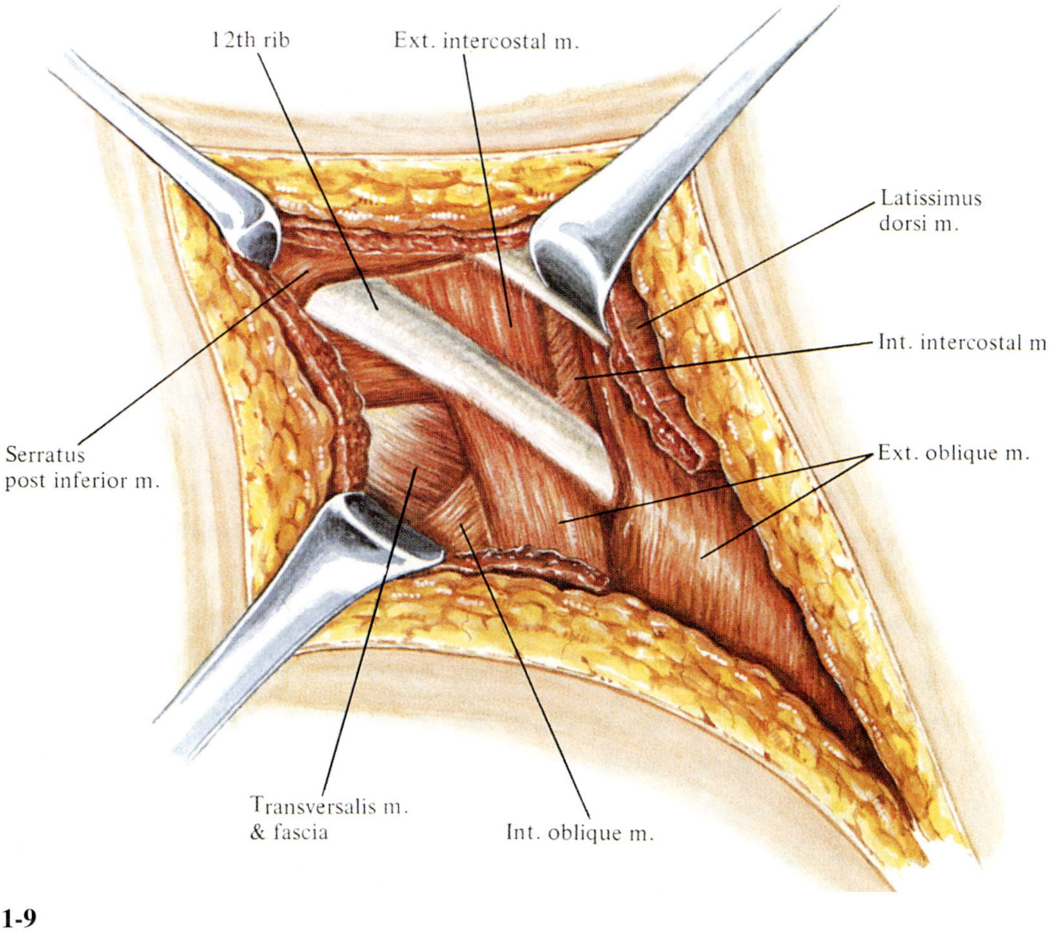

1-9

1-12. The proximal end of *the rib is transected and lifted from the underlying subperiosteal bed.* The distal portion of the rib is similarly transected.

1-13. The rib is moved and *the flank muscles are incised,* exposing the retroperitoneal fat.

An alternative may be useful to the surgeon: After the rib has been removed, the distal periosteal bed can be used to develop an avascular blunt plane of dissection beneath the medial abdominal muscles. This maneuver also allows the peritoneal wall located near the rib to be pushed medially by several fingers and allows the index and middle fingers to increase tension anteriorly on the muscles for further dissection and hemostatic control. The kidney can now be visualized, enclosed by Gerota's fascia and surrounded by pararenal fat.

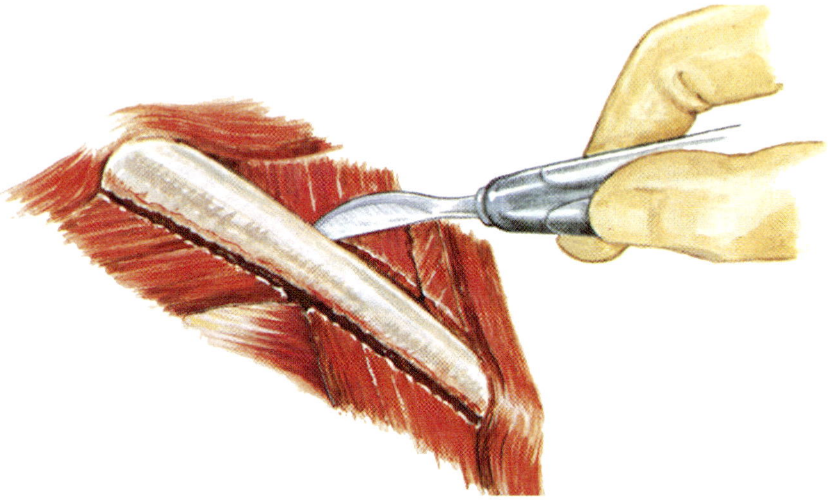

1-10

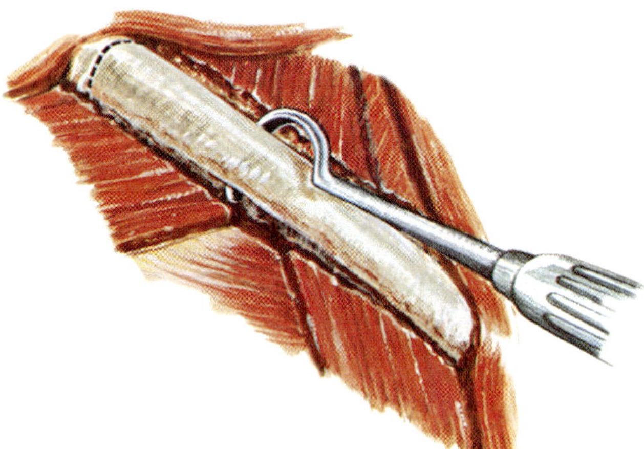

1-11

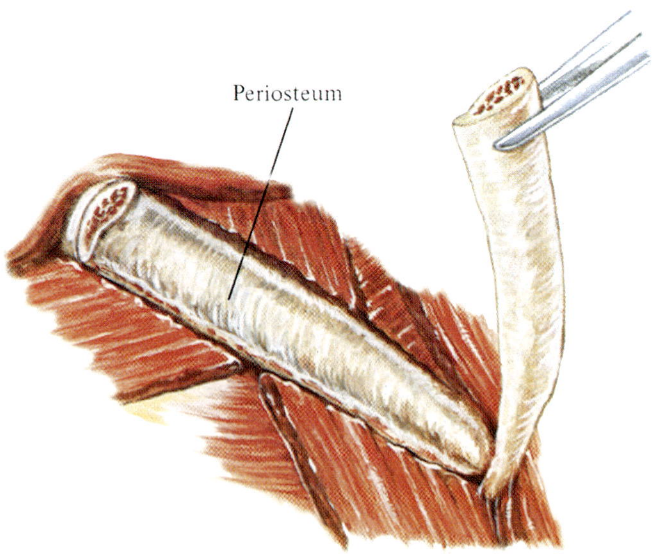

1-12

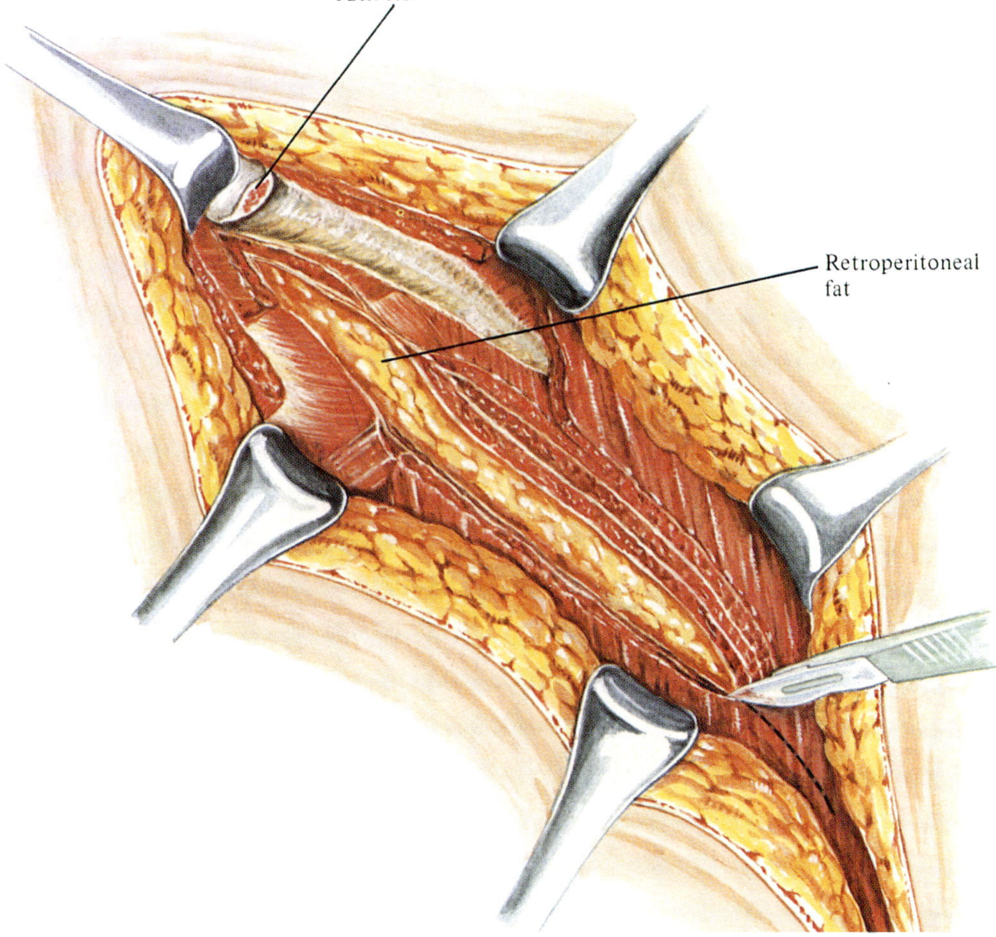

1-13

2. Anterior Abdominal-Transperitoneal (Transabdominal) Approach

On occasion, a much wider exposure and field may be required than is permissible by the approaches that have been described. When a patient has significant pulmonary insufficiency, the supine position allows for more efficient respiratory exchange and more effective monitoring by the anesthesiologist. This approach is also useful when a large kidney mass is present. Renal vessels can be more readily exposed and controlled near their site of origin. The anterior route, for example, is favored by general surgeons who are operating on patients with intra-abdominal pathology because it permits excellent exposure and easy access to the appropriate organ.

2-1. *A vertical midline incision of the skin is made.* A subcostal oblique line of incision, similar to that used in approaches to the gallbladder, can be employed and is one that we favor.

2-2. The peritoneal cavity is entered. Routine inspection and palpation of the abdominal contents is carried out. *The right kidney and fascial attachments are exposed* by incising the lateral attachments of the ascending colon and reflecting the colon medially. A neoplasm is identifiable through Gerota's fascia in the lower pole of the right kidney. The duodenum has been retracted medially after kocherization of its lateral border, exposing the inferior vena cava and right renal vein. The renal artery is barely visible in the illustration because it lies posteriorly to the right renal vein and inferior vena cava. The renal artery must be controlled at the outset. This can be accomplished in several ways: 1) Identify the medial border of both the inferior vena cava and abdominal aorta. 2) Pass an umbilical tape under the vena cava superior to the renal vein; blunt dissection will usually circumvent a posterior lumbar vein. 3) Gently lift the vena cava to allow dissection of the right renal artery distal to its origin but between the great vessels. 4) Several ligatures are passed (1–0 silk) around the renal artery. Prior to excision, the ureter has been identified and retracted medially.

Another approach to the right renal artery may be advantageous if the kidney mass is of moderate size. The renal vein is freed and an umbilical tape is passed. Inferior traction of the vein will expose a portion of the renal artery. Careful dissection will allow the placement of ligatures around the artery. Early branching of the renal artery is fairly common at this site. Therefore, this maneuver may not permit the surgeon to have a full visual field, and only partial arterial hemostasis may be achieved.

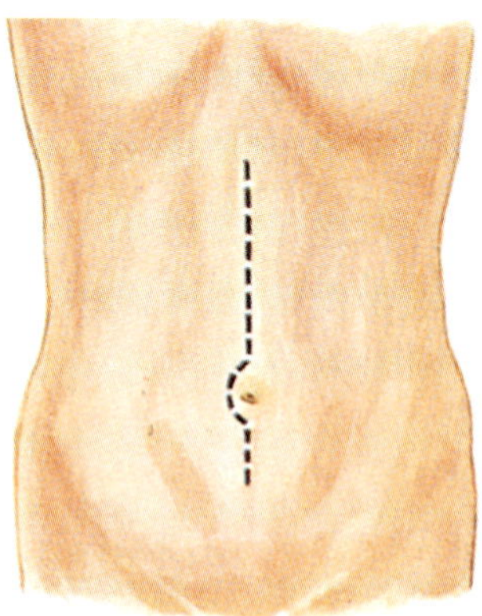

2-1

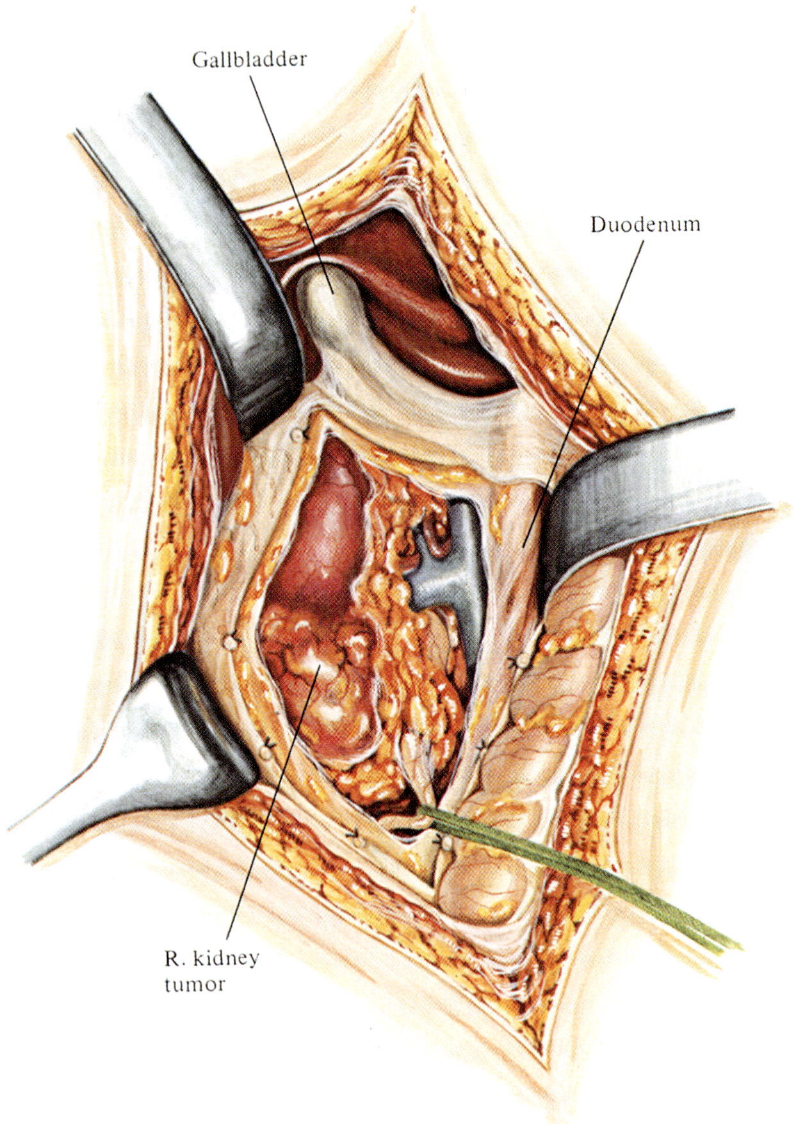

2-2

A third approach to the renal artery can be considered. The kidney and its investments can be dissected posteriorly, starting at the periphery and extending to the hilus. The renal artery can now be palpated and carefully dissected. Gently lifting the kidney can place slight tension on the renal artery and its course can be traced to the appropriate point of ligature.

We strongly suggest individual ligation of the artery and vein, respectively, rather than mass pedicle ligation, which is often performed blindly. The renal artery and vein are individually ligated and divided between ties. The ureter is similarly ligated and cut. The kidney and tumor mass can be further dissected and removed.

2-3. *In the anterior transabdominal approach to the left kidney, the descending colon is retracted medially.* The procedures described for the approach to the right kidney are surgically performed. The renal vessels are individually ligated on the proximal half. The distal vessels are secured with a clamp. The ureter is ligated inferiorly and the superior portion is secured with a clamp. The illustration depicts total nephrectomy with en bloc removal of Gerota's fascia, except for the upper pole of the left kidney.

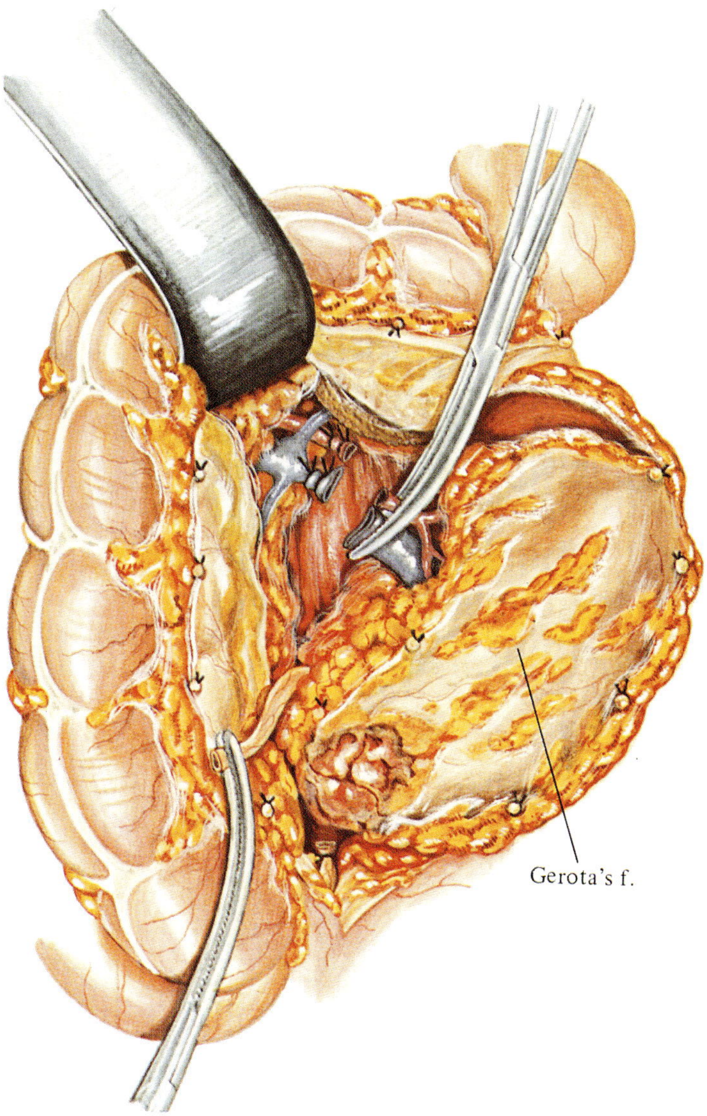

2-3

3. Thoracoabdominal Approach

When the kidney tumor engulfing the upper pole is large (greater than 10 to 15 cm), and malignancy is suspected, a planned thoracoabdominal approach is best considered. This provides the wide exposure necessary for radical en bloc resection of the tumor that may involve removal of the ipsilateral adrenal gland.

A preoperative workup is mandatory. An intravenous urogram is essential to diagnose and to verify the presence of a contralateral functioning kidney. Selective renal arteriography is helpful in planning operative strategy. Computerized axial tomographic (CAT) scanning is also helpful diagnostically. An inferior venacavogram may provide information relevant to local resectability of the tumor. High vena caval invasion may dictate unresectability or using cardiopulmonary bypass.

The following sequence of illustrations demonstrates the operative approach after a diagnosis of right renal neoplasm.

3-1. The patient is positioned on the table in a recumbent position with the right side elevated 40° by sandbags or pillows. *The planned incision* is *indicated by the broken line.* The abdominal component of the incision extends transversely and slightly inferiorly across the midline from the lateral edge of the left rectus muscle to the right costal margin opposite the tenth interspace. The rectus muscle on the right side is divided, and the incision is carried down through the peritoneum to enter the abdomen.

3-2. Through a thoracic incision exposing the tenth interspace, *the latissimus dorsi muscle is incised,* exposing the external and internal intercostal muscles.

3-3. *The thoracic component of the incision is extended across the costal margin* and through the tenth intercostal space *into the right pleural cavity.* The diaphragm is divided in the direction of the chest incision. The liver edge and retroperitoneal fat are seen, along with the hepatic flexure of the colon.

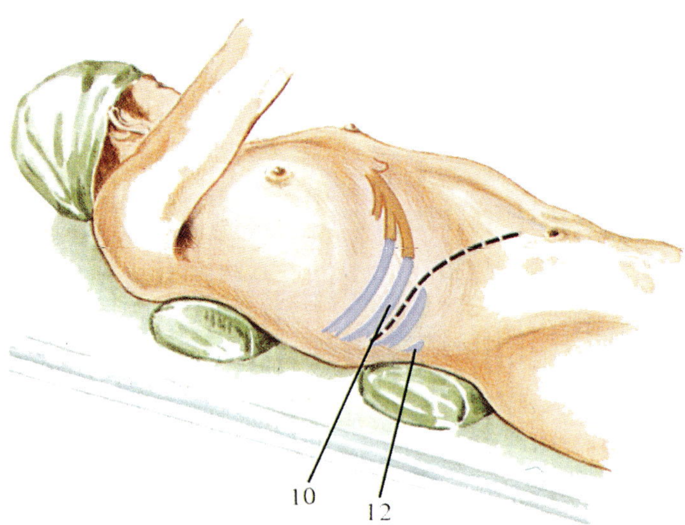

3-1

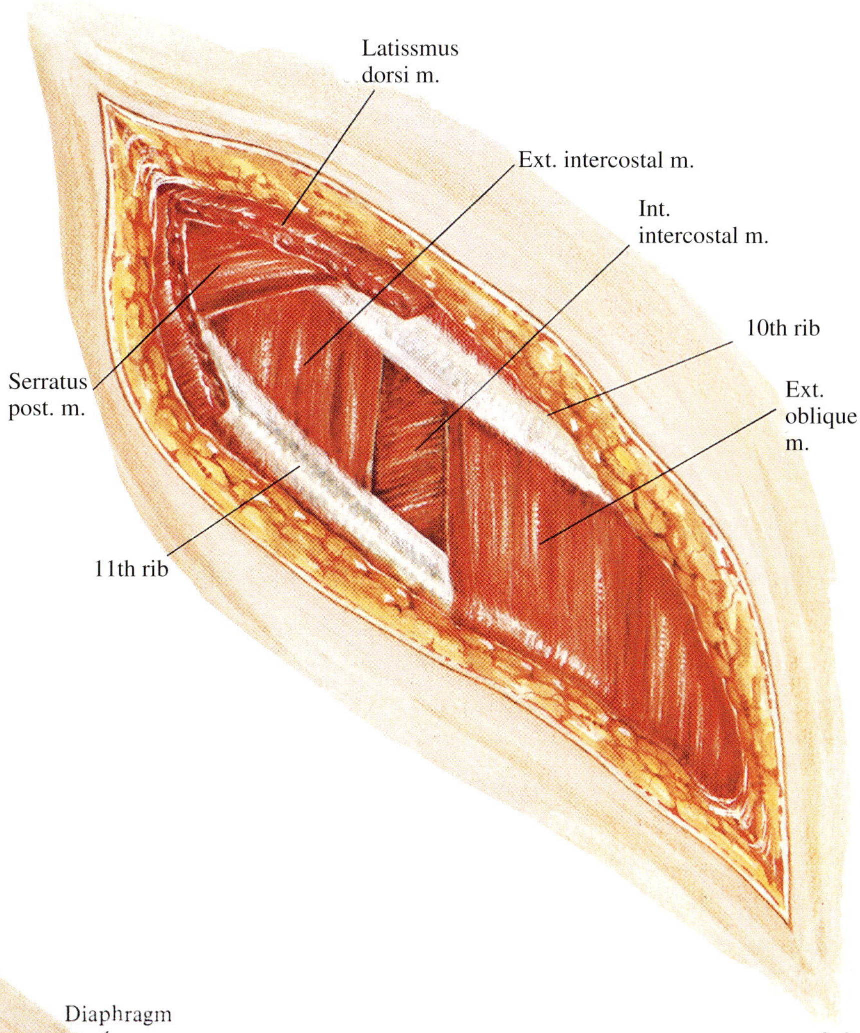
Latissmus
dorsi m.
Ext. intercostal m.
Int.
intercostal m.
10th rib
Serratus
post. m.
Ext.
oblique
m.
11th rib

3-2

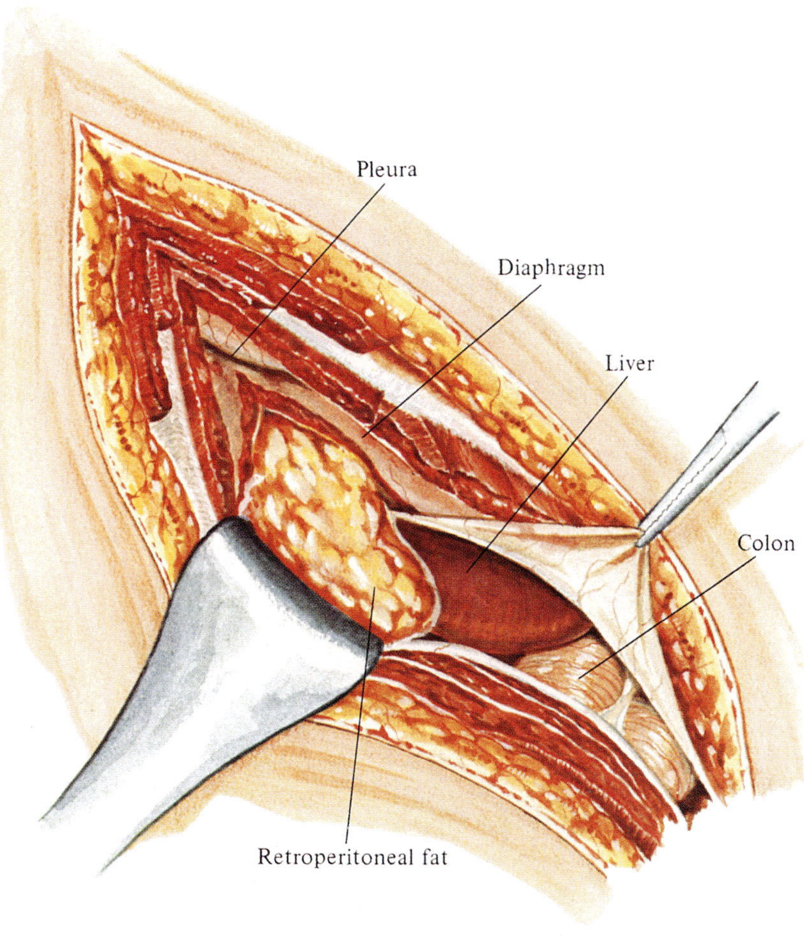
Pleura
Diaphragm
Liver
Colon
Retroperitoneal fat

3-3

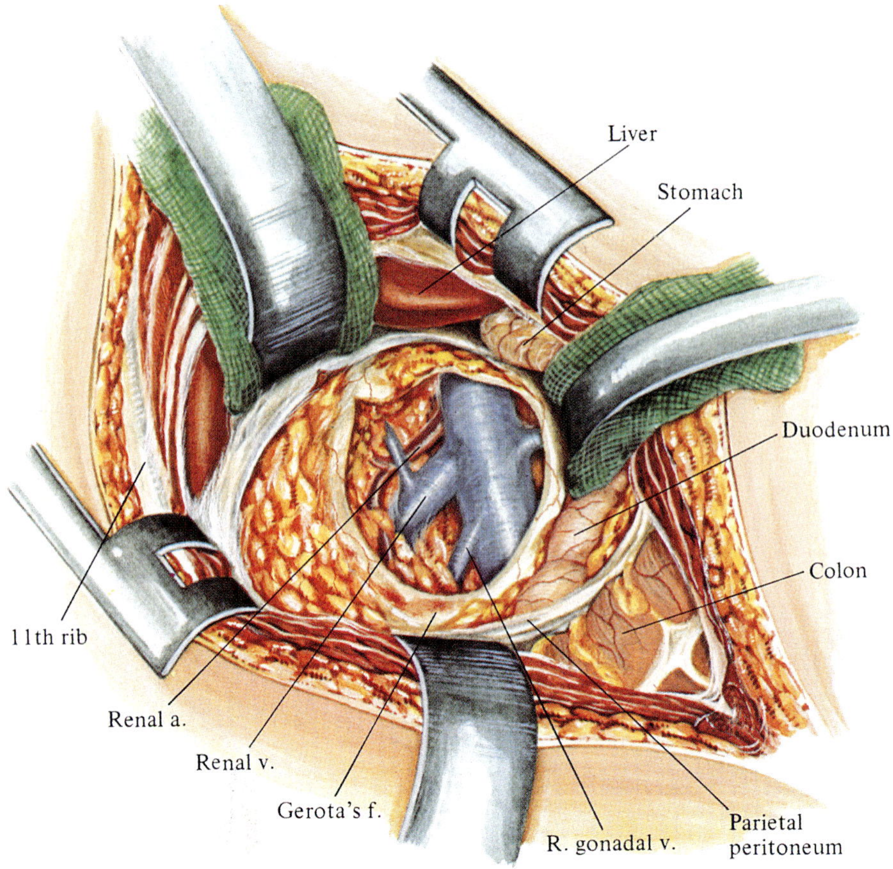

3-4

3-4. In this portion of the incision (abdominal) are the *inferior vena cava, renal artery and vein, and Gerota's fascia* surrounding the kidney, as well as portions of liver, stomach, duodenum, and colon. The duodenum has been mobilized and retracted medially exposing the vena cava and right renal vein. The renal artery is exposed, dissected, and doubly ligated behind the vena cava. The renal vein is also doubly ligated and transected in between. The ureter is exposed, doubly ligated, and divided. Fascial attachments of the kidney to the undersurface of the liver are removed by incising the peritoneum superiorly. The tumor mass and kidney are then removed. The adrenal gland (at right) is removed with the mass if tumor extension is noted.

NEPHRECTOMY

4. Standard Nephrectomy

For a routine nephrectomy procedure, any of the previously described surgical approaches can be used. In the following sequence, the right anterior transabdominal approach is employed.

4-1. *The ascending colon is retracted medially;* the duodenum is then freed and similarly retracted. Gerota's fascia is opened, exposing the right kidney. If a renal adenocarcinoma is suspected, the fascia is left intact.

4-2. *The lesion at the lower right pole of the kidney is exposed* along with its vascular supply. The ureter has been isolated and retracted inferiorly by a tape.

4-3. *The double-clamp technique is used on the proximal end of the renal vasculature.* (Usually we elect to isolate and clamp each vessel individually.) The renal artery is isolated and ligated first (see 2–3); this is followed by ligation of the right renal vein.

4-4. *The right renal vessels are doubly ligated.*

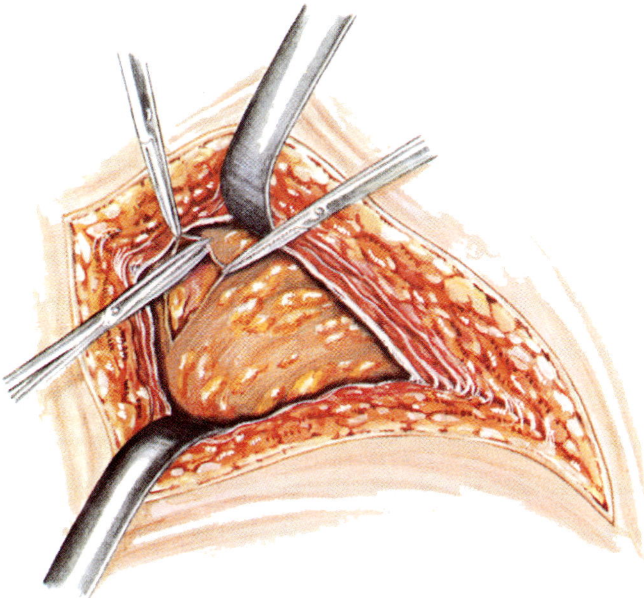

4-1

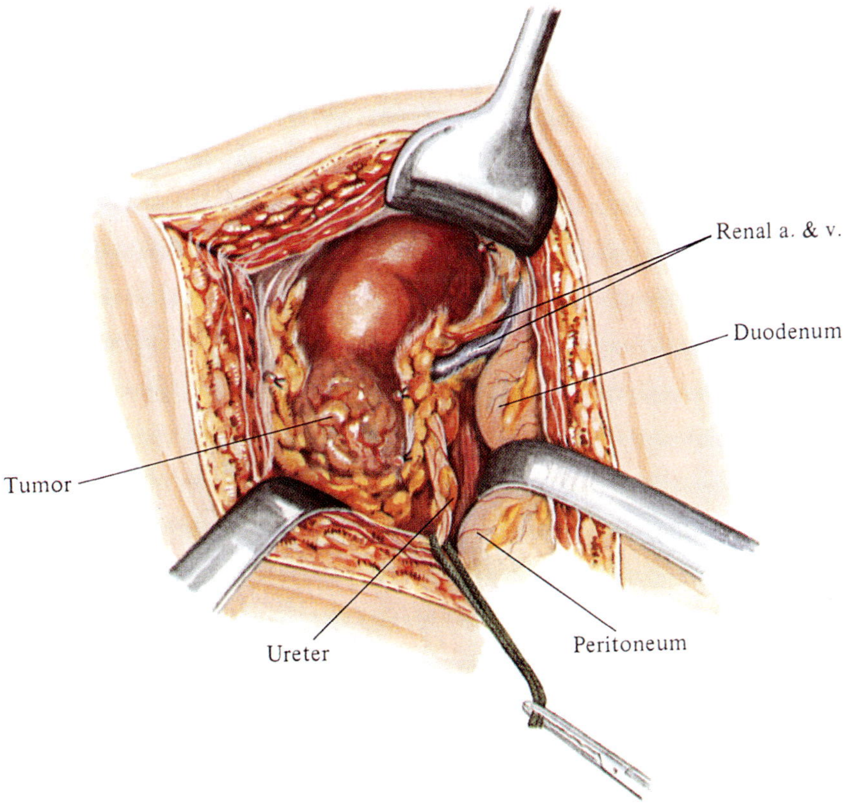

4-2

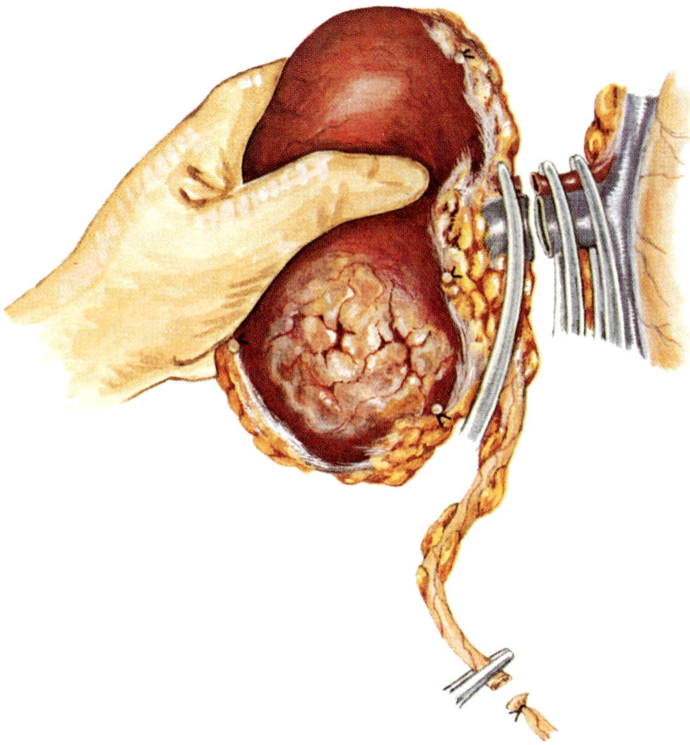

4-3

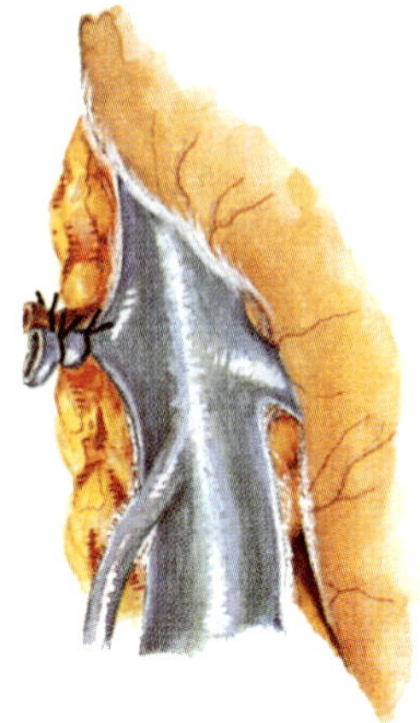

4-4

5. Subcapsular Nephrectomy

The kidney is depicted outside the operative field for clarity.

5-1. A subcapsular nephrectomy is performed since the kidney is immobile and adherent to surrounding fascial structures. *The anterior renal capsule is removed* to allow further dissection.

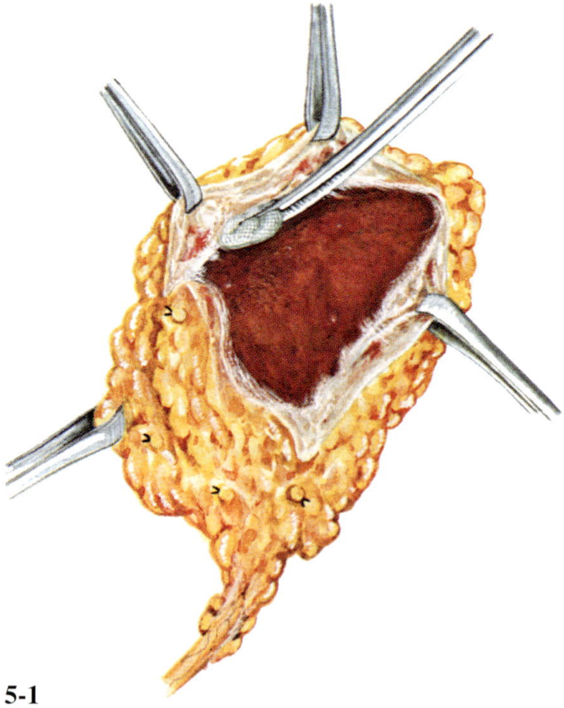

5-1

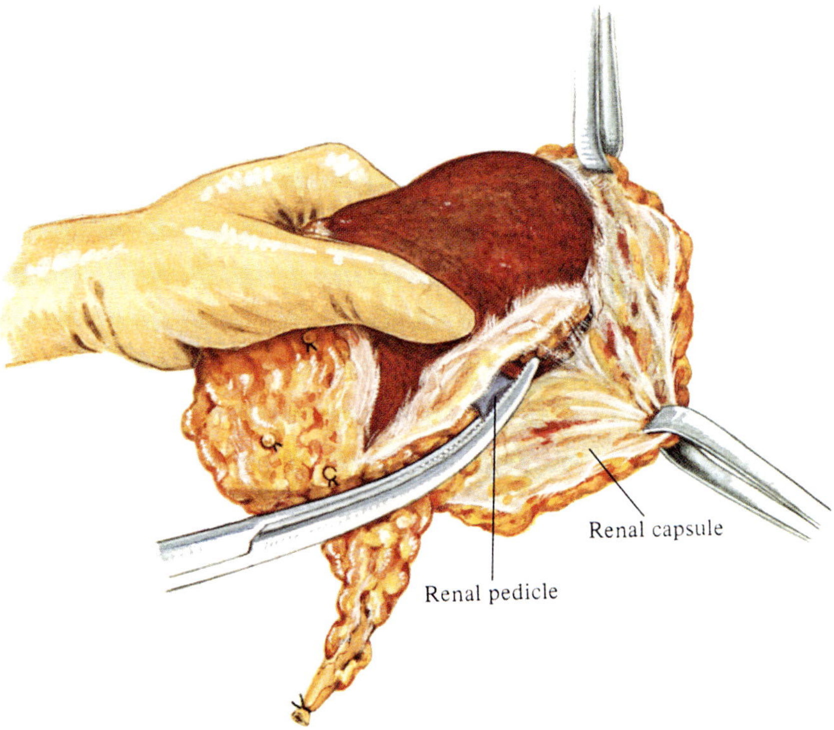

5-2

5-2. *The renal hilus beneath the capsule is exposed to allow a pedicle clamp to engage the renal vessels.* The renal pedicle is doubly ligated before the vessels are transected beneath the capsule. The ureter is isolated, ligated, and tied.

Final kidney removal is best accomplished by sharp dissection through fascial investments but avoiding the proximal renal pedicle.

6. Standard Partial Nephrectomy

In the following sequences, the left kidney is exposed through a lumbar-flank approach.

6-1. The left renal artery lies posterior and slightly superior to the renal vein. *A vascular clamp is used to interrupt arterial blood flow* temporarily. The kidney is shown raised from the operative field. A circumferential incision is made at least 1.5 cm from the diseased margin. A frozen section of the border can be useful in determining the margin of clearance if necessary. Bleeding from the free parenchymal edge is reduced because of the vascular clamp on the renal artery. Regional cooling (15° C) of the kidney (see 8–3) can prolong the period of functional preservation up to approximately 2 hours. A kidney should not remain ischemic at normal temperatures beyond 20 to 30 minutes. Intermittent clamping may extend the safe period for another 20 minutes.

6-2. *During closure of the caliceal structures, we use running continuous locking sutures with 4–0 chromic catgut. Bleeding points are located by intermittent unclamping of the renal artery.*

6-3. *Closure of the renal capsule is accomplished by using mattress type sutures* (3–0 chromic catgut).

6-4. If bleeding persists after closure, *a deep through-and-through suture (2–0 chromic catgut) can be used to obtain hemostasis.*

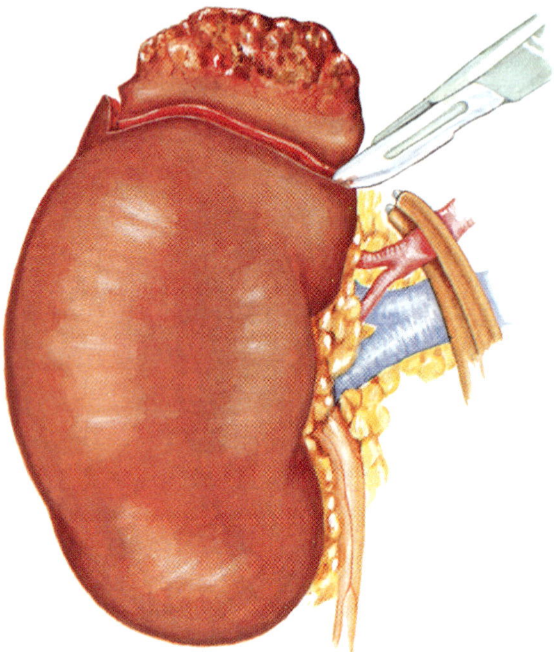

6-1

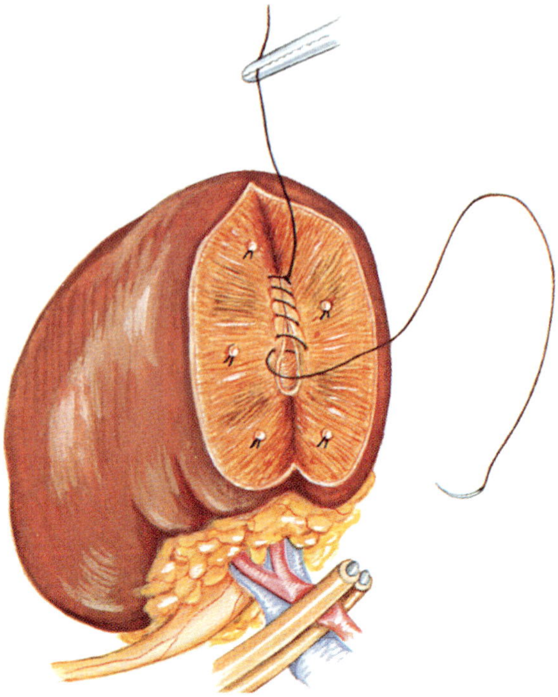

6-2

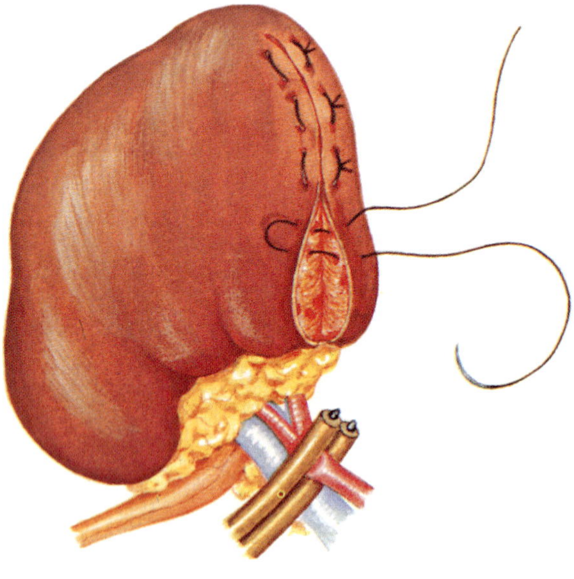

6-3

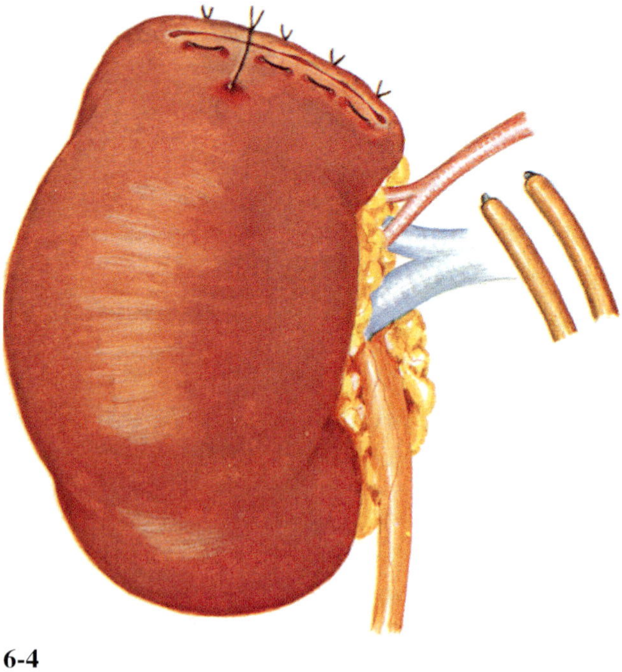

6-4

7. Tie Technique for Partial Nephrectomy

In the following sequence, the left kidney lower pole is exposed through a lumbar flank approach. The tie technique permits rapid removal of the diseased segment; renal arterial clamping is usually not necessary. Exposure of the renal artery, however, is important.

7-1. *A circumferential incision is made through the renal capsule* 1.5 to 2 cm distal to the diseased margin. The proximal margin of the renal capsule is carefully peeled back to expose the tie area.

7-2. *A superficial circumferential incision is made.*

7-3. *A noose with a half tie* (No. 1 nylon) is secured directly into the circular, superficial incision area.

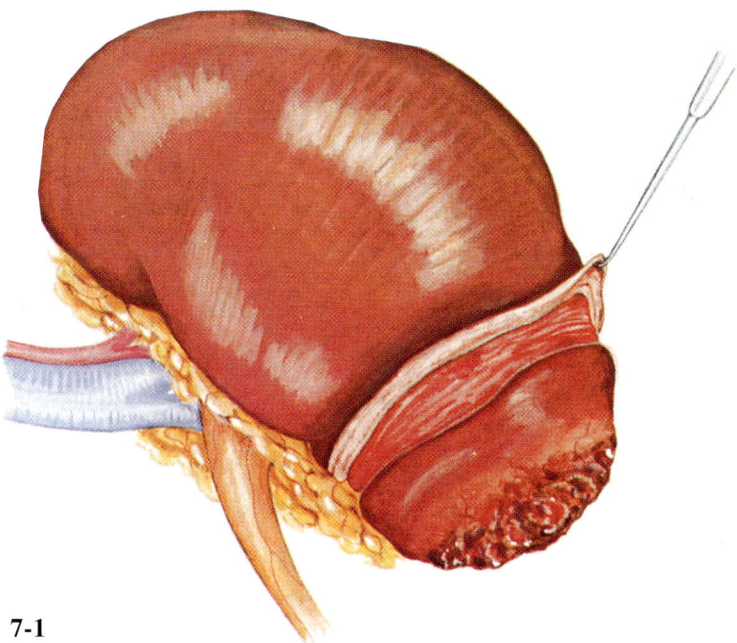

7-1

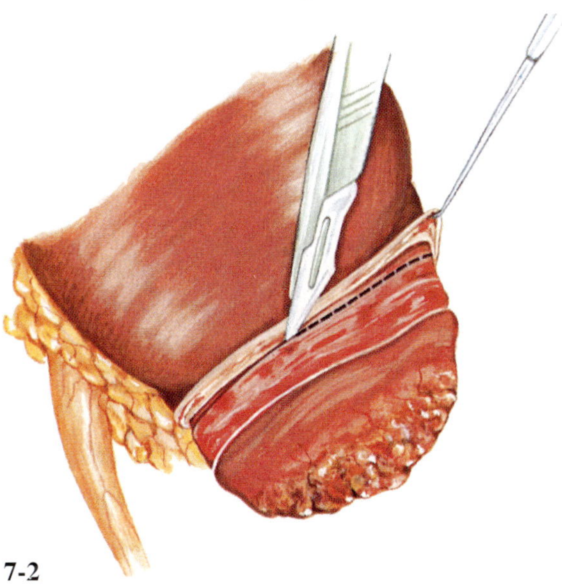

7-2

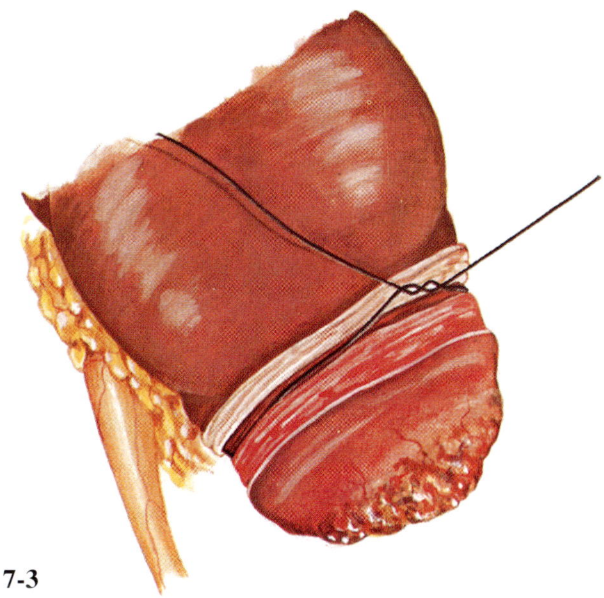

7-3

7-4. *The noose is tightened* until a core of parenchymal tissue measuring approximately 1.5 cm remains; it is finally secured.

7-5. *The diseased parenchyma and its free margin are excised by sharp dissection*, taking care to leave a small portion of ligated parenchymal stump.

7-6. *The base of the stump is secured with a suture ligature* (1–0 chromic catgut). It is then grasped and elevated by a surgical clamp.

7-7. After the distal stump is excised, *the original noose will fall free or is removed.* If necessary, hemostasis can be further secured by individual suture ligatures (4–0 chromic catgut).

7-8. *The renal capsule is reapproximated* after any redundant tissue has been removed.

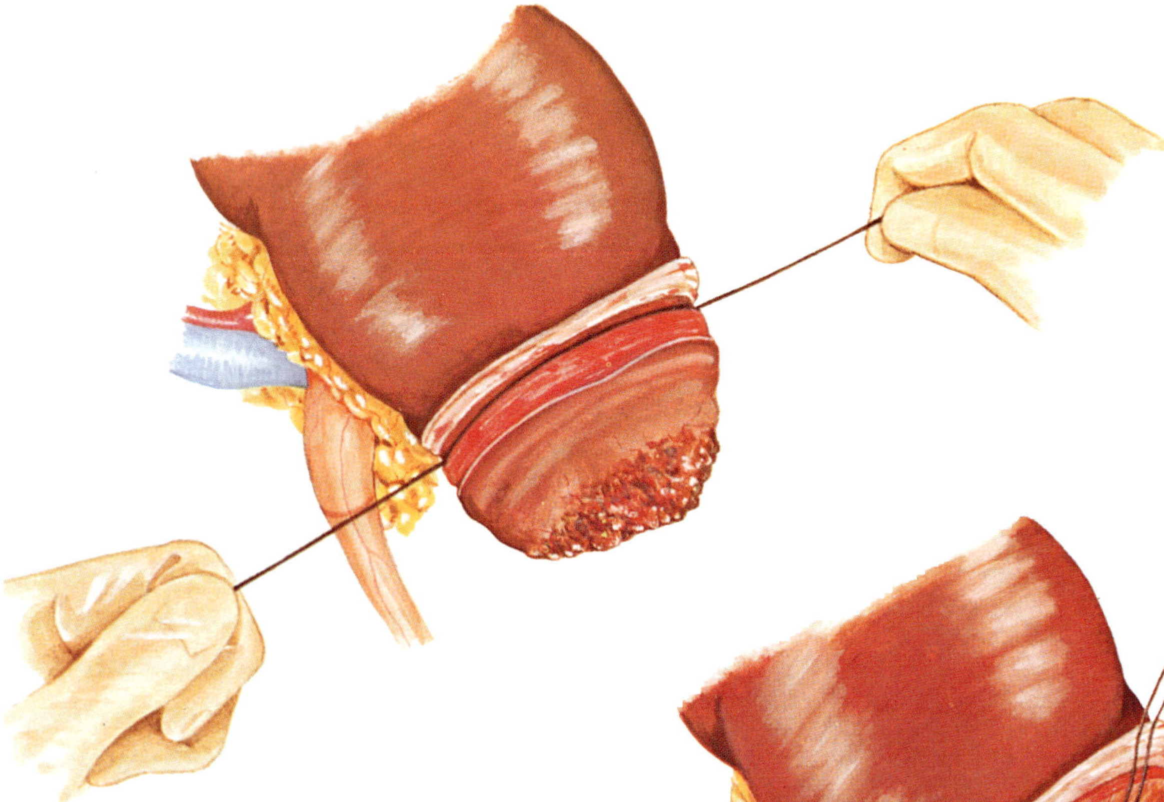

7-4

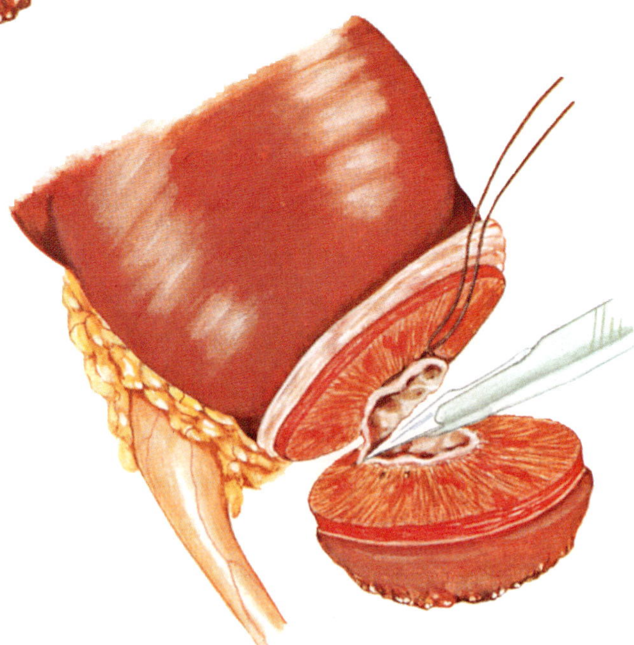

7-5

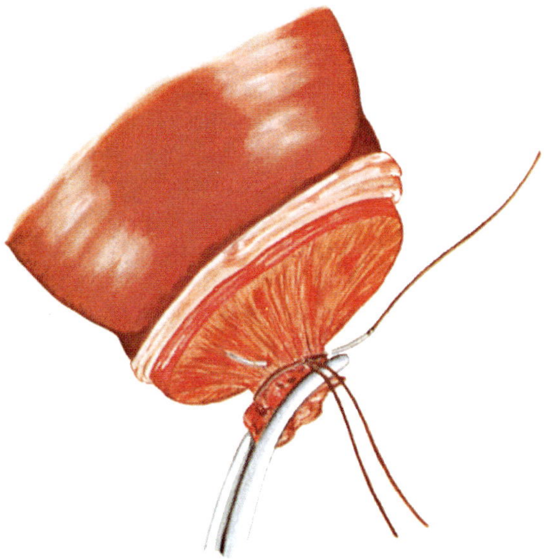

7-6

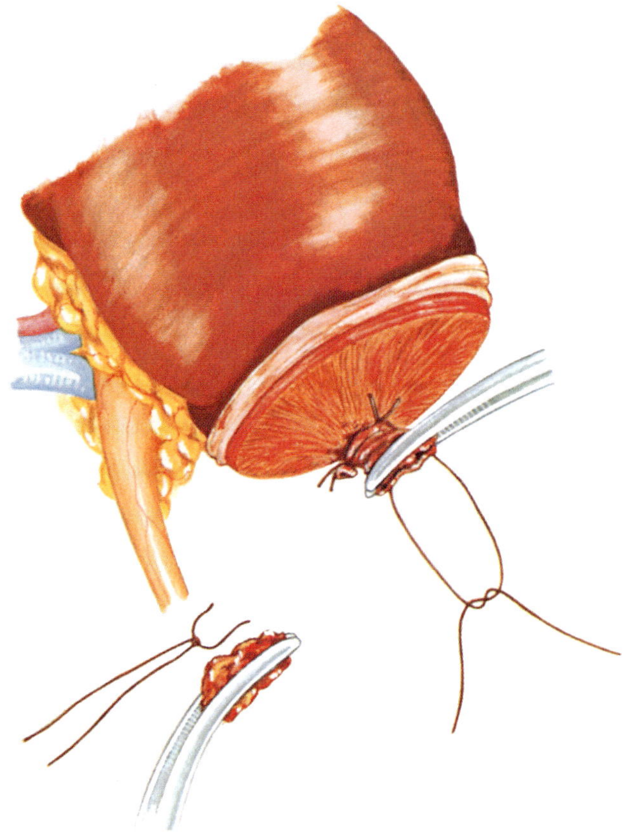

7-7

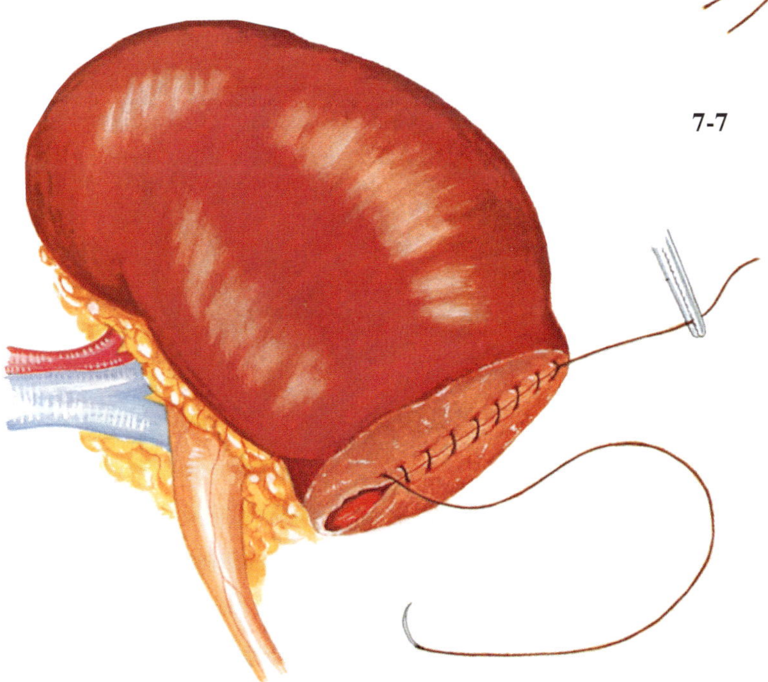

7-8

8. Renal Cell Carcinoma

8-1. Removal of tumor thrombus in the vena cava from right renal cell carcinoma. Renal cell carcinoma involving and extending into the vena cava: tumor extension to the superior vena cava, but below the diaphragm.
Renal cell carcinoma confined to one kidney is usually best diagnosed by a CT scan. Hematuria is often present as an important sign. A right renal carcinoma can progress to include tumor extension into the lumen of the vena cava. In this situation, we obtained an abdominal aortogram with selected arteriography to allow mapping of the vascular structures. An inferior vena cavogram was also performed to evaluate the extent of tumor progression superiorly in the vena cava.

We have had experience with several large right renal carcinomas extending into the superior vena cava. The assistance of a general vascular or cardiothoracic surgeon is important, and a team approach is used. A transabdominal approach with a long vertical midline incision from 4 inches below the umbilicus to the xiphoid process is used. The sternum is also surgically prepared and draped. The surgery is performed in a large room where cardiothoracic surgery is performed. Cardiopulmonary bypass is available on

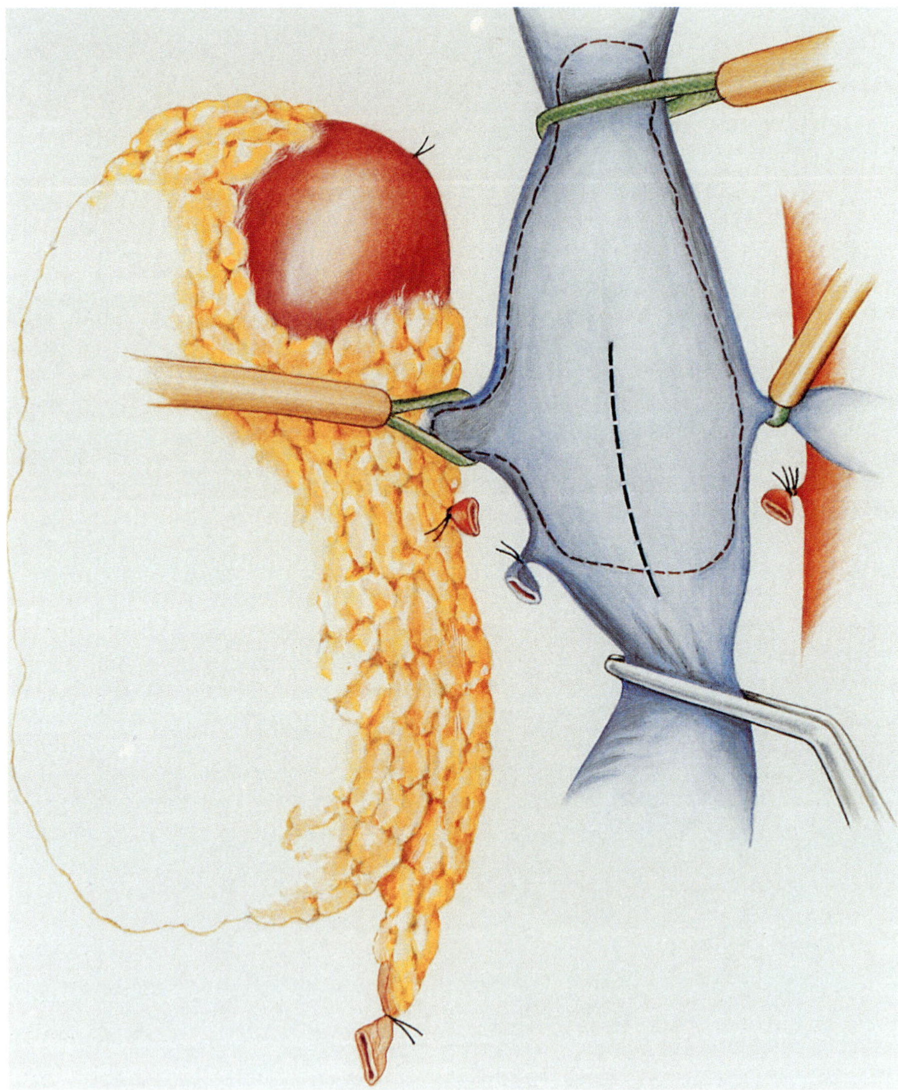

8-1

standby. The cosurgeon is the cardiothoracic-vascular surgeon. The cardiac bypass machine is readied and made available with the appropriate team members.

In one of our cases (see 8–1), the kidney was carefully freed as shown. The vena cava was surgically exposed as demonstrated. The tumor thrombus could be carefully palpated extending up the abdominal portion of the vena cava. By careful palpation, the superior extent of the tumor was noted to be above the diaphragm. The thrombus-tumor was manipulated inferiorly by careful finger manipulation. A vascular loop was placed around the vena cava at its upper extent (see 8–1), superior to the tumor thrombus. The inferior vena cava was clamped as shown. The left renal vein was temporarily clamped with a surgical vascular loop inside a short rubber catheter to allow tension and closure of the loop.

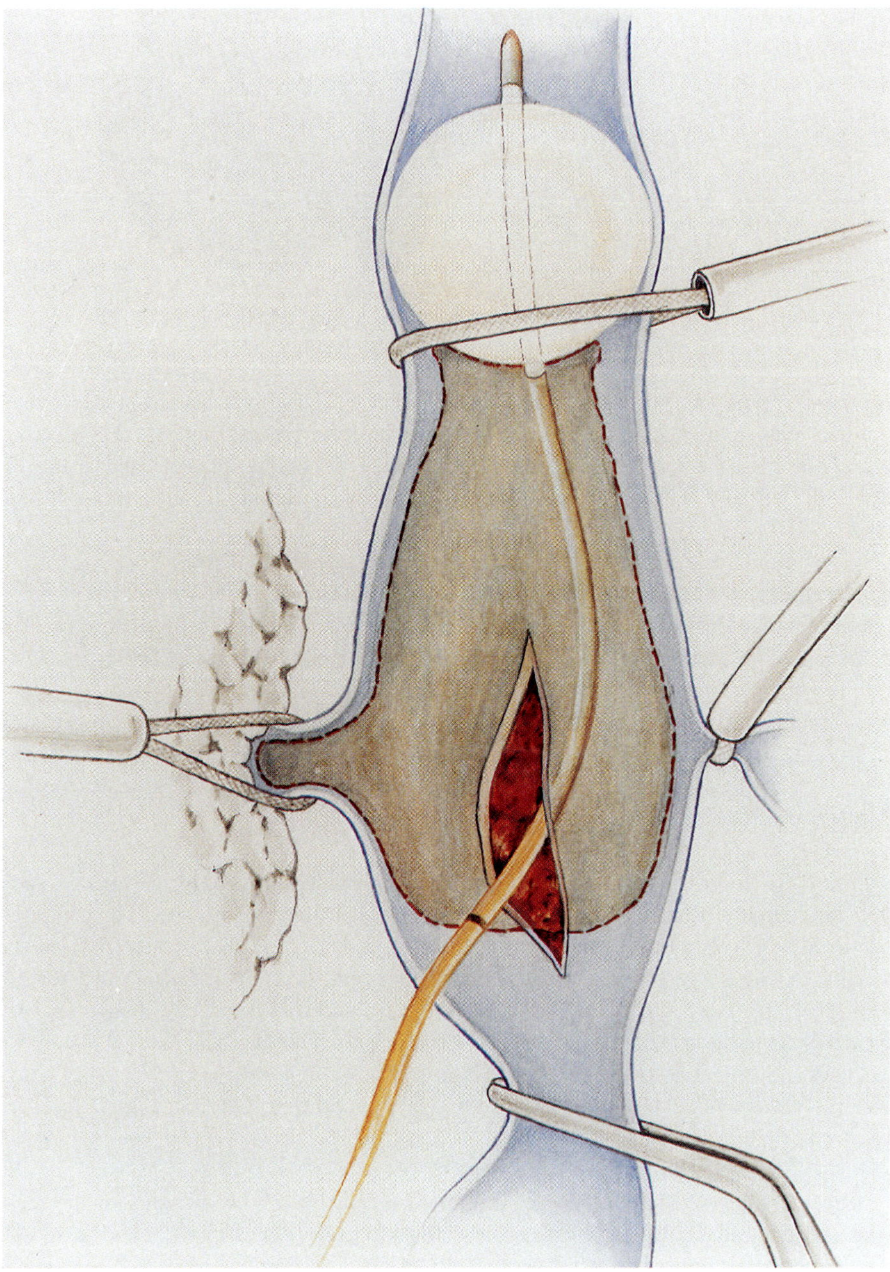

8-2

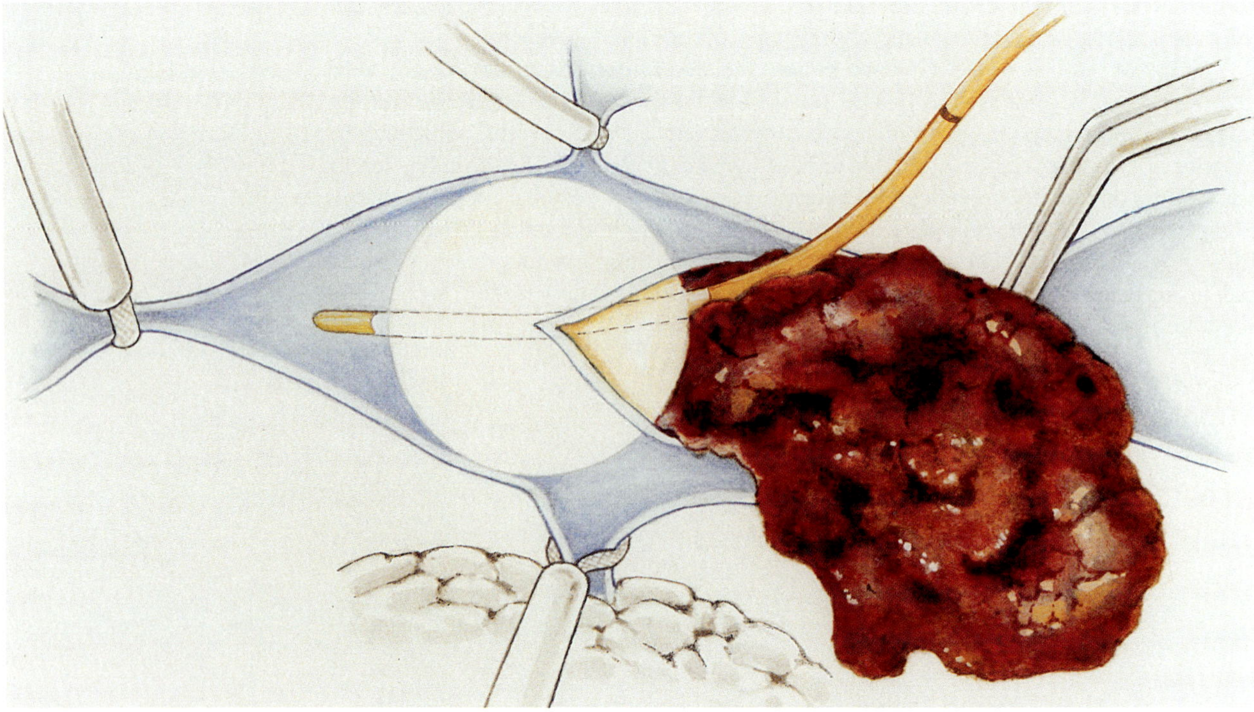

8-3

8-2. and 8-3. The first illustration shows the bulk of the tumor exposed inside the lumen of the vena cava. A Fogarty balloon catheter has been passed superior to the tumor mass and the balloon is inflated as shown. With the tip of the catheter above the diaphragm, the inflated balloon is used to extract the tumor as shown in the second illustration.

The vena cava is surgically repaired with vascular sutures. Blood flow is reestablished. A radical nephrectomy is performed including a long segment of proximal ureter. The radical nephrectomy is completed. Vascular sutures (5–0) were used to close the vena cava. Before the final closure, the lower vascular clamp was carefully opened to remove the air. The vascular loop around the left renal vein was also opened. The vena cava was finally closed by suturing the venotomy. A nasogastric tube for decompression of the stomach and small bowel may be needed for several days.

9. Nephropexy

A nephroptotic kidney, often on the right side and in a thin, young to middle-aged woman can lead to obstruction of the kidney at the ureteropelvic junction. The usual patient is in her 40s. When she assumes the upright position, she will notice pain in the right flank. A careful history can bring out the fact that the right kidney in the upright position drops perhaps 1 to 2.5 inches (2.5 to 6 cm), and this change in anatomical location will lead to an ureteropelvic junction obstruction. The diagnosis can also be confirmed using intravenous pyelography. It is important when obtaining this x-ray study to have the patient also stand so that the change in anatomic location with severe obstruction can be demonstrated on x-ray.

9-1. The incision is made following the anatomic order of the muscles in the right flank as demonstrated. Gerota's fascia of the right kidney is carefully opened. The kidney is pushed cephalad so that its normal anatomic position is assured. Then, a 1-0 Vicryl suture is used and is placed through the capsule of the lower kidney as demon-

9-1

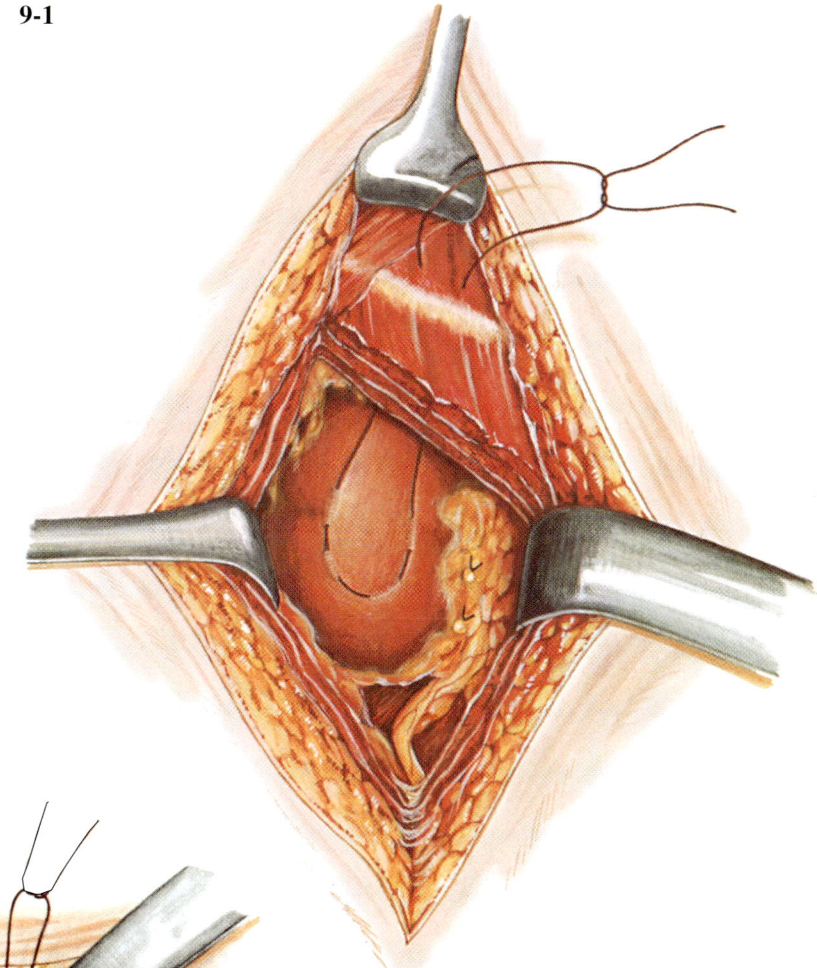

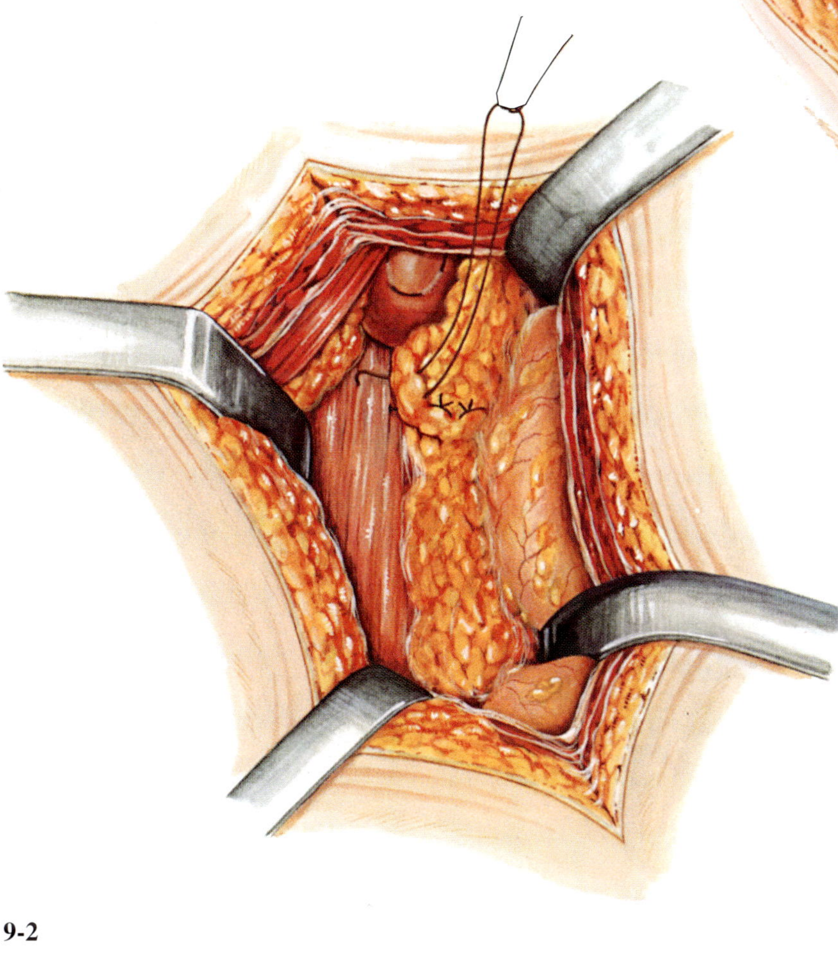

9-2

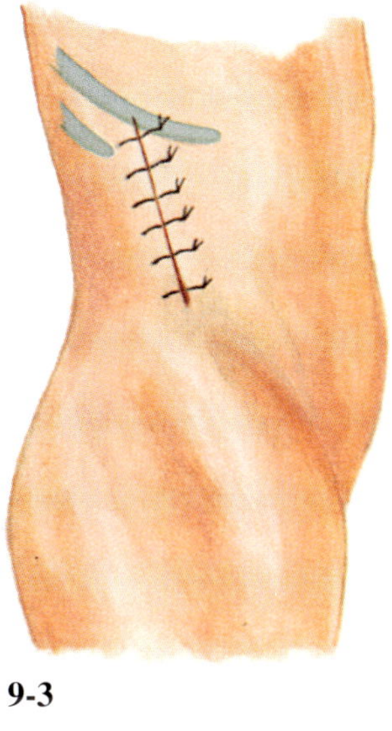

9-3

strated. The two loose ends of this long suture are placed above the 12th rib and secured so that kidney nephroptosis will not occur when the patient is in the standing position.

9-2. This clearly demonstrates the new location of the kidney after the second tie is placed as demonstrated.

9-3. The incision with the sutures in place. The patient is asked to avoid horseback riding or any vigorous physical exercises, such as aerobics or tap dancing, for at least 5 to 6 weeks.

10. Pyelolithotomy

For extrarenal pyelolithotomy, the renal pelvis of the right kidney is approached anteriorly through a transabdominal incision. We have generally obtained superior preoperative and operative x-ray films of the kidney with the patient in the supine position.

10-1. *Stay sutures expose the ureteropelvic junction.* A Randall's stone forcep is inserted to remove the calculus. The kidney is maintained in the operative field by gentle traction of the fascial attachments at the lower pole.

10-2. After removal of the calculus it is advisable to insert an 8 Fr red rubber ureteral catheter to wash out small residual stones and debris. An x-ray film taken at this time can be useful. A second ureteral catheter (5 or 6 Fr) is inserted inferiorly and passed into the bladder (20 to 23 cm). The purpose of this maneuver is to rule out the possible pres-

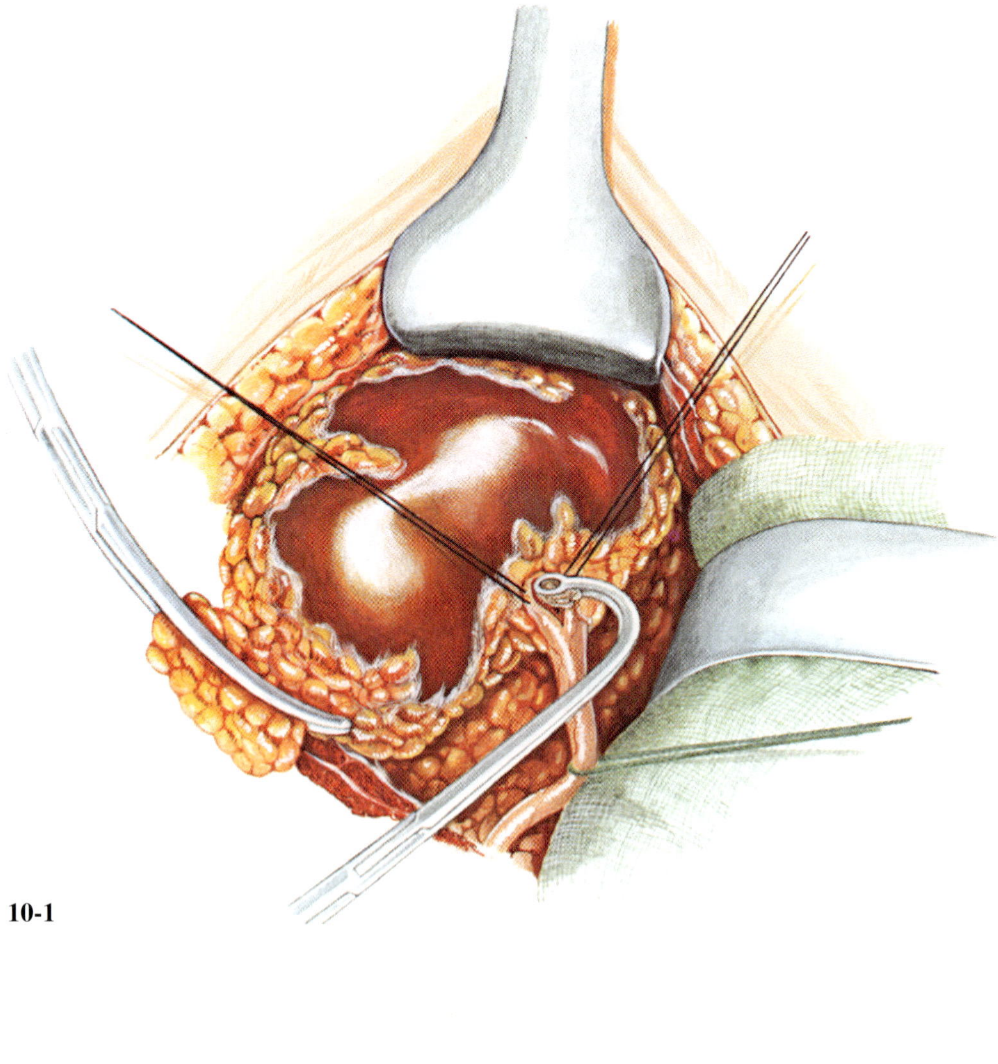

10-1

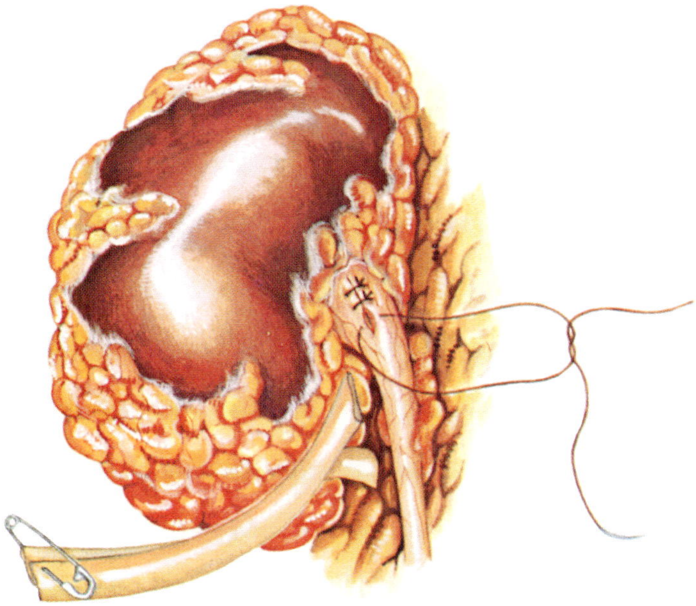

10-2

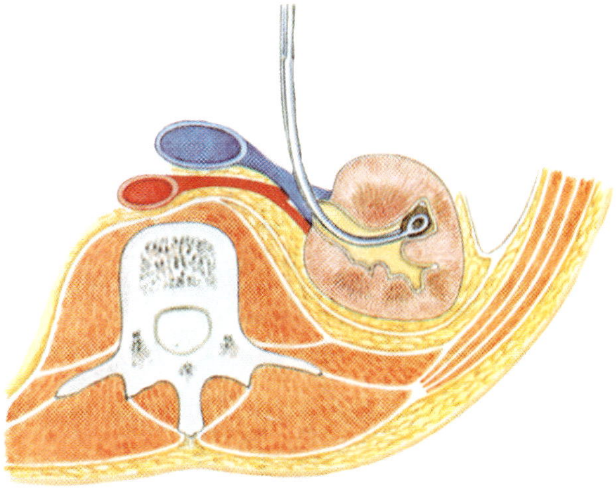

10-3

ence of a stony fragment that has migrated at the time of manipulation. *Ureteral reapproximation is accomplished by periadventitial sutures* (4–0 chromic catgut). *Two flat tubular drains are secured in place.*

10-3. A cross section. The *stone forceps is used to grasp a calculus* lodged in a major calix. This maneuver is more easily accomplished with the patient in a supine position or with the anterolateral area over the kidney elevated.

INTRARENAL PYELOLITHOTOMY

In the following sequence, two techniques are described to remove the calculus.

11. Gil-Vernet Technique

11-1. *A moderate-sized calculus is lodged in the intrarenal pelvis of the right kidney.*

11-2. A standard incision is made to approach the posterior right kidney. In this instance *a flank incision and dissection exposes the renal pelvis.* A posterior dissecting plane is developed between the pelvis and the renal hilus. The renal artery is isolated but not clamped.

11-3. Blunt dissection between posterior pelvis and renal hilus is continued within the kidney to allow significant *exposure of the pelvis and major calices.* Special long-handled retractors (similar to vein retractors) are useful to expose this surgical field (*dotted line*). Stay sutures are inserted for exposure of the pelvis. The incision in the pelvis is made and the calculus can now be removed. Catheter irrigation (8 Fr) is useful to remove debris. A ureteral catheter is passed inferiorly into the bladder. Stay sutures are removed. Standard closure of the pelvis is performed. As a standard precaution, a flat tubular drain is placed near the pelvis and secured for 3 to 5 days before shortening it. A multiperforated flat tube connected to a closed drainage tube and reservoir may be substituted.

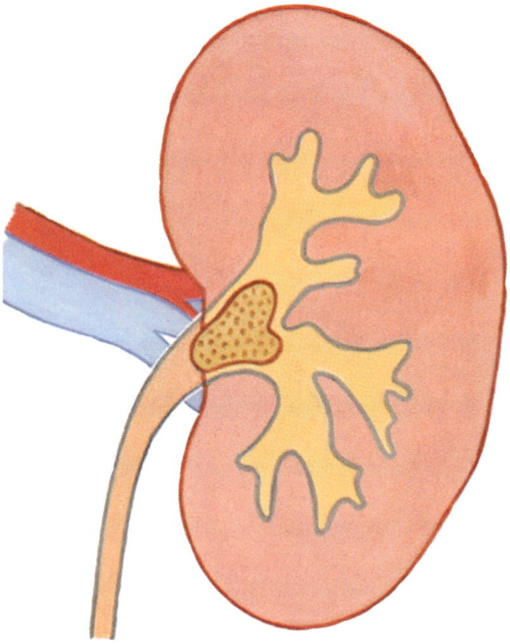

11-1

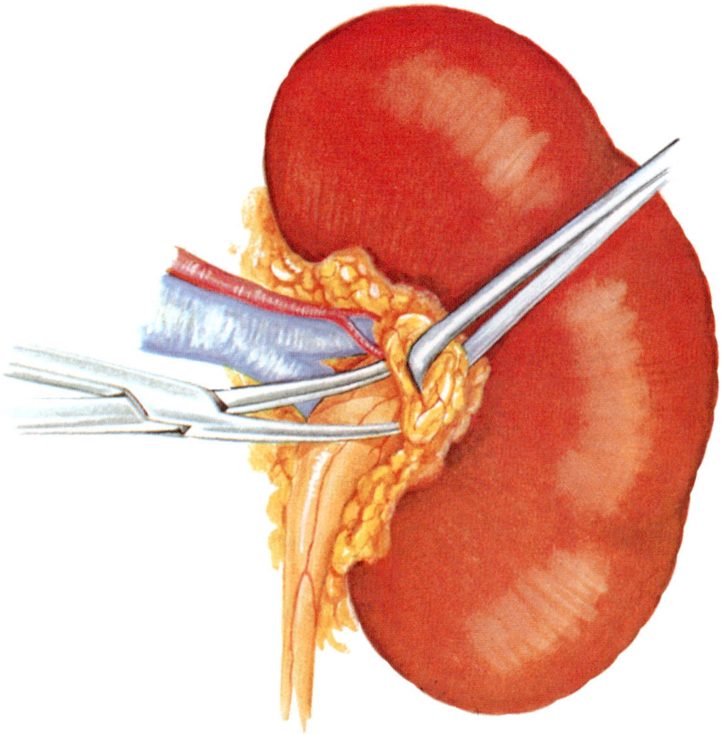

11-2

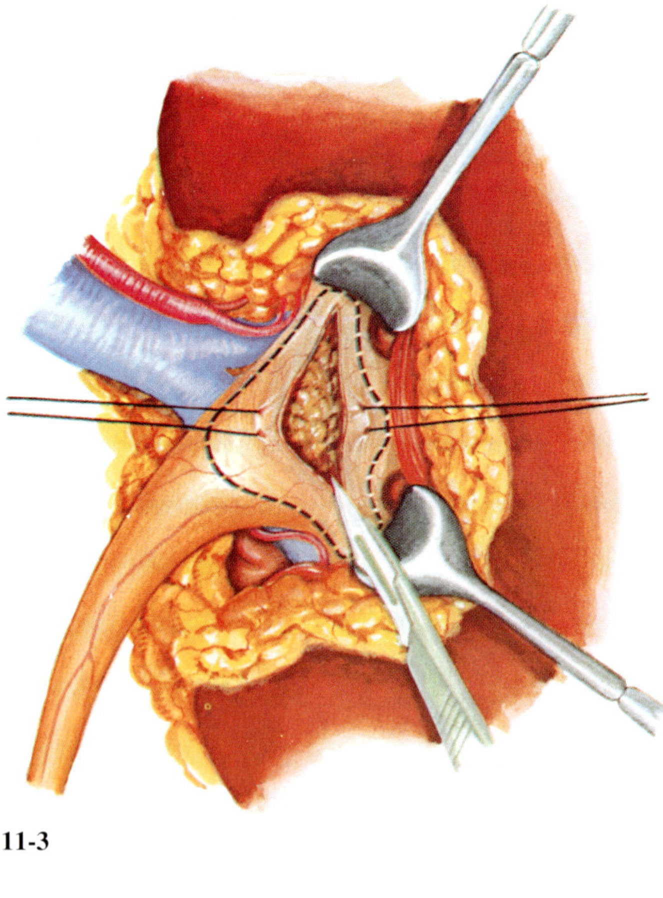

11-3

12. Subcapsular Technique

12-1. An alternative operative approach to the posterior right kidney is similar to the previously described Gil-Vernet method. The *dotted line depicts the line of incision through the renal capsule.*

12-2. *The capsule is incised and peeled* back to expose the intrarenal pelvis. Vein retractors help to expose the surgical field.

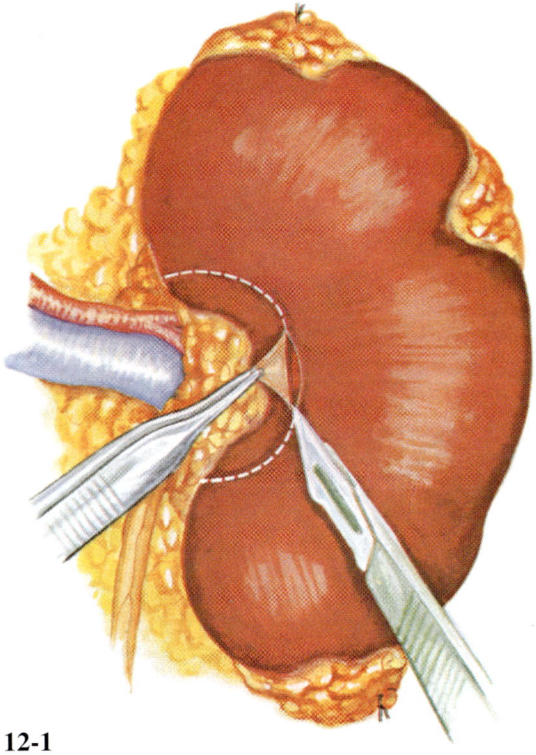

12-1

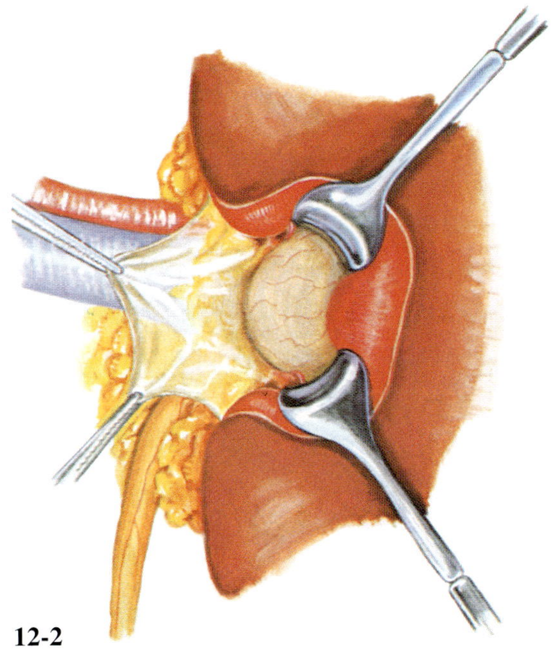

12-2

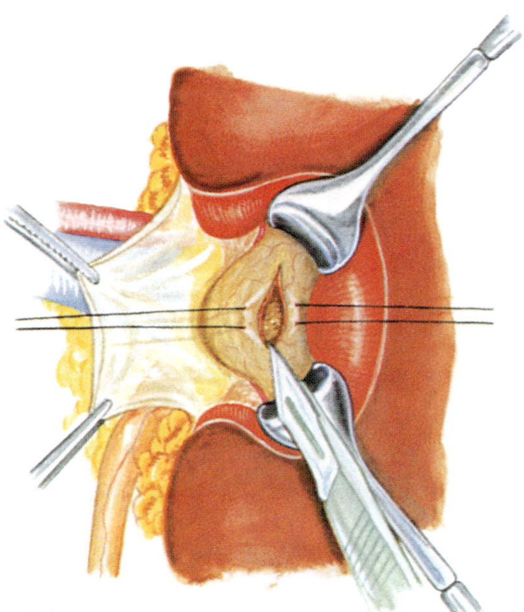

12-3

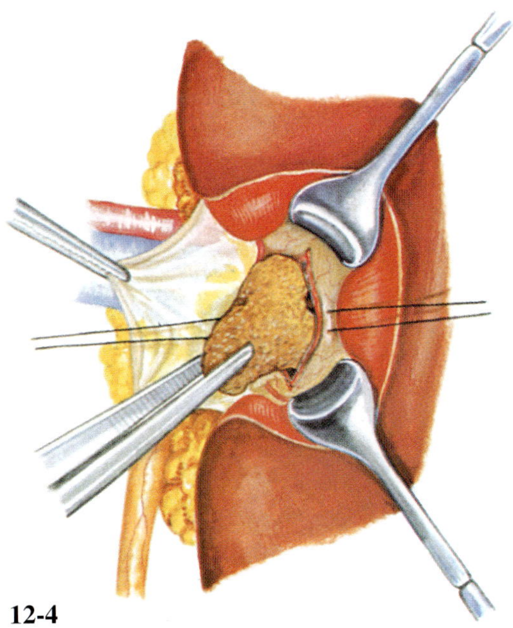

12-4

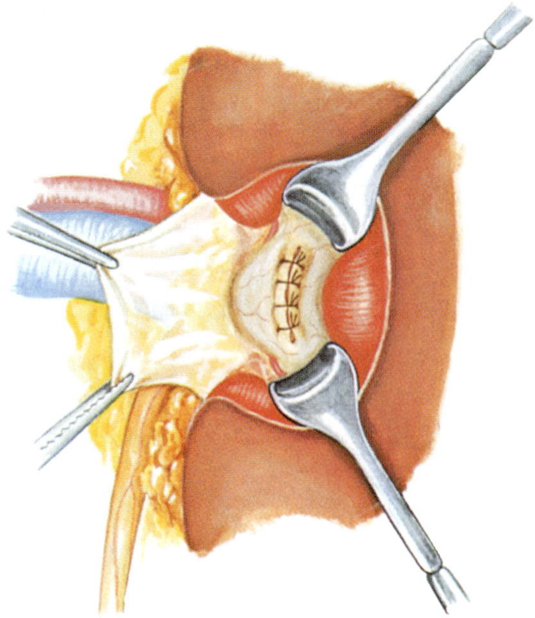

12-5

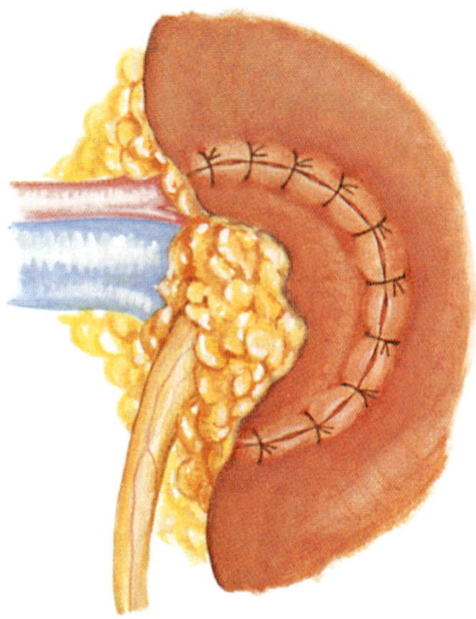

12-6

12-3. *Stay sutures are placed in the renal pelvis.* An incision is made into the lumen of the pelvis.

12-4. *The calculus is removed.*

12-5. Before closure, catheter irrigation is performed within the pelvis. *A ureteral catheter is passed inferiorly to the bladder.* Standard closure of the pelvis is performed.

12-6. *The renal capsule is reapproximated.* A multiperforated flat tube connected to a closed drainage tube and reservoir is inserted prior to closure of muscle and skin.

13. Combined Pyelolithotomy–Nephrolithotomy

In the following sequence, a technique for a stone lodged in a major calix is demonstrated. A standard incision is made to approach, in this case, the left kidney (anterior transabdominal technique).

13-1. *Extrarenal pelvic insertion of the index finger immobilizes the stone by pressure.* In certain instances a Randall's stone forceps can be substituted for the finger.

13-2. *The calculus is readily removed from the incision site.* Through-and-through irrigation is performed.

13-3. For kidney closure, *insertion of a nephrostomy tube may be indicated,* e.g., pyeloplasty or nephrolithotomy. We favor the use of a red rubber straight Robinson catheter (16–22 Fr). Extra holes are cut in the end of the catheter remaining in the renal pelvis.

We have had success with a simple atraumatic method for inserting the nephrostomy tube from skin opening through renal parenchyma, lower dependent calix, and renal pelvis. The use of a male VanBuren sound, (16 Fr), with an opening previously drilled through its curved tip is helpful.

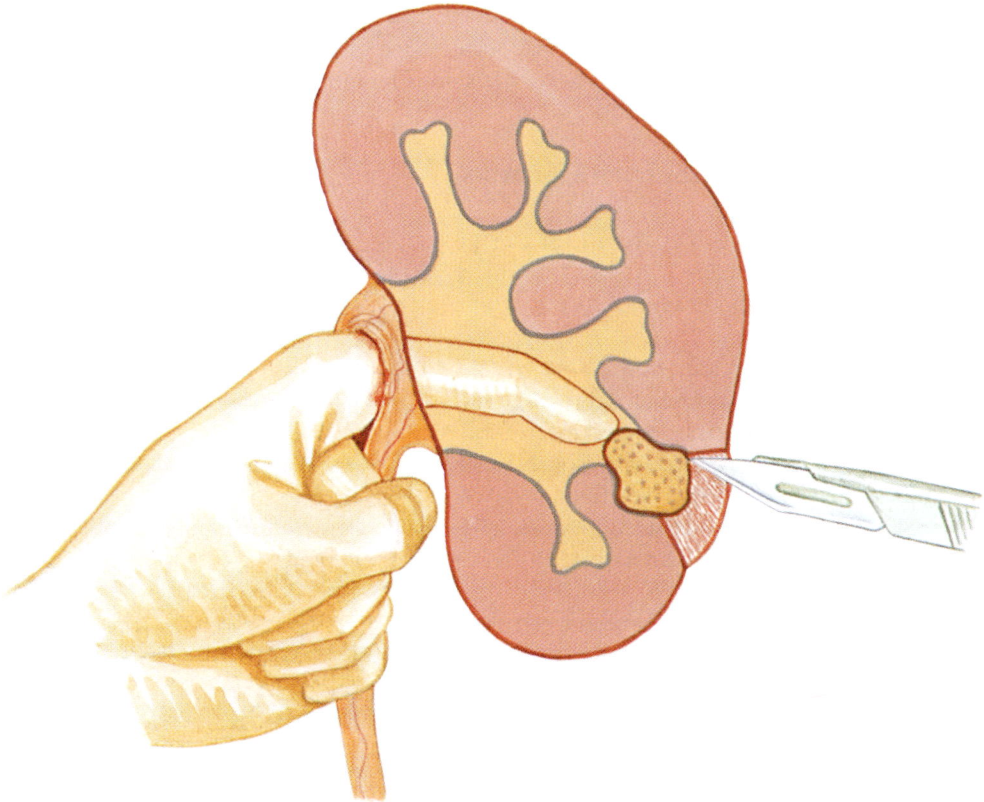

13-1

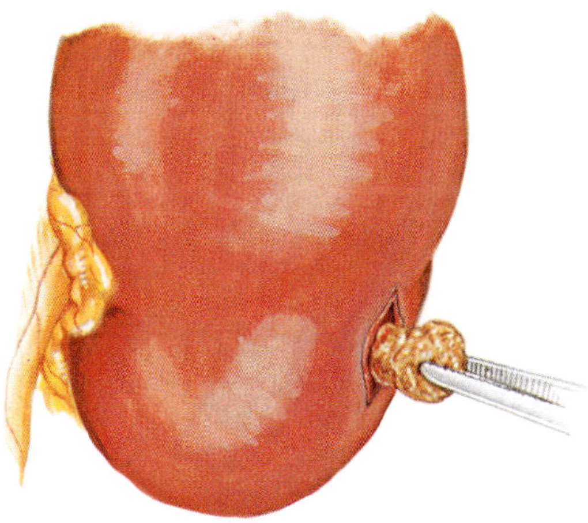

13-2

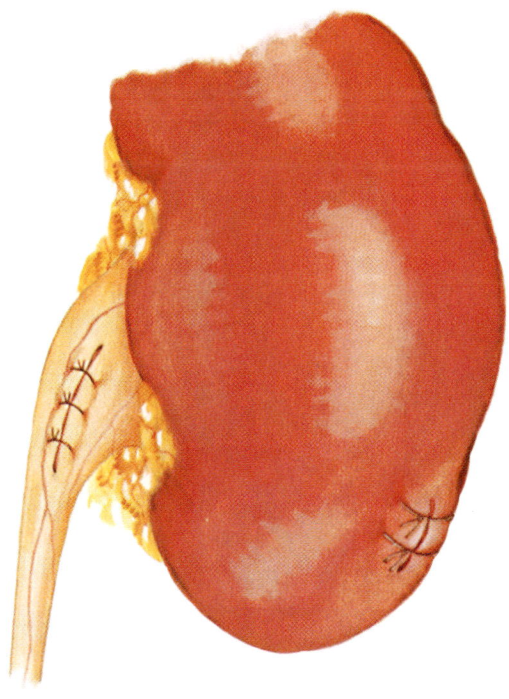

13-3

The tip of the sound is inserted through the renal pelvis and into the dependent calix. Gentle lifting of the sound will provide localization of the sound's tip at the periphery of the renal parenchyma. Only a small incision is required for the sound to be exposed at the renal periphery.

14. Removal of Staghorn Calculus

The preferred surgical approach for this procedure is the lumbar flank method (described earlier), because it provides satisfactory exposure of the kidney surface and posterior renal pelvis and easy access to the renal artery.

14-1. In the schematic showing the *preferred avascular line of incision,* there are two major branches of the renal artery, anterior and posterior. The small area of relative avascularity (*arrow*) is best determined at surgery by injecting 3 mL methylene blue dye into one major arterial branch. Boyce and Elkins prefer the administration of 20 mL methylene blue injected intravenously. We believe the posterior or anterior arterial branch can be briefly occluded. A small 25-gauge needle with 3 mL dye can then be injected in the major renal artery branch (posterior or anterior).

14-2. After the kidney has been freed and lifted from its bed, *the renal artery is temporarily occluded with a vascular clamp.* Cooling of the kidney can be accomplished in several ways. We prefer the method and procedure described in 8–2 and 8–4. Other methods include the use of sterilized ice packs, refrigerated saline, or sterile saline slush in a plastic envelope. On a rare occasion, frank removal of the kidney and "workbench" surgery may be elected by the surgeon. This requires renal artery perfusion of a hypothermic solution (7° C) to preserve function. The ureter is not severed in this procedure.

The following sequence of illustrations demonstrates the details of staghorn calculus removal by an intersegmental approach.

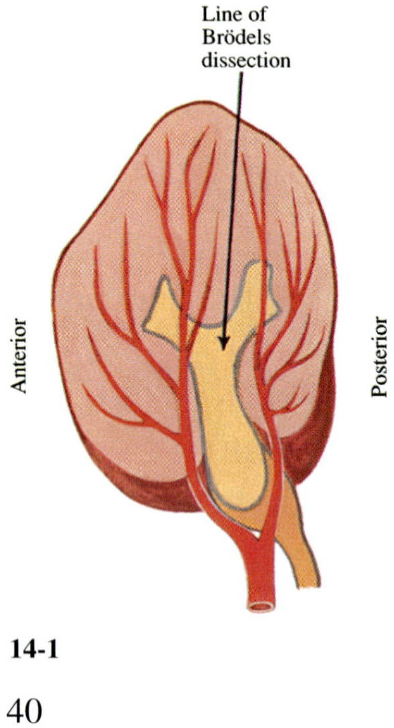

14-1

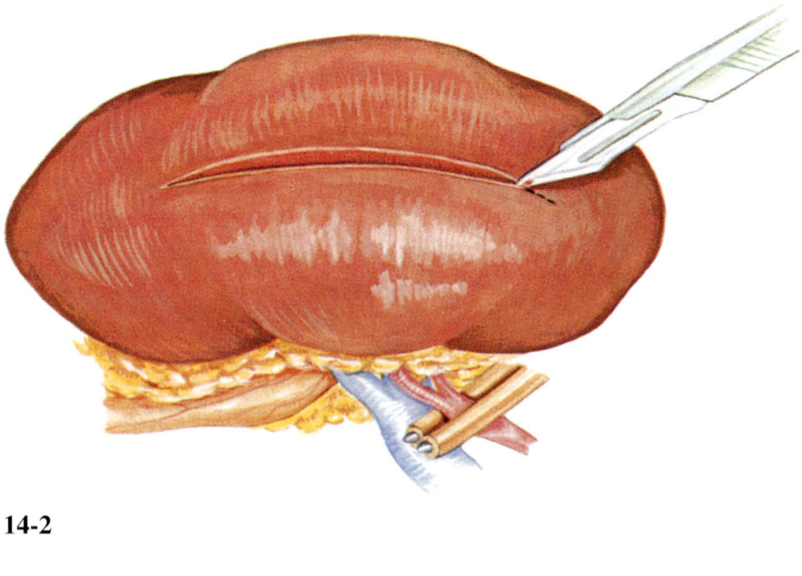

14-2

14-3. The *incision is extended* by blunt dissection *down to the surface tissue of the pelvis and calices.* The handle of the knife is used.

14-4. *Branches of the renal artery and vein* can be recognized and *are individually ligated.* The pelvis is entered between the anterior and posterior calices at the caudal end of the kidney. The peripelvic venous plexus is less well formed on this end.

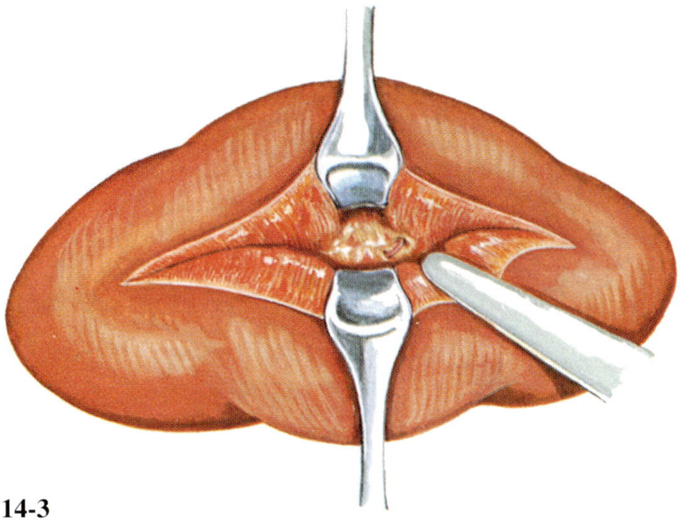

14-3

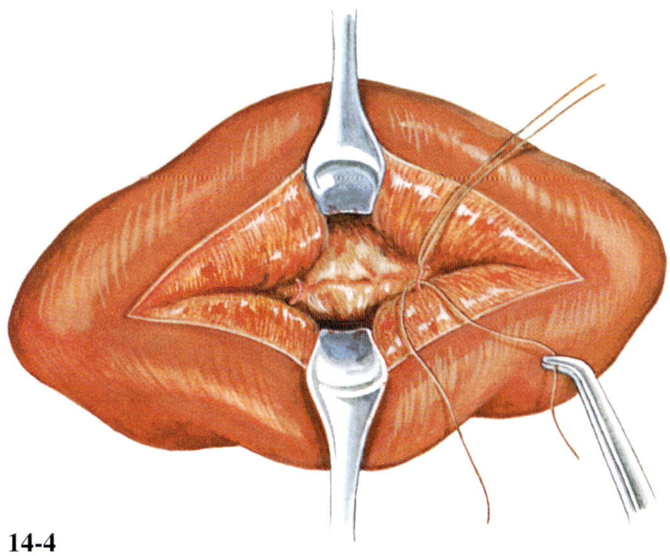

14-4

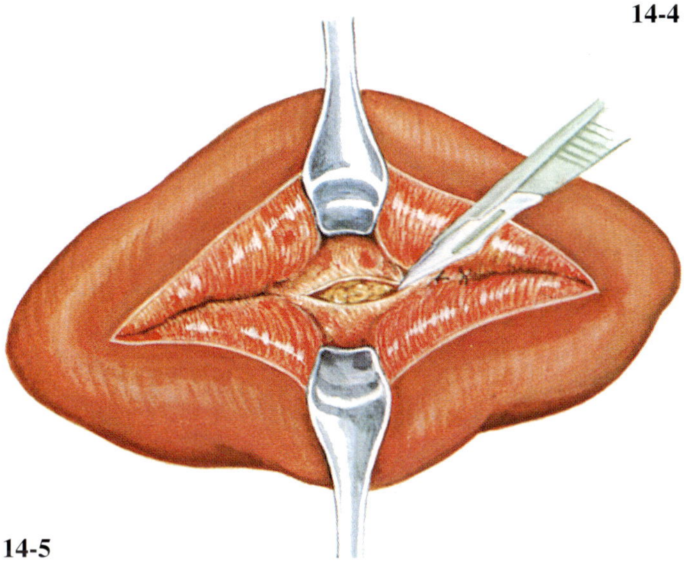

14-5

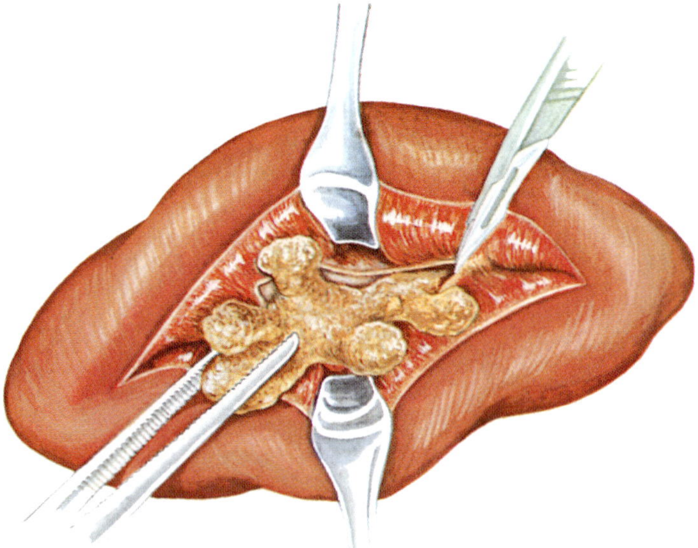

14-6

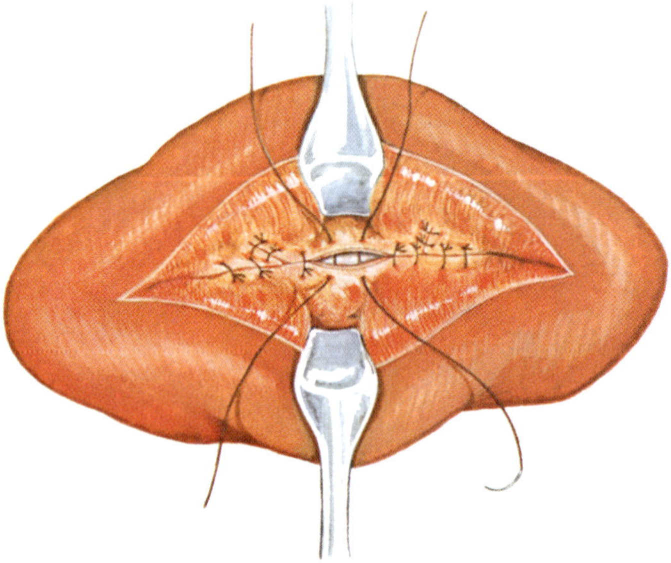

14-7

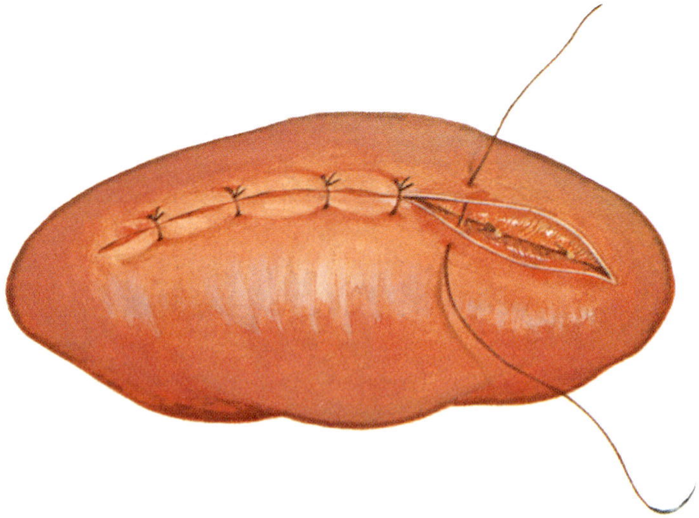

14-8

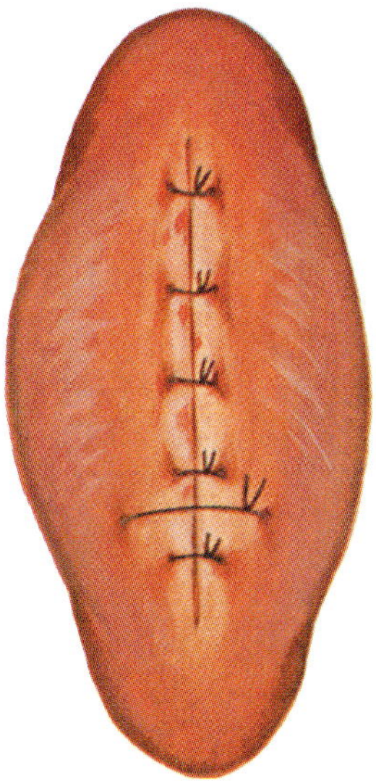

14-9

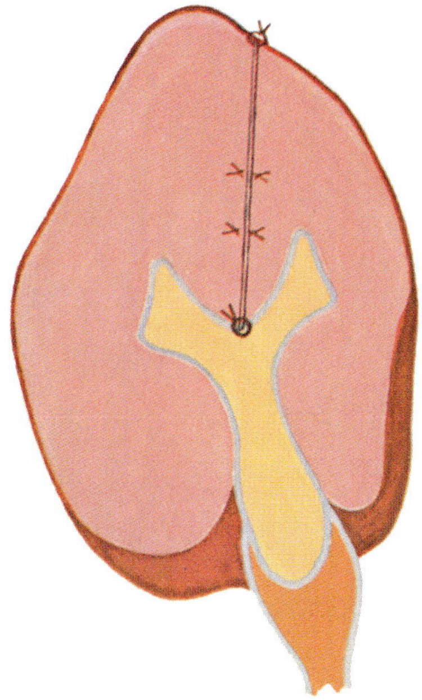

14-10

14-5. The *incision is* made and *gradually extended into the pelvis* to facilitate removal of the staghorn calculus. Each calix containing a branch of calculus is opened by extending the incision from the incised pelvis. The posterior calices are incised on their anterior surfaces, and if necessary, the anterior calices are opened on their posterior surface. All caliceal extensions are made in the transverse plane. This technique will generally avoid the transmedullary and interlobar arterial branches.

14-6. The calices are opened and dissected in a lateral and medial direction to allow *removal of the stone in a single piece.*

Closure

14-7. *Pelvic and caliceal closure is made with 5–0 chromic catgut.*

14-8. *The renal capsule is closed.*

14-9. *Continued vascular oozing can be controlled by one or more deeper sutures.*

14-10. *A schematic clarifies internal details of the closure.*

15. Hydronephrosis and Pyeloplasty

Either the lumbar flank or the transabdominal approach to the kidney can be used (see descriptions of these approaches earlier in this section). We do not prefer one approach over the other.

Diagnostic Workup. Before a patient undergoes an operation for unilateral, congenital hydronephrosis, selected studies are helpful in addition to the intravenous pyelogram. We believe that a voiding cystourethrogram is indicated to rule out vesicoureteral reflux. Renal split-function tests, noninvasive, are useful. We use the photoscintiscanner with the Anger camera. After injection of 300 μCi (adult dose) Hippuran ^{131}I, we can obtain renal plasma flow in each kidney. In many instances cystoscopy and retrograde pyelography may be required to demonstrate the ureteropelvic junction obstruc-

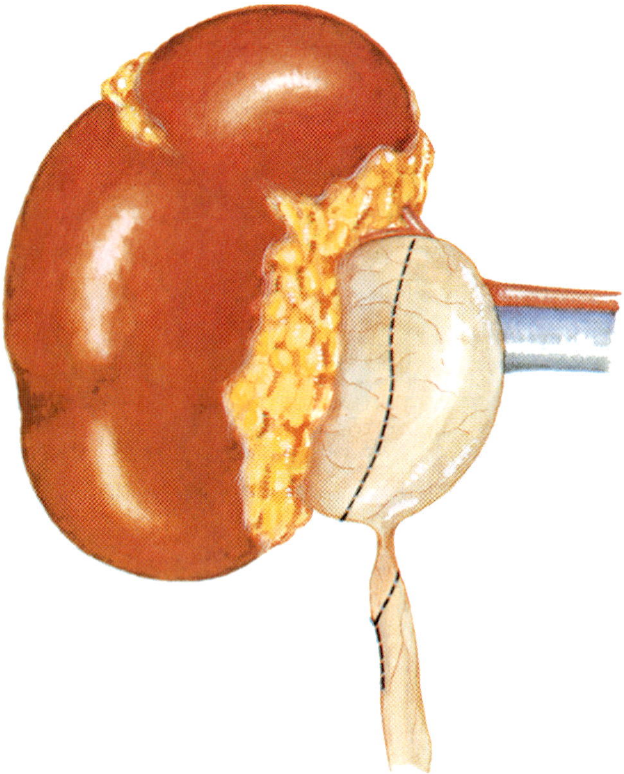

15-1

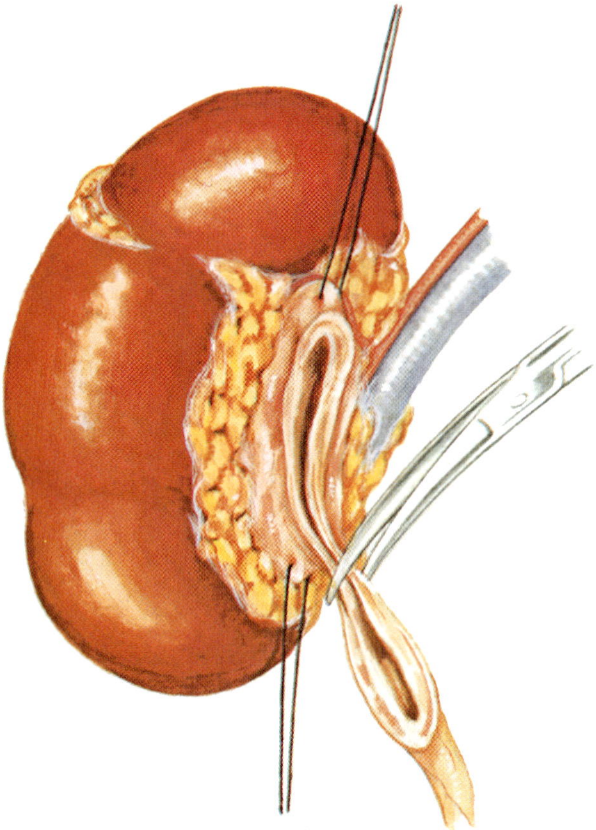

15-2

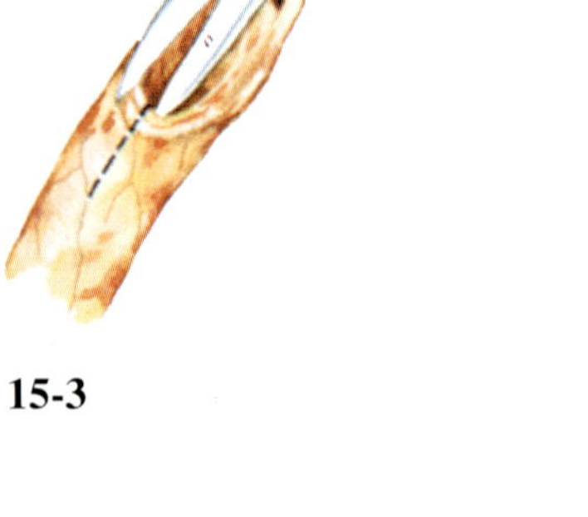

15-3

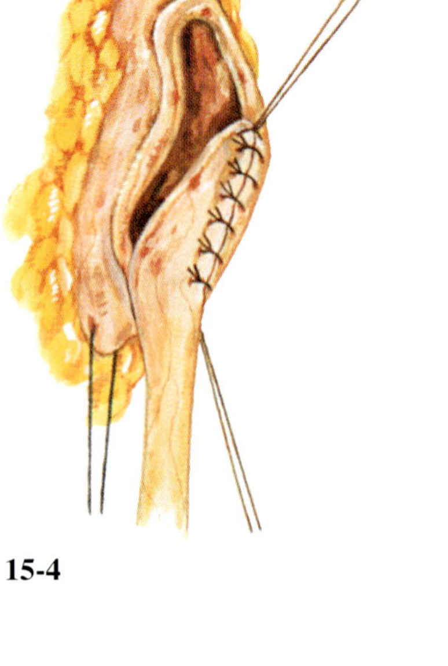

15-4

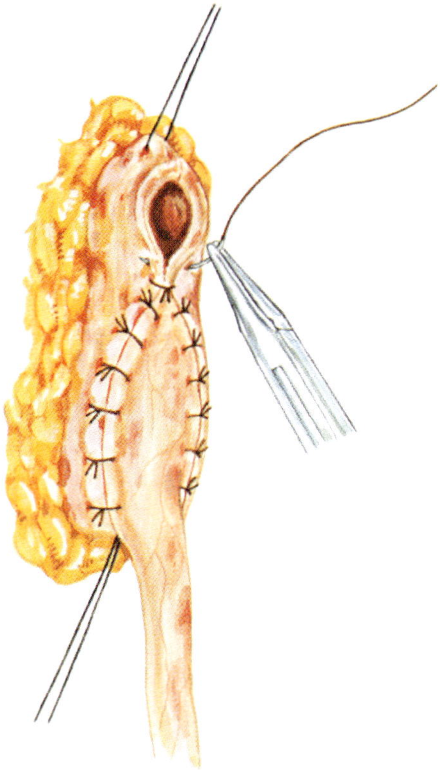

15-5

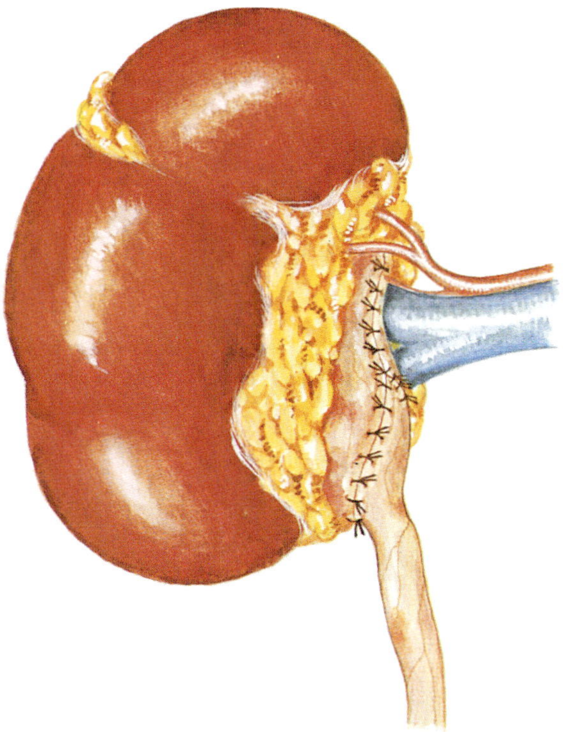

15-6

tion. We schedule this last procedure in the adult patient during late afternoon of the day prior to surgery.

15-1. In the *isolated posterior left kidney, the vein is anterior to the artery.* Both lines of incision are shown for a dismembered pyeloplasty.

15-2. *Stay sutures guide the excision of excessive renal pelvis.*

15-3. *The severed ureteral stoma is widened* by a longitudinal cut. One can avoid twisting the ureter by using a stay suture.

15-4. *One edge of the pyeloplasty has been accomplished by means of interrupted 4–0 chromic catgut sutures.*

15–5. The pyeloplasty has been completed and *the remaining renal pelvis is reapproximated and sutured.*

15-6. *Pyeloplasty and pelvic closure are completed.*

When the abdominal incision is closed, if the urine is uninfected, a nephrostomy tube is not used. A flat tubular drain is placed near the pyeloplasty. This drain is connected to a tube that leads to the exterior. The distal end is capped by a bulb that creates negative pressure. A ureteral stent can be inserted, extending across the anastomotic junction and brought out as a nephrostomy. Extra holes in the stent, positioned at the renal pelvis, are helpful. Closure of the musculature and skin is performed in the usual fashion.

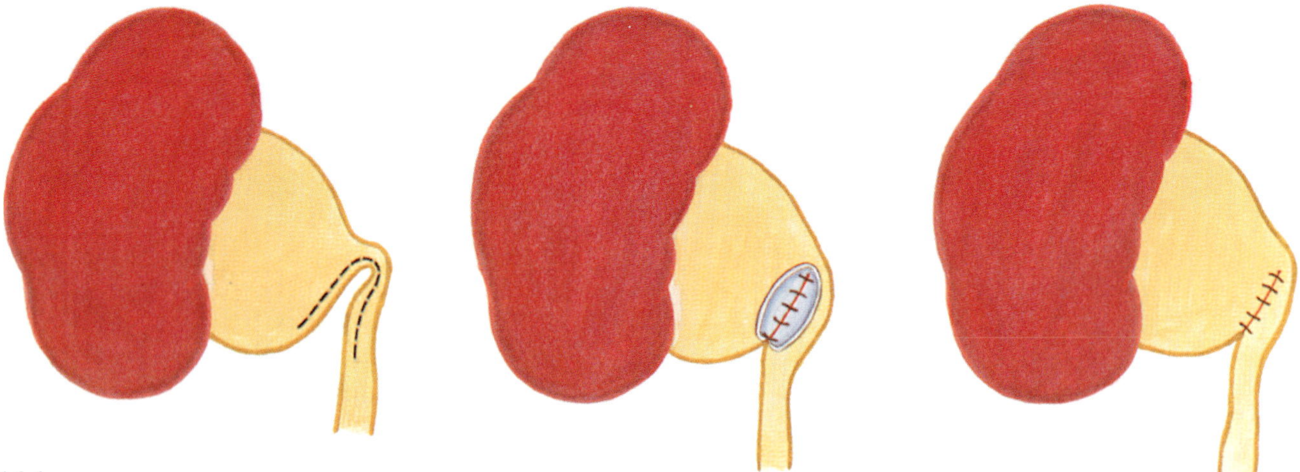

16-1

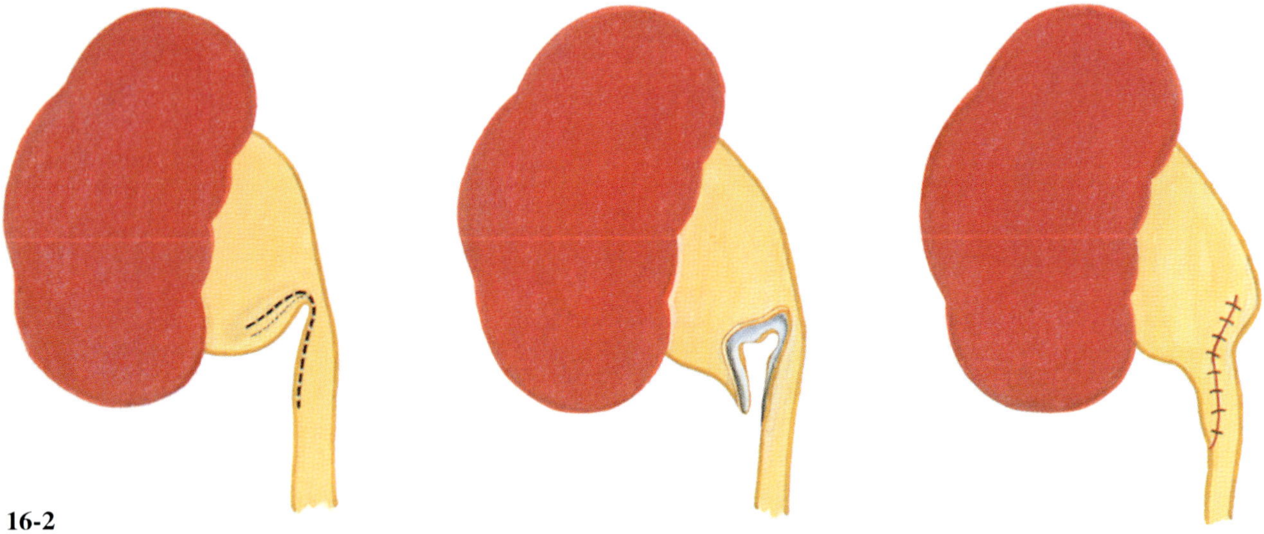

16-2

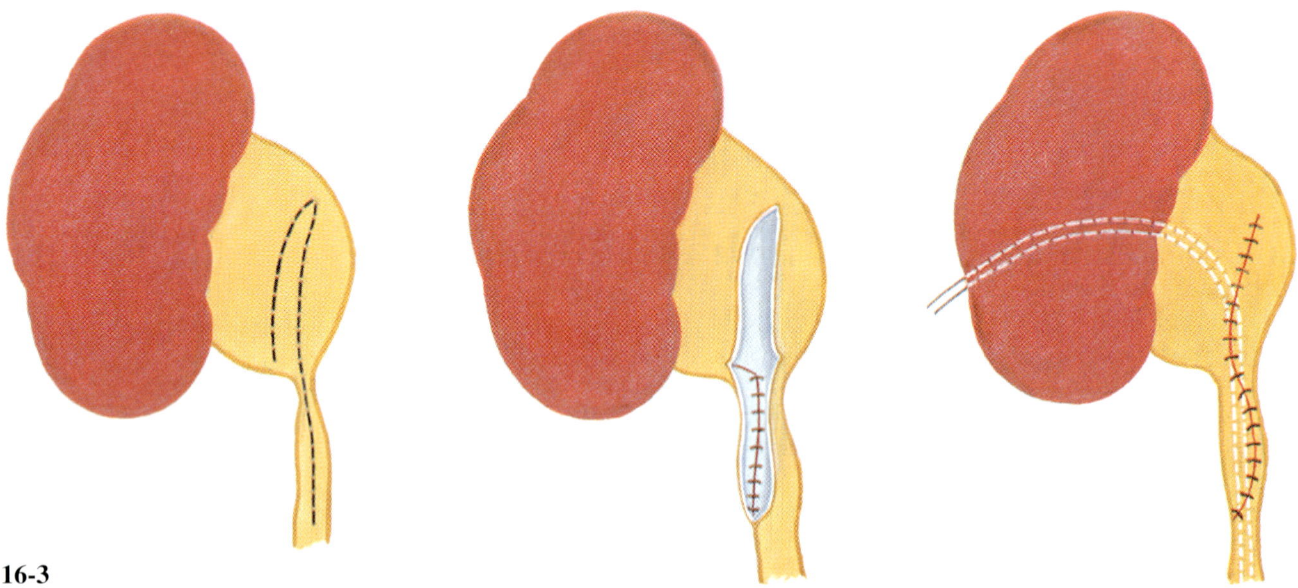

16-3

16. Variations of Technique for Hydronephrosis.

The following illustrations show variations in surgical treatment.

16-1. *von Lichtenberg pyeloplasty* (Finney principle for pyloroplasty)

16-2. *Foley-Y type pyeloplasty*

16-3. *Culp-Scardino pyeloplasty*

17. Surgical Treatment of Renal Cyst

The procedure is demonstrated on the left kidney lower pole. Either a flank or transabdominal incision can be used to reach the diseased organ. We prefer the flank approach.

17-1. *Fluid is aspirated* and submitted for cytology. If malignant cells are found, a nephrectomy is indicated at a later date.

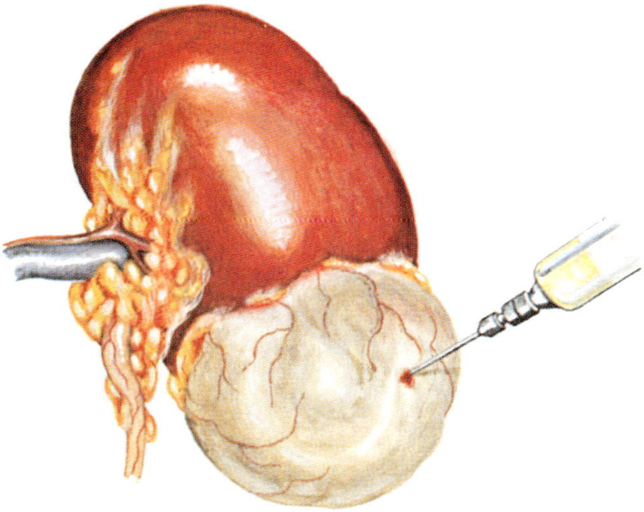

17-1

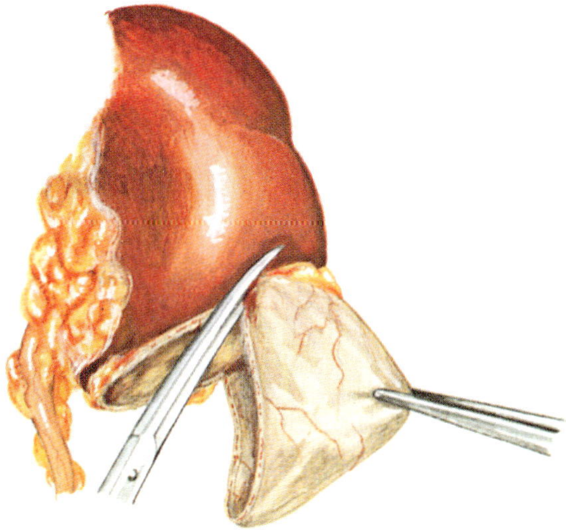

17-2

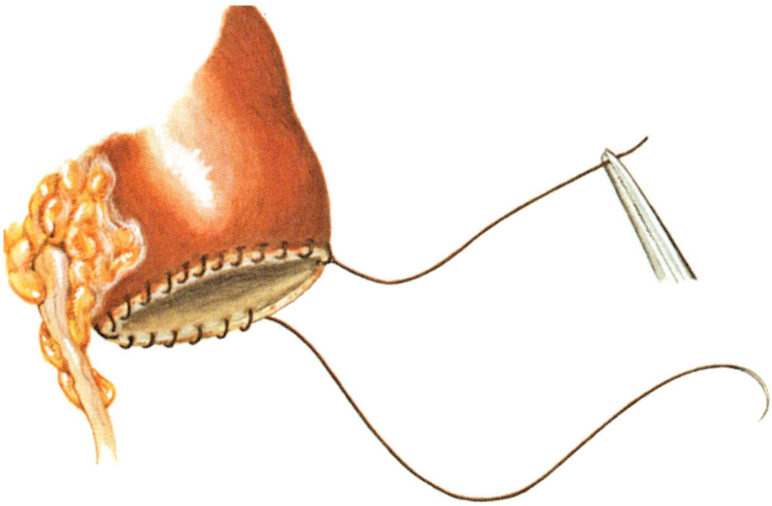

17-3

17-2. The *cyst is circumferentially excised,* leaving a 1 to 2 mm cuff.

17-3. A *continuous hemostatic stitch* is used.

18. Trauma to the Genitourinary System

Kidney Injuries

18-1. A diseased or anomalous kidney (congenital anomaly, or a hydronephrotic kidney) is more easily injured than a normal kidney following an auto accident or physical trauma. Penetration of soft tissues is not necessary.

The most common causes of kidney injury are a severe fall, an auto accident, or a gunshot wound. Penetrating injuries usually involve multiple organs and a point of entry may be present with or without a point of exit. A bullet can ricochet and cause multiple organ injuries. A team approach is used, and the urologist is usually involved because of gross hematuria, or a pelvic injury involving the bladder, and bladder neck-urethral area.

Gross painless hematuria is the key sign of urinary tract injury. The associated organ injuries (for example, the spleen or a liver laceration) will, of course, provide pain and possibly shock due to blood loss. To define the extent of kidney injury, a CT scan should be performed as an emergency if the patient's vital signs are stable. Intravenous contrast media can be injected when gross hematuria has been verified. An emergency CT scan is a definitive study and should be performed to define the magnitude of the intra-abdominal injury. If renal injury is present, the CT scan will define the severity and extent of the renal trauma. A left renal injury will often involve trauma to the spleen. A right renal injury may be present along with injury or laceration of the liver.

If the above studies confirm the urologic injuries, then surgical exploration may be

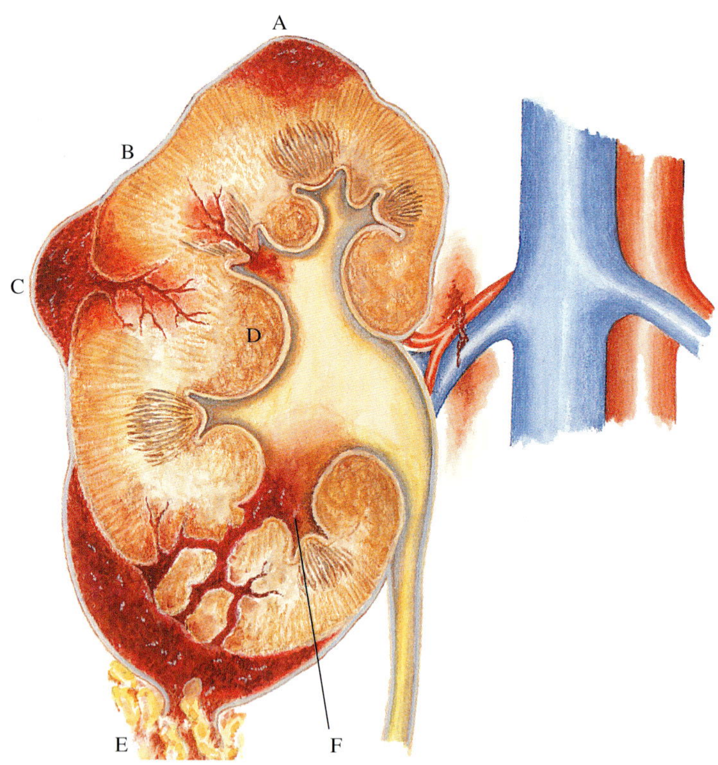

18-1

necessary. Because multiple organ system injury may be present, the trauma surgeon and the urologist should explore the patient together. The abdomen and retroperitoneal space must be carefully examined. Bowel injury must be ruled out before proceeding retroperitoneally. Every attempt is made to salvage the kidney. A partial injury—contusion or minor laceration—need not be explored after the CT scan. A major laceration at the pole of the kidney with significant retroperitoneal hemorrhage may necessitate a partial nephrectomy. Only as a last resort should a nephrectomy be performed—usually to stop persistent hemorrhage from a severely lacerated kidney. At exploration it is usually best not to open Gerota's fascia at the site of injury. Exposure often leads to brisk bleeding and loss of the entire kidney. Minimal exposure to warrant a partial nephrectomy is appropriate in some instances.

The figure in this section (see 18–1) illustrates the various types of renal injuries that can be sustained in a motor vehicle accident. The injured person can be a pedestrian. In most instances the passenger has not buckled his/her seat belt and the passenger is thrown against the inner wall or seat of the automobile, sustaining a significant bruise to his/her upper abdomen.

In 18–1, A to F illustrate the types of injuries that a kidney can sustain. A subcapsular hemorrhage is shown at the upper pole (A). An intrarenal laceration with rupture to the renal pelvis is demonstrated (B). Laterally, and just superior to the mid-kidney is a demonstration of a subcapsular hematoma (C). If bed rest is not mandated, the subcapsular hemorrhage can progress and extend. We have seen hypertension of an episodic nature due to renal cortical compression from the hematoma. Deep to the subcapsular hematoma is evidence of some disruption of parenchyma (D). At the lower pole are demonstrations of two different types of injuries. A capsular rupture can be seen (E) and a complete capsular rupture into the calix (F) is demonstrated.

Bladder Injuries

Auto accidents or a fall from a significant height may cause a bladder rupture. A full bladder at the time of injury will usually coexist and the rupture may be quite severe. Hematuria may be present as a diagnostic sign. If an isolated injury to the bladder has occurred, a cystogram performed by inserting a urethral catheter and injecting, under low pressure, 100–200 mL of contrast media will confirm the injury. A major bladder laceration, usually with intraperitoneal extravasation of urine, must be explored. Surgical repair of the bladder is indicated using two layers of chromic catgut (2–0) for closure. A suprapubic cystostomy is mandatory for 7 to 12 days, depending on the severity of injury.

Urethral Injuries

A ruptured urethra can occur after a fall or an auto accident where the perineal area has been injured. If the disruption is severe and includes pubic rami fractures, the urethra in the bulbous area may be completely transected. The diagnosis of urethral disruption is made by a retrograde urethrogram. Urethral continuity needs to be established by surgery. At the time of surgery, a combined approach may be necessary. After preparing the patient and placing him into the lithotomy position a flexible cystoscope or ureteroscope may be passed via the urethra after the bladder has been fully exposed surgically. At surgery, visualization of the bladder neck and prostatic urethra and observation and visualization of the light coming from the distal urethra at the site of interruption may allow passage of a cannula or small catheter across the disrupted urethra. Reestablishment of urethral continuity using the least amount of trauma is important. A silicone 20–22 Fr catheter is used in adults; a smaller catheter will be needed in a child after reestablishing continuity. The silicone catheter is kept in place for at least 4 weeks.

Scrotal-Testicular Injury

Injury to the testicles can occur as a result of trauma. Every attempt should be made to save the testicle. Ultrasonography of the testicles can provide actual visualization of the injured site in the testicle. Salvaging the testicle on surgical exploration is mandatory. Exploration is best carried out within the first 1 to 2 hours after injury.

19. Diagnosis and Treatment of Perirenal Abscesses

Perirenal abscesses are not common, but they are potentially a very lethal complication due to bacterial infection or progression of the infection with migration of the abscess to critical retroperitoneal areas.

Several decades ago, the mortality rate following the development of perirenal abscesses was about 50%. The patient usually developed a bacterial infection due to Staphylococcus aureus. Many of these patients were immunologically compromised. Uncontrolled diabetes mellitus with periods of noncompliance by the patient is a common scenario.

Most collections of perirenal abscesses occur within or adjacent to the kidney. The illustrations demonstrate the route of spread. The abscesses can best be demonstrated by CT scan. The major clinical consideration is to be suspicious of an abscess in order to make a prompt diagnosis and start treatment. The patients often have diabetes mellitus.

Perirenal abscesses can develop from the mouth, the skin, or respiratory infections. In today's clinical arena, the disease usually begins as a kidney infection, probably in a drug abuser. The abscesses are due to bacterial infection in a patient who has diabetes mellitus or who is partially immunocompetent. The offending organisms are usually Eschericia coli or Proteus mirabilis.

The infection can develop if a small obstructive stone in an upper pole of the kidney is present. The progressive obstruction of urine leads to infection, particularly in a patient with severe diabetes mellitus. The infection can be progressive so that the spread can be into the perirenal area. The abscess takes more than a few days to enlarge and progress, and the patient may actually present 7 to 10 days later. With bacterial spread the interstitium—the medulla and cortex of the kidney—may form small abscesses. At this interval in time, antibiotic therapy can still usually deal with and eradicate the infection. However, in our experience, and in reviewing the last 22 cases at our major hospital, the patient is often a diabetic who is somewhat malnourished, and with infection the abscess develops and may spread in a variety of ways. As mentioned above, the key diagnostic test is a CT scan. Blood cultures and urinary tract cultures should be obtained so that appropriate antibiotic treatment may be started.

Making the diagnosis, as mentioned, can be difficult. The patient's complaint may be a vague flank or abdominal pain. The fever may only be in the 101° F range. A significant leukocytosis is not present. We have noted that the increase in white cell count is only in the 12,000 range. Clinical findings which can suggest the presence of an abscess are as follows:

1. The patient is compromised, and has been on a very poor therapeutic regimen for the diabetes mellitus.
2. The discomfort and pain on one side has been present for at least 7 days.
3. An abdominal mass or flank mass may be present with tenderness.
4. A positive blood culture due to E. coli or P. mirabilis has been identified.
5. Even though appropriate antibiotic therapy including an aminoglycoside and intravenous ampicillin has been started, 48 hours later the clinical response has not been beneficial.

The clinical findings that should raise the suspicion of perirenal abscess include the following workup: on chest x-ray, the diaphragm on the side of the abscess may be elevated; a pleural effusion on the same side may be present; the psoas muscle margin may reveal a very indistinct kidney border, or a mass effect may be present. On ultrasonography, intrarenal and perirenal abscesses appear as hypoechoic masses; gas within the abscess may be present and is echogenic. The CT scan is the most helpful diagnostic test.

Management of Renal Abscess

19-1 and 19-2. The cross section and longitudinal section shown delineate the spread of the abscess. Therefore, drainage must address these pockets of abscess. Drainage by surgery necessitates eradicating these purulent sites extraperitoneally.

Patients with kidney infections require hospitalization. The drainage of the abscess is obviously necessary. The aminoglycoside and ampicillin intravenous therapies must be started and continued. The use of floxacins by the intravenous route is another good choice. Care must be taken to be sure that kidney function is still not altered significantly. The procedure will probably include a nephrectomy on one side, and the remaining kidney must be able to sustain life.

Although antibiotic treatment followed by percutaneous drainage of an abscess is an attractive approach, we believe that surgical exploration is mandatory (19–1 and 19–2). The appropriate antibiotics must be continued. The drainage route in our hands has been to use an extraperitoneal approach to carefully drain the major abscess cavities. A subcostal incision which is extraperitoneal is a good location focusing on the 12th rib. Loculations may be present and blunt dissection is used to allow evacuation of the ab-

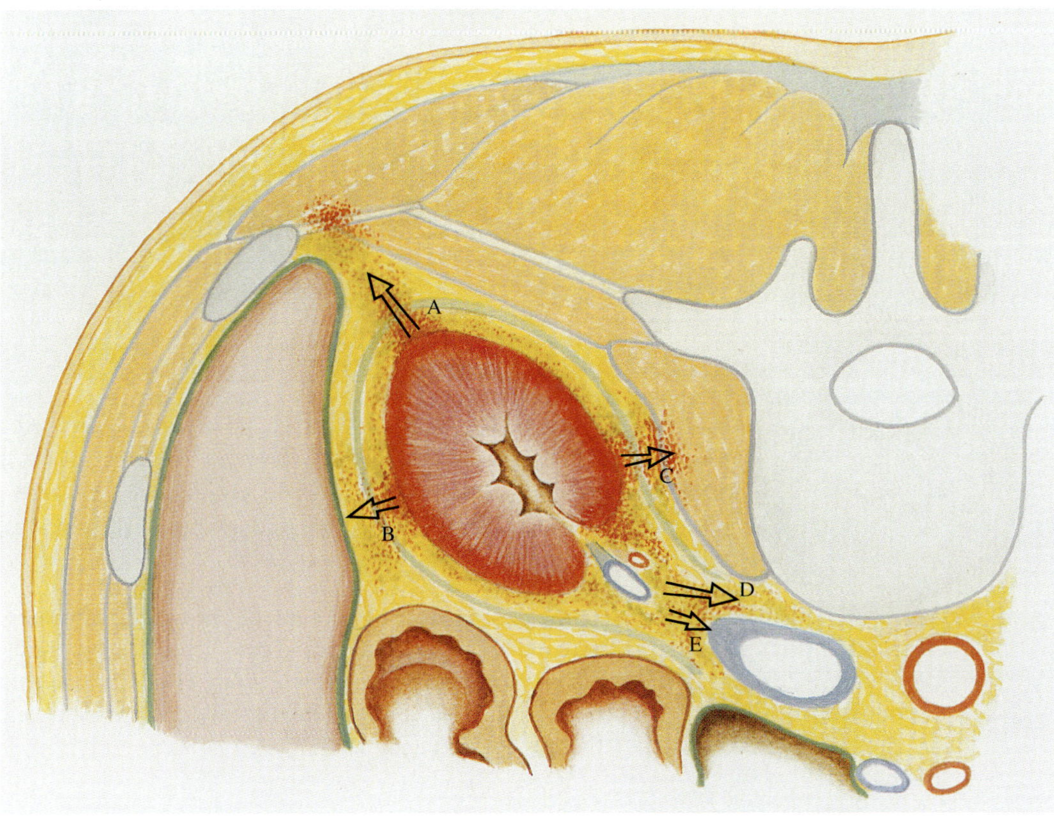

19-1. Perirenal Abscess (I) (after Netter). A: to flank through PCN wound; B: to retroperitoneal tissue through renal fascia of Gerota; C: to psoas muscle; D: to midline—prevertebral; E: to inferior vena cava.

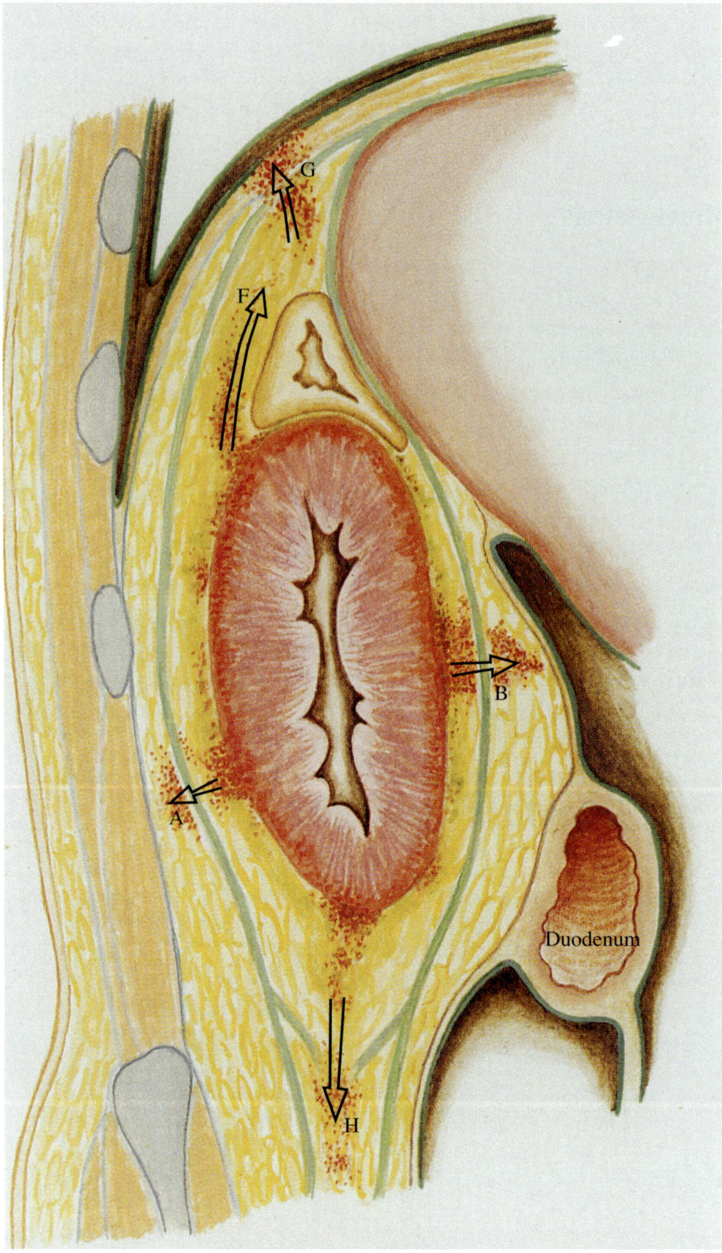

19-2. Perirenal abscess (II) (after Netter). F: to retrohepatic and subphrenic area; G: to pleural cavity through diaphragm; H: to pelvic retroperitoneal tissues.

scess. One should avoid entry into the peritoneal cavity or into the chest cavity. Primary nephrectomy in the instances where the abscess is widespread may be necessary, but, if possible, viable tissue should be maintained and partial nephrectomy is a better route to follow. If the kidney is nonfunctioning, then, of course, nephrectomy may be required.

Postoperatively, antibiotic therapy is continued. Renal function is carefully monitored.

Kidney Transplantation

The operative approach for kidney transplantation will vary according to the patient—adult or child.

Indications for the procedure are determined by the presence of bilateral end-stage kidney disease necessitating chronic hemodialysis. Although it is unproved, we believe that tissue typing with matching of antigens between an unrelated donor and the recipient is important. Blood groups must be compatible and without evidence of elevated blood antibody titers in the recipient against the incoming donor lymphocytes (antigens). Reports suggest that multiple blood transfusions to the recipient prior to transplantation are beneficial.

For cadaver kidney transplantation, the organ must be carefully harvested and perfused under hypothermia for preservation. We prefer en bloc dissection of both donor kidneys, including the adjacent aorta and vena cava. With donor kidneys meticulous care also must be taken to preserve the vascular supply to the ureters.

If a choice exists, a donor left kidney is reversed and implanted into the recipient's right iliac fossa. Hypothermic flushing of the donor kidney at the time of harvest, using an intracellular solution, can preserve function up to 18 hours.

20. Adult

20-1. *The line of incision* for an adult patient is oblique and extraperitoneal.

20-2. The peritoneum is reflected medially. *The inferior epigastric artery and vein are individually ligated and divided.* In the male the vas deferens and spermatic cord on the side of the allograft are divided to prevent ureteral obstruction.

20-3. *The external iliac vein and internal iliac artery are exposed.* Care is taken to ligate all major lymphatic vessels to prevent fluid accumulation (the use of silver clips ex-

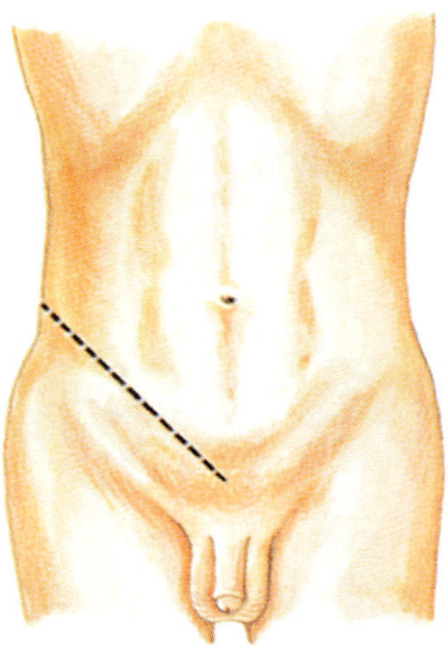

20-1

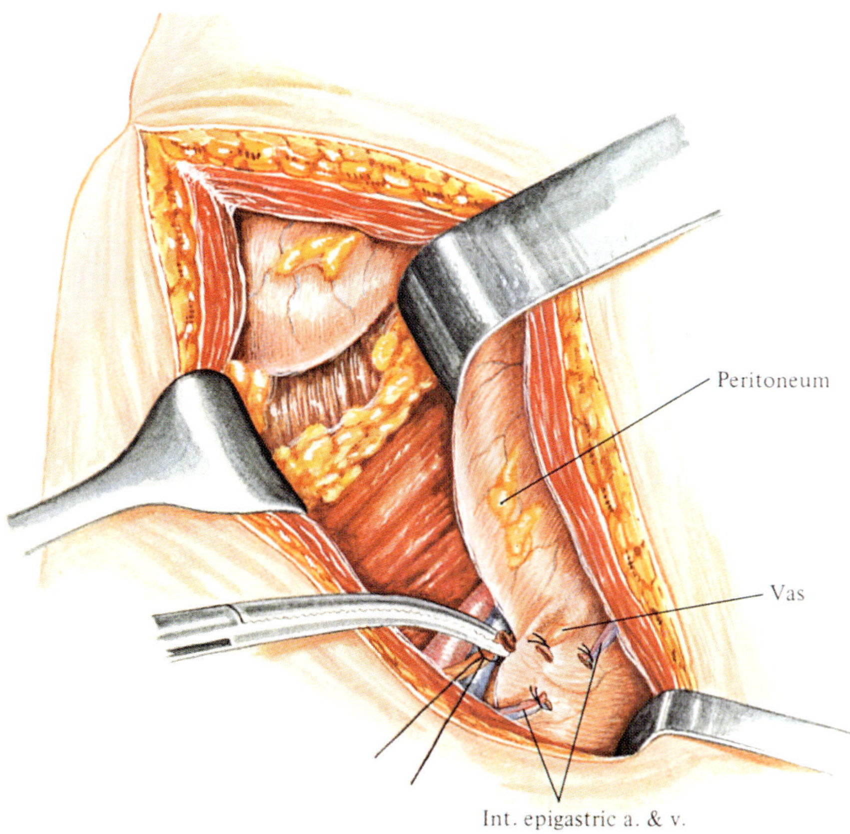

20-2

pedites this maneuver). Using an umbilical tape around the hypogastric artery facilitates isolation of its major branches. At this point in the procedure the proximal hypogastric artery is freed and prepared for use. The distal branches are doubly ligated in continuity (2–0 silk) and transected between ties. A bulldog vascular clamp is placed at its origin. The external iliac vein is freed prior to the venotomy.

20-4. *Vascular clamps are placed on the external iliac vein superior and inferior to the venotomy site.* An elliptical venous window is created that approximates the size of the donor renal vein. The elliptical opening lies slightly anterolaterally. If a valve in the external iliac vein is noted, it must be made nonfunctional by sharp dissection.

The venous anastomosis is completed end-to-side prior to arterial anastomosis. Continuous vascular sutures (5–0 nylon) are used from end to end. Heparinized saline is used several times to irrigate the lumens of both recipient and donor veins prior to closure.

20-5. *Venous anastomosis (top) and arterial end-to-end anastomosis (bottom) are performed.* Heparinized saline is used to irrigate the arterial lumens prior to completion

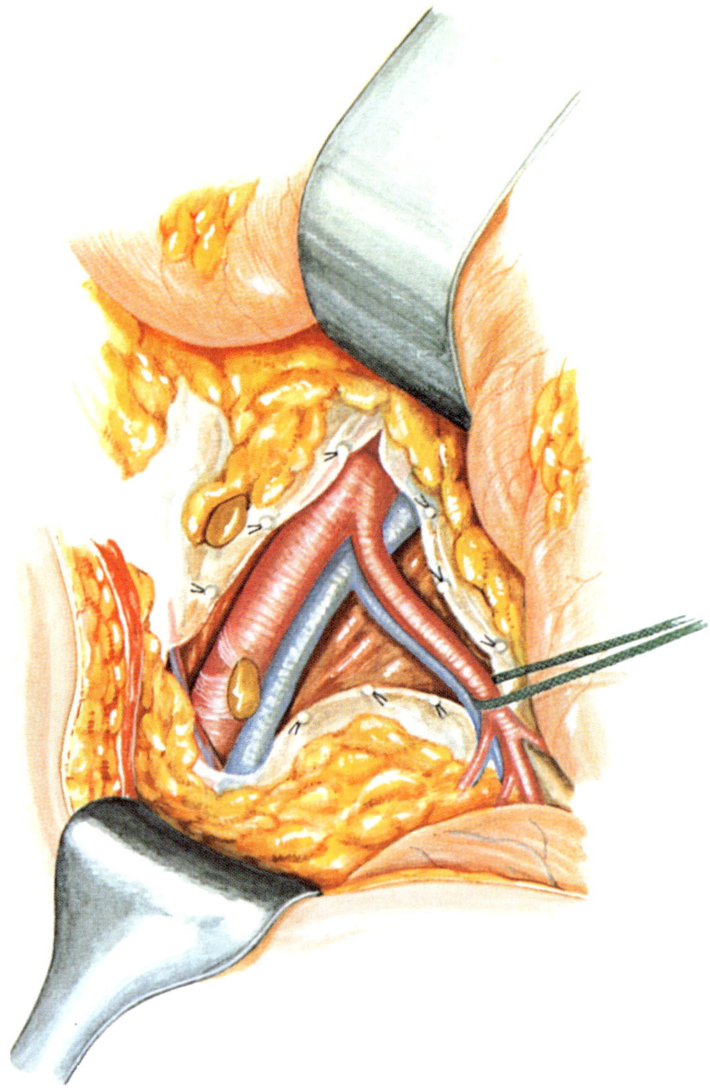

20-3

20-4

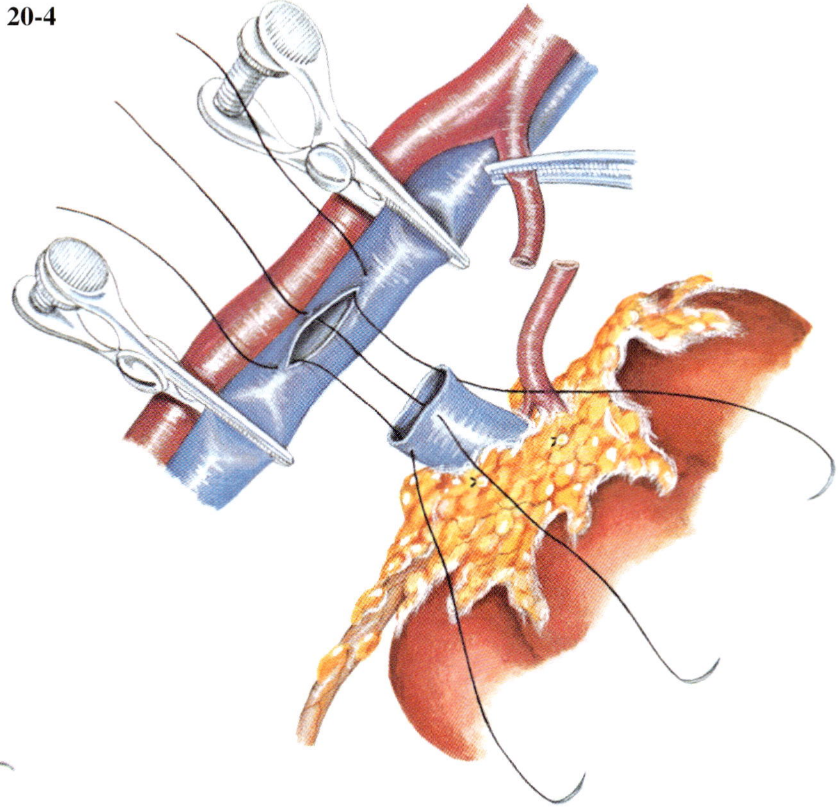

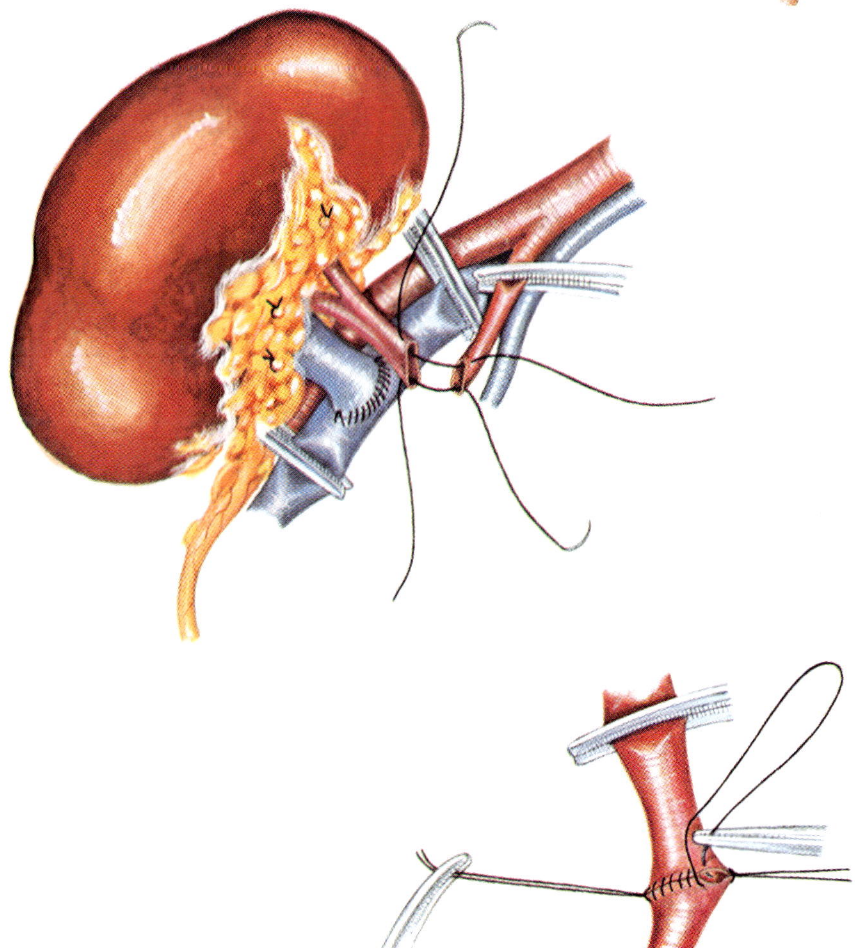

20-5

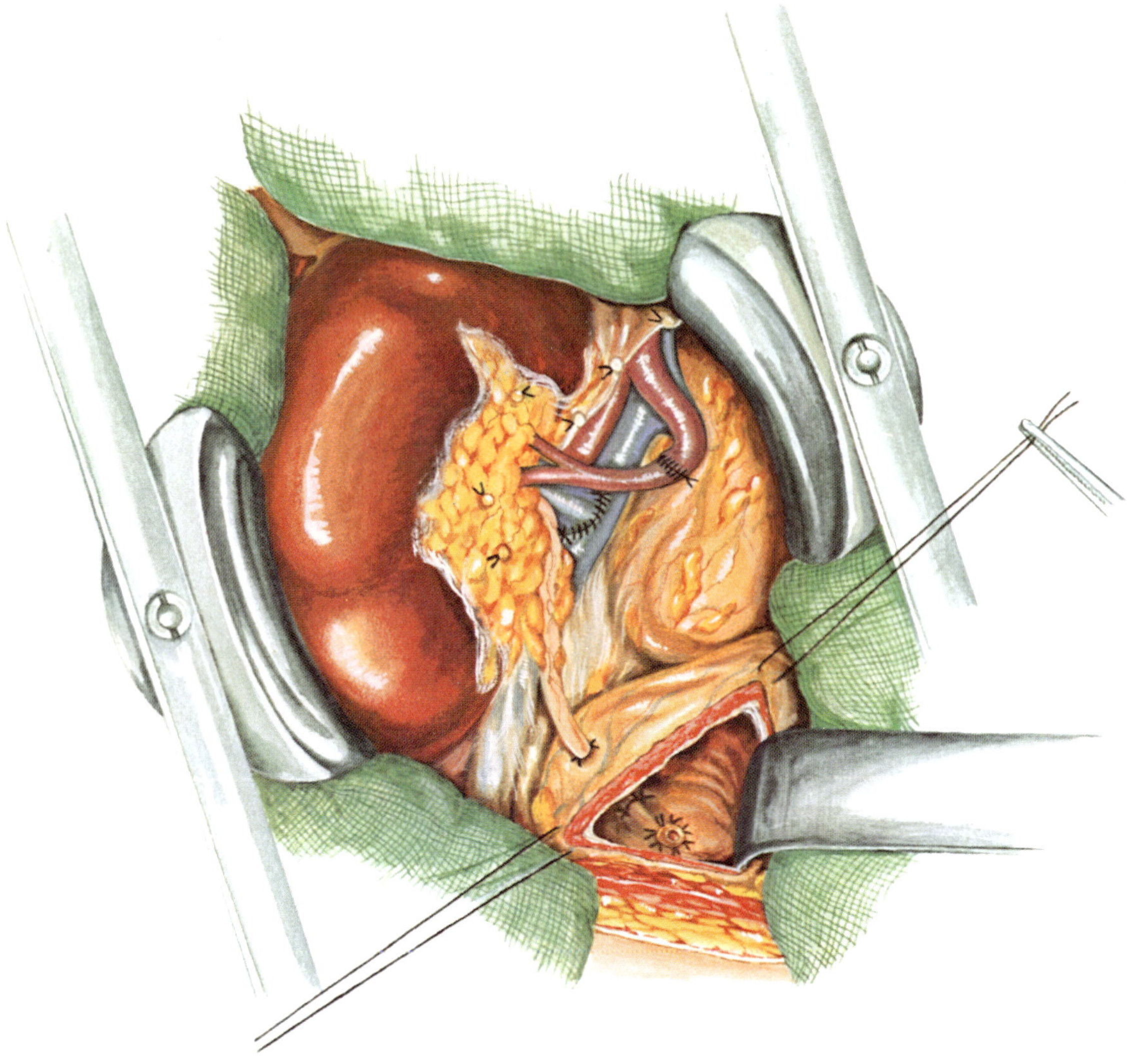

20-6

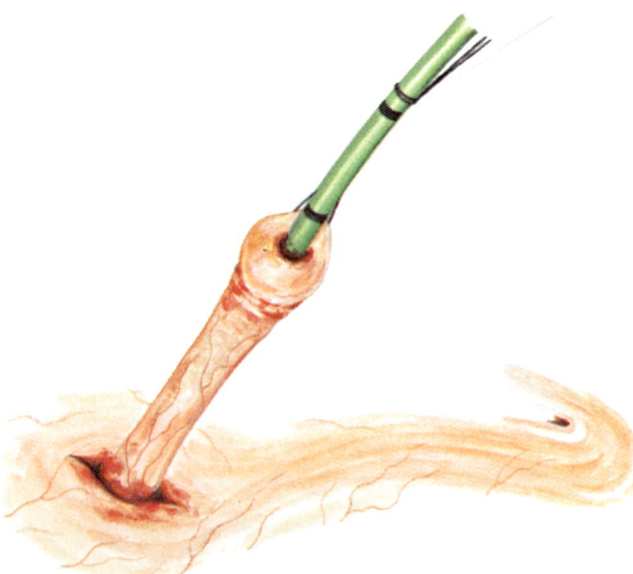

20-7

and suturing of the arterial ends. (During this interval the kidney is maintained at hypothermic levels—15° C—by cooling the capsular surface with refrigerated sterile saline.)

Vascular clamps are removed prior to proceeding with the ureteral neocystostomy. The superior venous clamp is removed before the inferior venous clamp. The arterial bulldog clamp is removed last.

20-6. *Anastomosis of donor ureter into recipient bladder.* The Politano-Leadbetter technique is used.

20-7. Briefly, *the ureter is inserted into the bladder* through a submucosal tunnel. Excessive ureter is excised. The ureteral stoma is secured to bladder mucosa by interrupted 4–0 chromic catgut sutures. The inferior sutures include bladder muscle and the mucosa at the inferior medial end of the tunnel. Closure of the bladder wall is accomplished in two layers (3–0 chromic catgut). A watertight closure is important. A flat tubular drain lateral to the bladder wall is inserted and maintained for 5 to 7 days. A Hemovac multiperforated tube may be substituted for the flat tubular drain. A urethral indwelling Foley catheter (18 Fr) is introduced and maintained for 5 days.

21. Child

It is usually difficult to transplant an adult donor kidney into a child. Therefore the incision is different from that used in an adult. A vertical or paramedian midline incision al-

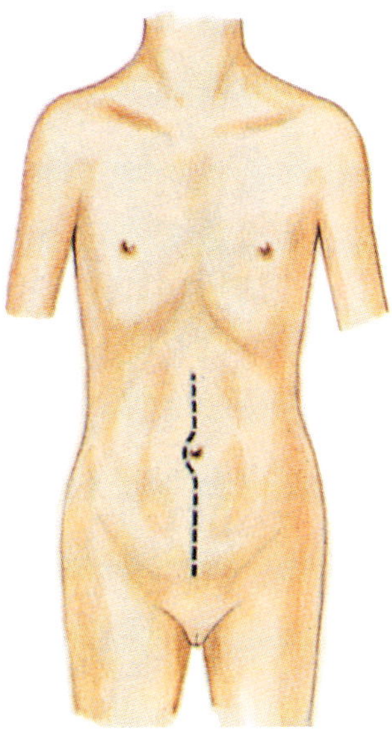

21-1

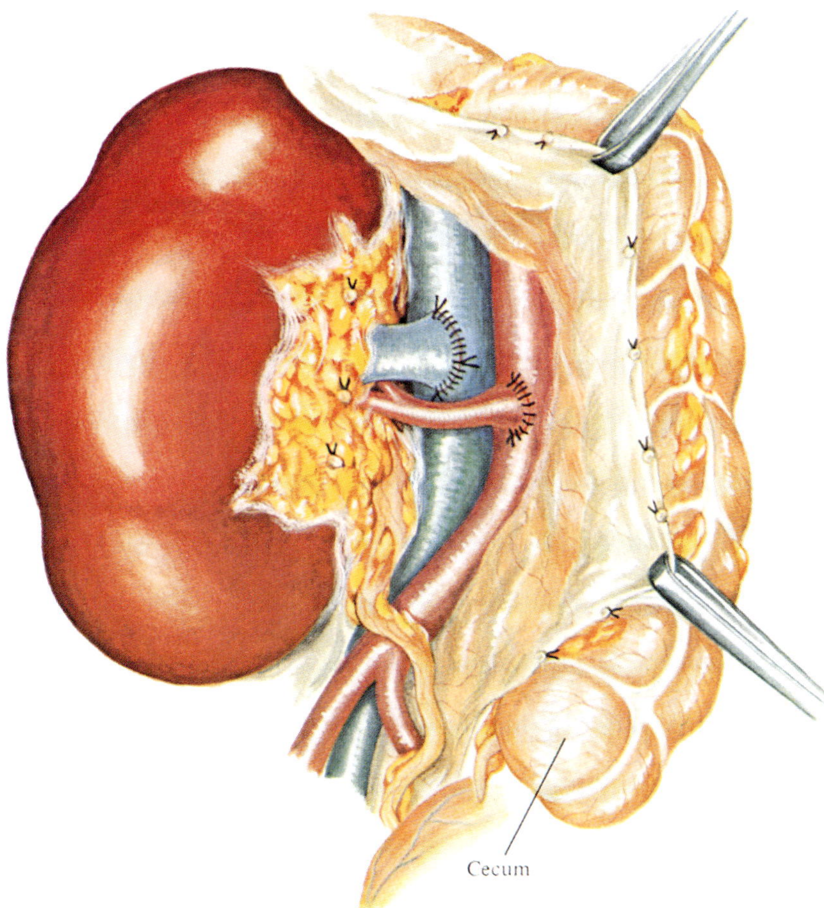

21-2

lows the cecum and ascending colon to be freed and retracted medially, exposing the great vessels.

21-1. The appropriate *line of incision for a young recipient.*

21-2. Donor-recipient anastomosis varies from that normally used in an adult. *The donor renal artery is anastomosed to the abdominal aorta,* end to side. A Satinsky vascular clamp facilitates this anastomosis. The donor renal vein is anastomosed to the inferior vena cava, end to side. The ureter is implanted into the bladder by means of a submucosal tunnel.

22. Autotransplantation of the Kidney

The following illustrations schematically present a procedural technique to accomplish autotransplantation. A long vertical midline transabdominal incision is used. It extends from the mid-epigastrium to the symphysis pubis.

Case Report. RB is a 15-year-old white female who was observed to be hypertensive during a routine examination at high school in September 1976. A suspicion of renovascular hypertensive disease led to a complete workup. The intravenous pyelogram revealed a delay in appearance time of contrast material in the right kidney. In the upright position nephroptosis of the right kidney was noted. Selective renal arteriography revealed 75% stenosis of the main right renal artery due to fibromuscular hyperplasia (Fig. 22-A). In addition, secondary stenosis was seen in the primary arterial branch supplying the right lower pole. Renal vein blood samples were obtained for renin-angiotensin I assays. The right renal vein sample revealed a level of 38 ng/mL/hour (normal, 2.5 ng/mL/hour). The vein draining the right lower pole had an elevated level of renin-angiotensin I, 94.5 ng/mL/hour.

An autotransplant of the right kidney was performed in April 1977. Renal hypothermia was employed because of the known benefits of cooling. The ureter was not transected. The lower pole renal arterial branch was dilated (coronary dilators) after the kidney was cooled outside the abdominal wall.

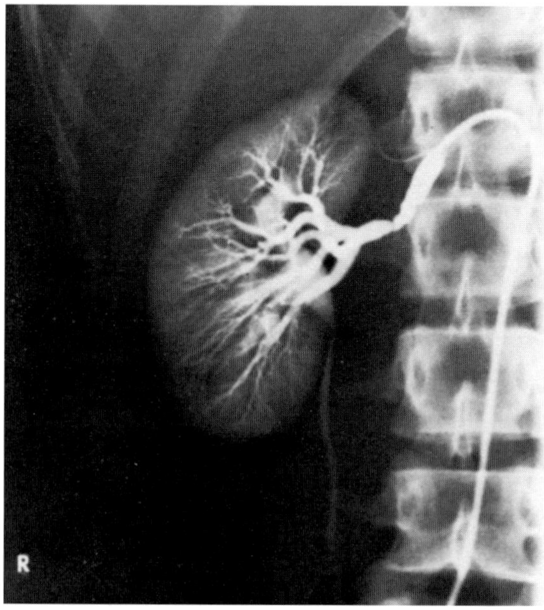

22-A

Her postoperative course in the past 20 months has revealed two normal peripheral vein renin levels. In addition, her blood pressure is 120/80 supine.

22-1. *Early fibromuscular hyperplasia in the proximal right renal artery* and its inferior branch.

22-2. *The right renal artery and right renal vein (not shown) have been transected.* Care is taken so that the ureter remains in continuity, and its blood supply maintained. The kidney is removed from its bed and is cooled outside the incision line by the method described in the case report. The hypothermic kidney is conveniently positioned so that

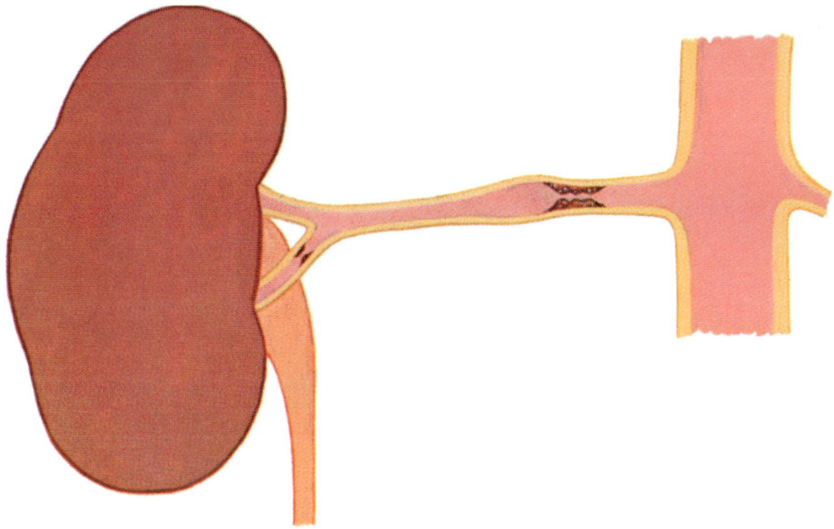

22-1

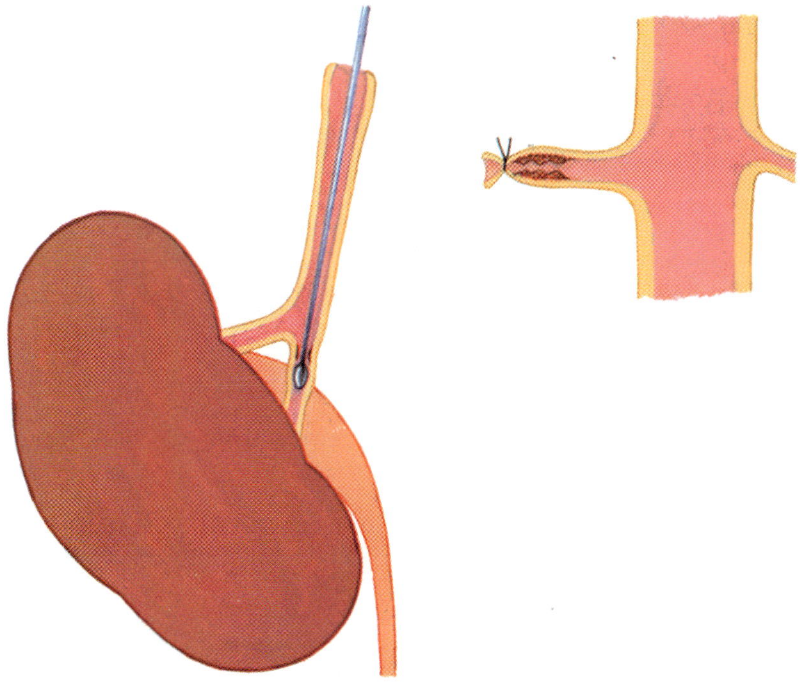

22-2

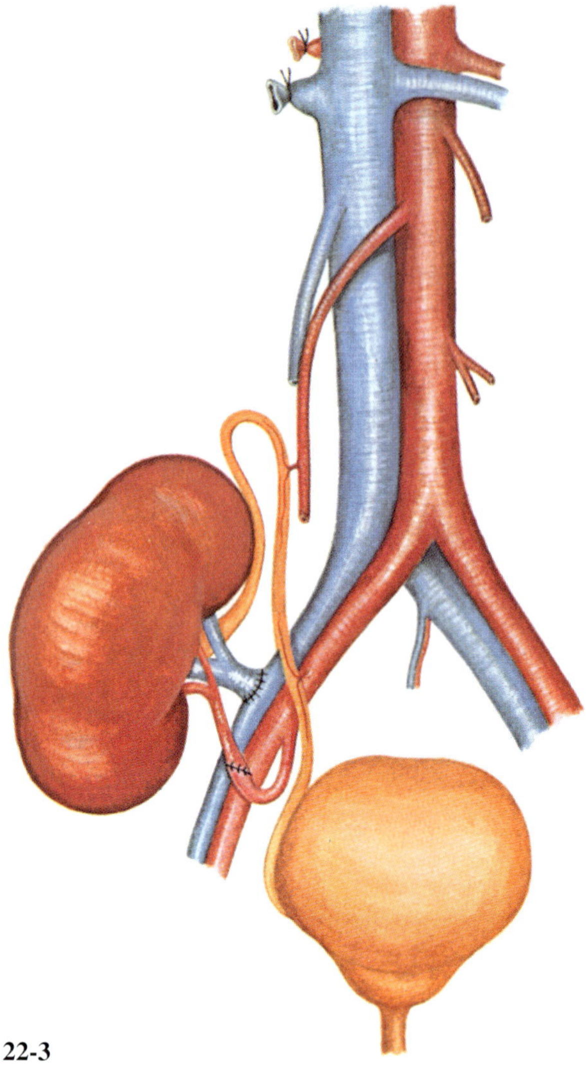

22-3

a coronary dilator (increasing sizes) can be inserted into the arterial lumen, in this case to reach the inferior branch of the renal artery, dilating the lesion.

22-3. After the stenosis is corrected, autotransplantation can be completed. *The kidney is rotated so that the poles are reversed.* The renal vein is anastomosed to the external iliac vein, end to side, and the renal artery is anastomosed to the hypogastric artery, end to end.

23. John Barry Technique for Extending Right Renal Vein Length in Renal Transplantation

23-1. John Barry technique.
On some occasions in harvesting the right renal cadaveric kidney it is obvious that the renal vein is short, and probably will not reach the iliac vein on the opposite side in the recipient.

The illustration clearly shows a very good technique for lengthening the short right renal vein. As demonstrated, a cuff of vena cava still attached to the right renal vein is isolated. The opposite renal vein (left) is divided from the vena cava leaving a small cuff as shown.

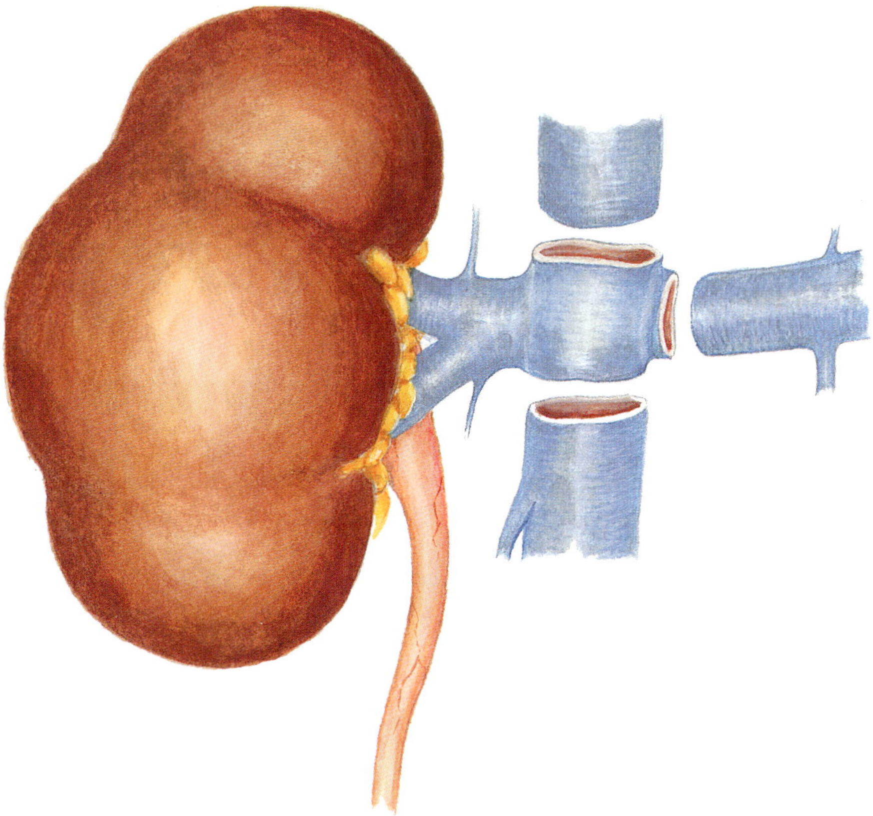

23-1

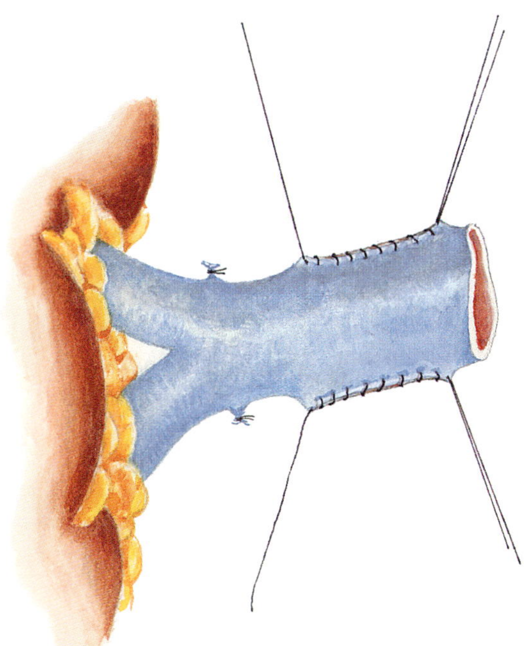

23-2

23-2. Right renal extension in a cadaver kidney.

Two running 5-0 chromic or Prolene sutures are used to close the superior opening and the inferior opening of the vena cava respectively. The renal allograft can now be implanted into the opposite iliac fossa.

Renovascular Surgery

Hypertension has recently attracted wide medical attention. Perhaps 28 million people in the United States have hypertension. The estimate is that in 3 to 5% of those suffering hypertensive disease, the kidney is the source of the elevated blood pressure. A few centers specializing in renovascular surgery claim that the kidney can be implicated in 5 to 15% of cases, but this figure is probably high and misleading.

Today, renovascular hypertension can be diagnosed in the main by noninvasive procedures. A patient should undergo further investigation if there is a recent onset of hypertension in a young adult or worsening of hypertension in an adult (under 50 years of age). A negative family history in a patient with recent hypertension should spur the physician to obtain at least a rapid-sequence intravenous pyelogram and a renogram-renal scan-imaging study.

If patients previously responsive to medications for maintenance of normotension develop severe hypertension, then further diagnostic study is indicated to rule out renovascular ischemia.

A history of trauma to the flank or the occurrence of emboli to the lower extremities should alert the physician to the possibility of recent renal ischemia and hypertension.

Diagnostic Workup. The physical examination will document the presence of hypertension. In a child, the appropriate blood pressure reading is quite different from the adult normal pressure of 120/80 mm Hg. Similarly, a blood pressure of 135/90 may be normal in the patient in his fifth decade of life. An upper abdominal bruit is present in 80% of patients with severe renovascular disease. The murmur is heard just lateral to the midline of the epigastrium, particularly in fibromuscular disease.

Laboratory and X-ray Studies. The intravenous pyelogram, when performed in rapid sequence following the injection of contrast media, is still the most useful and practical test for identifying the affected kidney. Kidney size, disparity, and abnormalities in configuration, can be noted. The early appearance of contrast media in each kidney is noted. Delay in appearance time is noted in renal ischemic kidneys. Hyperconcentration of contrast media approximately 15 to 20 minutes following intravenous injection is also observed on the affected side. We discontinue antihypertensive medications for 3 weeks in all patients undergoing a diagnostic workup. We start these patients on a low-salt diet. On the day of study we ambulate the patient and keep the patient in the upright position for several hours before withdrawing peripheral venous blood for study of renin-angiotensin I levels. If the pressor levels determined by radioimmunoassay are elevated, then arteriography is performed, and renal vein blood samples are obtained for measurement of pressor substances.

We believe the use of the Anger camera attached as part of the photoscintiscanner apparatus is useful. We use a four-probe system that feeds data to a computer. Iodohippurate ^{131}I is injected intravenously after the kidney surfaces have been localized by using Technetium pertechnetate 99m. We have obtained renal plasma flow rates in each kidney by means of the four-probe system.

Renal arteriography is indicated to determine the severity and extent of renovascular disease. This study serves as a useful roadmap to the kidney proper. The two most common lesions demonstrated by arteriography are fibromuscular dysplasia and atherosclerotic plaques. The plaques occur in the more elderly patients and are located near the origin of the main renal arteries. The proximal one-third of both renal arteries or the aorta at its origin may be involved. Medial fibroplasia (fibromuscular dysplasia) is the most common type of mural dysplasia (75%) encountered. It often involves both arteries; if unilateral, it appears more often on the right side. The characteristic beading is seen in the female patient in the second, third, and fourth decades of life. The location of arterial dysplasia is in the distal two-thirds of the arterial tree and its primary branches.

Contraindications to Surgery. Renovascular surgery may be contraindicated in an older patient with multiple system disease, including the cardiovascular system. If renal insufficiency is present, then surgery may be contraindicated. Finally, widespread and extensive renal arterial disease, if present, may preclude reconstructive surgery. Nephrectomy may also be contraindicated.

24. Anatomy of the Renal Artery and Its Major Intrarenal Branches

The renal arteries arise from the lateral aspect of the abdominal aorta opposite the superior border of the second lumbar vertebra. They course toward the renal hilus on each side. The right renal artery courses posterior to the inferior vena cava. Both renal veins lie anterior and slightly inferior to the renal artery. The left renal vein courses anterior to the aorta in the majority of cases.

Each kidney is supplied by a single renal artery in approximately 75% of cases. Other variants are possible, including multiple renal arteries to each kidney. The single renal artery divides into an anterior and posterior branch near the midpoint of the aorta and renal hilus or in the hilar region.

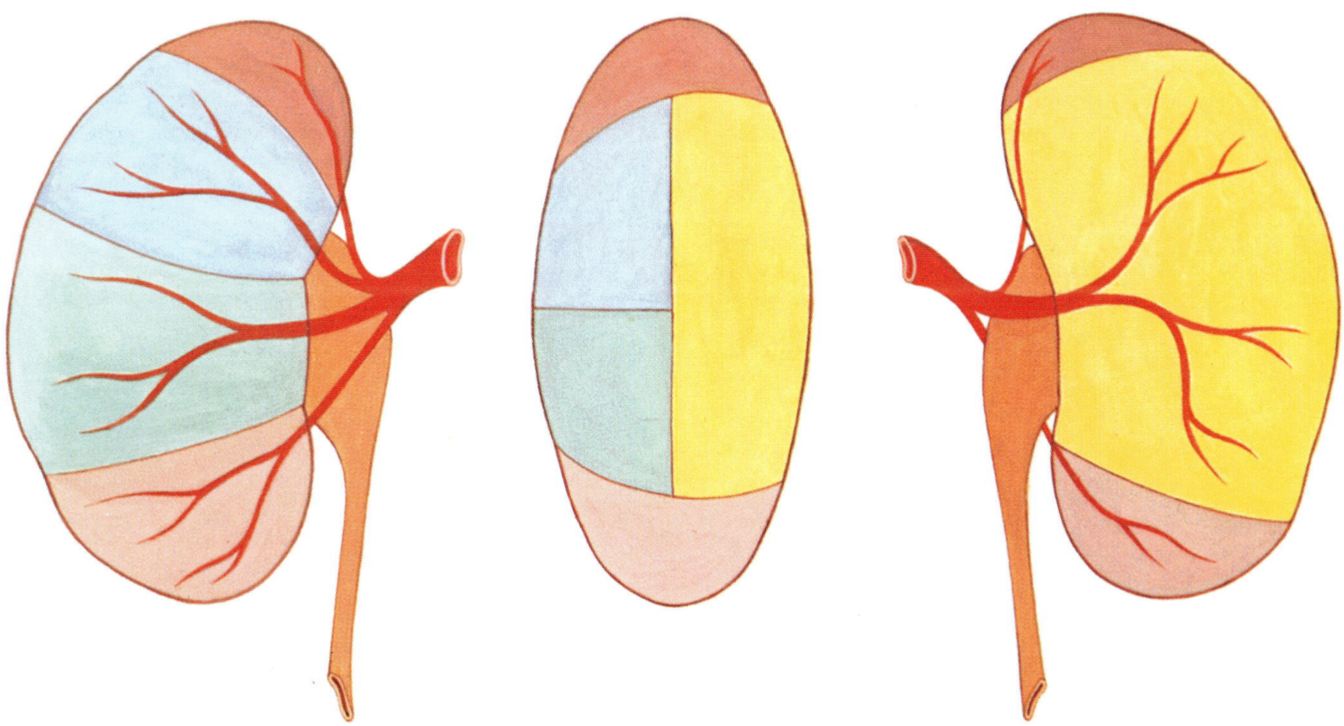

a. Anterior view of right kidney **b.** View: opposite hilus **c.** Posterior view of right kidney

24-1

24-1. The number of major branches coming off the renal artery varies from two to five. The schematic illustrates the usual trunks found on the anterior and posterior surface and the areas of kidney supplied by each major branch.

25. Transabdominal-Transperitoneal Approach to the Left Renal Artery and Left Kidney

The patient is in a supine position and the table is hyperextended so the bend is at the second lumbar spine area. A sandbag or elevation of the kidney rest will assist in the hyperextension. An anterior vertical midline incision is made from the xiphoid process and curves around the umbilicus in an obese patient to the mid-lower abdomen. A transverse chevron-type incision, starting as a subcostal incision, is an excellent alternative.

The transverse colon can be lifted out of the wound onto the anterior superior abdominal wall and protected by a moist lap pad. The small bowel can be packed away into the right upper quadrant or placed into a plastic bag and lifted out of the wound onto the right lateral abdominal wall.

25-1. The approach to the left renal artery is affected by *mobilizing the splenic flexure of the colon and the descending colon.* The colon is freed by incising the paracolic peri-

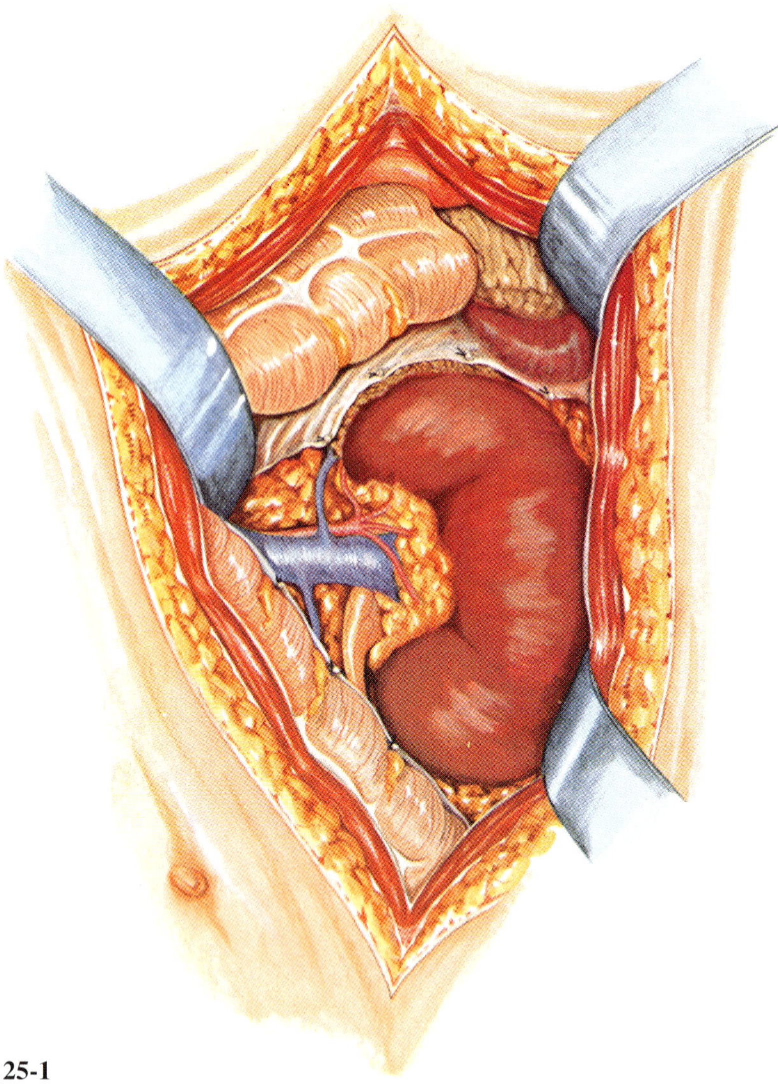

25-1

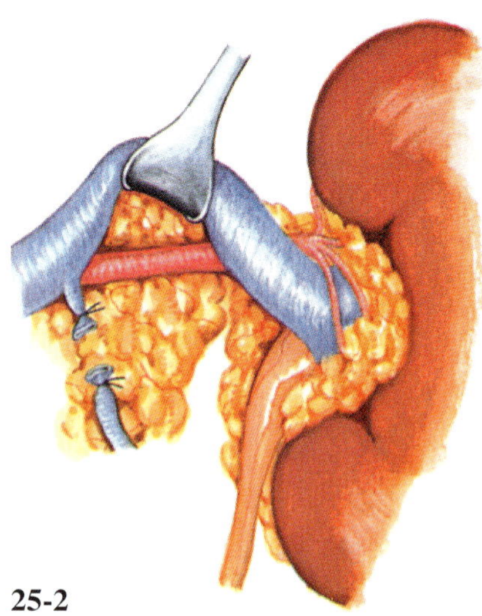

25-2

toneal attachments. The lienocolic ligament must be severed before medial retraction of the upper descending colon is possible. After Gerota's fascia and the underlying kidney have been exposed, the renal hilar area is dissected by blunt and sharp dissection. The key anatomic landmark is the left renal vein coursing anterior to the aorta. Careful dissection of the renal vein will expose the adrenal vein and the spermatic vein. The renal artery is posterior to the vein and slightly superior. The major trunks of the left renal artery can be dissected near their origin.

25-2. *Elevation of the vein by a retractor.* The left renal artery is exposed.

26. Transperitoneal Approach to the Right Renal Artery and Right Kidney

The incision and operative approach into the peritoneal cavity are as described for the left kidney. The ascending colon is mobilized by incising the paracolic reflection. The

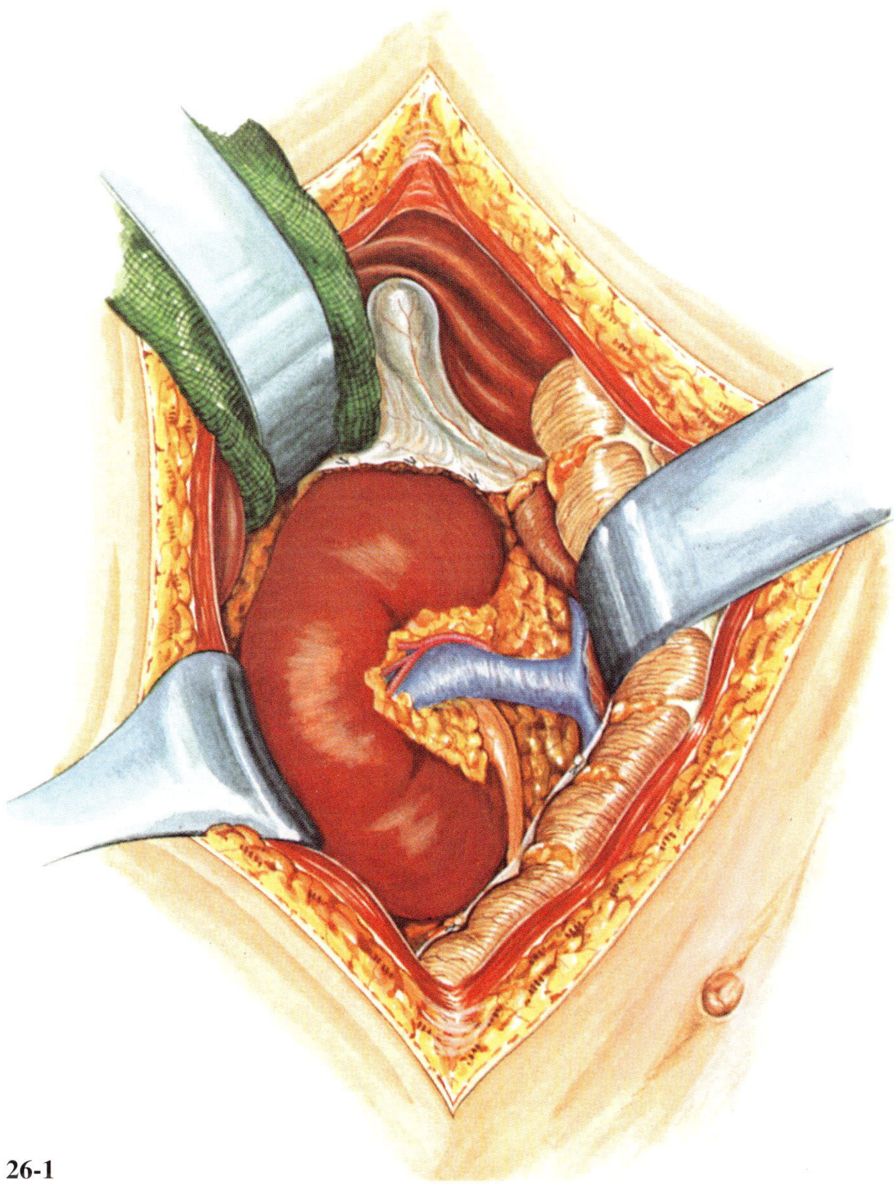

26-1

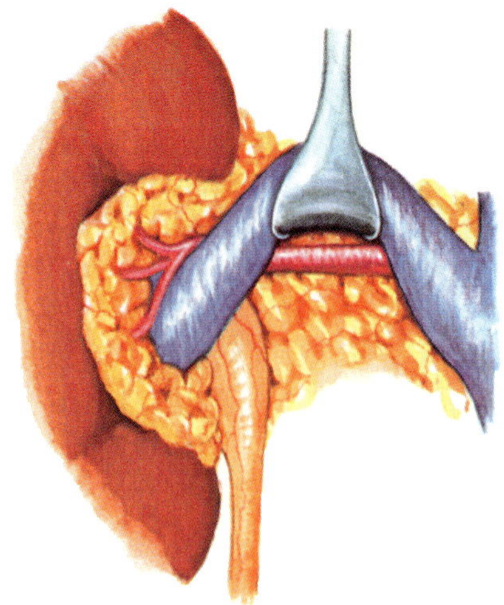

26-2

hepatocolic ligament is cut to free the hepatic flexure. The hepatic flexure and ascending colon can be retracted medially.

26-1. The *right renal vein is exposed* after Gerota's fascia has been opened and the renal hilus has been carefully exposed by dissection. The vein and ureter are exposed. The duodenum still overlies most of the inferior vena cava.

26-2. *Elevation of the renal vein and final exposure of the distal right renal artery* and its major extrarenal branches.

27. Exposure of Both Renal Arteries

For a more direct approach to the proximal renal arteries, vena cava, and aorta, the duodenum must be mobilized and retracted medially and superiorly.

After the peritoneal cavity has been entered, the transverse colon is lifted out of the wound onto the superior portion of the incision. The small bowel is carefully placed into a plastic bag and lifted out of the right margin of the wound. The posterior parietal peritoneum is incised under the duodenum.

27-1. *Duodenal mobilization* is begun by incising or kocherizing the inferior and lateral border of the duodenum. The ascending portion of duodenum must also be freed before the duodenum can be rotated and lifted upward. The retroperitoneum can now be widened, and the major renal vessels can be dissected. The inferior mesenteric vein may be sacrificed to allow wider exposure. On the left side, the spermatic vein may be doubly ligated and transected.

Once the inferior vena cava and renal veins are exposed, the underlying renal arteries can be easily reached and visualized.

The inferior vena cava is mobilized by blunt dissection. Even when the right renal artery is exposed at its origin, the left renal vein must be exposed and freed to allow lateral retraction of the vena cava. A large, blunt, right-angle clamp or vascular clamp can be passed behind the vena cava. Umbilical tapes are then passed above and below the renal veins to allow control and mobilization. Ligating the spermatic vein on one or both sides assists in the exposure. Lumbar veins may be encountered behind the vena cava, and they can be controlled by a silver clip distally and a ligature proximally. The proximal one-third of the right renal artery can be exposed by retracting the vena cava later-

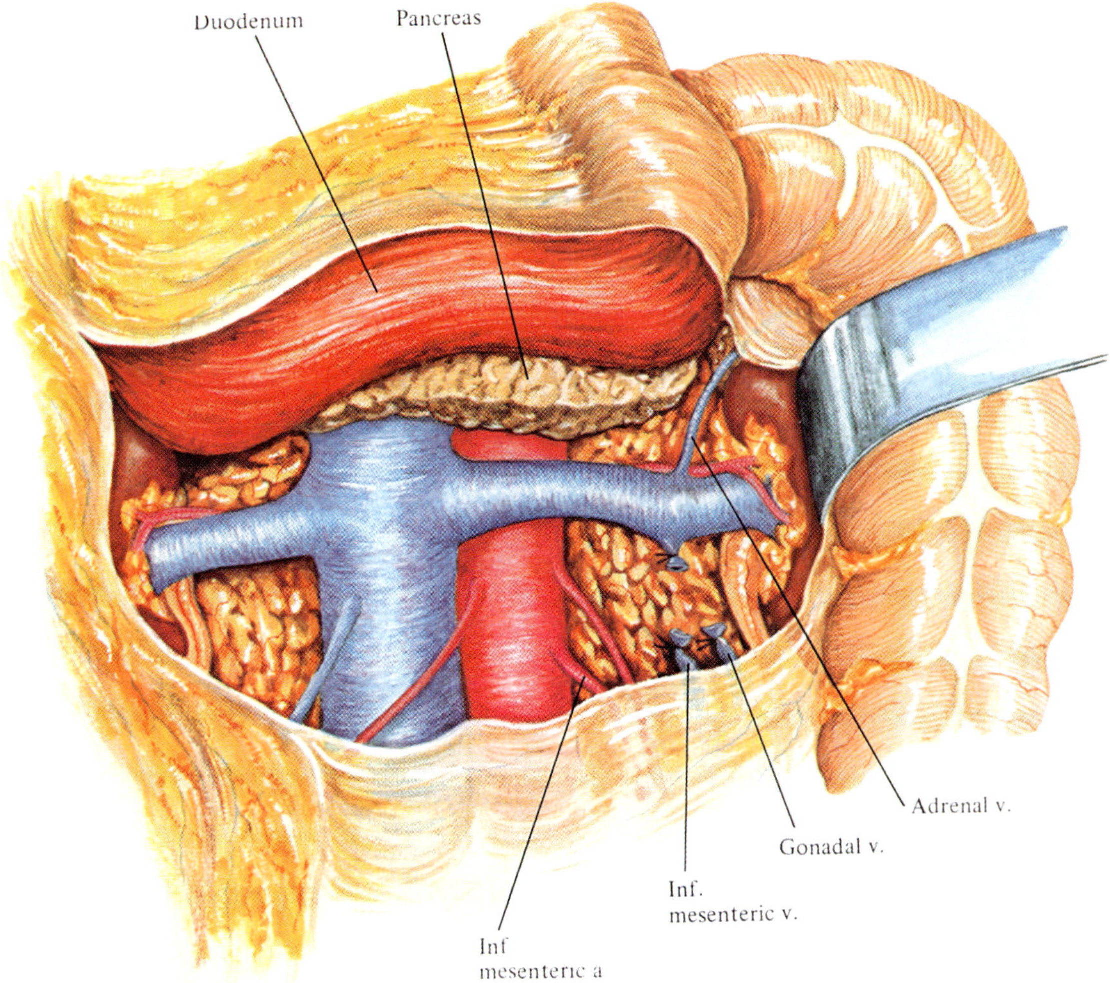

27-1

ally. For lesions of the distal two-thirds the vena cava is retracted medially and the right renal vein is raised superiorly or inferiorly as indicated. If the renal artery is clamped for more than 20 minutes, regional hypothermia may be indicated.

When one is operating on the proximal one-third of the renal arteries, the abdominal aorta should be mobilized. Abdominal tapes are passed behind the aorta superior and inferior to the renal arteries. This maneuver provides control of the major vessel should the vascular clamps slip from the proximal artery or part of the aorta.

Heparin is usually administered before the renal artery or the aorta is clamped. Mannitol, 10% in Ringer's lactate, can be given 15 minutes prior to renal artery ischemia. It is continued during surgery and after the operation if renal hypothermia has not been employed. Approximately 1 liter can be administered over a 6-hour period with relative safety.

28. Endarterectomy of the Right Proximal Renal Artery

Endarterectomy of the right proximal renal artery may be performed when a plaque obstructing the renal vessel is found.

28-1. The *left renal vein is retracted superiorly,* and the vena cava is retracted laterally. An occlusive clamp is placed around part of the aorta to include the origin of the

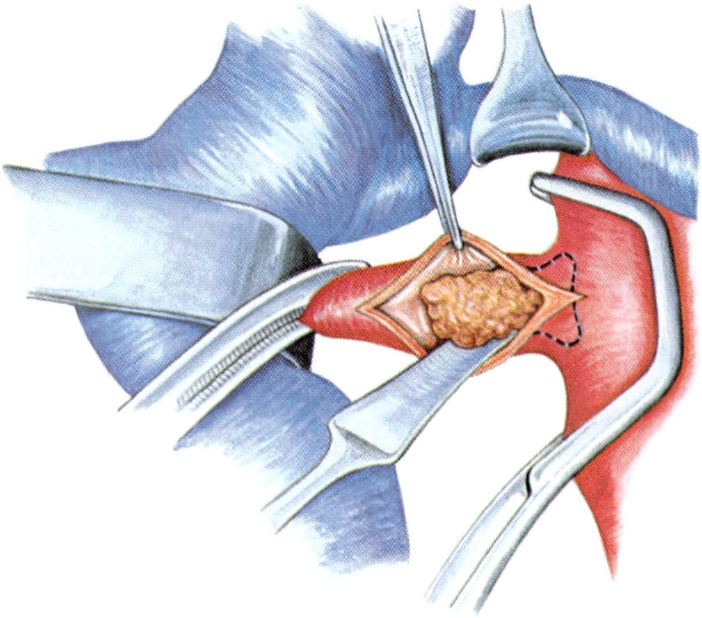

28-1

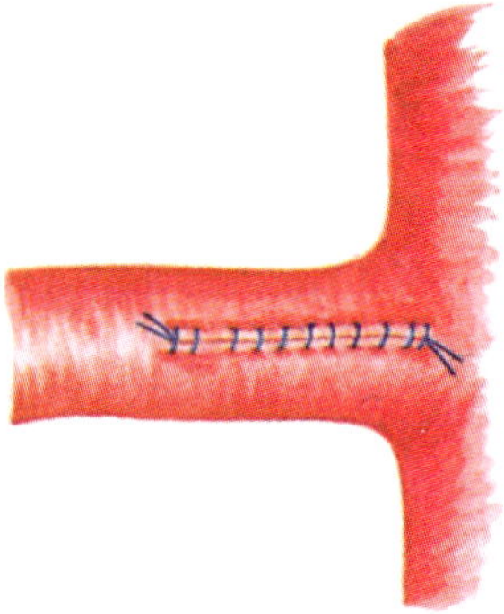

28-2

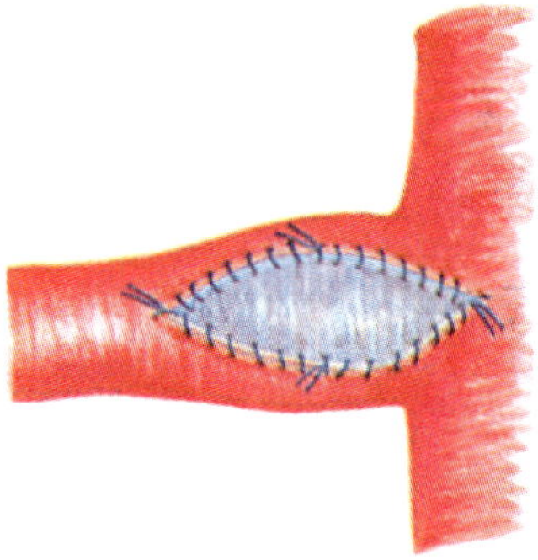

28-3

renal artery, but the aorta is not occluded completely. The distal renal artery is also clamped. An arteriotomy is made and can be extended into the aorta. A Cannon arterial dissector is used to dissect the plaque in a meticulous but complete fashion.

28-2. The *open renal artery may be closed* by a 5–0 continuous polypropylene or vascular nylon suture.

28-3. *A vein patch from the saphenous vein may be sutured in place to cover the defect.*

29. Segmental Removal of a Stenosed or Fibromuscular Segment

29-1. The left renal vein is retracted inferiorly. The adrenal vein and left spermatic vein are ligated. A vascular clamp is placed over part of the aorta, excluding the origin of the left renal artery. Flow through the aorta is not interrupted. A vascular clamp is placed on the distal renal artery and the lesion (*dotted lines*) may then be removed.

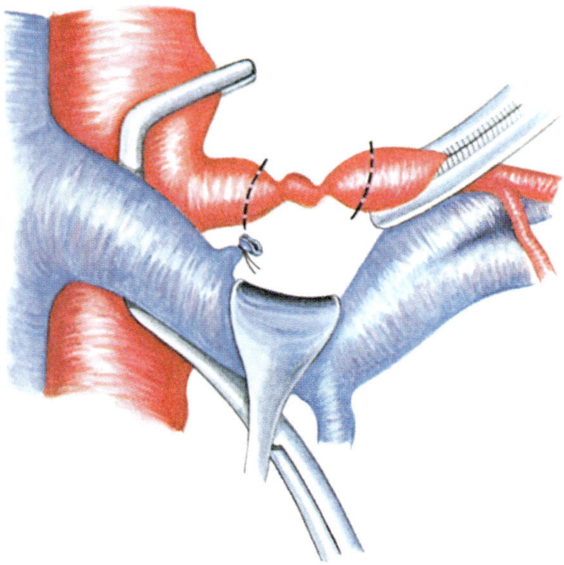

29-1

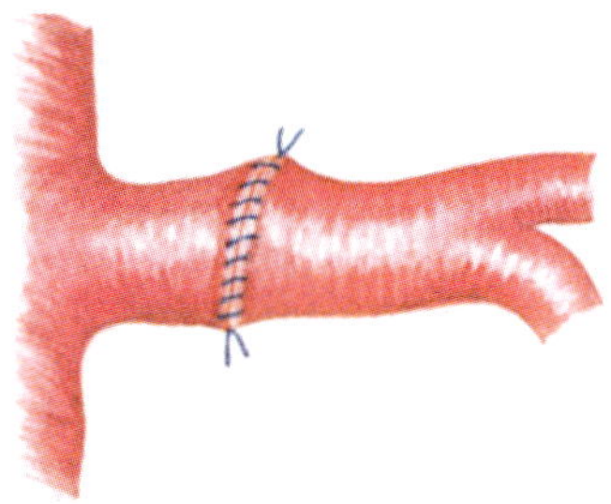

29-2

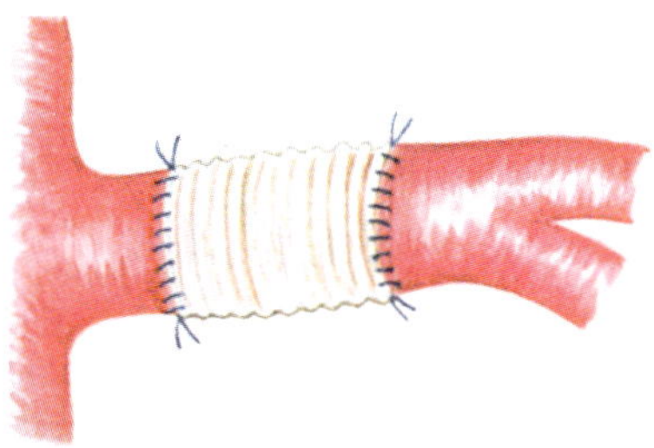

29-3

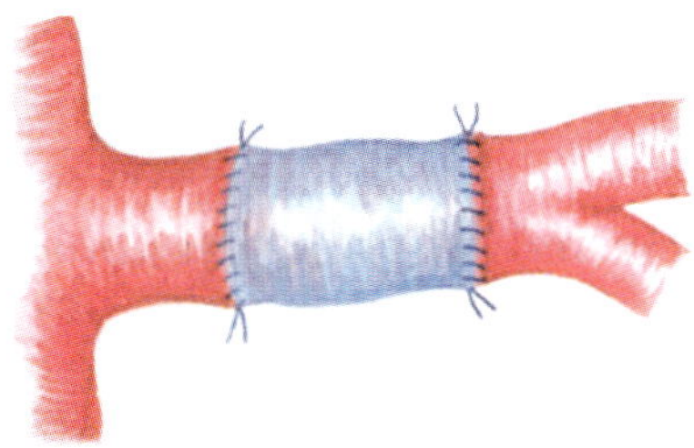

29-4

Reanastomosis of the renal artery is performed by one of three acceptable techniques.

29-2. *End-to-end anastomosis.*

29-3. *Interposition of a Dacron tubular graft to reestablish flow.*

29-4. *Saphenous vein graft to complete continuity.*

30. Aortorenal Dacron Bypass Graft from Mid-right Renal Artery to More Inferior Abdominal Aorta

30-1. The stenotic diseased proximal artery is seen on the right. *A Dacron graft (end to side) is interposed.* The anastomosis of the artery to the graft is performed initially. Before the final sutures are placed, heparinized saline is used to fill the graft. Blood flow can also be initiated to seal the interstices of the graft.

30-2. *After the proximal renal artery has been freed of any diseased segment, it is reanastomosed to the aorta.* The vena cava is retracted laterally by a small flat tubular drain used as a tape to allow adequate exposure. The aorta is temporarily occluded to permit the anastomosis (end to side) in a bloodless field. Heparinizing the patient is important. Renal hypothermia can be used to protect kidney function.

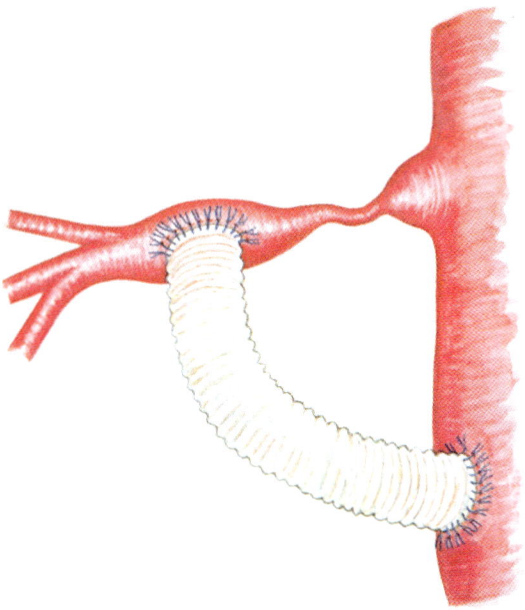

30-1

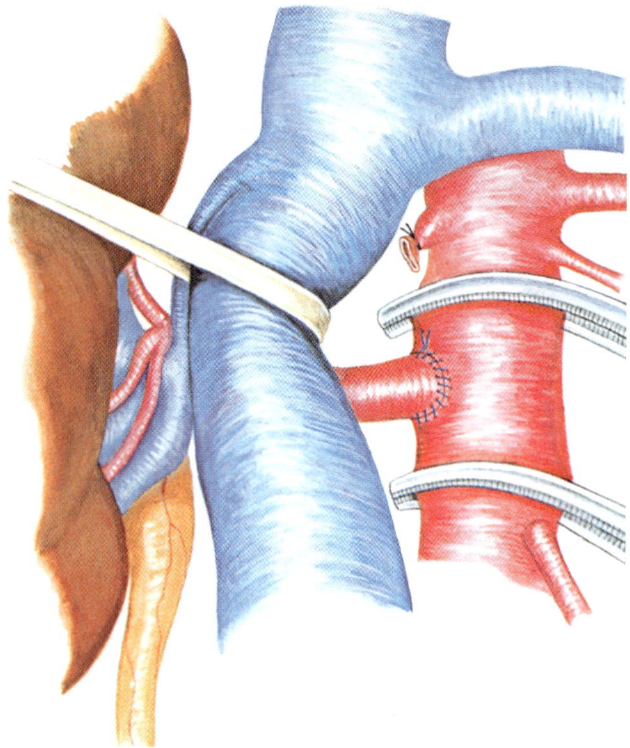

30-2

31. Splenorenal Arterial Anastomosis

Before formal plans are made to use the splenic artery, it is important that the splenic branch of the celiac axis be visualized. Atherosclerosis in the vessel will preclude its use. Oblique arteriograms of the splenic artery are useful.

The splenorenal bypass procedure is more difficult than other renovascular procedures. This is particularly pertinent if one uses the surgical approach consisting of an anterior duodenal mobilization.

We prefer a slight flank abdominal approach through the bed of the 11th rib. We usually can avoid entrance into the pleural cavity. If the pleura is entered, then a tube is used to empty the pleural cavity of air prior to closure.

Using the approach posterior to the left kidney and flank area, we can dissect the renal artery from its midrenal portion. By entering the peritoneal cavity it is now possible to identify the splenic artery and vein.

An excellent guide to the splenic vein is the inferior mesenteric vein near its entrance into the vena cava. The splenic artery can be isolated adjacent to the vein. The artery is isolated by a tape and carefully dissected to prevent injury to the pancreas. Sufficient mobilization must be carried out so that the artery can reach the renal artery without tension.

Arterial branches supplying the pancreas and adjacent viscera must be ligated. The adrenal vein to the left renal vein is also doubly ligated. Now the proximal splenic artery is occluded with a vascular clamp. It is not necessary to remove the spleen because of excellent collaterals from the short gastric arteries.

Most vascular surgeons prefer an end-to-side anastomosis. The renal artery is mobilized and heparin and intravenous mannitol (10%) are administered. The renal artery is occluded on both sides of the anastomosis. The divided splenic artery (distal side has been ligated) is brought to the site of anastomosis. An arteriotomy in the renal artery is made.

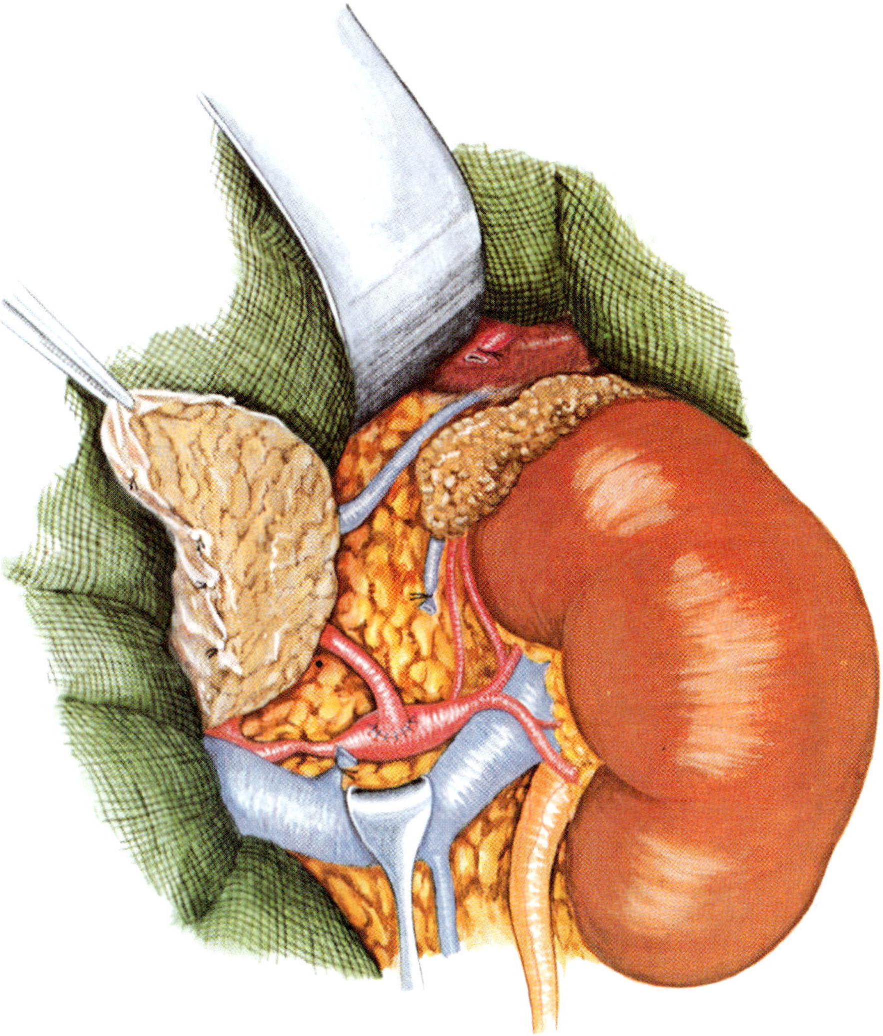

31-1

31-1. *The end of the splenic artery is approximated to the open renal artery by vascular sutures* (5–0) on each end. The splenic artery can be dilated or spatulated to accommodate the arteriotomy if necessary. The posterior row is sutured first. The anastomosis is then completed.

32. Renal Artery Aneurysm Involving Entire Right Renal Artery at Major Bifurcation into Posterior and Anterior Branches

A midline approach to the kidney, using a transperitoneal exposure, is satisfactory. The paracolic space on the right is exposed by retracting the ascending colon medially. The renal artery is exposed proximal and distal to the aneurysm. This exposure is enhanced by retracting the vena cava medially. Renal hypothermia (15° C) is useful and protects renal function during the period of renal ischemia. We use a surface cooler.

An alternative to the procedure we describe in situ is the use of "workbench" surgery. It is important that the ureter be protected. In this technique, the kidney is removed from its bed after the proximal renal artery and renal vein are divided. The kidney is cooled by immersing the organ in cold saline slush. The aneurysm is excised, and

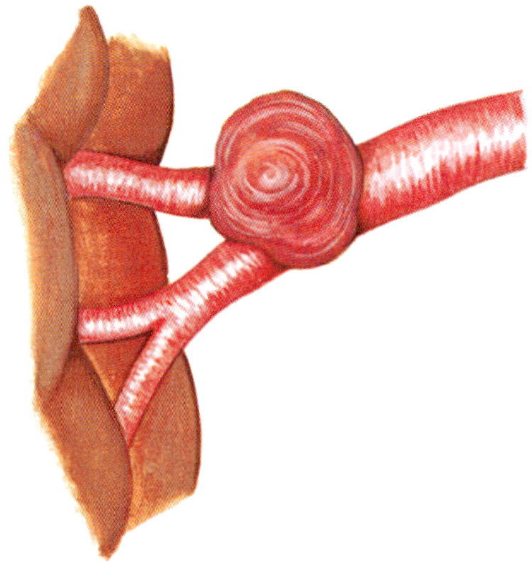

32-1

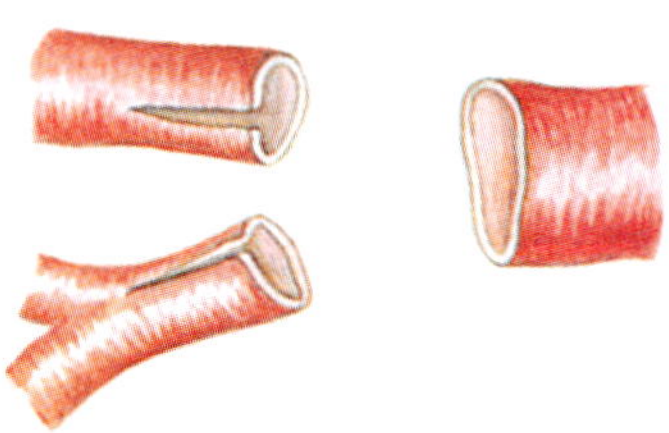

32-2

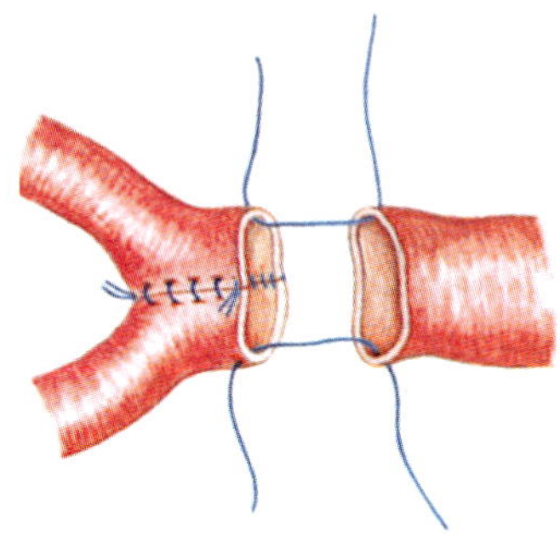

32-3

the renal artery can be further cooled by cannulating both distal artery branches and infusing a hypothermic 7° C solution (250 mL) into each branch.

32-1. *The aneurysm is exposed* after the renal artery and its distal major branches are carefully dissected and exposed. A vascular clamp is placed proximally. Two small bulldog clamps are placed distally. The aneurysm is excised.

32-2. *Reestablishment of continuity is effected by incising both distal branches* in longitudinal fashion at a site where they would lie in apposition. The incision is about 8 mm in length. The side-to-side anastomosis distally is completed first, thus widening the stoma.

32-3. *End-to-end anastomosis* (5–0 nylon vascular suture) is completed.

33. Extracorporeal Shock Wave Lithotripsy (ESWL)

ESWL is a noninvasive method for treatment of renal and ureteral stones. This method of focused "shock waves" has been in wide use for more than 10 years, and it is now standard treatment for obstructive stone disease (5 mm or more in the ureter or 3 to 5 cm in the kidney). Our experience includes more than 6000 patients.

Professors Chaussy, Eisenberger, and Schmiedt are the three German urologists who deserve the most credit for helping Dornier to develop this new treatment modality for renal stones in patients.

Today, the HM3-Dornier apparatus is still in wide use. A general anesthetic or a regional block—epidural or spinal anesthesia—is still needed if the Kv to be generated is more than 19 to 22 Kv. For a renal stone measuring 7 × 14 mm or larger, 2000 shocks with excellent focusing on the stone is needed for stone disintegration. New reports from many centers suggest that an energy potential in the 14 Kv range can break stones measuring 6 to 12 mm without significant anesthesia (general or spinal–epidural anesthesia).

The ESWL shock wave consists of a broad but single positive pressure front with multiple frequencies; a steep onset with a gradual decline in the pressure waves is noted. Compared with ultrasonic waves, the shock waves can be transmitted through water without loss of energy. Tissue damage is not seen when one uses the parameters described above.

Indications for ESWL

The indications as suggested by Chaussy can be used in 70% of stone cases, and they are as follows:

1. Single stones in the renal pelvic collecting system, <2.5 cm.
2. Multiple stones in the renal collecting system or pelvis, <3.0 cm.
3. Ureteral stone in lower ureter or superior half of the ureter (5 mm or more); a stent is useful in promoting disintegration. If the calculus lies over the sacral bone, a prone position of the patient is employed; again a stent is helpful in the treatment procedure.
4. Infected stones; the patient should be pretreated with antibiotics and it should be continued during the ESWL procedure. An overnight stay is indicated in only a few cases and allows close monitoring and continuation of antibiotics and fluids in selected cases. Most patients can be discharged after ESWL.
5. Partial staghorn stones; with a nondilated collecting system, several treatments may be needed.

Approximately 20% of the nonselected patient population harboring stones are eligible for ESWL. A high success rate can be achieved without complications. At the present, due to refinements, approximately 70% of unselected patients will benefit from ESWL as the sole therapeutic modality.

33-1. The team members using the ESWL machine are seen. Drs. Erdal Erturk, Abraham T.K. Cockett, and Louis L. Glass, on the gantry, are shown.

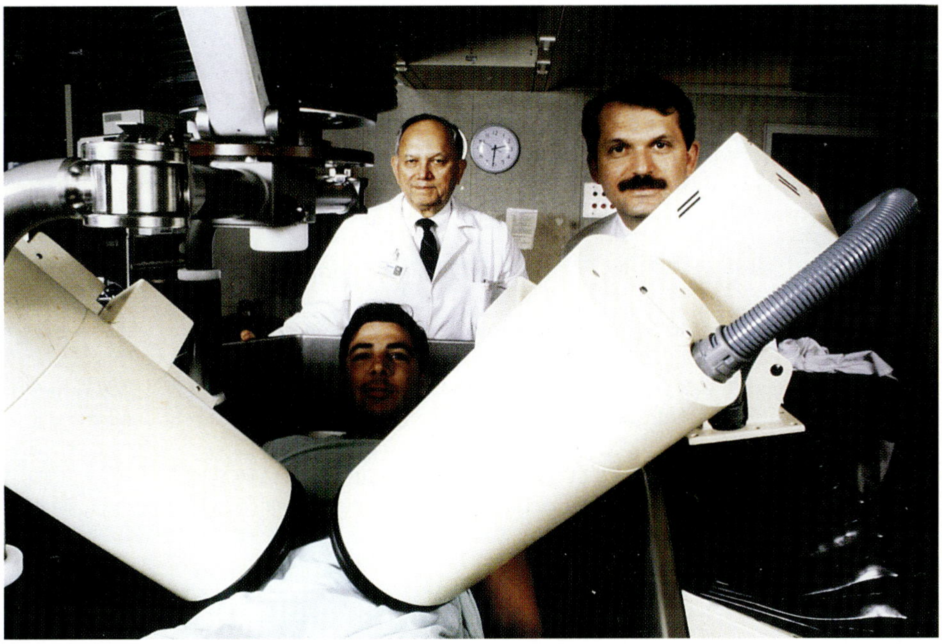

33-1

The remaining 20% of complicated cases are eligible for ESWL and endourologic procedures. If the occasional patient has a bleeding disorder, ESWL is not used. Aspirin, prophylactic therapy in the United States, must be discontinued for approximately 12 days before scheduling ESWL treatment. The bleeding time should be normal prior to the procedure. Weight limitations still apply to the HM3 apparatus. A patient weighing 300 lbs. cannot be treated on the Dornier machine because of weight limitations on the gantry.

Staghorn Stones: Treatment by Percutaneous Nephroscopic Insertion of Instrument

Treatment with percutaneous nephroscopic insertion of the tube followed by stone disintegration and removal is still the major treatment of choice.

ESWL in combination with nephroscopic stone disintegration to fragment the remaining large fragment is often useful.

Today most urologists who have access to an ESWL machine will obtain the assistance of a uroradiologist with expertise in the renal area. A urologist working in a stone center may have sufficient experience to insert a long needle with an obturator into a dependent calix harboring stone. Ultrasonography is exceedingly useful in some instances to localize the dilated calyx.

Suggested Readings

Anderson JC, Hynes W. Retrocaval ureter: case diagnosed preoperatively and treated successfully by plastic operation. Br J Urol 21:209, 1949.

Basso AG, Netto ICV, Cockett ATK. Renal preservation with a modified intracellular hypothermic solution. Invest Urol 11:136, 1973.

Boyce WH, Elkins IB. Reconstructive renal surgery following anatrophic nephrolithotomy: follow up of 100 consecutive cases. J Urol 111:307, 1974.

Culp OS, DeWeerd JH. A pelvic flap operation for certain types of ureteropelvic obstruction: preliminary report. Mayo Clin Proc 28:483, 1951.

Deming CL. Nephroptosis: relation to liver, spleen and stomach. Correction by new operation. Am J Surg 9:218, 1930.

Erturk E, Sheinfeld J, DiMarco PL, Cockett ATK. Renal trauma: evaluation by computerized tomography. J Urol 133:946, 1985.

Finney JMT. A new method of pyloroplasty. Johns Hopkins Bull 13:155, 1902.

Foley FEB. A new plastic operation for stricture at the ureteropelvic junction. Report of 20 operations. J Urol 38:643, 1937.

Gil-Vernet J. New surgical concepts in removing renal calculi. Urol Int 20:255, 1965.

Linke CA, Linke CL, Davis RS. Cadaver donor nephrectomy. Urology 6:133, 1975.

Netto ICV, Basso AG, Cockett ATK. Renal preservation: a modified solution for 18 hours of protection. Urology 2:389, 1973.

Politano VA, Leadbetter WF. An operative technique for correction of vesicoureteral reflex. J Urol 79:932, 1958.

Rob C, Frank IN. Renal artery occlusive disease with hypertension. In: Hardy JD, ed. Rhoads Textbook of Surgery, 5th ed. Philadelphia: JB Lippincott, 1977.

Scardino PL, Prince CL. Vertical flap ureteropelvioplasty. South Med J 46:325, 1953.

Sheinfeld J, Erturk E, Spataro RF, Cockett ATK. Perinephric abscess: current concepts. J Urol 137:191, 1987.

von Lichtenberg A. Plastic surgery of the renal pelvis and ureter. JAMA 93:1704, 1929.

Yoho A, Stueber P, Koletsky S. Further experiences with intermittent occlusion of the renal pedicle. Surg Forum 11:499, 1960.

The Ureter

2

Surgical Anatomy

STRUCTURE AND LOCATION

The ureters are fibromuscular structures that transport urine from the kidney pelvis to the bladder; the ureters begin at ureteropelvic junction as a continuation of renal pelvis and extend to the ureteral orifices. Their lengths in the adult are 25 to 34 cm. The left ureter is about 1 cm longer than the right one. Both ureters are retroperitoneal in their course and attach loosely to the posterior layer of peritoneum with the exception of the upper 4 to 5 cm.

From the ureteropelvic junction to the iliac vessels, the ureters lie on the anterior surface of the left and right psoas major muscles (Fig. 1). The right ureter courses lateral to the inferior vena cava. The upper portion is covered by duodenum. The left ureter can be located lateral to the inferior mesenteric vein. The spermatic or ovarian vessels lie medial to the ureter for the superior half, then cross over to continue downward in a lateral location to ureter.

SURGICAL RECOGNITION

The ureter is a fibromuscular structure that demonstrates peristaltic activity when compressed with atraumatic forceps. The best method to locate the midureter is to find this structure as it crosses anterior to the common iliac artery at the origin of the hypogastric artery. The ureter can be palpated at this junction. The ureteral surface has an increased capillary and arteriolar network which will aid in recognition.

In gynecologic surgery, the lower ureter may be traumatized. Ureteral catheterization facilitates identification of the ureter. A fiberoptic ureteroscope entails the use of a 7 or 8 French catheter. We do not use this instrument because of possible trauma to the ureteral wall.

The pelvic ureter crosses the common iliac vessels at its bifurcation, passes along the lower border of the internal iliac artery, and crosses its anterior branches. As the ureter approaches the bladder, it is retroperitoneal. The lower ureter is surrounded by a plexus of veins; the terminal ureter passes obliquely through the bladder wall for about 2 cm (Fig. 2).

In the female, the terminal ureter passes the supravaginal part of the cervix, about

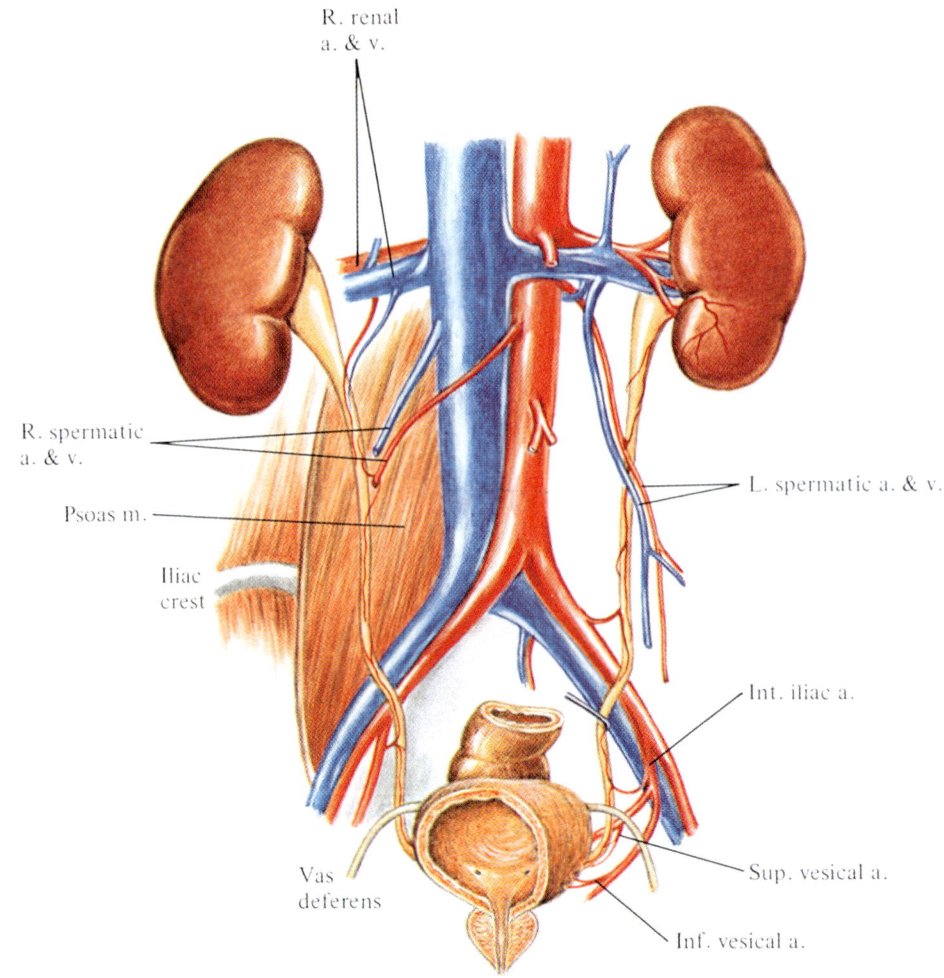

FIG. 1.
The ureters and vascular supply in the male.

1.5–2.5 cm in a lateral position, and is covered by the uterine artery and veins; it enters the posterior vesical wall obliquely (Fig. 3).

In the male, the terminal ureter is crossed by the vas deferens above the ureterovesical junction and is nearly overlapped by the upper end of the seminal vesicle (Fig. 4).

Three narrow areas are recognized along the course of each ureter: The uppermost is at the ureteropelvic junction. The second occurs where the ureter crosses the iliac vessels at the pelvic brim. The third is within the bladder wall (ureterovesical junction). These narrow areas often impede passage of urinary calculi. The intravesical portion of the ureter is the narrowest; it has only a longitudinal muscle layer and is an important topographic point with regard to ureteral reflux.

Insertion of a small fiberoptic ureteroscope up the appropriate ureter obviates the need for a 7 Fr or 8 Fr ureteral catheter. The fiberoptic ureteroscope has a strong illuminating light at the tip of the instrument and it helps to identify the exact location of the appropriate ureter when many adhesions are present. The same technique can be used at the time of laparoscopy to identify the appropriate ureter prior to laparoscopic nephrectomy.

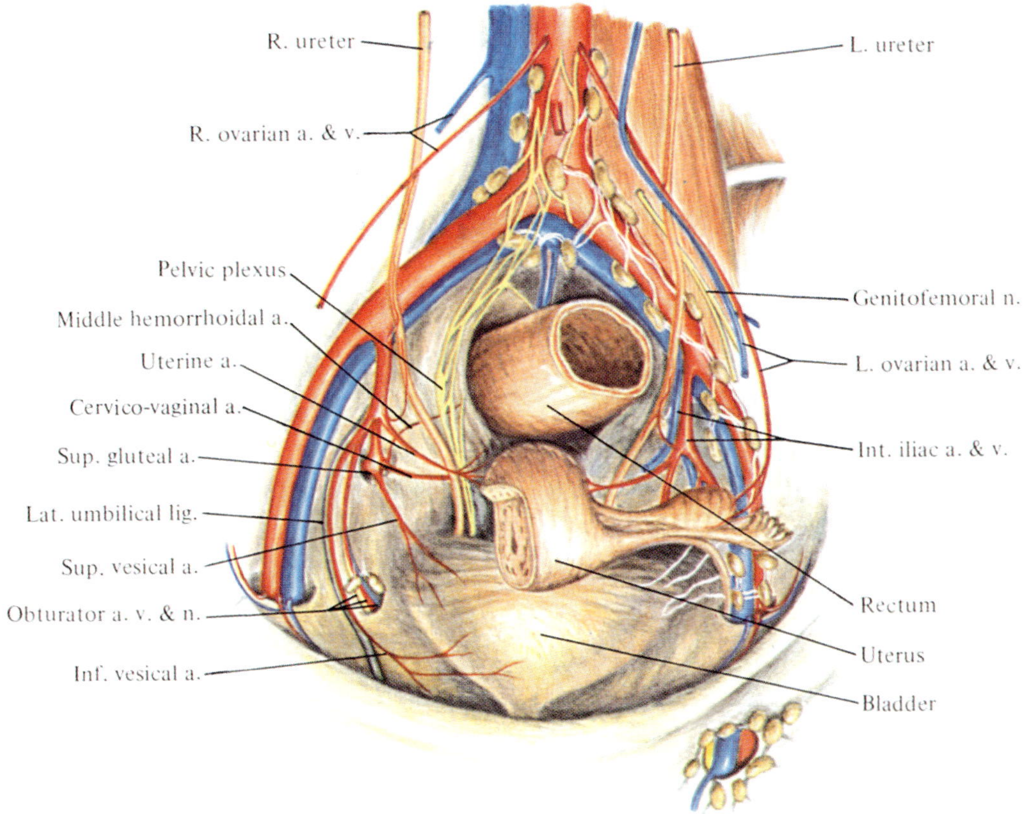

FIG. 2.
Pelvic portion of ureter in the female.

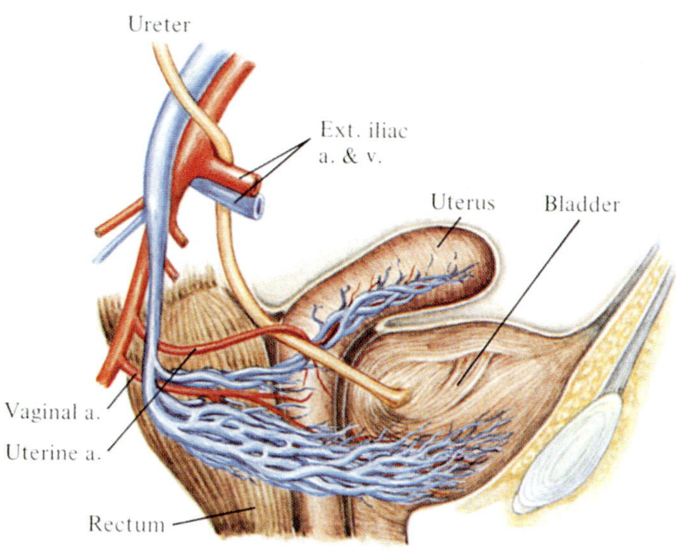

FIG. 3.
Deep pelvic part of ureter in the female, lateral view.

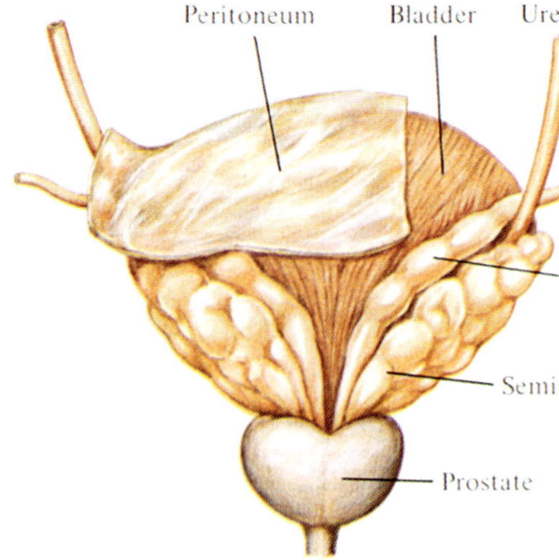

FIG. 4.
Posterior view of the prostate, seminal vesicles, and vas deferens.

VASCULAR SUPPLY

The arterial supply to the ureters is derived from several sources. The extrarenal pelvis and upper ureter are supplied by branches from the renal artery. The middle one-third of the ureter derives its supply from branches of the gonadal, the colic, and the common iliac or hypogastric arteries. The lower third of the ureter is supplied by arteries arising from the superior vesical, middle hemorrhoidal, and inferior vesical arteries (Figs. 1 and 2).

These vessels from several sources anastomose freely, forming a fine network covering the ureter. Because of this vascular network, the ureter can withstand a considerable amount of surgical trauma without fear of sloughing.

The veins begin as a fine meshwork and empty into the main veins, which correspond largely to the adjacent arteries.

Lymphatics communicate with the lymph nodes nearest the ureter in the abdomen and pelvis.

NERVE SUPPLY

Nerves supplying the upper ureter are mostly from the plexus accompanying the ovarian or spermatic artery. The lower ureter derives its supply from the hypogastric and pelvic plexus. The nerves are derived mostly from sympathetic trunks and are independent of the renal pelvis and bladder (Fig. 5).

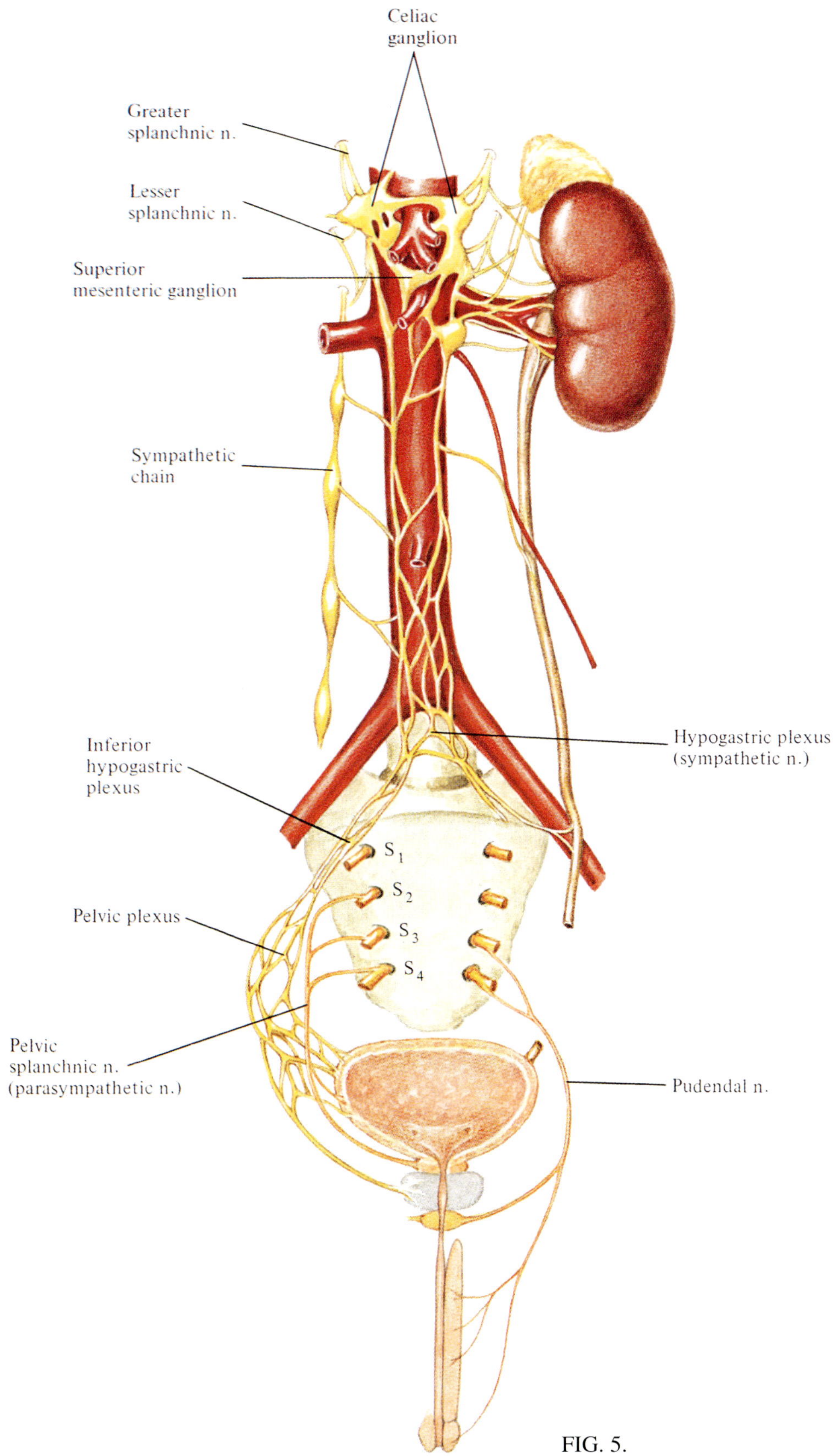

FIG. 5.
Autonomic and somatic nerve supply to the male urogenital system.

Operative Techniques

34. Foley "Muscle Splitting" Incision

As the following sequence of illustrations depicts, muscle splitting could be more appropriately termed muscle separation.

34-1. The *line of incision is oblique* from the midportion of the 12th rib to the anterosuperior spine of the iliac crest. The operating table is slightly flexed and the lumbar muscles underlying the operative area are under only slight tension.

34-2. The *muscles forming Petit's triangle*—latissimus dorsi (posterior border) and external oblique (anterior border)—*are bluntly separated* to expose first the internal oblique and, once through this layer, the transversalis fascia. The fascia is incised to expose adipose tissue in the retroperitoneal space.

34-3. *The upper ureter containing the calculus is exposed and isolated.* A small flat tubular drain or umbilical tape is placed around the ureter superior to the calculus to prevent retrograde migration of the calculus. The ureteral incision as indicated by a dotted line is made over the calculus. When the calculus is withdrawn by forceps, a ureteral catheter (5 Fr) is passed in both directions to the level of the renal pelvis and bladder.

Periadventitial ureteral sutures (4–0 chromic catgut) are used to reapproximate the edges only if a gaping ureteral incision is observed. Insertion of a Jackson-Pratt closed drainage tube before final closure is mandatory. The drain can be removed after several days.

An alternative approach to the midureter is extraperitoneal and can be started by using an incision that is also used for left varicocelectomy (high left spermatic vein ligation). On the right, a nearly horizontal skin incision may be employed. The abdominal muscles are separated along the lines of their fibers. External oblique, internal oblique, and transverse abdominal muscles are separated bluntly with large curved clamps or with the fingertips. The peritoneum is reflected medially with a Deaver retractor or a sponge on a ring forcep. As the dissection is carried medially across the psoas

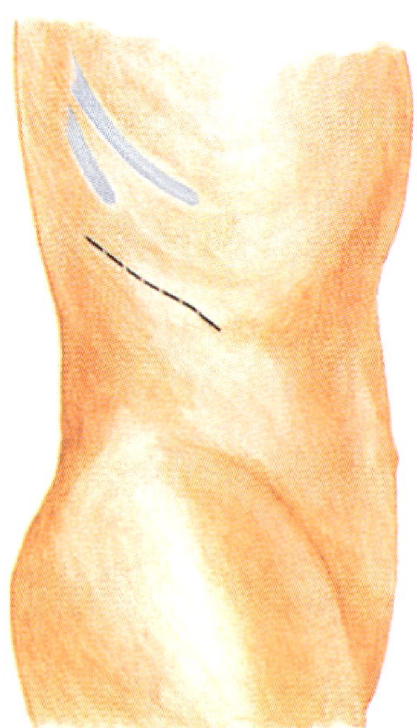

34-1

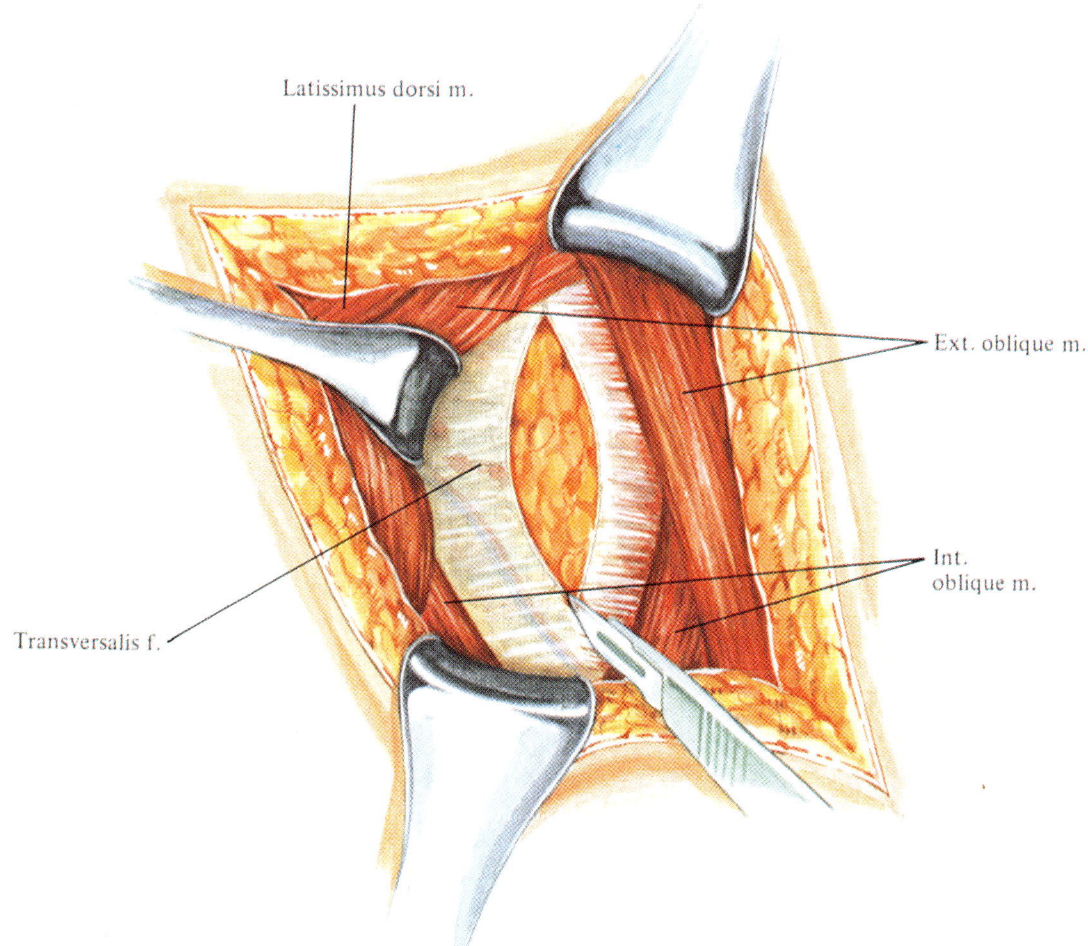
Latissimus dorsi m.
Ext. oblique m.
Int. oblique m.
Transversalis f.

34-2

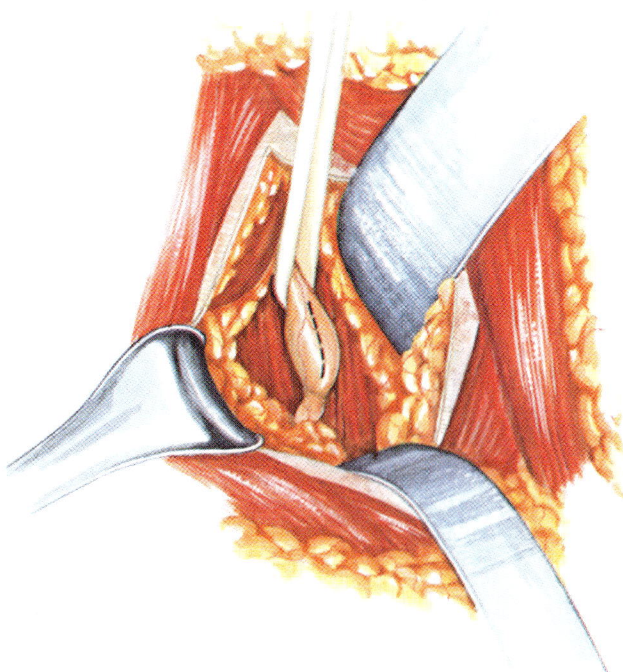

34-3

major muscle, the transversalis fascia surrounding the spermatic vein will be encountered first. More medial retraction and posterior dissection will expose the ureter. The calculus is palpated. A small flat tubular drain or a Babcock clamp is passed around the ureter superior to the calculus to prevent upward migration.

35. Vertical Lumbar Approach with Minimal Dissection for Upper Ureteral Calculus

The following sequence of illustrations demonstrates the operative approach described by Minami focusing on the upper ureter. This approach was first described by Simon and Czerny and modified by Minami.

35-1. The skin incision is started below the lower edge of the 11th rib and a little anterior to the tip of the 12th rib; it is carried straight downward until one reaches the iliac crest.

35-2. Minami approach. Cross section at level of mid-right kidney. The arrow indicates the route of minimal muscle dissection. Transversalis fascia is exposed by reflecting the latissimus dorsi muscle backward and the external oblique muscle forward.

35-3. Transversalis fascia is incised vertically and one now enters into the retroperitoneal space. Care must be taken not to injure the 12th intercostal nerve and vessels. Gerota's fascia is opened, and the dilated ureter containing the calculus is exposed. An umbilical tape is placed superior to the calculus to prevent retrograde migration to the renal pelvis. The procedure for removing the calculus and effecting closure have been described in the techniques for the Foley "muscle splitting" incision.

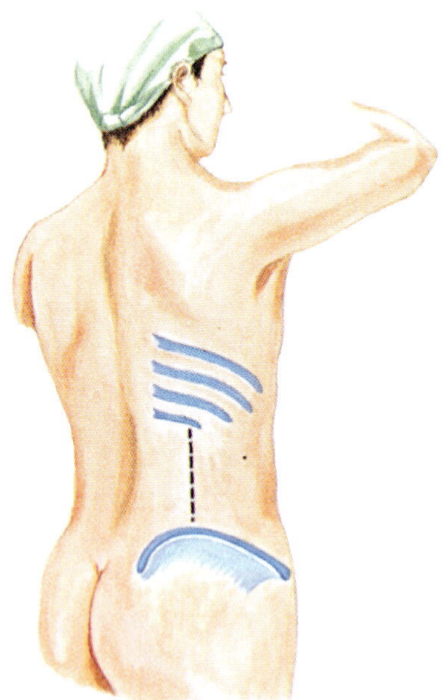

35-1

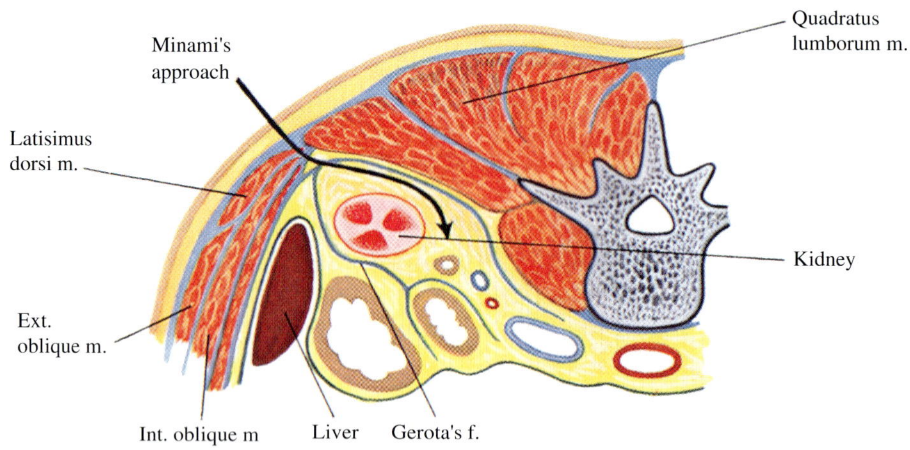

35-2

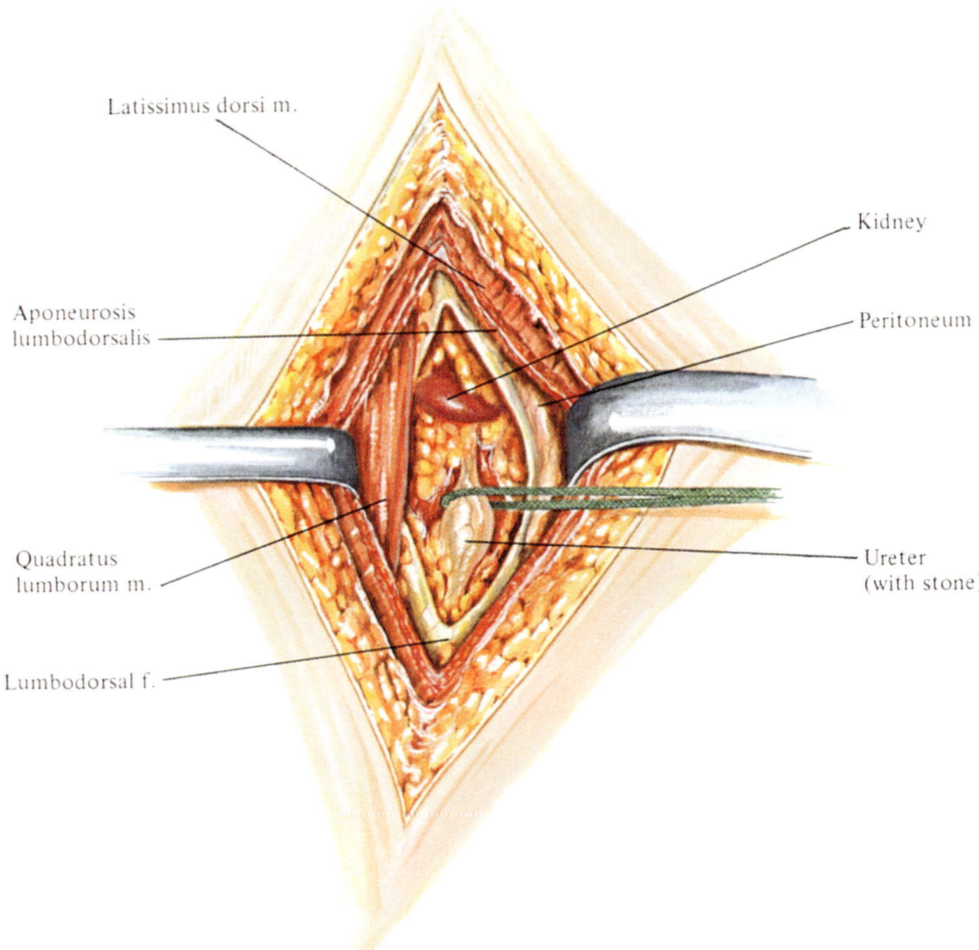

35-3

36. Ureterolithotomies of Lower Ureter

36-1. The following *lines of incision* can be used depending on the location of the calculus: 1) vertical midline, 2) paramedian, 3) oblique, or 4) transverse.

A discussion of the anterior abdominal wall is appropriate at this point. The rectus abdominis muscle extends from the thorax on each side to the pubis. It originates from the pubic crest and anterior pubic ligament. It inserts along the anterior surface of the fifth, sixth, and seventh costal cartilages. The medial border is separated from that of its fellow by the linea alba. The anterior surface of the muscle has three tendinous insertions which provide added strength. They are located at the costal cartilage, the umbilicus, and between the two.

The sheath of the rectus abdominis can best be discussed by regions, as follows:

1. Above the costal margin the sheath is incomplete; the anterior wall is the aponeurosis of the external oblique; no posterior wall exists. Therefore the muscle lies on cartilage.
2. From the rib margin to the midpoint between umbilicus and pubis, the sheath is

complete. The internal oblique aponeurosis divides at the lateral border of rectus muscle into anterior and posterior layers.

a. The anterior wall of the sheath consists of the aponeurosis of the external oblique plus the anterior layer of the internal oblique aponeurosis.
b. The posterior wall consists of the posterior layer, aponeurosis of internal oblique and the aponeurosis of the transversus abdominis muscle, and the transversalis fascia. The transversus abdominis muscle, which extends behind the rectus, is muscular to the midline.

The posterior sheath ends midway between the umbilicus and the pubis. The arched lower border or sheath is the line of Douglas. Inferior to this border, the internal oblique aponeurosis does not divide but goes anterior as a common sheath. The inferior epigastric artery enters the sheath of rectus abdominis by crossing this edge.

3. From midway between the umbilicus and the pubis to symphysis pubis, the anterior wall is formed by the aponeurosis of the external and internal oblique muscles plus the transversus abdominis muscle. The transversus abdominis and the internal oblique are fused. The external oblique does not fuse until it reaches midline. The posterior wall is formed by the transversalis fascia.

In a female patient an oblique or a transverse incision is probably the best approach to avoid the uterus and adjacent vascular supply (Figs. 2 and 3). The following illustrations depict the surgical approach to the right lower ureter.

36-2. *A vertical midline incision is carried through the fascia.*

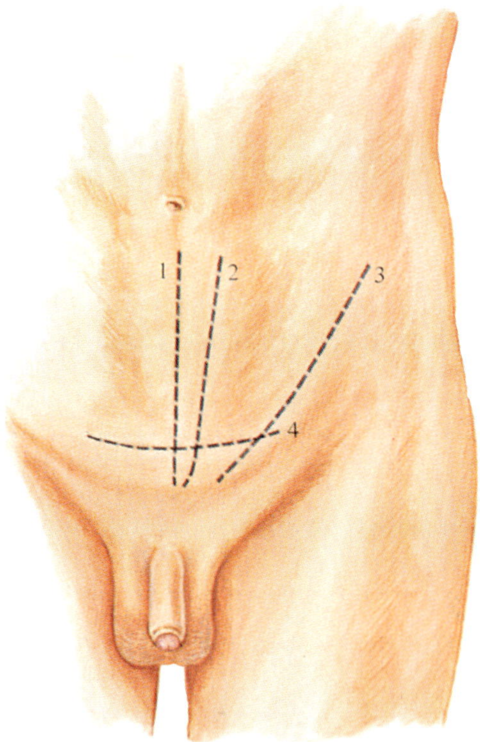

36-1

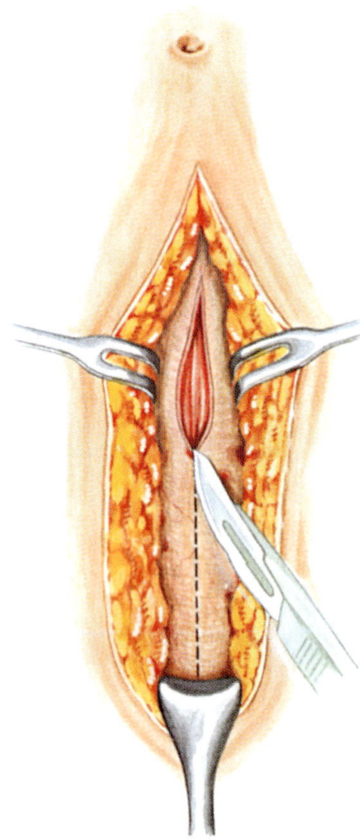

36-2

36-3. *The muscle and underlying peritoneum are retracted* medially, exposing the retroperitoneal fat.

36-4. *The dilated portion of the right ureter containing a calculus is exposed.*

36-5. Stay sutures improve exposure.

36-6. *The stone is removed.*

36-7. *The ureter is catheterized inferiorly.*

36-8. Interrupted 4–0 or 5–0 chromic catgut sutures are used for closure of the ureter.

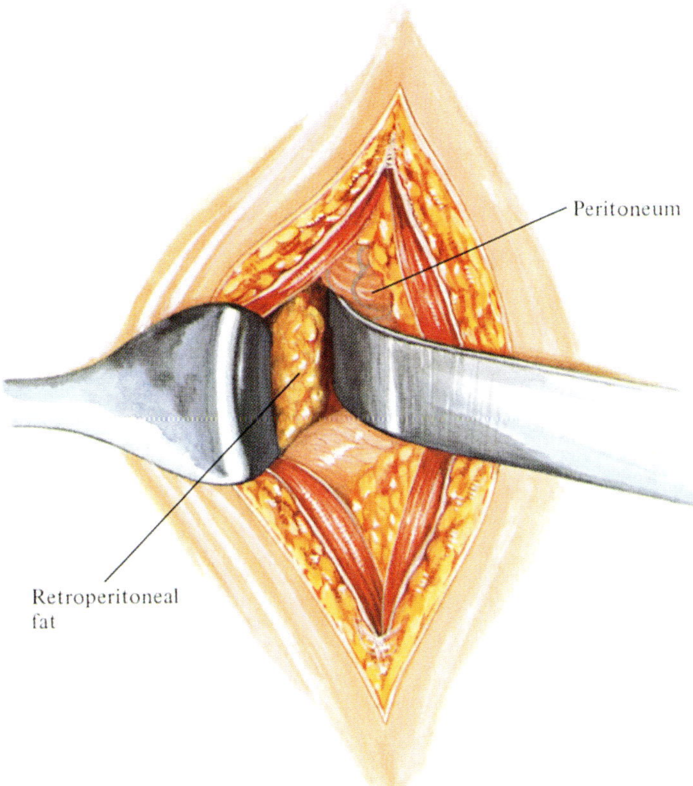

36-3

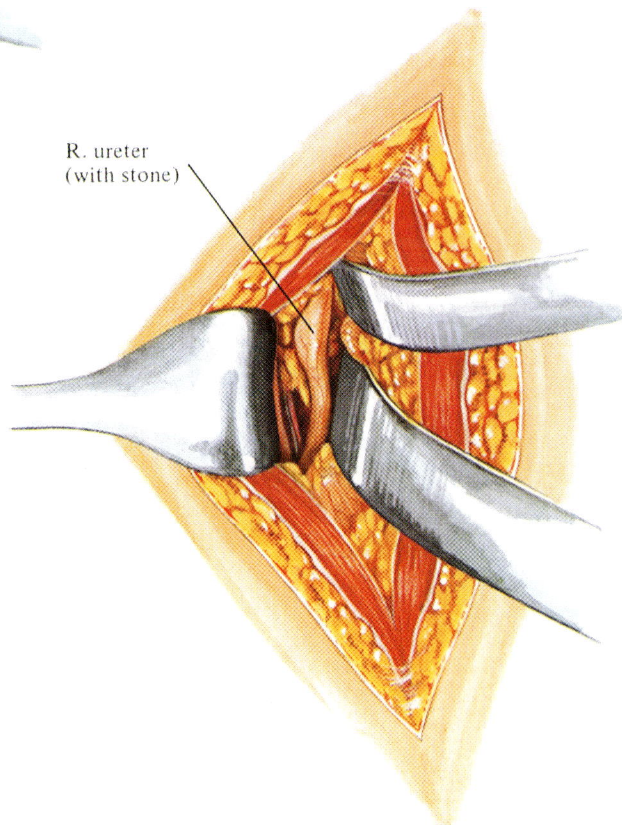

36-4

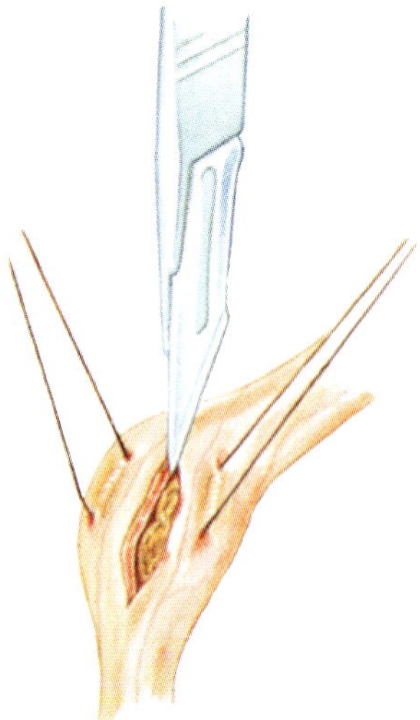
36-5

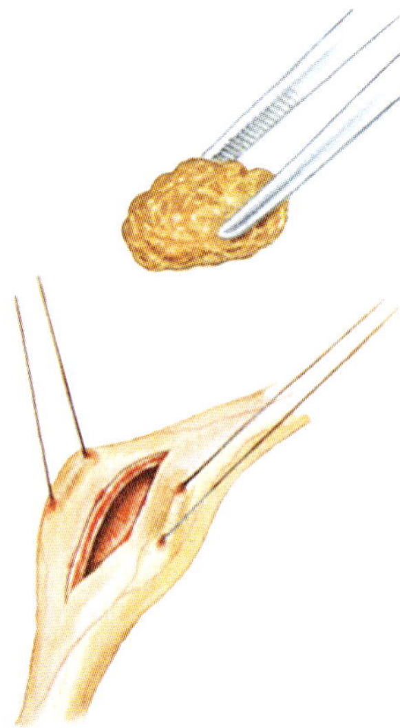
36-6

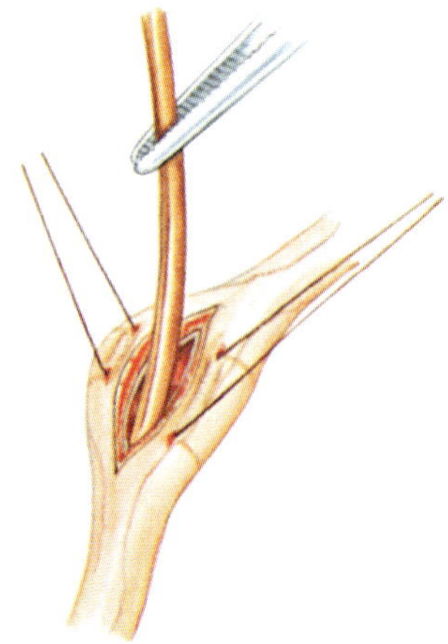
36-7

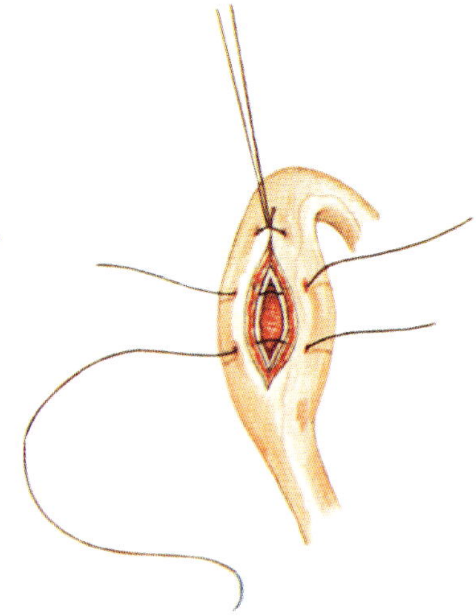
36-8

37. End-to-End Ureteroureterostomy

Damage to a ureter, inadvertently caused by previous surgery or due to penetrating wounds, may require excision of a short ureteral segment. Clinical experience has indicated a high incidence of ureteral damage in the female undergoing gynecologic surgery. The following illustrations demonstrate the two best methods of anastomotic repair.

37-1. *The short damaged ureteral segment is excised, the remaining ends are trimmed on a bias and reapproximated.* Anastomotic closure is accomplished with 4–0 or 5–0 chromic catgut sutures, depending on ureteral size.

37-2. In this alternative, *end-to-end anastomosis is affected by excising the short damaged ureteral segment, securing the remaining ends with stay sutures,* and examining the tissue. The ureteral lumen is widened on opposite ends (180° apart) by incising each

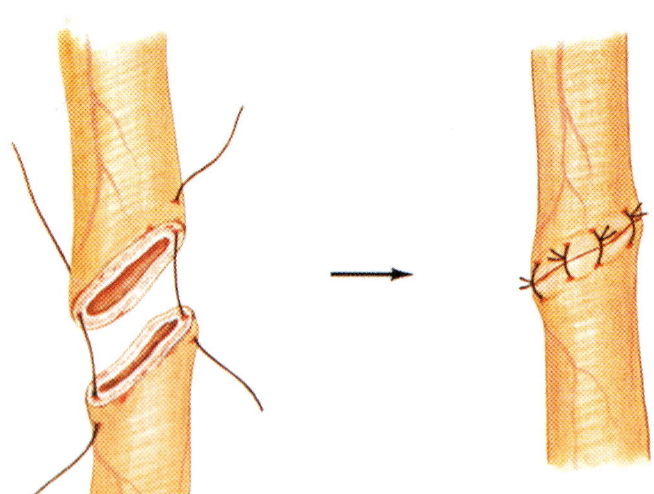
37-1

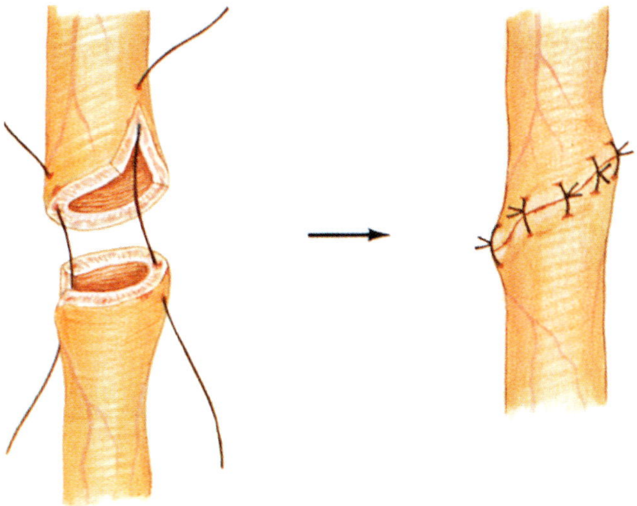

37-2

wall longtitudinally (approximately 8 mm). Ureteral ends are reapproximated and secured using 4–0 or 5–0 chromic catgut.

In all instances of ureteral repair, a Jackson-Pratt drainage tube is inserted and secured for 3 to 5 days.

38. Transureteroureterostomy

Unilateral damage to a long lower segment of ureter may occur. Under such circumstances anastomotic repair may be required.

38-1. This *schematic shows crossover of the upper right ureter* after removal or ligation of the damaged segment. Note that this is done by an end-to-side anastomosis.

Transureteroureterostomy

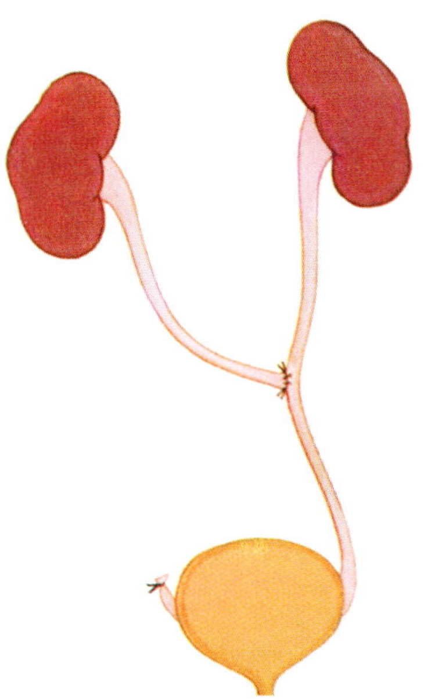

38-1

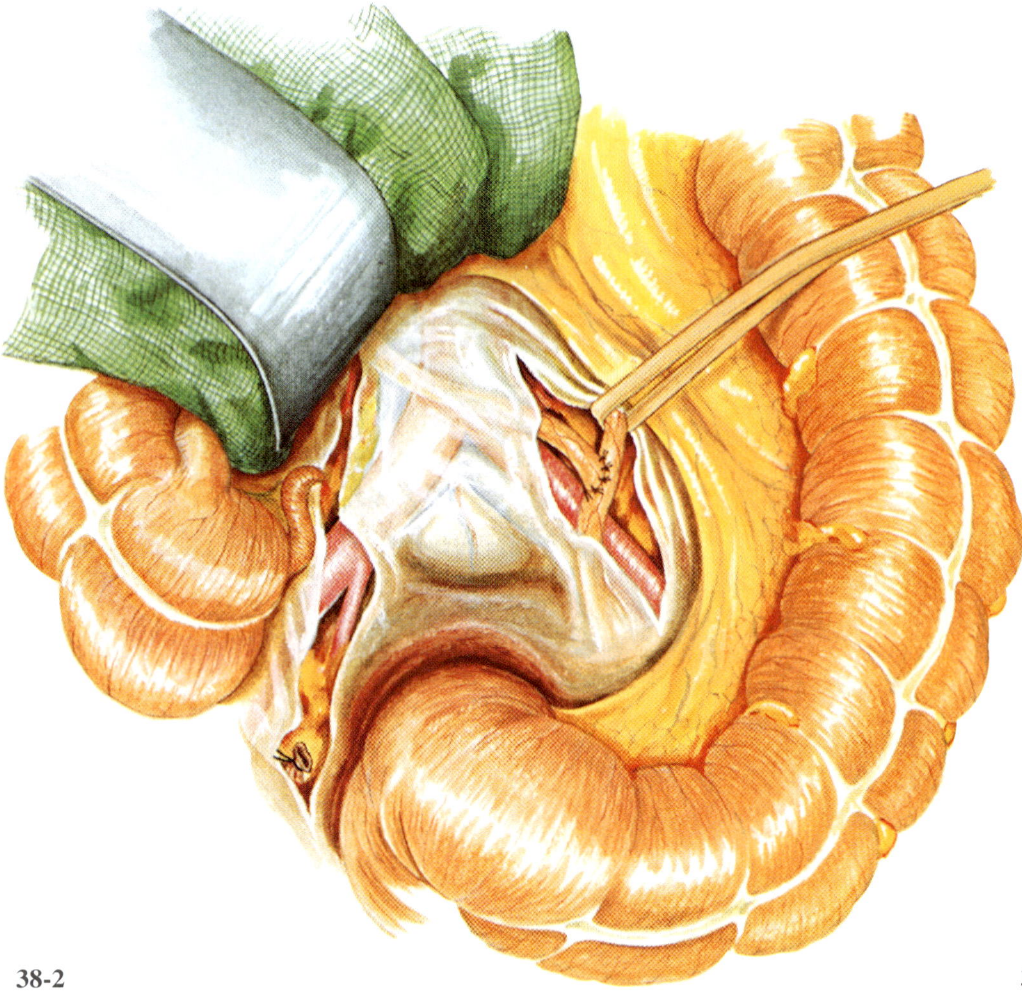

38-2

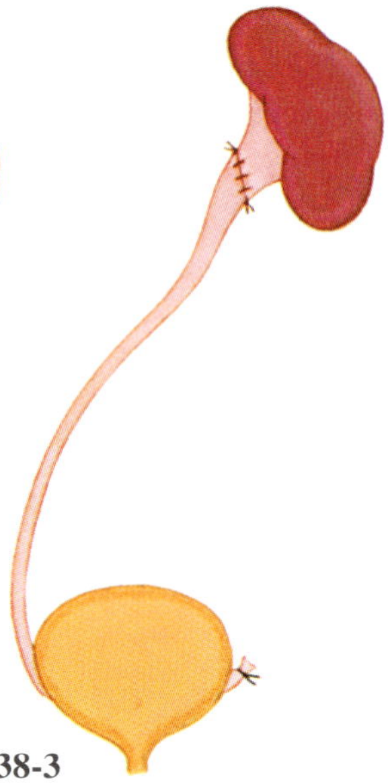

38-3

38-2. The surgical field is reached through a transabdominal approach. *Both middle ureters are located by separate retroperitoneal dissections.* The end-to-side transureteroureteral anastomosis is performed in the retroperitoneal space. A small flat tubular drain facilitates the isolation of the left ureter and assists in exposing the anastomotic junction.

38-3. If necessary, *the anastomosis of a contralateral ureter to the healthy kidney may be used.* A situation such as this could be surgically handled by autotransplantation, by placing the left kidney in the right iliac fossa.

39. Total Nephroureterectomy for a Ureteral Carcinoma

General Considerations. A ureteral tumor extending through ureteral muscle and producing nonfunction or poor function of a kidney on one side is generally treated by nephroureterectomy including a cuff of bladder wall. The diagnostic work-up of such a patient deserves mention.

Symptoms of pain, ureteral colic, or back pain (dull ache due to hydronephrosis and distention of the renal capsule) may bring the patient to a physician. The finding of gross or microscopic hematuria associated with pain should prompt the physician or urologist to obtain an intravenous pyelogram. If the appropriate kidney is not functioning, then cystoscopy and a bulb retrograde pyelographic study should be performed to assist in the diagnosis. Ureteral brushing of the tumor and appropriate examination of the cells may also confirm the diagnosis.

Finding a filling defect in the ureter at the site of obstruction after an intravenous pyelogram is often diagnostic. The differential diagnosis will include 1) ureteral tumor, 2) blood clot, or 3) nonopaque calculi. The uric acid level in the blood may assist in the diagnostic work-up of the patient.

In selected instances, performing antegrade pyelography has assisted significantly in the work-up. This has been useful in delineating the site of the lesion and the contour of the lesion from the superior side.

39-1. The patient lies supine, and *a sandbag is placed beneath the patient* on the appropriate side. The broken lines indicate the lines of incision. A transverse abdominal incision is first made.

39-2. *The transversus abdominis muscle is separated* and hemostasis is controlled by coagulation.

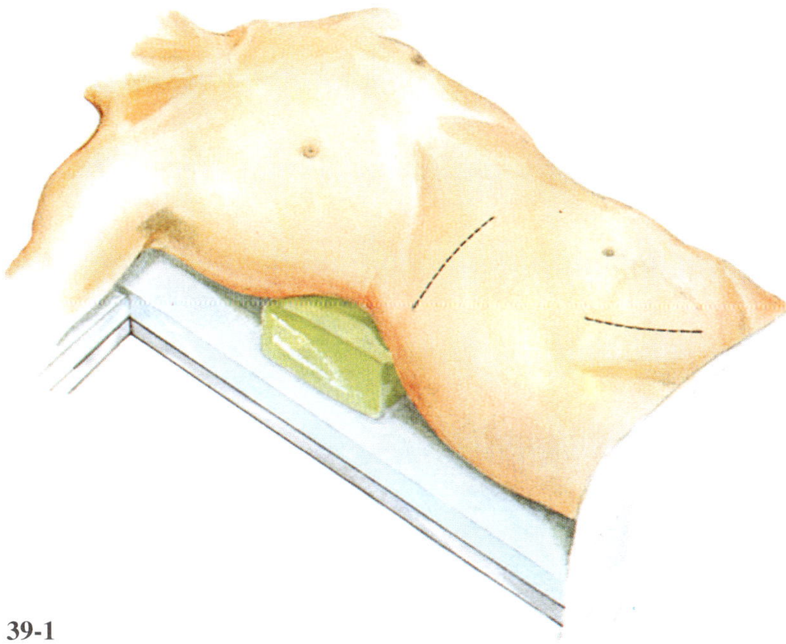

39-1

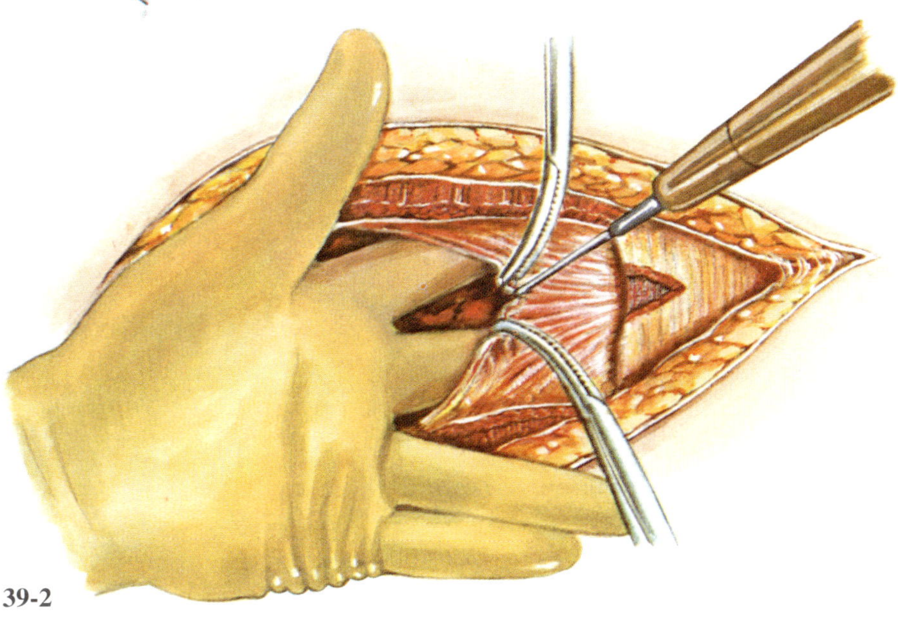

39-2

39-3. *Preperitoneal fat and extraperitoneal fat are exposed.*

39-4. *The renal pedicle is exposed.* The renal artery is doubly ligated on the proximal side (1–0 silk) and severed. A tie has been placed around the renal vein prior to double ligation.

39-5. *The ischemic kidney is lifted out of its bed.* The ureter is still in continuity.

39-6. *The lower abdominal oblique incision is now initiated* (see 39–1).

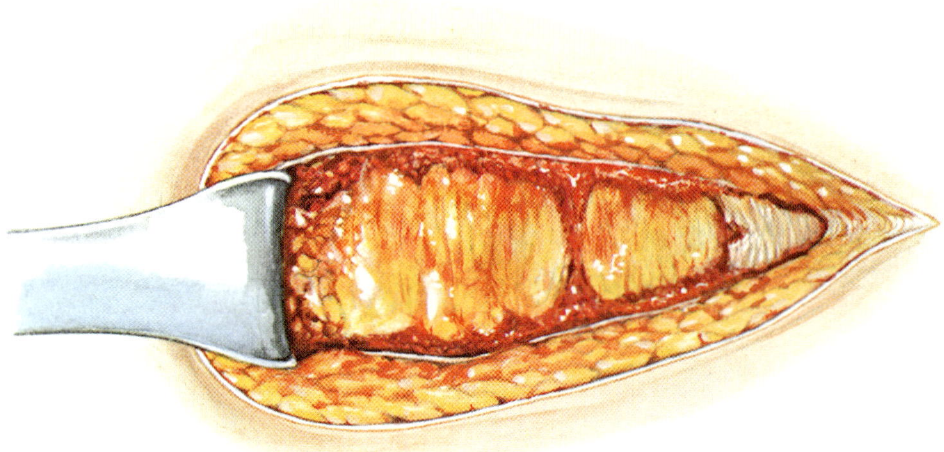

39-3

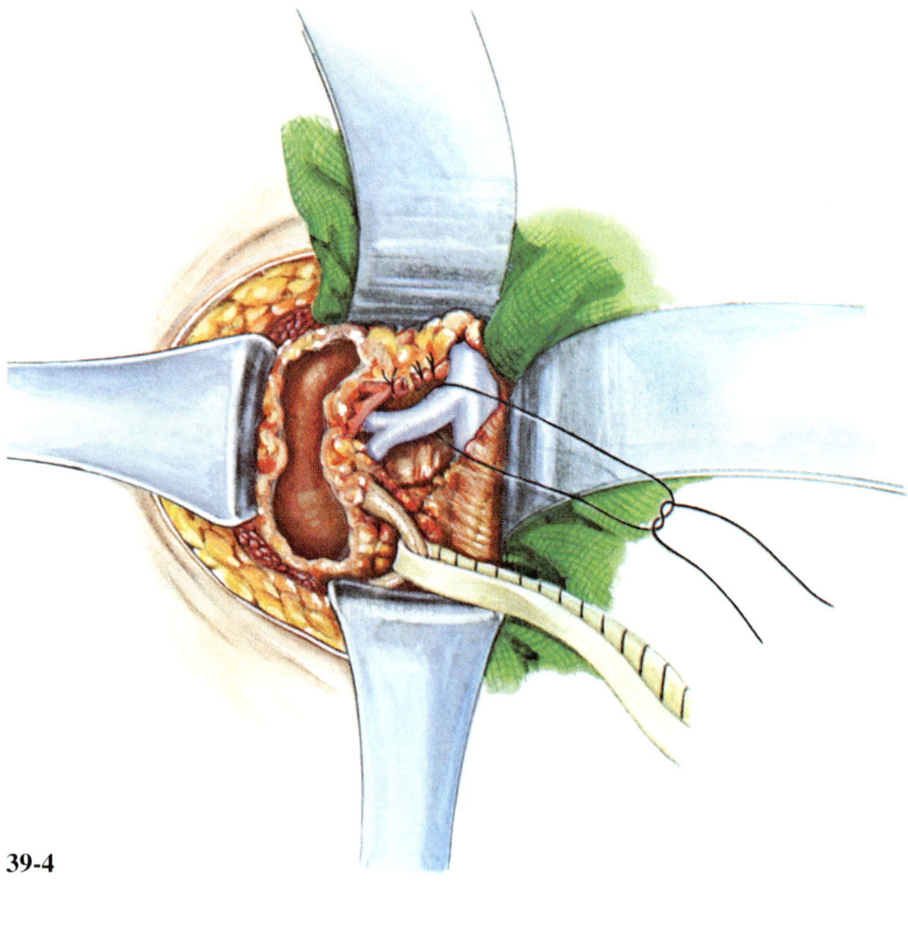

39-4

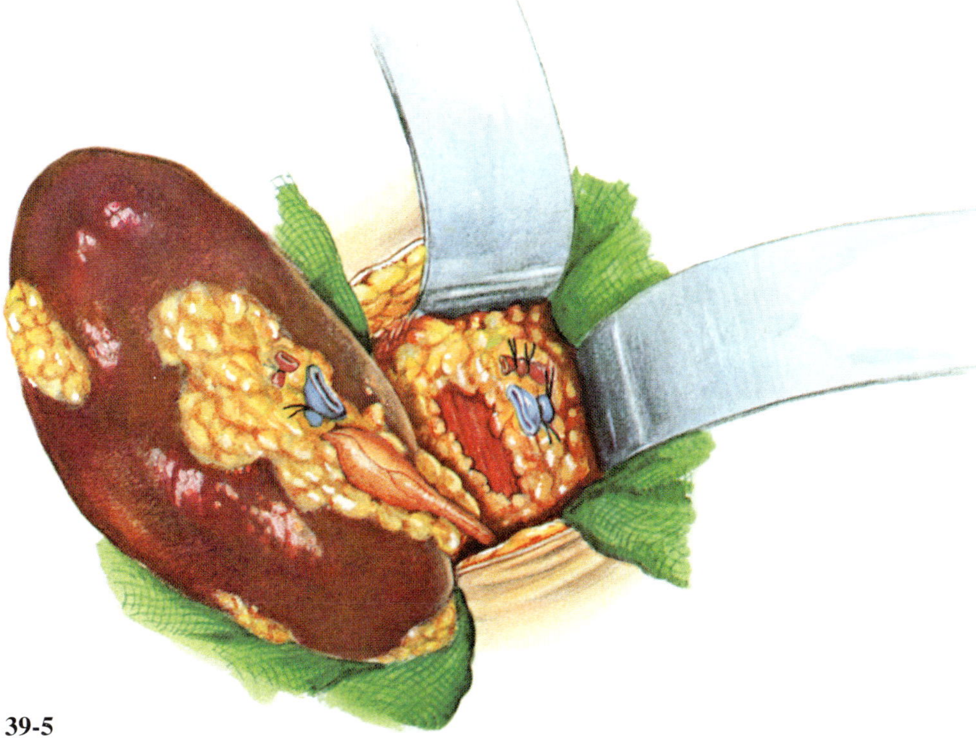

39-5

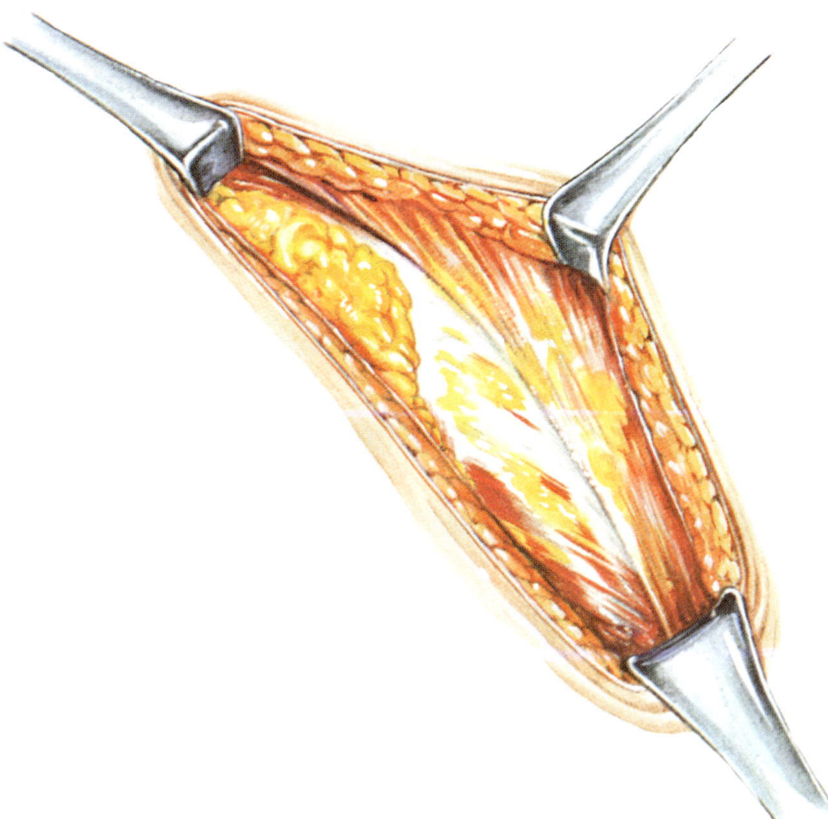

39-6

39-7. After the muscle layers are incised and the peritoneum is retracted medially, *the ureter and* the tumor are exposed. The bladder has been retracted medially.

The extraperitoneal space between both incisions is developed by blunt dissection to allow passage of the kidney to the site of the inferior surgical field.

39-8. *A cuff of bladder including the distal ureter is removed* to complete the nephroureterectomy. The tumor is removed. The bladder opening is reapproximated in two layers (3–0 chromic catgut sutures).

Closure of both wounds can be performed simultaneously by members of the the surgical team. A Penrose drain is not necessary in the upper incision. A small Jackson-Pratt drain can be led from the bladder area and maintained for 2–4 days.

The muscular layers are reapproximated.

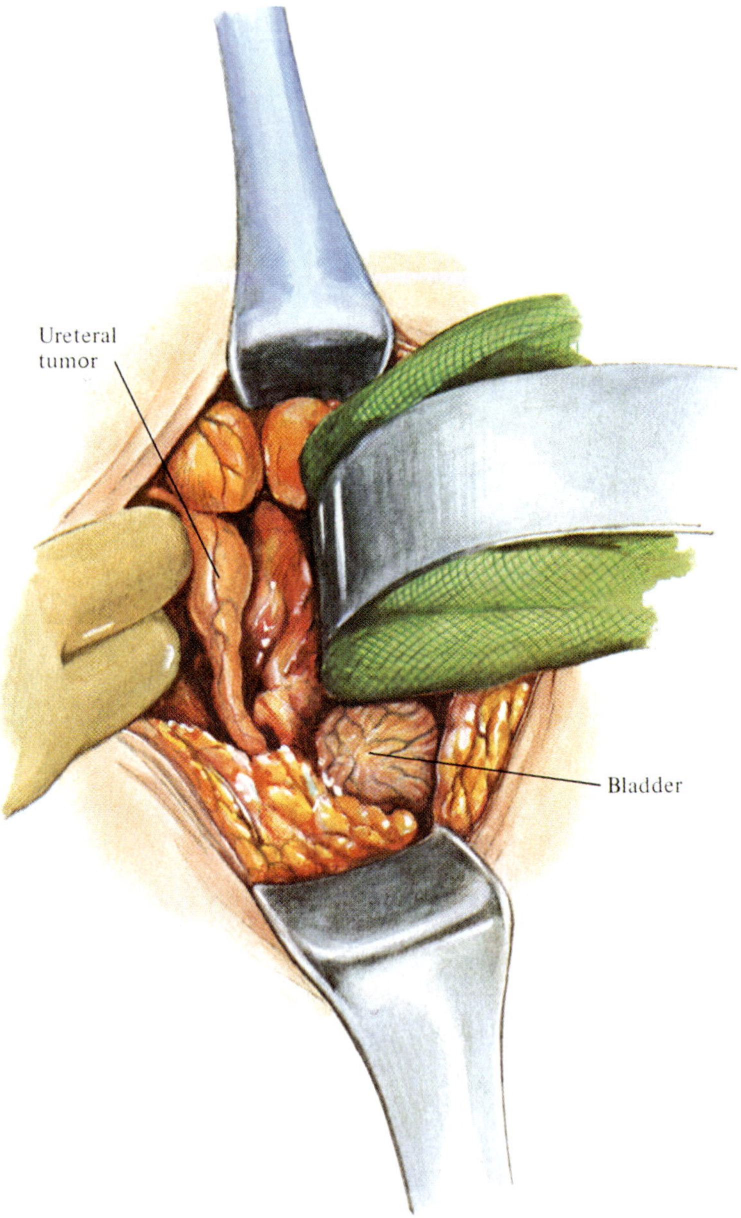

39-7

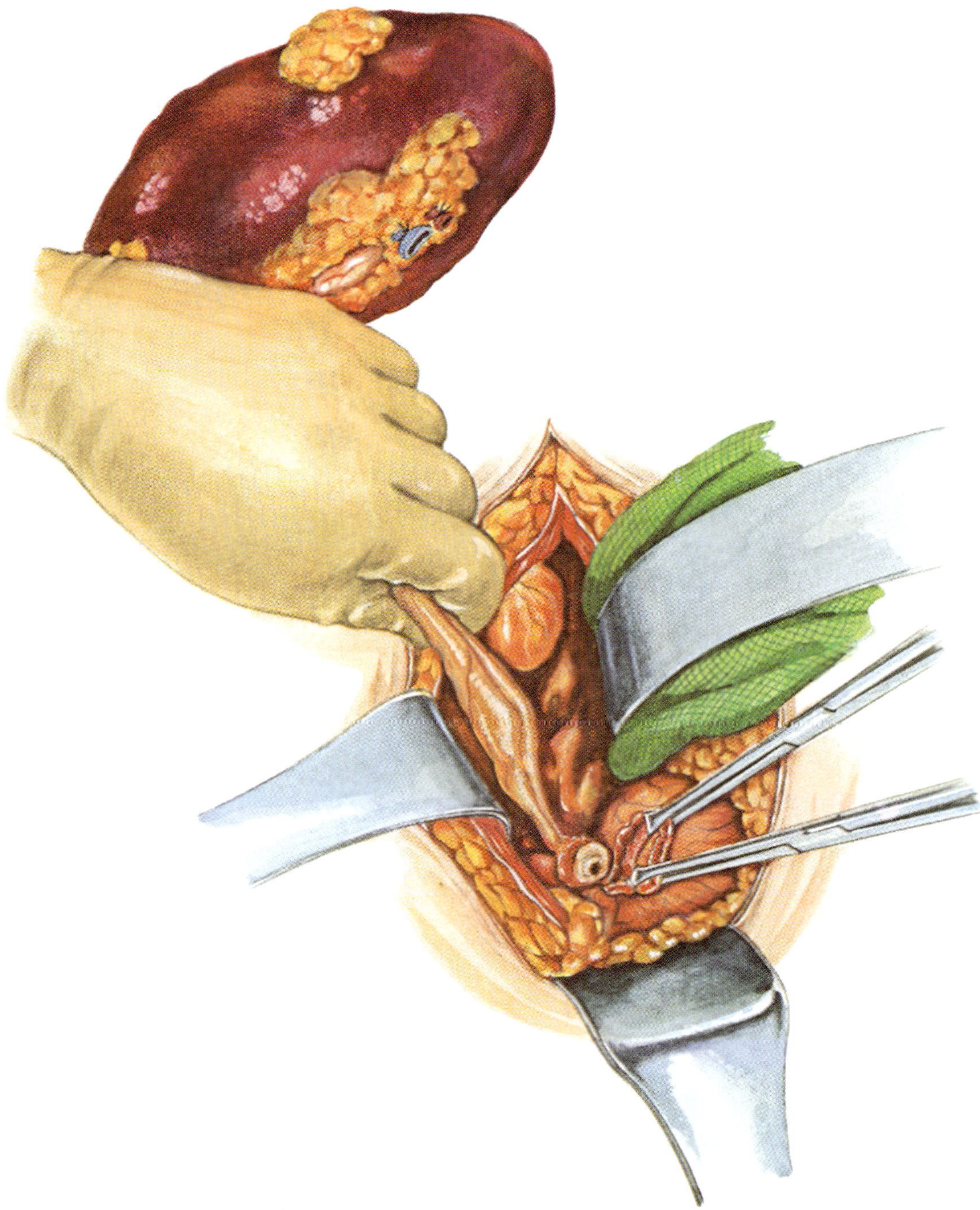

39-8

40. Transurethral Ureterectomy Using Intussusception of the Distal Ureter

Prior to open surgery, the patient is cystoscoped, and a ureteral bougie with a cobra head or a bulb head on the tip is inserted up the proximal ureter. The ureteral catheter with a balloon has been placed up the ureter where the transection is to be made.

40-1. The radical nephrectomy and freeing the upper half of the ureter is completed. The superior one-half of the appropriate ureter is isolated and a tie of chromic catgut is placed around the distal part of the freed, proximal ureter. A second tie is placed around the distal ureter that will allow transection with the cautery between both ties. The tip of the catheter with the cobra head is placed next to the site of transection and then a tie is placed around the neck of the cobra head to prevent the catheter from pulling out. One can also use a ureteral catheter with a balloon.

40-2. The ligature is shown.

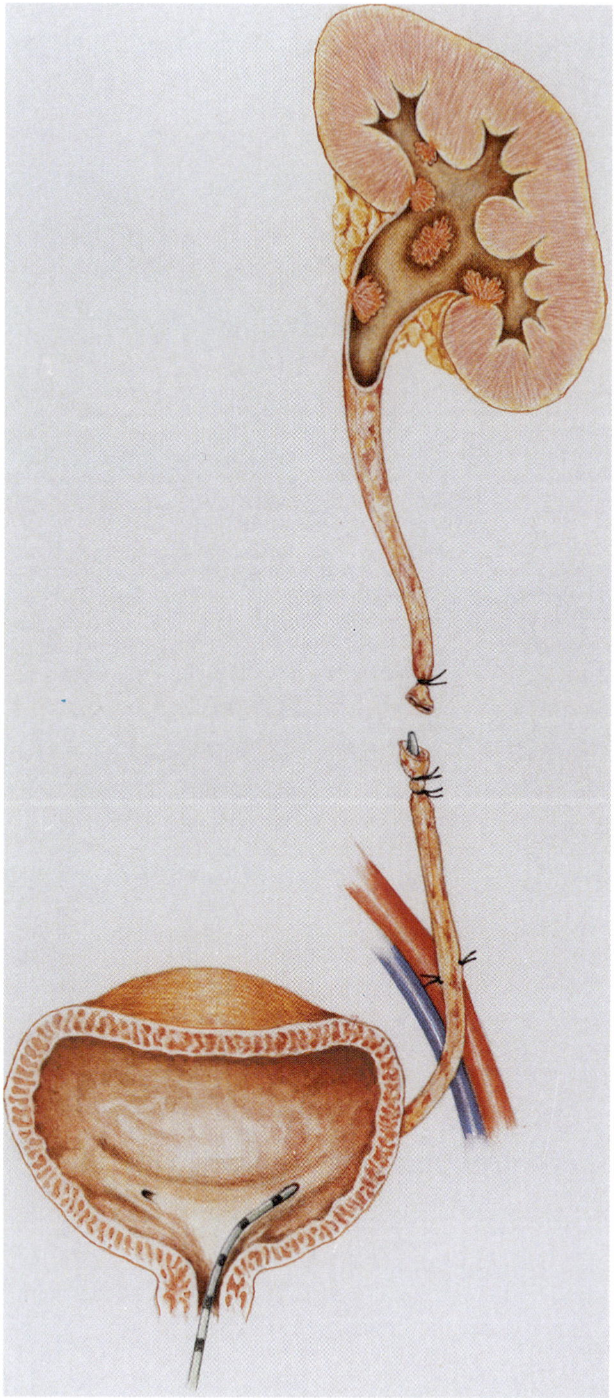

40-1

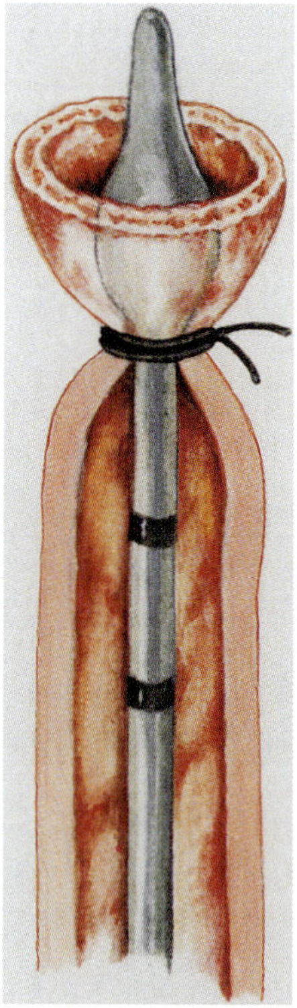

40-2

40-3. Before closing the abdominal wound, the bougie is carefully withdrawn intussuscepting the ureter as shown.

40-4. Further retraction of the catheter out through the urethra can be seen and the entire ureter is intussuscepted as shown.

The cautery and cutting element is then inserted through the obturator sheath using endoscopic visualization, and the distal ureter is transected and fulgurated as shown. A catheter is placed into the bladder for 24 hours after all of the endoscopic instruments have been removed.

It is possible that the surgeon may wish to remove the distal ureter with the balloon catheter, but with the incision open so that the midureter can still be controlled. The anterior approach with a subcostal incision allows removal of the kidney and exposure of the mid-ureter. The patient is in position for cystoscopy and appropriate draping has been used. After midureteral transection, the expanded cobra head ureteral bougie is

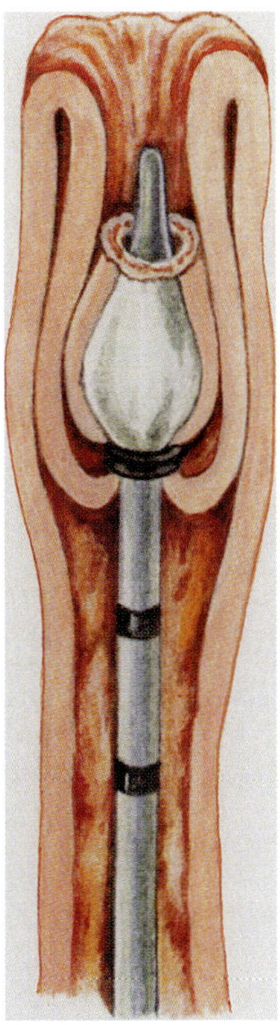

40-3

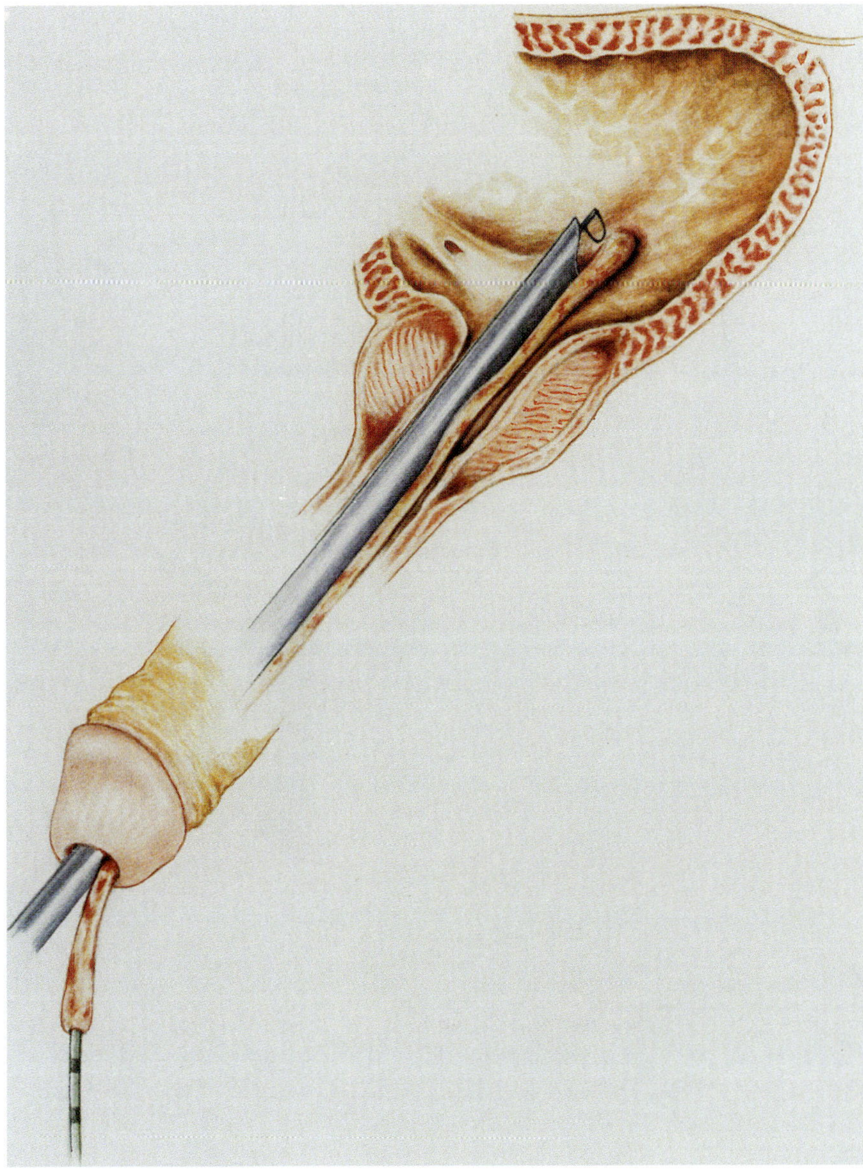

40-4

shown. The muscle around the appropriate ureteral orifice is incised using the cutting current, and the bougie and the lower half of the ureter is intussuscepted and removed. Bleeding is not a problem in the bladder although cystoscopic control is possible.

Vesicoureteral Antireflux Procedure

41. Politano-Leadbetter Technique

General Considerations. This procedure is most often performed in children. The child usually has suffered recurrent urinary tract infections. While the child is undergoing treatment, the voiding cystourethrogram (VCU) will demonstrate low-pressure reflux. An intravenous urogram (IVU) is obtained to rule out obstruction due to congenital anomalies. Urethral calibration and cystoscopy (urethroscopy) are carried out as a separate procedure under anesthesia to rule out significant urethral outlet obstruction. Such obstruction is dilated or treated at this time.

Recurrent urinary tract infection is treated by continuous antibacterial therapy. Sulfamethoxazole-trimethroprim or nitrofurantoin can be used for 1 year as part of a thera-

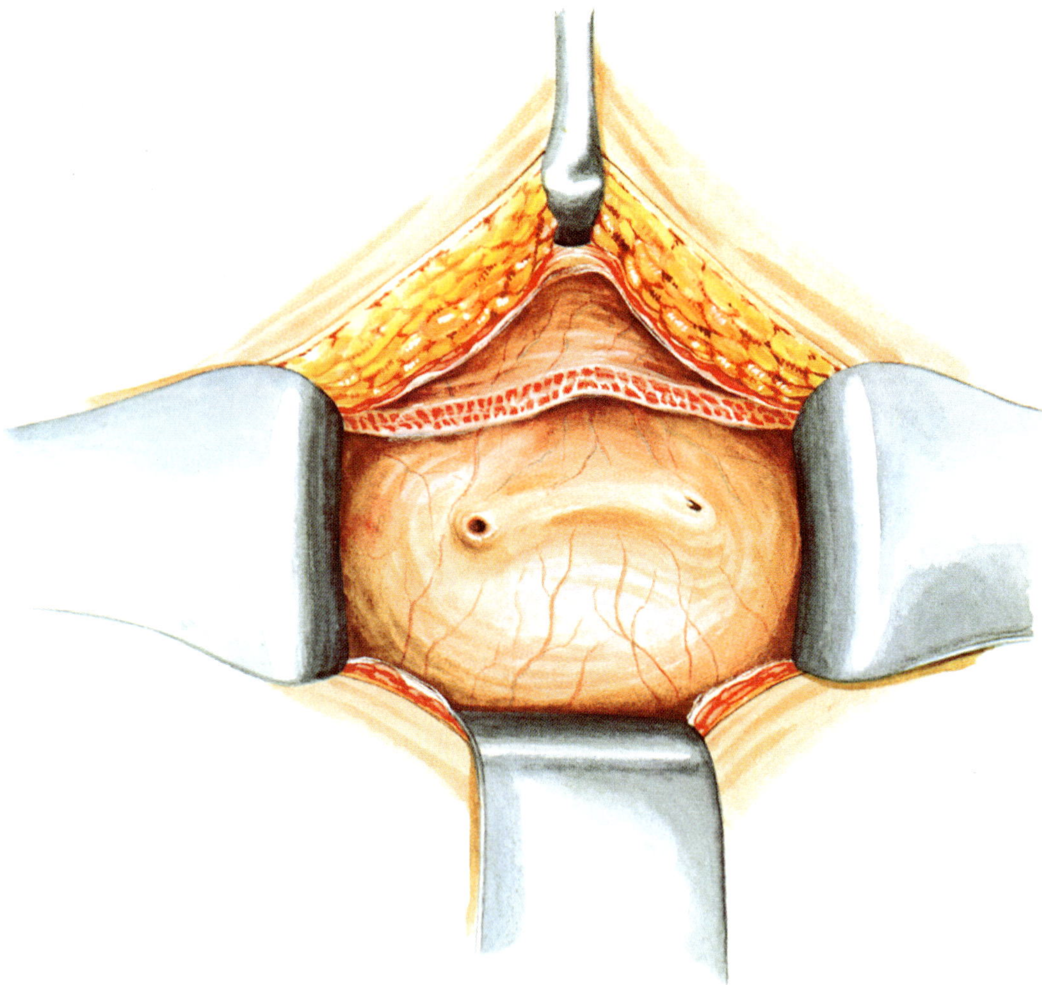

41-1

peutic trial. An interval VCU is performed at 6 months and 1 year to reassess the presence of reflux. If the low-pressure reflux persists, then the Politano-Leadbetter procedure is indicated.

Incision and Surgical Approach. A transverse lower abdominal incision is made (see 36–1). The fascia is similarly incised. The rectus abdominus muscles are retracted from the midline in a lateral direction, exposing the bladder and perivesical tissues.

41-1. *The bladder is opened.* Two narrow pediatric Deaver retractors may be substituted for the self-retaining retractors. A third Deaver retractor can be placed at the superior end of the bladder. The incompetent ureteral orifice is quite easily seen on the left side.

41-2. *A 5–0 feeding tube is inserted approximately 12 to 15 cm,* then a 3–0 silk stay suture is placed on one side of the ureteral orifice. Care is taken to include ureteral wall.

41-3. *The stay suture is tied around the tube* to allow traction on the orifice. A circumferential incision is made approximately 2 to 3 mm from the orifice.

41-4. *The ureter is freed from its supporting structures* for approximately 4–6 cm. Sharp and blunt dissection are used. A plastic iris-type scissor is useful during this maneuver. Occasionally, bleeding may be encountered. Hemostasis is important.

41-5. When the dissection is completed, *the ureter can be lifted with ease* through the opening in the bladder floor for at least 6 to 8 cm.

41-6. *Placement of the ureter into a new location* in the more superior and lateral aspect of the bladder wall is easily accomplished with the aid of a vein retractor to left mucosa and bladder musculature. By using the vein retractor, it is possible to visualize the posterior outside bladder wall where the new tunnel will be started. This maneuver will eliminate possible adhesions or inadvertent intraperitoneal dissection.

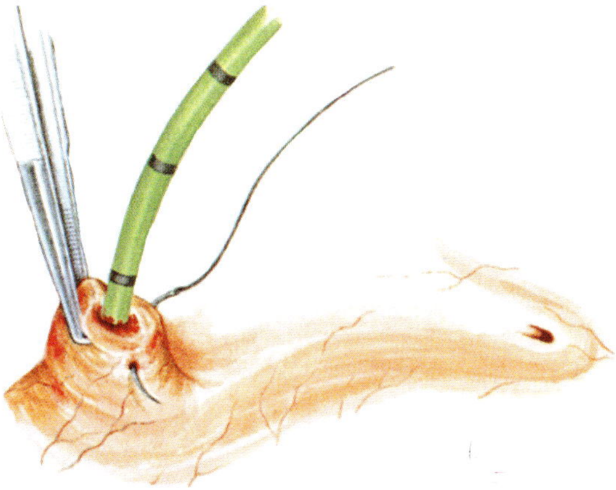

41-2

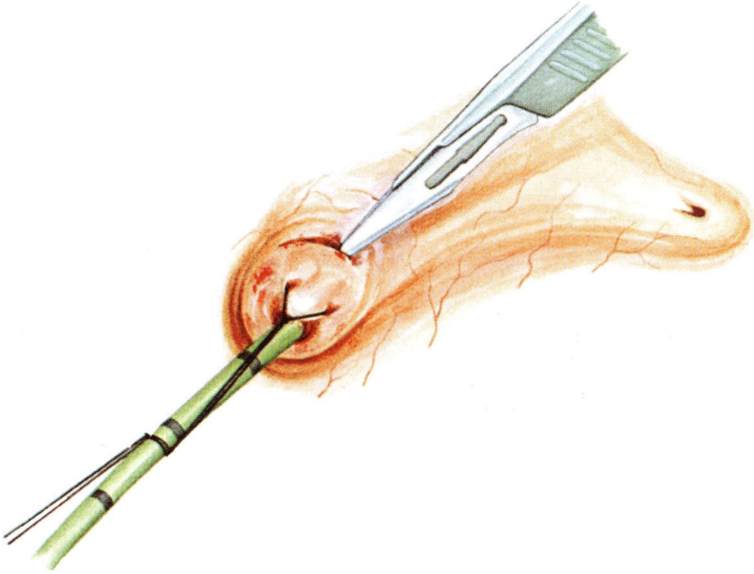

41-3

41-7. From the site of the old orifice *a right-angle clamp is passed behind the bladder in a superior lateral fashion* and pushed through the outer bladder wall to the mucosa, allowing an incision to be made through mucosa. The stay suture on the ureteral end is used to reroute the ureter through this new opening. The muscle layers at the site of the original ureteral orifice are reapproximated and sutured with 3–0 chromic catgut.

41-8. *The submucosal tunnel is created.* The stay suture is grasped and the ureter is

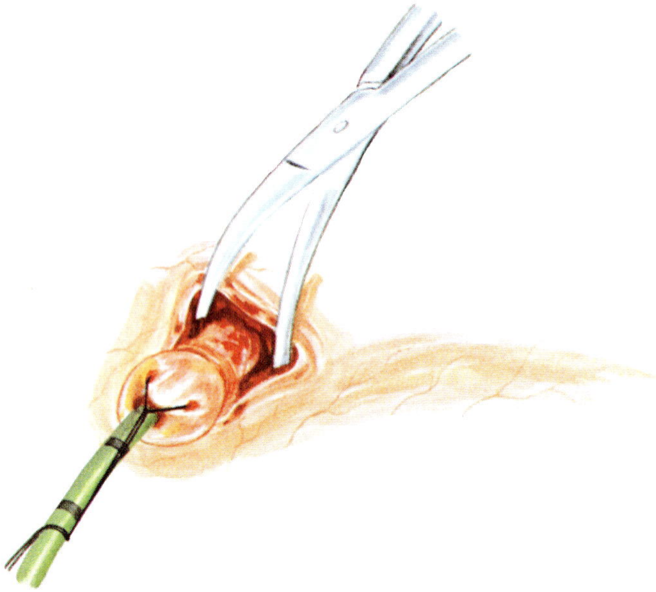

41-4

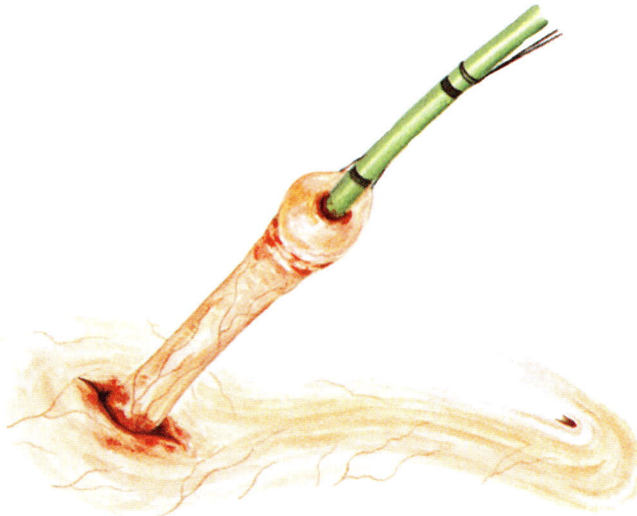

41-5

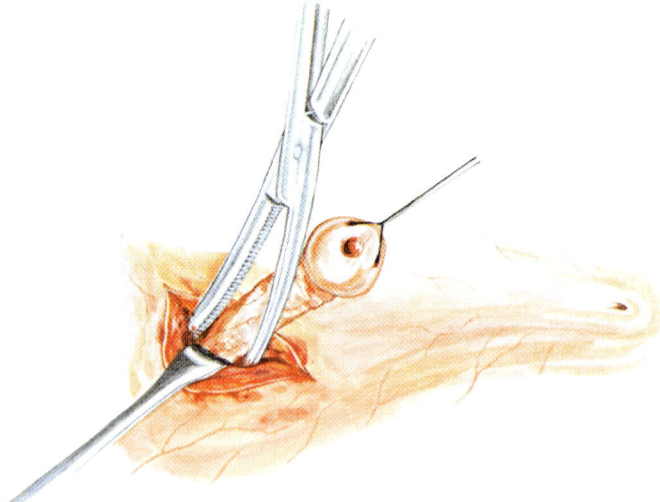

41-6

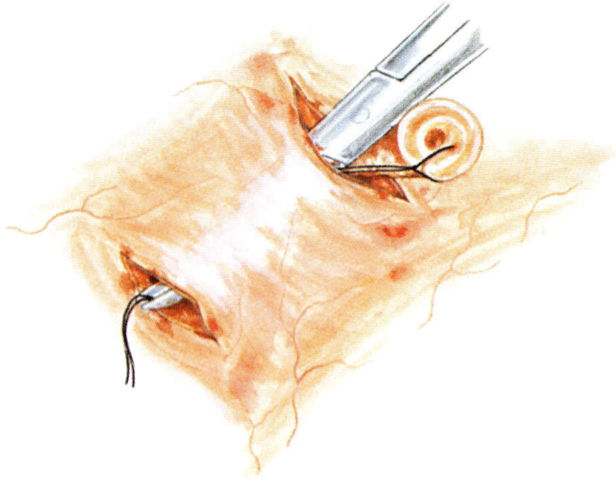

41-7

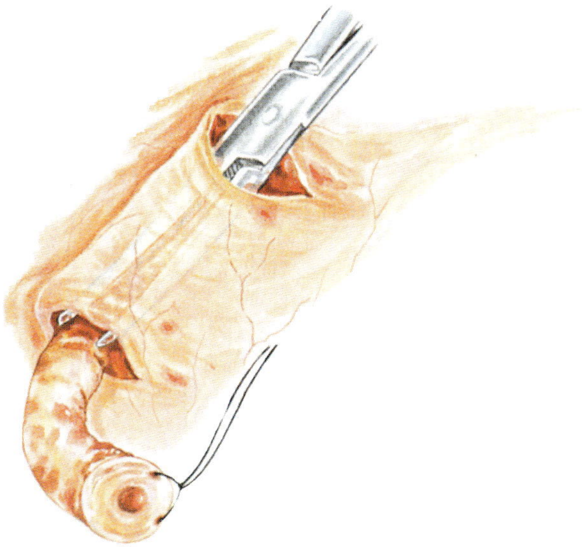

41-8

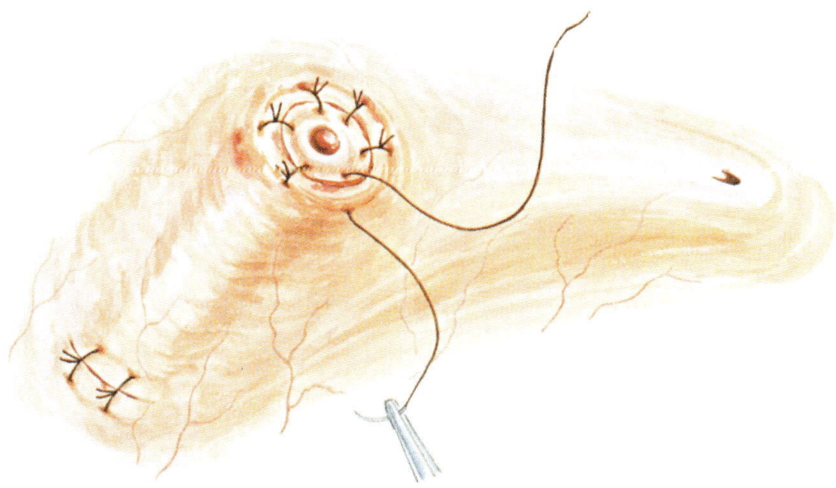

41-9

gently pulled through the new submucosal tunnel. The 5 Fr feeding tube is inserted for 6–8 cm to rule out any obstruction, kinking, or twisting of the ureter.

41-9. *The ureteral orifice is sutured to the bladder mucosa* with interrupted 4–0 chromic catgut sutures. Inferior sutures are placed to include bladder muscle. The mucosal incision at the superior lateral end of the tunnel is sutured. A ureteral stent is left up the ureter and is brought out through the bladder through a separate anterior opening. The stent is removed after 3 to 4 days.

The identical surgical procedure is performed if the other orifice is also incompetent.

The bladder is closed in the usual manner. Two layers of chromic catgut are used (3–0). A suprapubic cystostomy tube is preferred over an indwelling urethral catheter. A Jackson-Pratt tube is inserted paravesically and brought out through a separate skin incision.

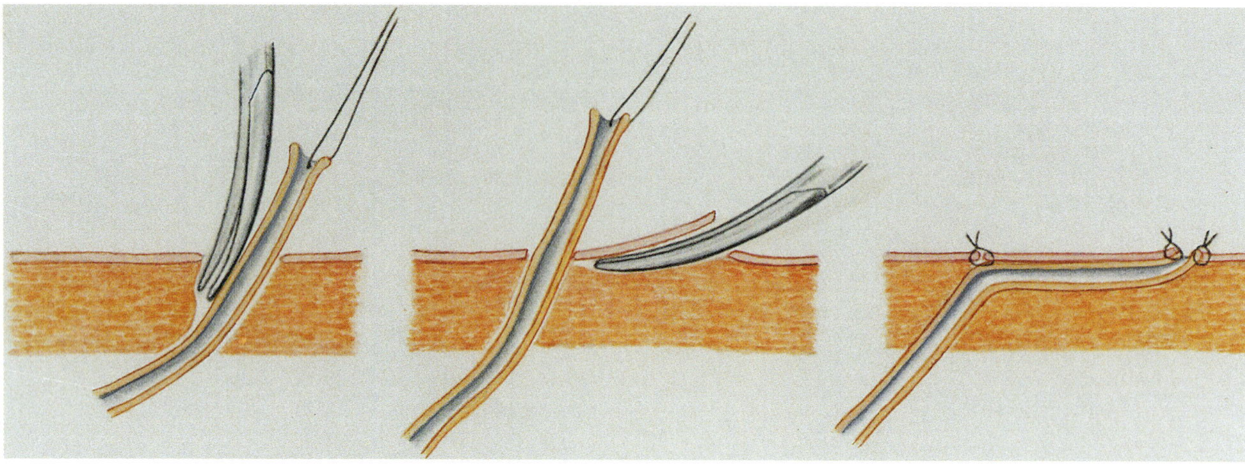

42-1 to 42-3

42. Glenn-Anderson Technique

The Glenn-Anderson technique for advancing the ureteral orifice is built upon the foundation of procedures which Drs. Hutch and Williams described some years ago. The procedure involves a submucosal tunnel which is fashioned medially and inferiorly toward the bladder neck. This is about 1.5 cm inferior and towards the site of the original hiatus.

42-1. The ureter is not moved extravesically, therefore, the risk of obstruction is nil.

42-2. What is useful in this technique is that the trigone should be larger than usual. The new ureterovesical anastomosis is quite near to the bladder neck and, therefore, more attention needs to be paid to the mucosal anastomosis.

42-3. It is possible to incise the muscular hiatus superiorly and medially and then close the detrusor muscle inferior to the ureter. This allows for a more limited distal tunnel, but a longer submucosal segment.

43. Cohen's Technique

Cohen's technique is a modification of the transtrigonal advancement approach. The advancement occurs transversely rather than inferiorly. It is technically easy and allows for a long submucosal tunnel. The ureterovesical anastomosis is also quite accessible. Should retrograde studies be advisable, several authorities in the field have criticized the technique because of the difficulty in catheterizing the ureter. Many pediatric urologists like the Cohen technique and, in fact, they prefer this approach as part of their routine in reimplanting the ureter to treat ureterovesical reflux.

43-1. The ureters have been isolated and freed.

43-2. The transverse tunnel has been formed.

43-3. Formation of the tunnel for the isolated distal left ureter is depicted.

43-4. The final closure of both tunnels and fixation of distal ureters to bladder mucosa.

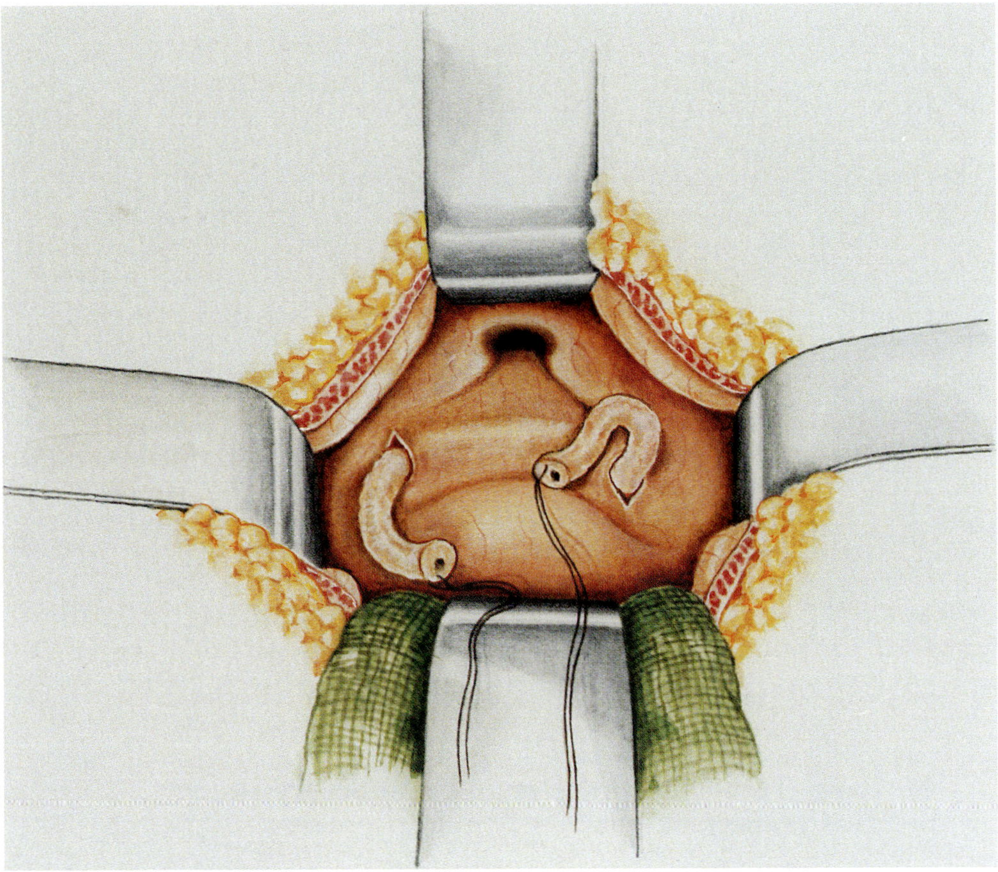

43-1

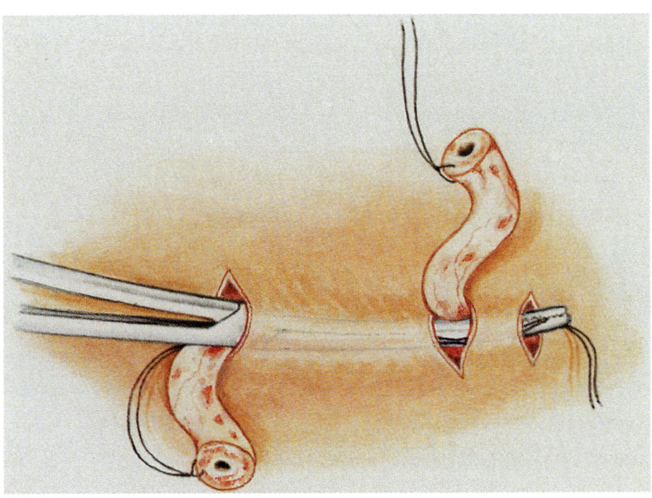

43-2

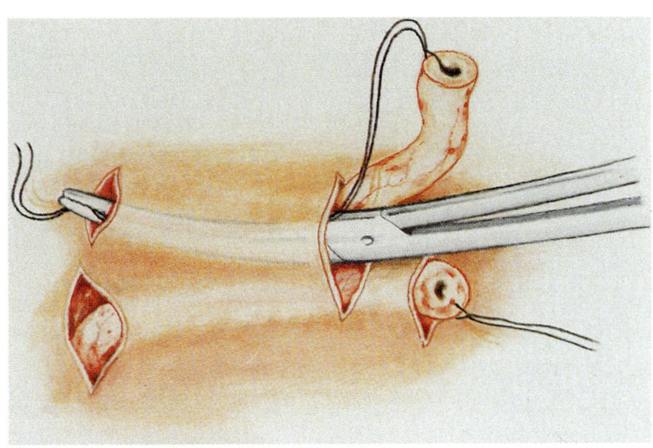

43-3

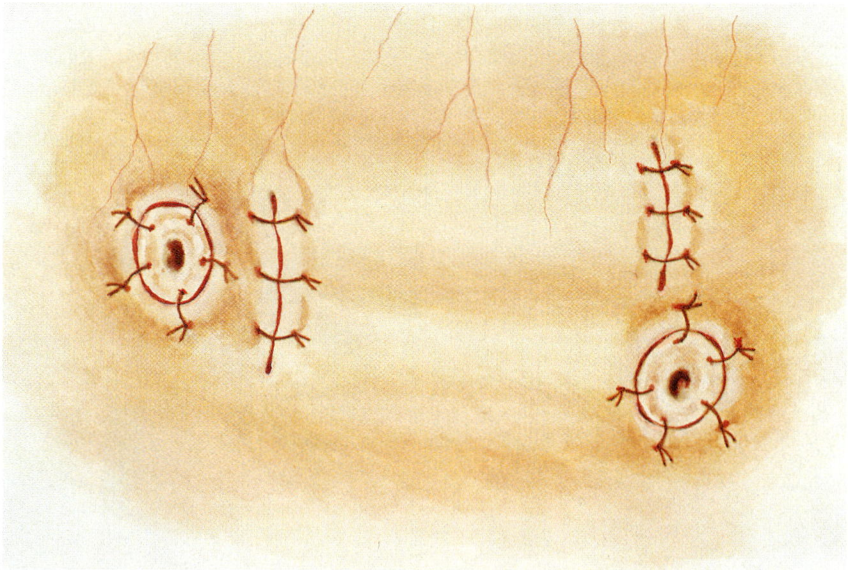

43-4

44. Barry Technique for External Ureteroneocystostomy in Renal Transplantation

Renal allograft implantation is often performed in the early morning hours when the surgeon has probably harvested both kidneys, and he/she is now involved in implanting the renal allograft. After the renal vein is anastomosed (end-side) to the iliac vein in the opposite fossa, the renal artery is anastomosed appropriately. The tired surgeon is now ready to implant the ureter into the bladder. The Barry technique allows a partially filled bladder to easily expose the anterior-superior anastomatic site.

44-1. Two vertical parallel incisions (2.5 cm) are made as shown. The implant is on the right side as shown.

44-2. A submucosal dissection is made medially, exposing the mucosal layer.

44-3. Blunt dissection laterally is carried out to provide an antireflux tunnel.

44-4. The ureter in the tunnel is being brought past the mucosal opening. Note the value of stay sutures to protect kinking and provide good visibility.

44-5. The anastomosis of bladder mucosa to the ureteral orifice is started.

44-6. 4–0 or 5–0 chromic catgut sutures are used, depending on the size of the ureter, and they are interrupted.

44-7. The bladder muscle layer is reapproximated over the two sites. Care is taken to be sure a kink in the ureter has not been created.

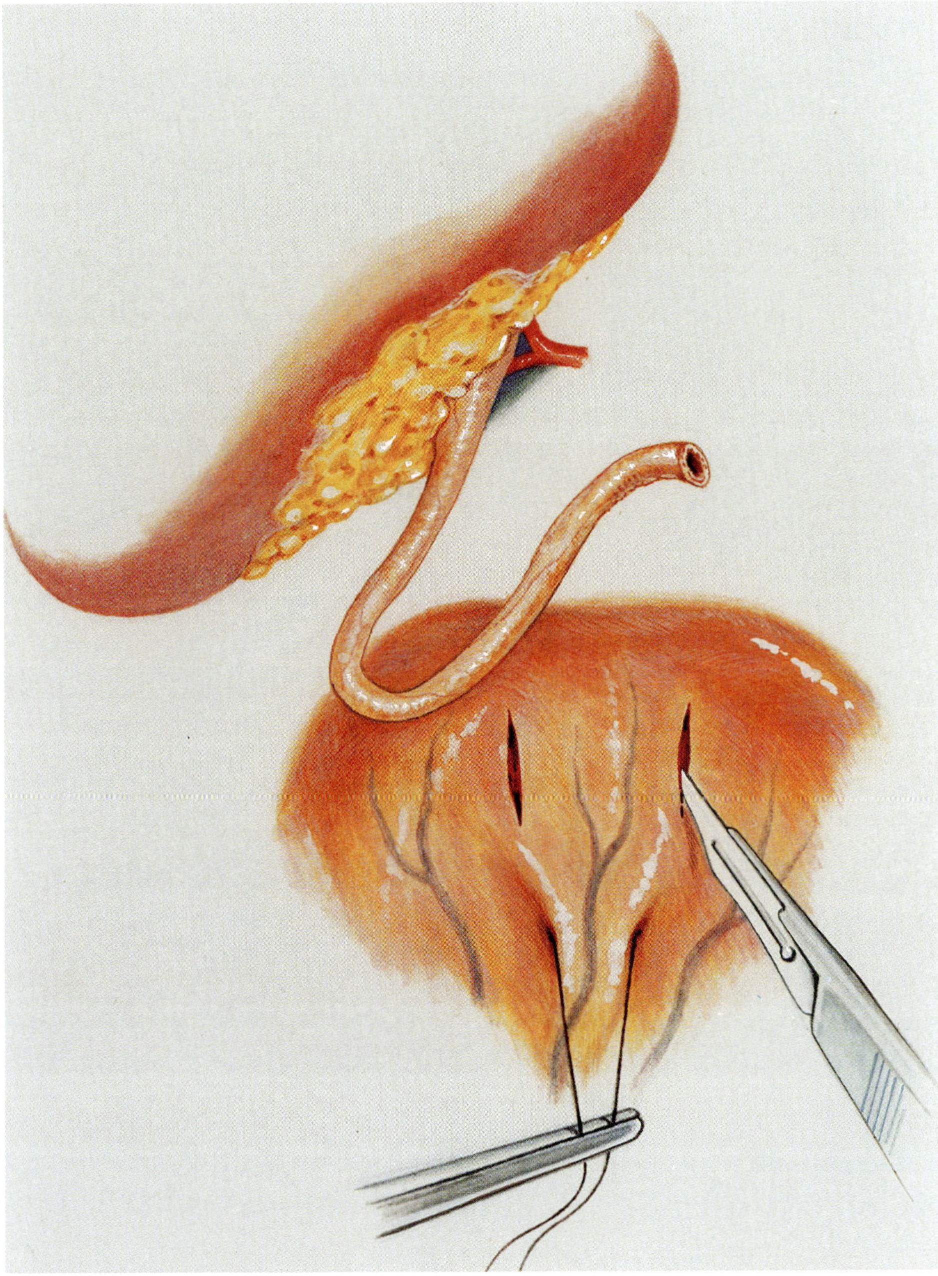

44-1

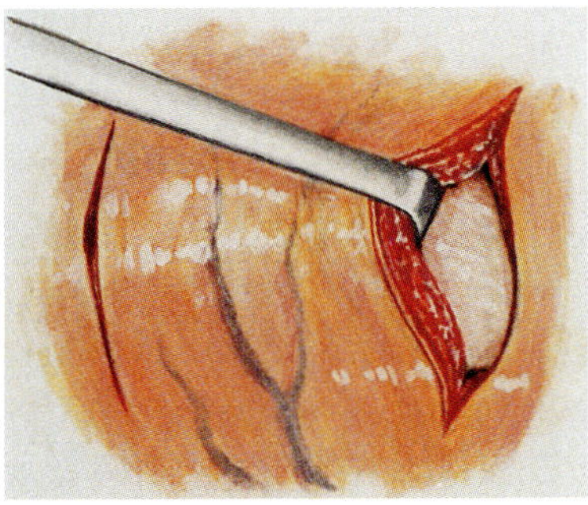

44-2

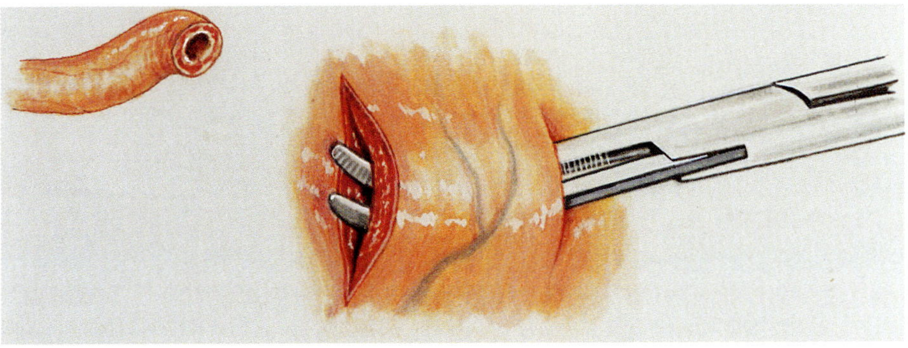

44-3

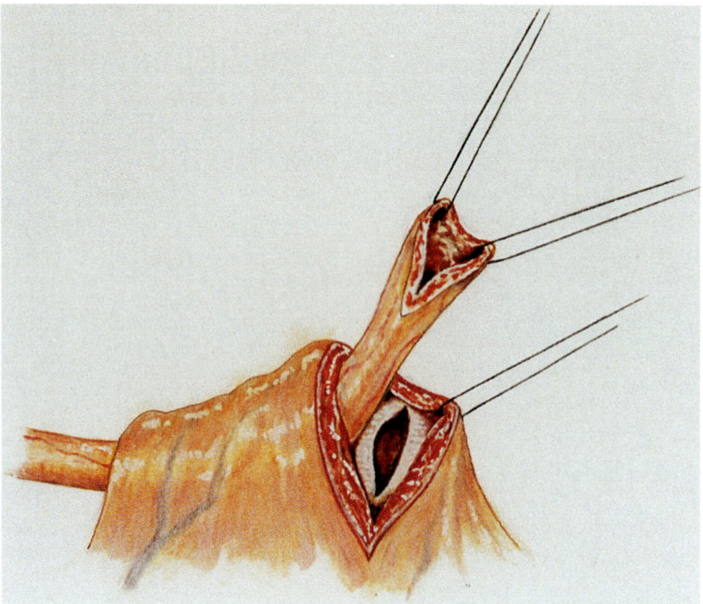

44-4

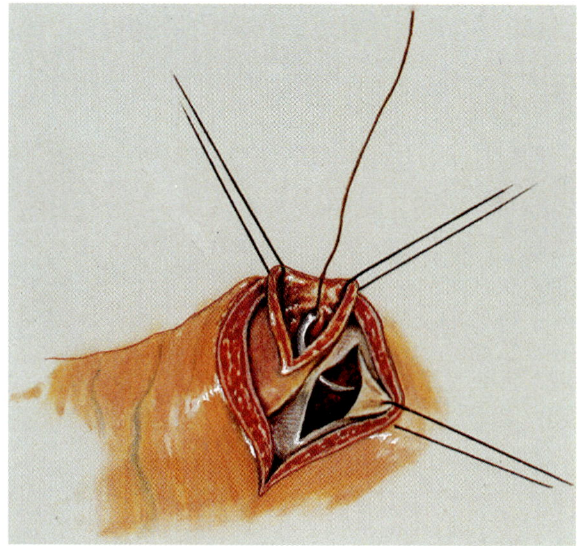

44-5

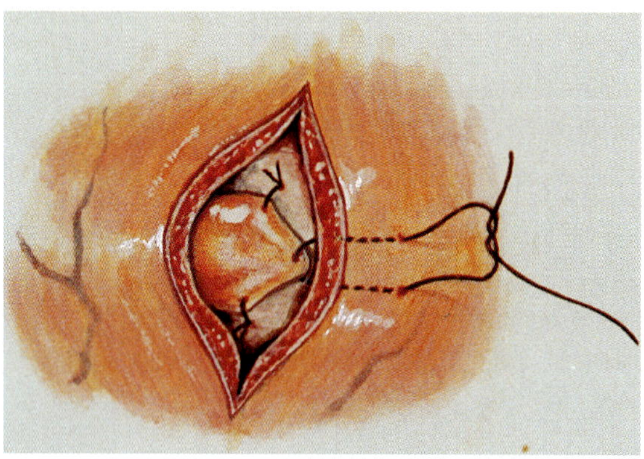

44-6

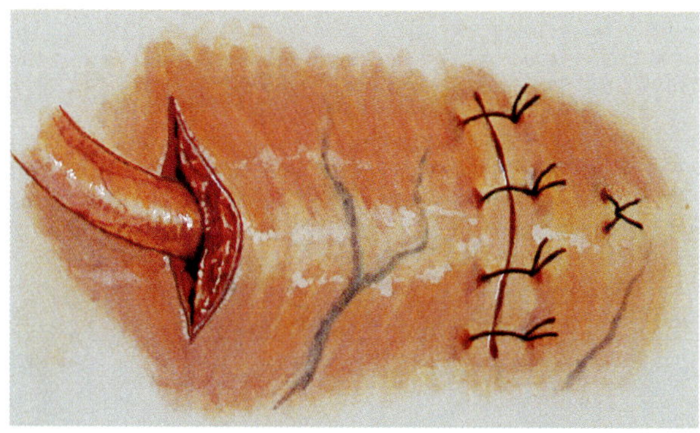

44-7

45. Other Procedures

45-1. In addition to the Politano-Leadbetter technique, *there are four alternative procedures:* the Lich-Gregoir extravesical submuscular trough; the Hutch technique; the Taguchi method; and the Bischoff technique.

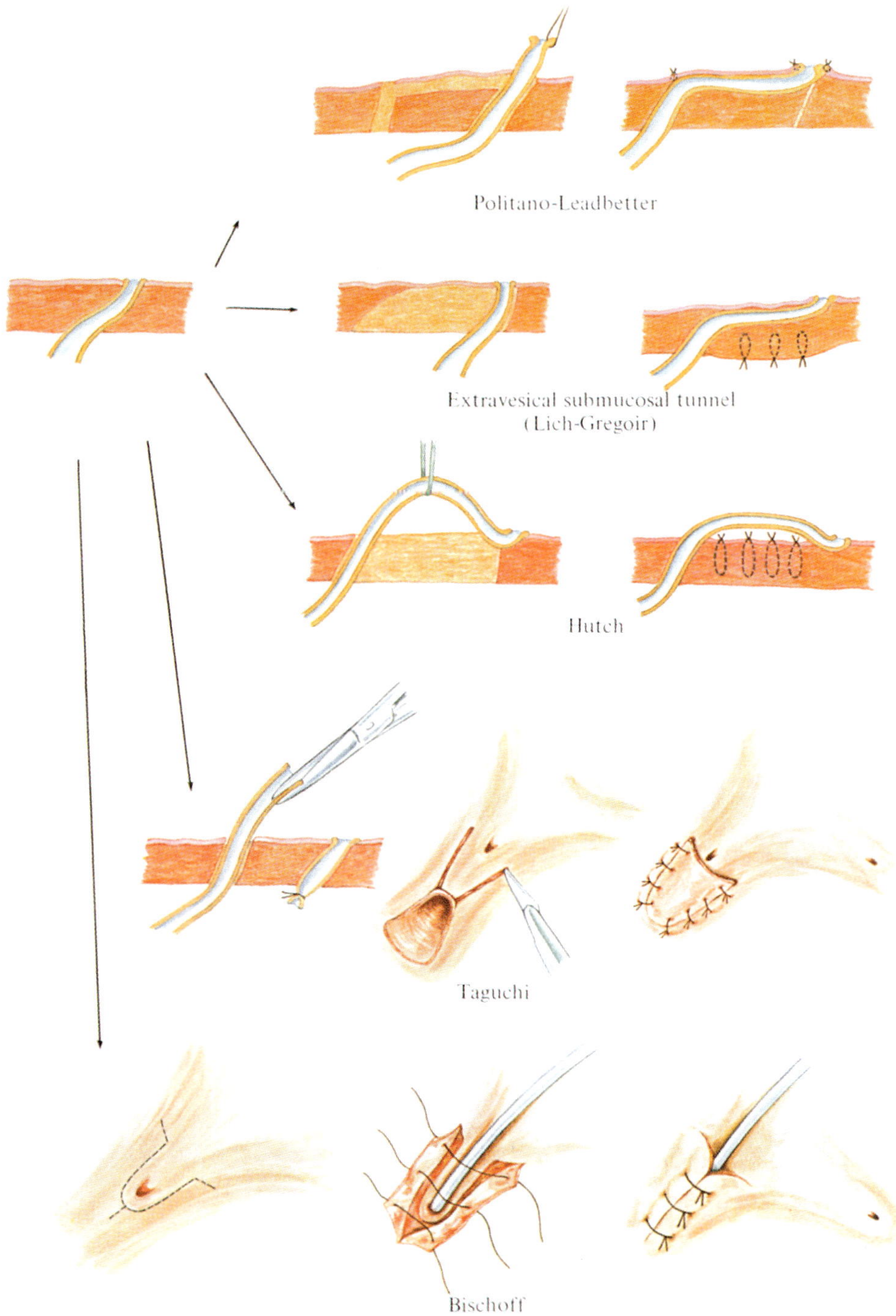

45-1

Suggested Readings

Anderson HV, Hodges CV, Behnam AM. Transureteroureterostomy (contralateral ureteroureterostomy): experimental and clinical experiences. J Urol 83:593, 1960.

Bischoff P. Megaureter. Br J Urol 29:416, 1957.

Dodson AI. Some improvements in the technique of ureterostomy. J Urol 55:225, 1946.

Goodwin WE, Harris AP, Kaufman JJ. Open transcolonic ureterointestinal anastomoses. A new approach. Surg Gynecol Obstet 97:295, 1953.

Goodwin WE, Scardino PT. Ureterosigmoidostomy. J Urol 118:169, 1977.

Gregoir W, Van Regemorter G. Le reflux vesicoureteral congenital. Urol Int 18:122, 1964.

Hutch JA. Vesicoureteral reflux in the paraplegic cause and correction. J Urol 68:457, 1952.

Lich R Jr, Howerton LW, Davis LA. Recurrent urosepsis in children. J Urol 86:554, 1961.

Minami T. Ureterilithotomy by vertical lumbar incision. Japanese J Urol 55:1071–1076, 1964.

Politano VA, Leadbetter WF. An operative technique for correction of vesicoureteral reflux. J Urol 79:932, 1958.

Simon, Czerny. Cited by Thomson-Walker's Genito-urinary Surgery, 3rd ed. New York: Paul B. Hoeber Inc, 1950:300.

Taguchi H, Saito K, Yamada T. Ureteroneocystostomy by means of a modified triangular flap method. J Urol 114:705, 1975.

The Bladder

3

Surgical Anatomy

STRUCTURE AND LOCATION

The adult urinary bladder is located anteriorly in the pelvic cavity, behind the pubic bones; in infancy the bladder is located in the suprapubic region. The resting, contracted bladder is a thick-walled organ, having superior and inferior walls, a fundus, and an apex. The urachus or median umbilical ligament, a strong fibrous cord, attaches to the apex; the right and left ureters attach to the posterolateral angles. The urethra attaches to the fundus.

As the bladder fills and becomes distended and ovoid, the fundus remains fixed; the apex and superior wall rise from the pelvis toward the abdominal cavity; the lateral walls stretch from the superior and inferior walls.

Peritoneum covers the superior and posterior walls of the bladder (Fig. 1).

The fundus of the bladder is fixed by continuity with the urethra. The neck of the bladder is fixed by pubovesical and puboprostatic ligaments that immobilize the bladder to the symphysis. The lateral umbilical ligaments, containing the atrophied supravesical portions of fetal umbilical arteries, also stabilize the bladder.

In the male, the posteroinferior aspect of the bladder is related to the rectum but is separated from it by seminal vesicles, ampullae of the vas deferens, and the rectovesical fascia of Denonvilliers (Fig. 2).

In the female, the posteroinferior aspect of the bladder rests against the upper part of the vagina and uterine cervix. The uterus extends and arches behind the posterosuperior aspect of the bladder but is separated by the pouch of covering peritoneum, forming the vesicouterine excavation.

The prevesical or space of Retzius is a division of the extraperitoneal space that extends from the pelvic floor to the umbilicus, bounded anteriorly by the posterior sheath of the rectus muscle and the posterior surface of the pubic rami. Urinary extravasation caused by extraperitoneal rupture of the bladder or by prostatic capsule perforations may extend rapidly into this space.

The bladder wall consists of several muscle layers. A layer of transitional cell epithelium covers the inner surface. The submucosal layer forms a loose connection between the muscle layer and the epithelium. The muscle layer consists of numerous bun-

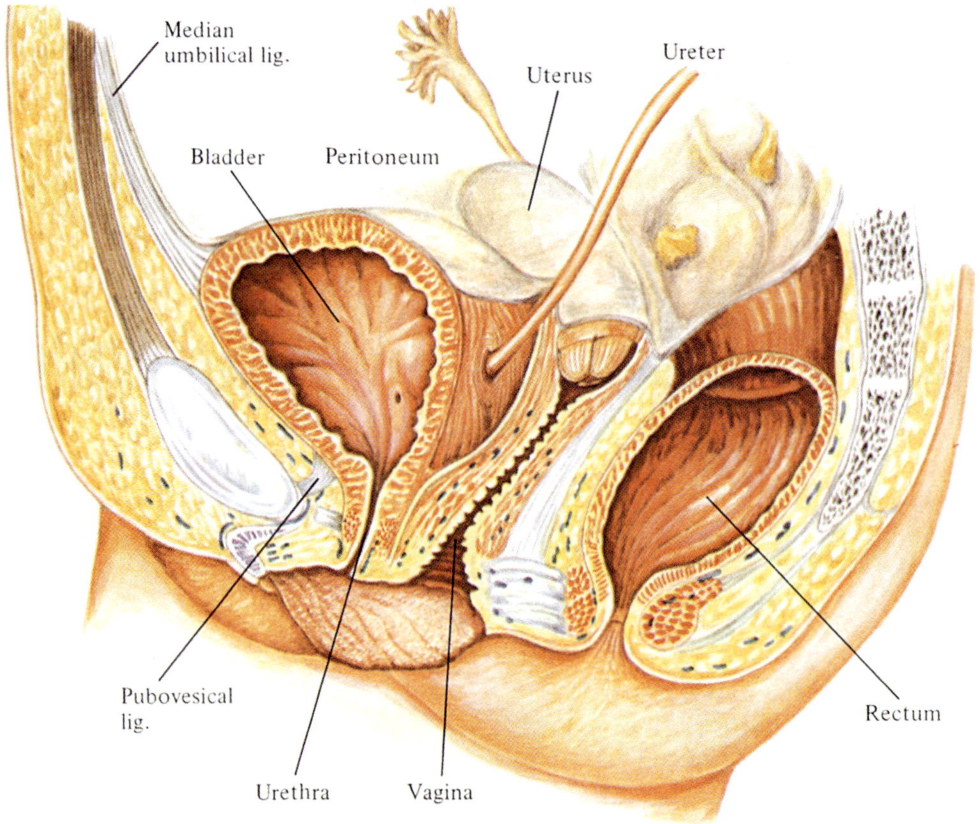

FIG. 1.
Midsagittal view showing structure and location of urinary bladder.

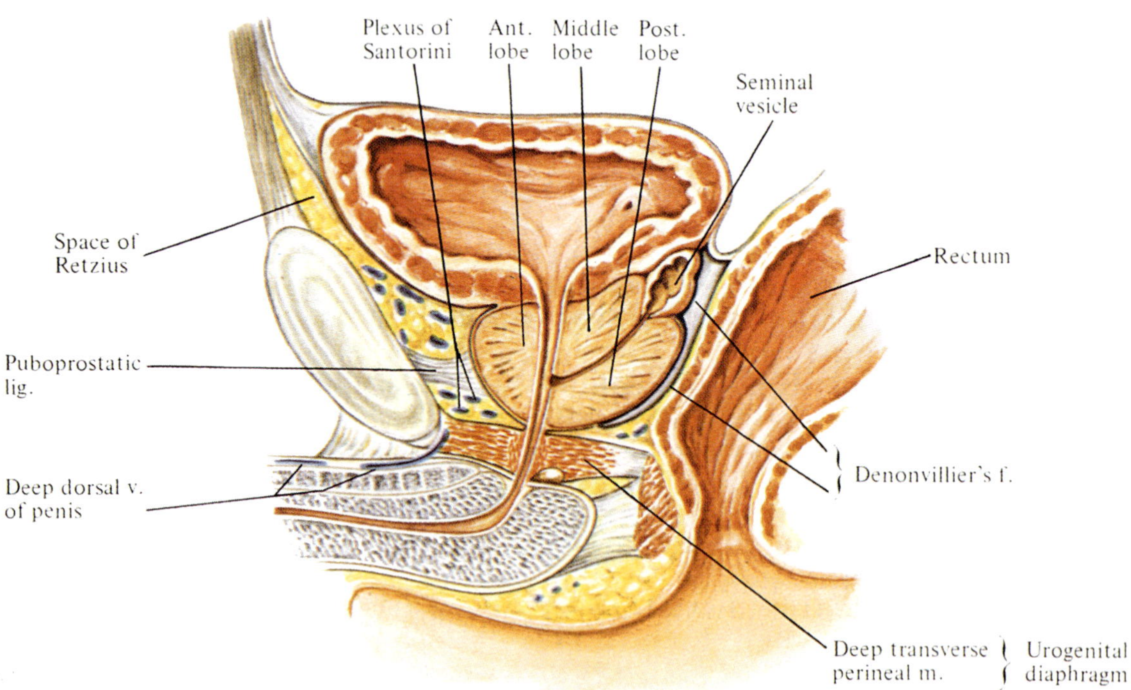

FIG. 2.
Midsagittal view at prostate, showing fascial relationships.

dles of nonstriated muscle traveling in different directions both obliquely and circularly around the bladder and forming a thick, elastic muscular wall. At the bladder neck these muscle bundles merge to form a ring called the internal vesical sphincter. A fascial layer loosely coats the muscle layers, except on the superior and upper part of the posterior surface, where it becomes very thin and is closely covered by a serous layer of peritoneum.

The appearance of the bladder interior varies, depending on the degree of bladder wall tension. When empty, the greater part of the bladder mucosa is thrown into folds and presents a wrinkled appearance. As the bladder distends, the mucosa becomes smoother, with fewer folds.

The trigone is a smooth-surfaced triangular area lying between the ureteral orifices at its basal angles and the internal urethral orifice at its apex (Fig. 3).

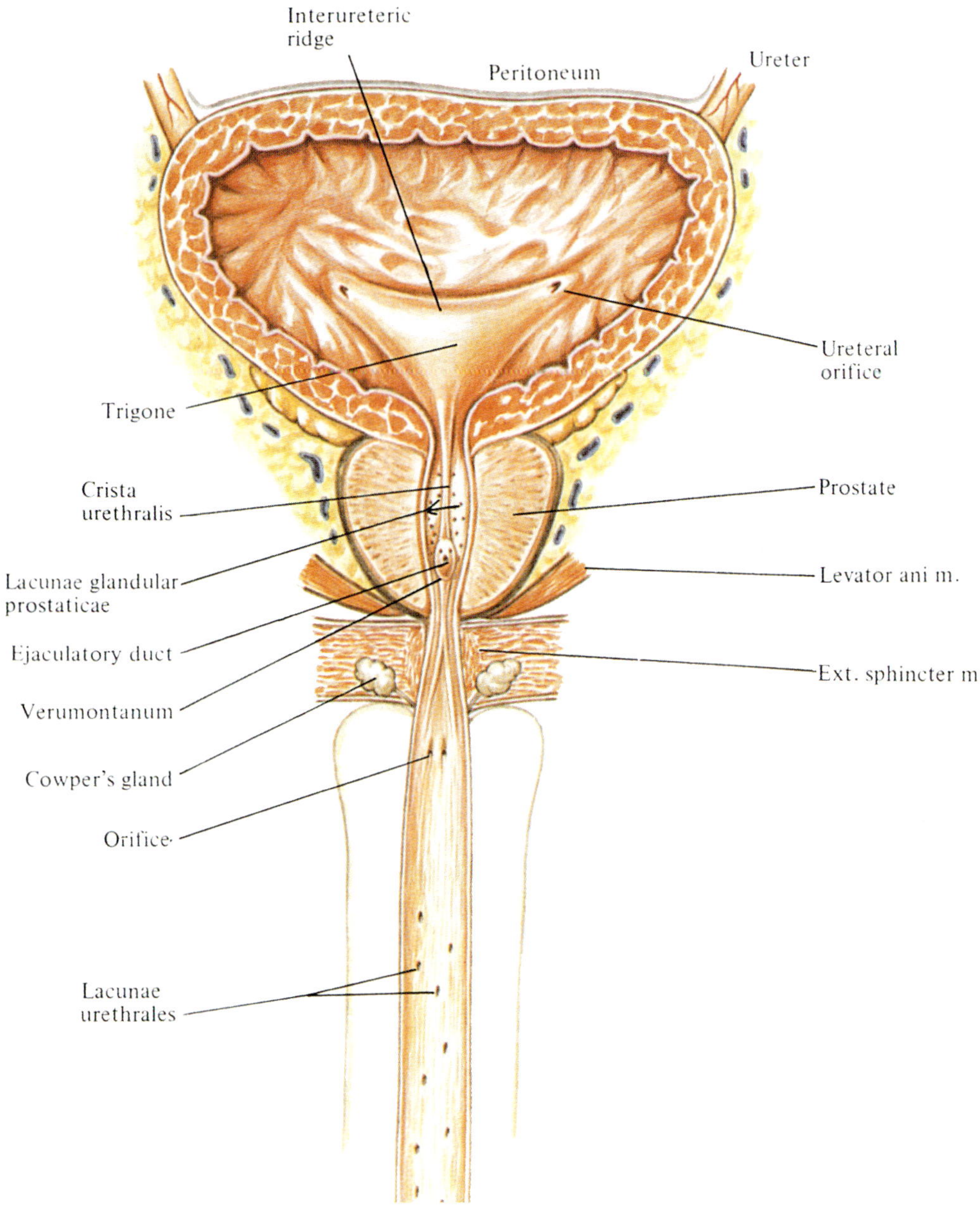

FIG. 3.
Interior of bladder, prostate, and proximal part of urethra in the male.

The interureteric ridge is a well-defined elevation between the ureteral orifices, which is raised by an underlying ridge of muscle.

VASCULAR SUPPLY

The arterial supply to the bladder derives mainly from the internal iliac artery and is composed of superior, middle, and inferior vesical arteries (Fig. 4). The superior vesical artery, which is the unobliterated part of the umbilical artery, supplies the superior and lateral walls of the bladder. The superior vesical artery reaches the bladder under the lateral reflection of pelvic peritoneum. The middle vesical artery is inconstant and may arise from the superior vesical artery or the internal iliac artery; often, it may be absent. The inferior vesical artery is derived from the internal iliac artery and is distributed between the fundus of the bladder, the seminal vesicles, and the prostate. Additional smaller arteries are derived from the middle hemorrhoidal and obturator arteries and, in the female, from the vaginal and uterine arteries.

The veins of the bladder anastomose freely to form perivesical plexuses, which are dense around the fundus of the bladder and drain into the internal iliac veins. In the male, the larger veins lie in the groove between the bladder and the prostate and form the vesicoprostatic plexus.

The lymphatics of the bladder (Fig. 5) begin in the submucosal layer of the bladder wall, collect in larger channels in the deep layer of muscle wall, follow the veins, and drain into lymph nodes along the internal and external iliac vessels.

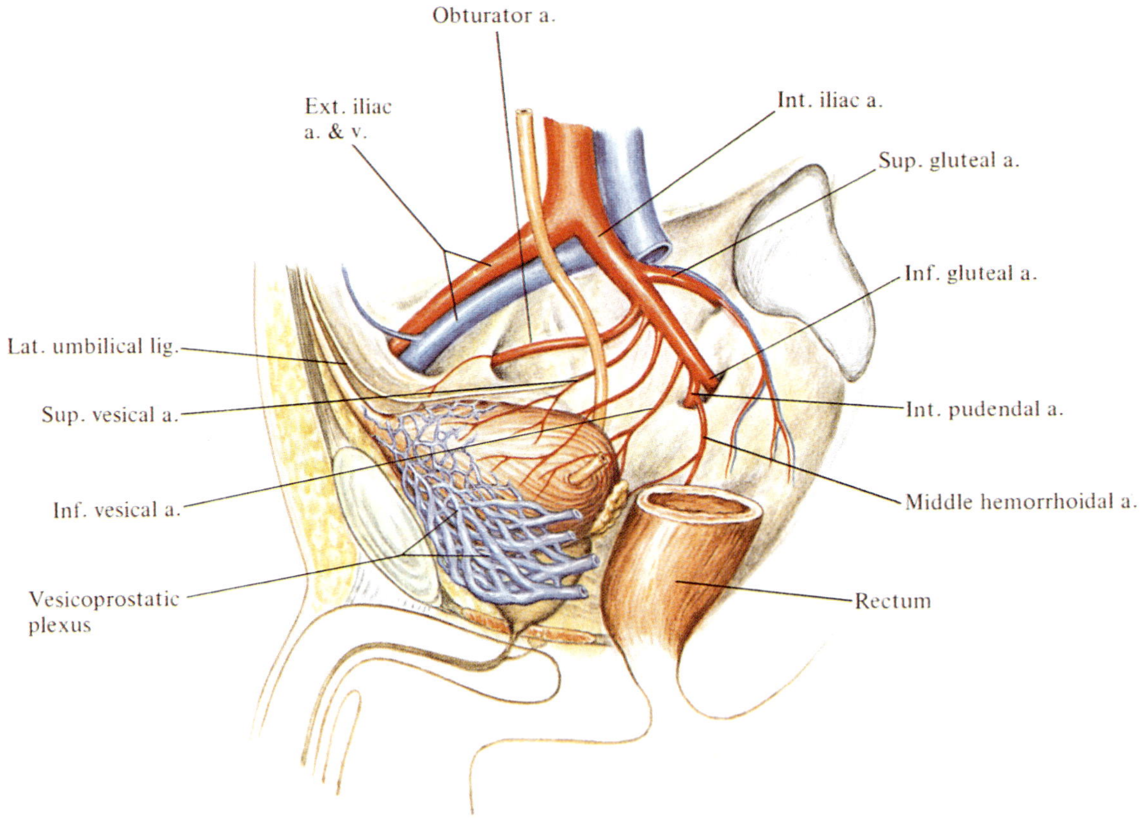

FIG. 4.
Arterial and venous supply to the bladder (sagittal view).

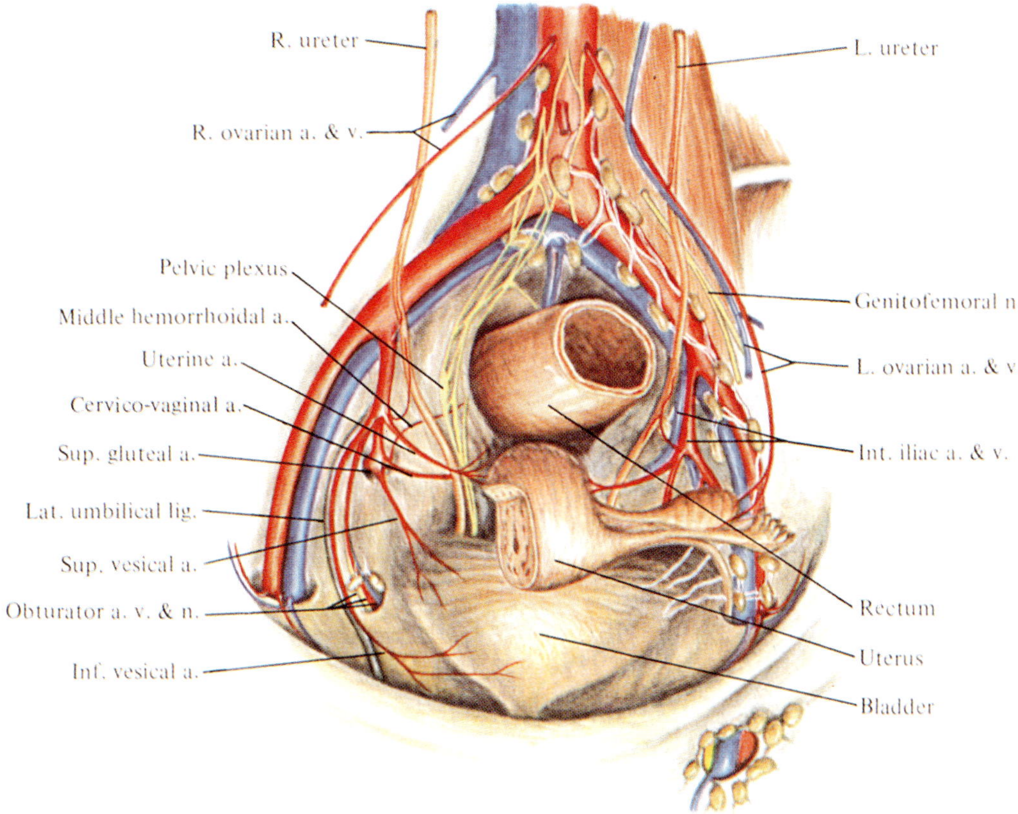

FIG. 5.
Pelvic portion of female ureter.

NERVE SUPPLY

The nerve supply to the bladder accompanies the supplying arteries and consists of nerves from both divisions of the autonomic system. Somatic nerves that control the sphincter are also present.

Sympathetic fibers are distributed to the bladder from the 11th thoracic to the second lumbar segments via the hypogastric and pelvic plexus. These nerves are stimulated during filling of the bladder and act to inhibit detrusor muscle tone; they also increase tension in the internal sphincter.

Parasympathetic fibers to the bladder arise from the pelvic splanchnic nerves, which are derived from the anterior primary divisions of the second to fourth sacral segments. These fibers stimulate "emptying" of the bladder and come into play during micturition by stimulating detrusor muscle contraction, elevating the trigone, and relaxing the internal sphincter. This event is accompanied by voluntary relaxation of the external sphincter by means of cerebral control via the pudendal nerve. The pudendal nerve arises from primary divisions of the third and fourth sacral segments and passes through the fatty tissue of the ischiorectal fossa (Fig. 6).

Introduction to Bladder Cancer

Bladder cancer is the sixth most common cancer among elderly males. A history of chronic cigarette smoking is usually seen. In the past, working in selected industries has resulted in finding cancer in males and females. The chemical industries, where beta

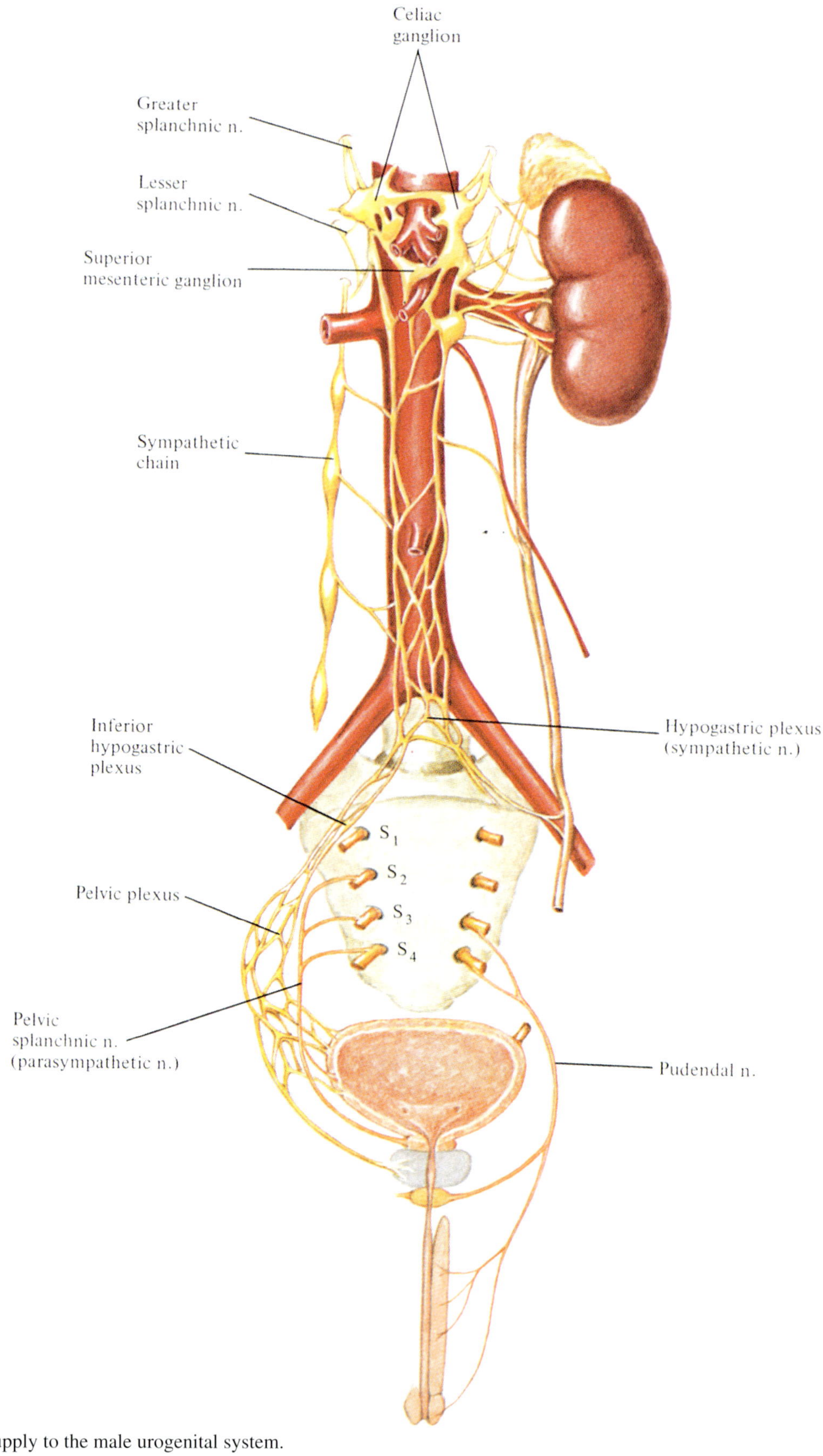

FIG. 6.
Autonomic and somatic nerve supply to the male urogenital system.

naphthylamines have been used during a long period have been particularly significant, and have resulted in the development of cancer.

Most primary bladder tumors are transitional cell carcinomas (TCCs). They may be either papillary or broad based in their configuration. In the majority of cases, staging and grading of the tumors, as described by Jewett and modified by Marshall, are probably the most important factors in allowing an accurate prognostic evaluation.

Staging of bladder tumors needs to be precise. The staging is based on the microscopic study of the tissue layers within the bladder wall. Accurate staging by pathologists is often subjective, although the information provided is clinically useful. What we, as urologists, need is accurate clinical staging for each case. An accurate assessment of depth of infiltration is crucial to providing appropriate therapy.

Bimanual pelvic examination under anesthesia, cystoscopy, cytopathology, and multiple biopsies are still essential to evaluate tumor staging and grading. If the tumor is palpable or the bladder is fixed, more radical therapy/surgery may be indicated. It is not difficult to separate between clearly superficial tumors and more deeply invasive bladder tumors. Careful observation of the neovascularity around the tumor is useful. This helps to provide a clinical diagnosis of the stage. Tumors with poor neovascularity are usually low grade tumors. Tumors with a very rich neovascular network are often high grade tumors.

According to our experience in Japan, nearly 79% of all bladder tumor cases are seen when they are in the superficial stage. About 86% of the patients treated by transurethral resection (TUR) biopsy—excision and fulguration—survive for 5 years.

Various imaging techniques are helpful in staging invasive tumors. Computed tomography (CT) scan and ultrasonography are exceedingly useful.

We have performed transurethral ultrasonography on 95 bladder tumor cases. The results were compared with pathologic staging of the tumors (Fig. 7).

Superficial tumors up to Stage T_1 (A) can be easily differentiated from the deeper staged cancer. Our accuracy rate is 100% for this stage. It is very difficult, however, to accurately stage tumors deeper than T_2 (B_1). Our clinical accuracy is less than 50%. Inaccurate staging is probably over staging. It is impossible to distinguish between T_a (O) and T_1 (A).

This illustration demonstrates the imaging techniques which are useful in today's clinical arena. Valuable objective information can be obtained regarding the depth of infiltration made by the bladder tumor. It is still impossible to distinguish between stage T_a (O) and T_1 (A). It is also very difficult to distinguish between T_2 (B_1) and T_3 (B_2), preoperatively. Usually this is only done by currently used imaging techniques.

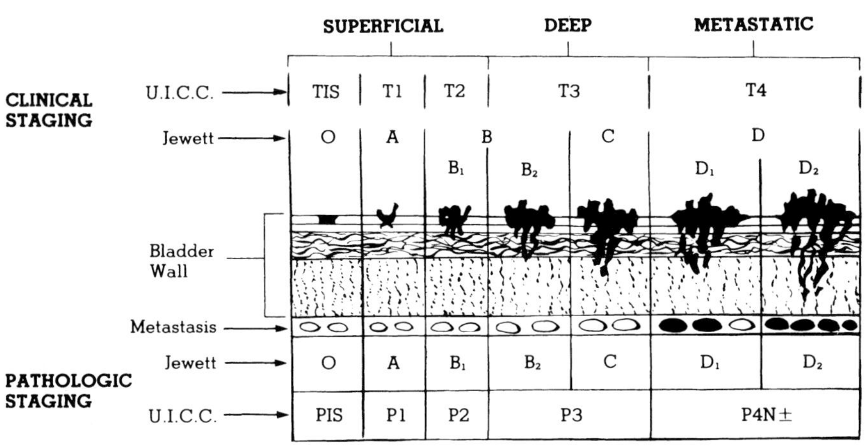

FIG. 7.
Bladder tumor infiltration into superficial and deeper depths of bladder wall.

NEWER TREATMENTS

Today, immunotherapy has been demonstrated to be effective in preventing bladder tumor recurrence after TUR and fulguration of the original tumors or TCC. Usually this tumor has not infiltrated into the muscle layer. Frequently the patient has a long history—more than 15 years of smoking one pack of cigarettes per day. We suggest that he/she stop smoking.

Our routine is to treat the patient with 1/2 dose (60 mg) bacillus Calmette-Guérin (BCG) for approximately 6 consecutive weeks after healing has taken place from the transurethral resection of bladder tumor (TURBT) (waiting period after transurethral resection of prostate gland [TURP] is 35 to 40 days). We treat the patients weekly for 6 consecutive weeks. We then follow with BCG 1 month later. The first posttreatment cystoscopic examination is performed at 3 months. Urinary cytology and random biopsies are obtained. If a recurrent tumor is present, which is rare, we repeat at least three of the weekly treatments before proceeding to monthly treatments. The monthly treatments are continued for 1 year. If no recurrences are documented at the end of 1 year of BCG treatment, we then proceed to BCG treatments every 2 months. Again, cystoscopy and bladder washes/biopsies are obtained at 3 month intervals. If the patient remains in remission, we proceed to BCG treatment at quarterly intervals (every 3 months). If successful, then we keep the patient on booster BCG treatments every 6 months for 10 years. At present we have many patients who received BCG and interleukin 2 (IL2) on the above schedule more than 7 years ago. In the United States we believe that BCG and IL2 may be superior to BCG alone. However, the Food and Drug Administration (FDA) has not approved IL2 for treatment of bladder tumors.

We have published extensively on the subject of immunotherapy for early infiltrative bladder cancer. We used a porcine-sensitive lymphocyte for treatment. This early protocol was developed by Dr. Michael O. Symes, an English immunologist from Bristol, U.K. Our combined experience with porcine cells goes back to 1976. We now believe that BCG and IL2 are a better combination. We use a 1/2 dose of BCG with the allogeneic IL2. We use 880 units of IL2 based on a tritiated thymidine assay which establishes potency against a known number of tumor cells. Our laboratory uses an established technique to make the allogeneic IL2.

The diagram lists both the International Union Internationale Contra Cancer (UICC) and the U.S. Clinical grading classification. This clearly shows the depth of penetration of the carcinoma with increasing grades. When TCC is superficially located in the epithelial surface, the tumor is of low grade (grade I). When the tumor invades superficial bladder muscle, then the tumor is probably grade I or II; with time the superficial cancer B can become a B_2 carcinoma. Extension to the bladder wall represents significant infiltration (stage C). If the tumor can not be controlled by BCG and IL2, then cystectomy may be the treatment of choice. In the male a total prostatectomy is also done. Other chemotherapies are available.

In our experience, a CT scan of the bladder and adjacent lymph node area is strongly recommended. We have reported a technique for bladder staging of TCC which uses 200–350 cc of diluted radiographic contrast fluid. When contrast is inserted into the bladder by a urethral catheter, the visualization of the stroma and muscle layers are clearly demonstrated. Extension of tumor to the outer bladder wall can be demonstrated by our CT technique.

Under anesthesia the patient is placed into the lithotomy position after a spinal anesthetic or general anesthesia. A bladder wash, using approximately 150–225 cc of saline, is used to vigorously barbotage the bladder epithelium and luminal wall. Professor Leon Wheeless and our group have published extensively on this subject. By careful screening, diploid, hyperdiploid, or aneuploid cells can be obtained before the biopsy procedure (TURBT). We gain information that informs the urologist that cancer is present or cancer will develop (aneuploid cells). A bimanual examination is important. If the tumor is palpable and the bladder wall is movable, then cystectomy is the treatment of choice.

When bladder cancer develops, gross, painless, total hematuria will be noticed. We have had excellent success in eradicating bladder TCC (grade I to II). When the tumor has not extended to the outer wall—serosal edge in some cases—we employ BCG and IL2. We have been able to eradicate TCC extending into the superficial and deep muscle layers by immunotherapy.

We use 60 mg of BCG (one half of the clinical dose) that contains 30 million colony forming units, and we place the BCG into saline (25 mL). IL2, produced by our research laboratory, is diluted with normal saline after thawing the test tube container. The mixture is inserted into the bladder by urethral catheter. The patient is asked to keep the solution in his/her bladder for 2 hours. Then he/she is requested to drink at least 2 liters of water or more so that he/she will expel the solution after 2 hours.

Our protocol for BCG and IL2 immunotherapy is as follows:

1. The patient is not bleeding from the bladder prior to insertion of the BCG and IL2. If bladder tumor biopsies were obtained, then we wait 4 weeks before starting the therapy.
2. We treat the patient weekly with BCG and IL2 for 6 consecutive weeks. After 6 weeks of therapy we start monthly immunotherapy treatment if the tumor is of a higher grade (grade II to III).
3. Monthly maintenance doses for 6 months can then be reduced to treatment every 2 months if the bladder wash and random biopsies at 6 1/2 months posttreatment show an excellent response.
4. Over the last 12 years we have kept 22 patients on BCG and IL2 inserting the solution every 6 months. If tumor recurs, then biopsies of the bladder are obtained and the patient is started on weekly BCG and IL2; in the few instances when a recurrence occurred we were able to obtain a remission over a long period—5 to 10 years during the second treatment cycle. Tumor recurrences are usually of a lower grade.

Figure 7 illustrates examples of bladder tumor with various degrees of infiltration into the bladder wall which can occur in humans. Bladder cancer has been staged accurately using two systems—the American System has an A, B_1, B_2, C, D, and D_2 classification particularly of TCCs. The tumor, node, metastasis (TNM) international classification system, along with the older U.S. classification, are included.

The most superficial cancer involves the transitional epithelium as shown. Carcinoma in situ (CIS) (tumor in situ [TIS]) is a much more serious problem. CIS can spread along the urothelium. More important is the fact that CIS can continue to proliferate and extend along the border between mucosa and superficial muscle. Muscle infiltration can occur over time if treatment is not initiated. Continued surveillance with biopsies and bladder washes are helpful in ascertaining the extent of infiltration. BCG is useful if a therapeutic protocol is warranted.

Operative Techniques

46. Open Repair of Bladder Neck Contracture

To approach the surgical field of the bladder, see **46–1** to **46–4**.

46-1. In our experience, the anatomic relationships of the bladder flap can be lost; therefore, it is advised that the area of incision be outlined with stay sutures and/or an electrocoagulating tip. *The line of incision and the final placement of the anterior bladder flap are indicated by the broken line near the center* of the illustration. Note that the bladder is filled prior to the operation.

46-2. The bladder incision is made transversely and follows the previously marked area. The bladder fluid is suctioned out. *Wedge resection of the posterior bladder neck* is made from 5 to 7 o'clock.

46-3. *Hemostatic sutures lateral to the edge of the posterior neck resection* (2–0 chromic catgut) *are helpful.*

46-4. *Bladder-widening flap placement and closure are completed.* The bladder neck contracture has been relieved. Before abdominal wall closure, an indwelling catheter is introduced and a flat tubular drain is positioned lateral to the site of bladder incision.

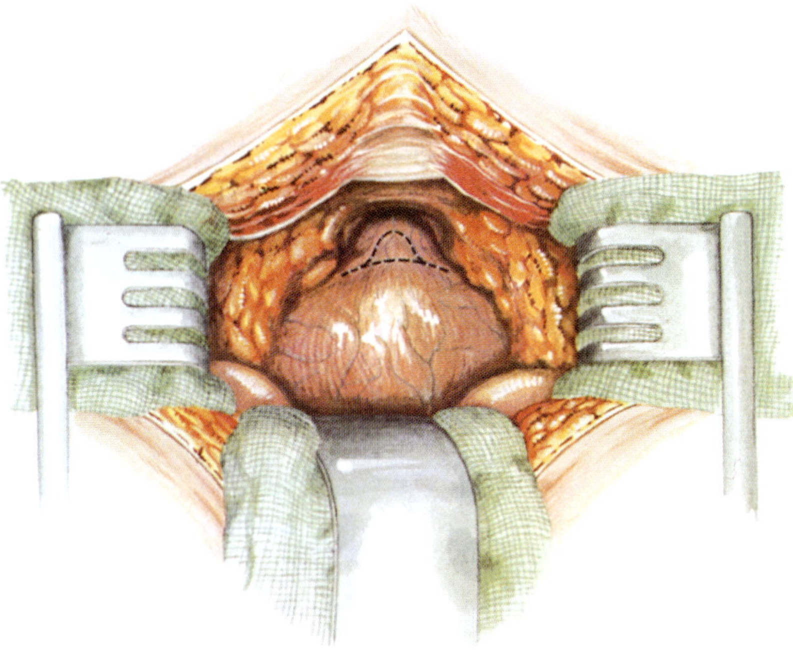

46-1

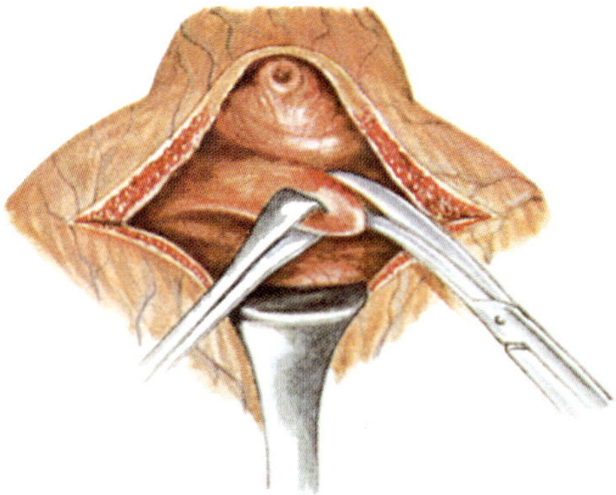

46-2

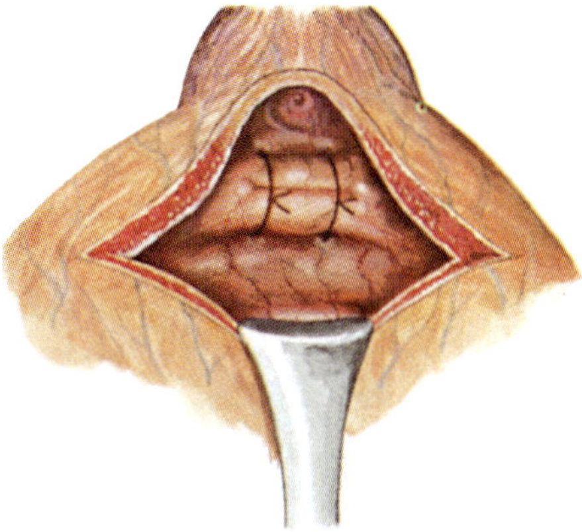

46-3

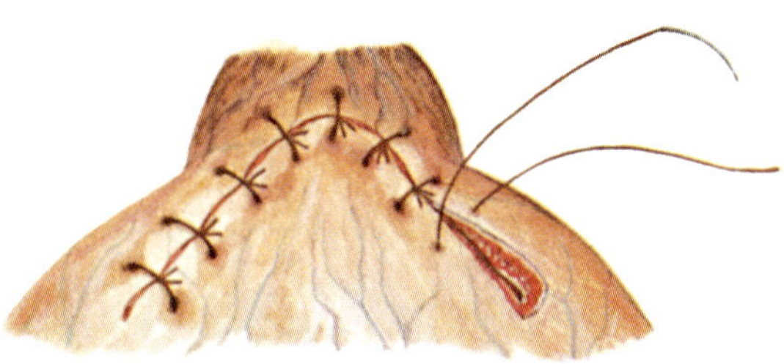

46-4

47. Boari-Ockerblad-Bischoff Bladder Flap for Ureteral Substitution

Indications for Procedure

When disease involving the lower third of the ureter has occurred, resulting in severe stricture formation or a megaureter, a Boariplasty should be considered. In many areas of the world tuberculosis can cause fibrosis with beading to a long segment of the lower ureter. In cadaver kidney transplantation procedures, kidney rejection, including fibrosis to the lower ureter, may also occur.

In any of the conditions cited, it is sometimes possible to hitch the superior-posterior portion of the bladder to the healthy ureter. If this is not possible then a Boari-plasty is an excellent alternative.

Other alternatives may be used in selected instances, for example, when the lower ureter on the appropriate side is not coursing through an inflammatory or infected bed of tissue. Renal autotransplantation is a possible solution in a few instances. Another possible alternative is transureteroureterostomy, as described in 38–1 and 38–2 in Chapter 2.

A vertical midline incision, extending from the symphysis to the umbilicus, is made. The anterior and lateral bladder surfaces are exposed. The ureter, which is diseased in its lower third, is transected and ligated, freeing the normal midureter.

47-1. *Stay sutures are placed on each side at the base of the selected bladder flap site.* The bladder flap is constructed; the extent of the flap is predicated on the length of the ureteral defect. The base of the flap curves posteriorly to the back bladder wall.

47-2. *The Bischoff antireflux Boariplasty.* Note that a flap of bladder mucosa—tongue-shaped—must be removed to expose a muscular trough for the antireflux proce-

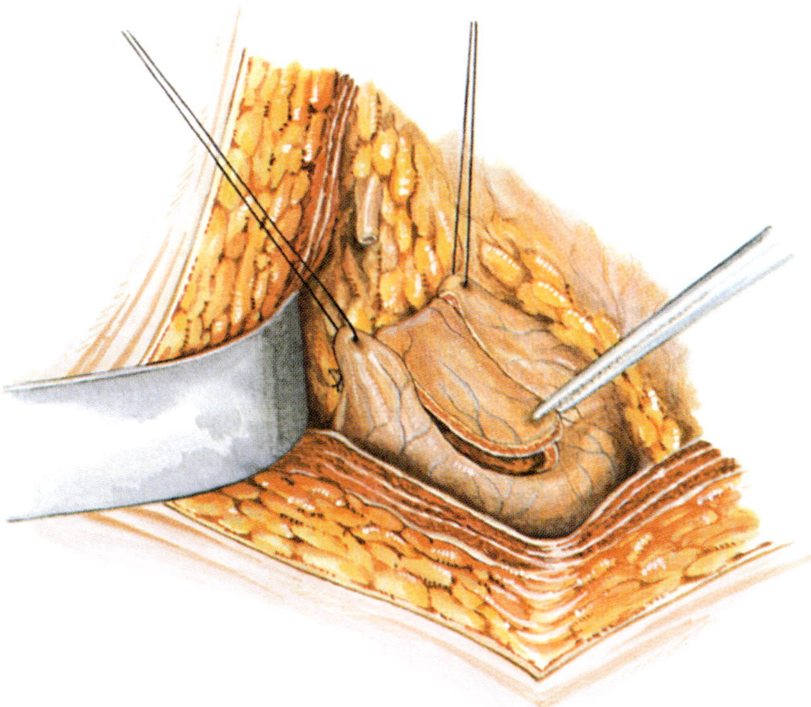

47-1

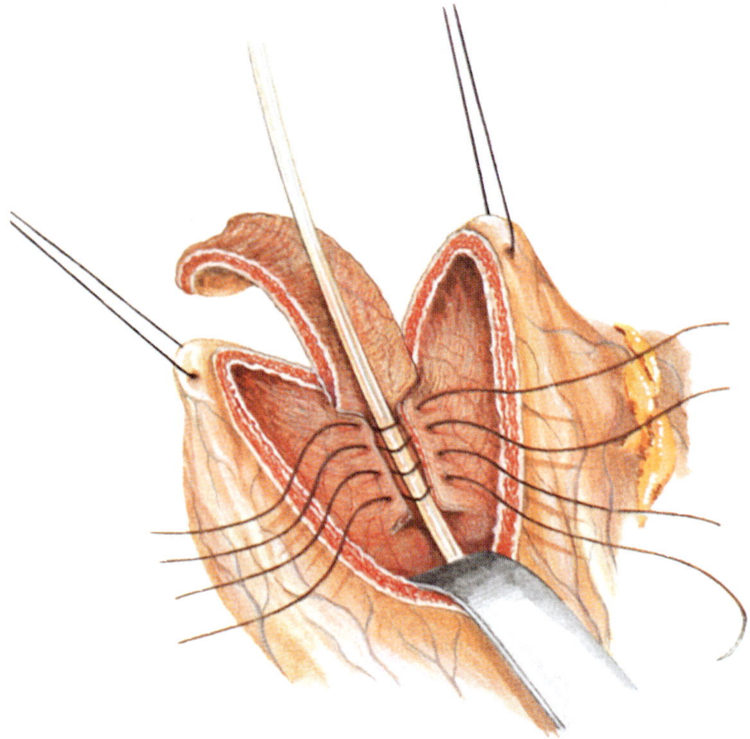

47-2

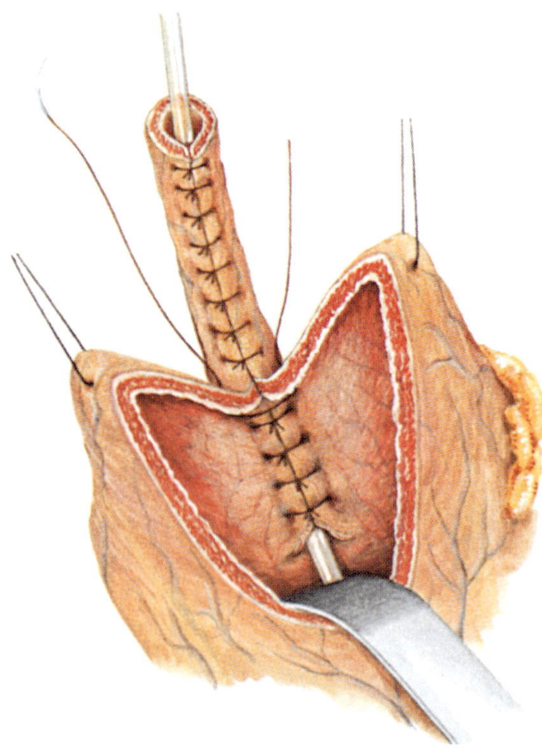

47-3

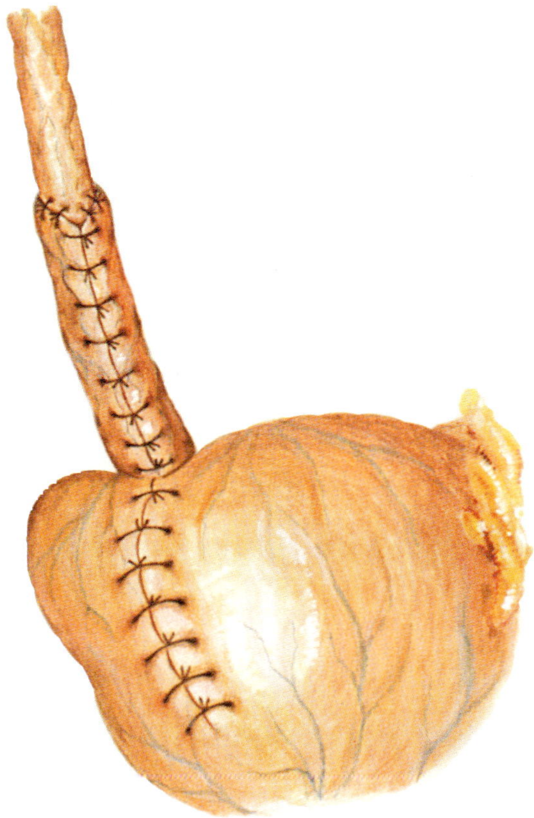

47-4

dure. The parallel incisions are approximately 8 mm apart and extend from the base of the Boari flap to a point 2 cm proximal to the bladder neck. The trough extends through one-half the bladder musculature. Care is taken to protect the opposite ureteral orifice. An 8 or 10 French stent is used. The lateral bladder edges are undermined to allow reapproximation of the antireflux tunnel. This tunnel is sutured; the most distal sutures are placed first, moving proximally. Each suture includes bladder mucosa and muscle. The most proximal suture (the last) is placed from outside the bladder to its interior and made ready for tying outside the bladder.

47-3. *The bladder flap (Boari flap) is tubularized* with 3–0 chromic catgut. The antireflux sutures are tied, moving superiorly or proximally. The most proximal antireflux suture is tied last, outside the bladder.

47-4. *The bladder is closed in two layers* with continuous and interrupted sutures (3–0 chromic catgut). The final step involves an end-to-end oblique anastomosis between the bladder flap and the ureter.

48. Psoas Hitch

The psoas bladder hitch procedure is used when ureteral length has been compromised due to distal ureteral obstruction. A shorter ureter lying superiorly can be used for ureterovesical reimplantation if the bladder is mobile and can be lifted.

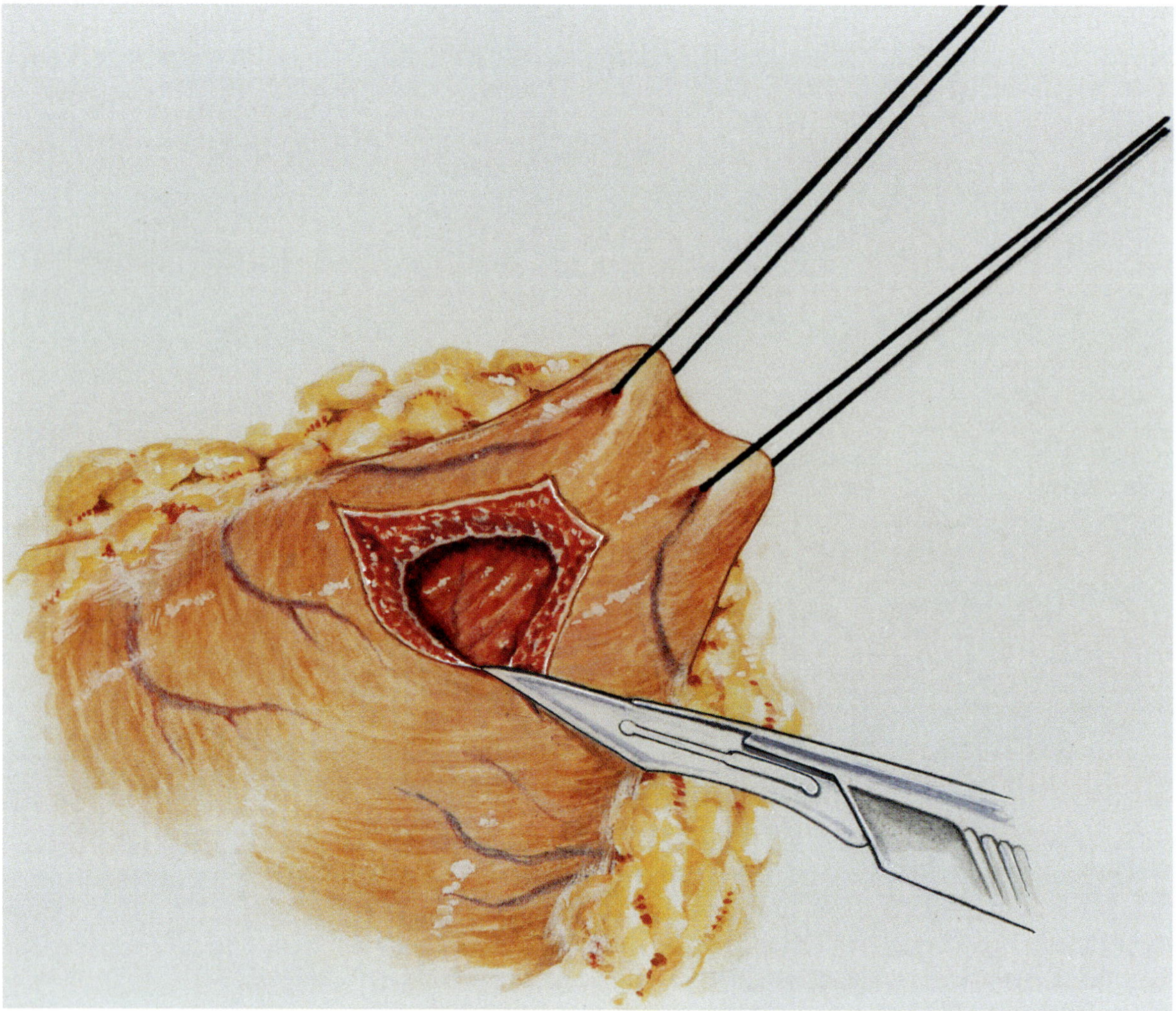

48-1

48-1. If the patient's bladder is mobile, it is possible to take the appropriate lateral bladder portion and fill it with saline. By carefully freeing the psoas muscle area anteriorly it is possible to prepare the floor on which the appropriate lateral bladder will be anchored. Before anchoring the bladder as part of the psoas hitch operation, it is best to perform the ureterovesical reimplantation. For the psoas hitch operation we use 0-Vicryl or 0-chromic sutures and make interrupted sutures so that the bladder is anchored appropriately. Care must be taken not to raise the anterior, lateral portion of the bladder in a superior fashion. This could make it virtually impossible for the patient to empty his or her bladder. The implantation of the ureter can be achieved after carefully dissecting the ureter towards the midline of the bladder.

48-2. It is possible to pass the ureter under direct vision. One of the criticisms of the psoas hitch technique is that it is performed in a blind fashion. However, one can open the bladder if needed and perform the actual ureterovesical anastomosis in a more precise fashion and under direct vision.

48-3 and **48-4.** Bivalving of the bladder anteriorly and performing a ureterovesical anastomosis after the bladder has been lifted to reach each ureter. The anastomosis must be performed without tension.

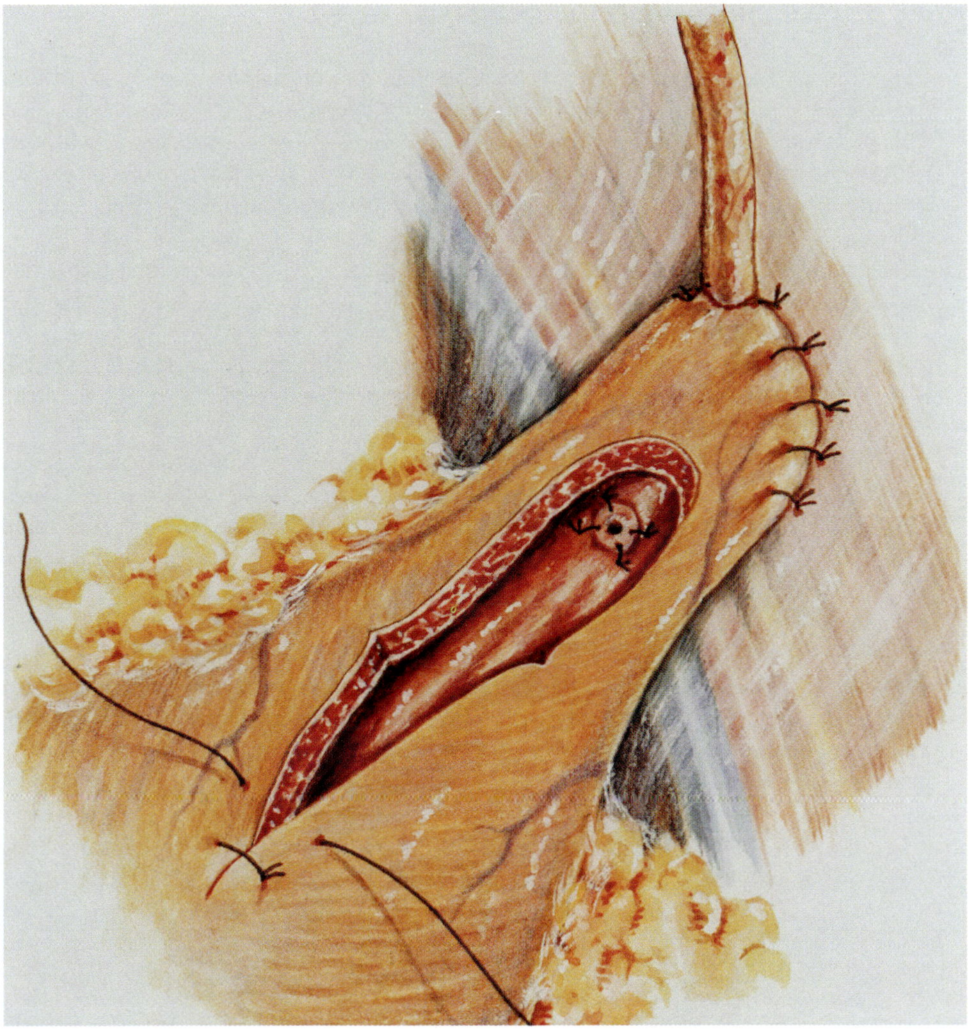

48-2

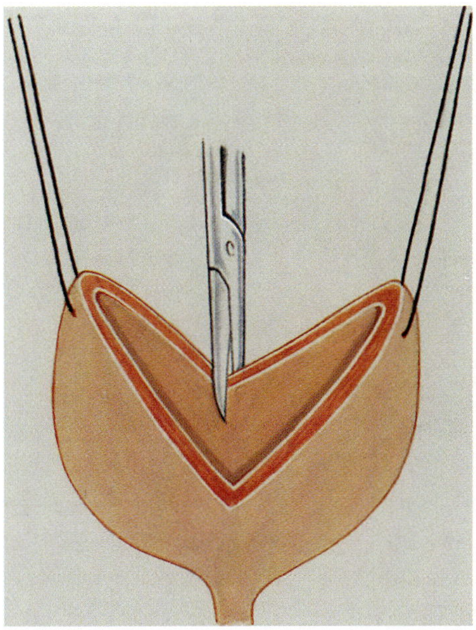

48-3

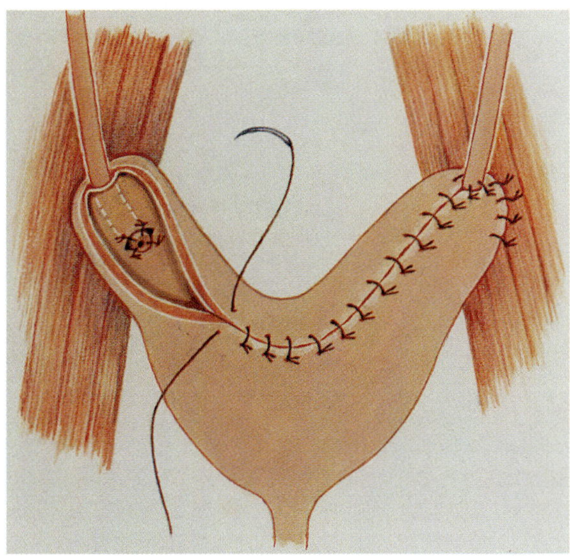

48-4

49. Partial (Segmental) Cystectomy

Careful patient selection for this procedure is important. Elderly patients with infiltrative bladder carcinoma located in the dome and/or lateral bladder wall are candidates. This procedure can be performed in poor-risk patients who probably cannot withstand radical cystectomy and urinary diversion. A segment of the bladder floor can be excised in continuity with the lateral aspect of the organ. Ureteral reimplantation is necessary in this instance.

An oblique lower abdominal incision is made to allow access to the lower ureter and appropriate bladder hemisphere (see 36–1).

49-1. *The bladder is opened widely* via an anterior midline incision. The bladder field is extended and maintained by the use of Allis clamps. The bladder tumor is seen on the right lateral wall. Because of tumor proximity to the right ureteral orifice, the ureter is transected and the distal tip ligated. A stay suture marks the proximal free end. An incision is made to approach the circumferential area which must be excised (dotted line). This includes removal of the right ureteral orifice, adjacent trigone, and ureteral stump.

49-2. *The line of excision is reapproximated and sutured in two layers.* The ureter is reimplanted on the posterior bladder.

49-3. *An indwelling urethral catheter (20–22 Fr) is inserted.* Anterior to the point of entry of the ureter, the bladder edges are reapproximated and sutured. Care is taken to avoid coagulation of the ureter, which lies posteriorly. The remaining portions of the bladder wall are doubly sutured with 2–0 chromic catgut.

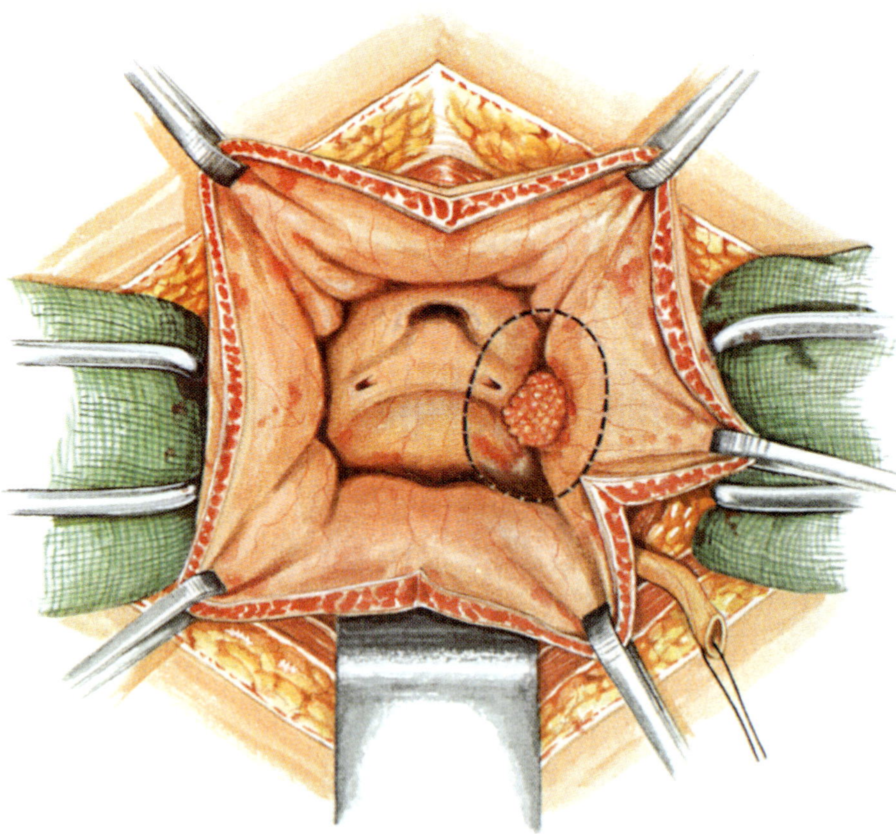

49-1

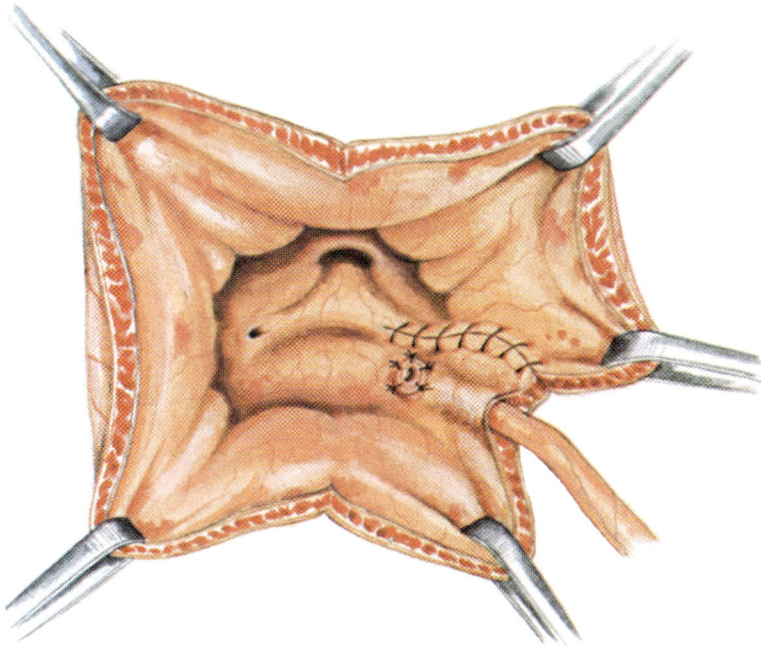

49-2

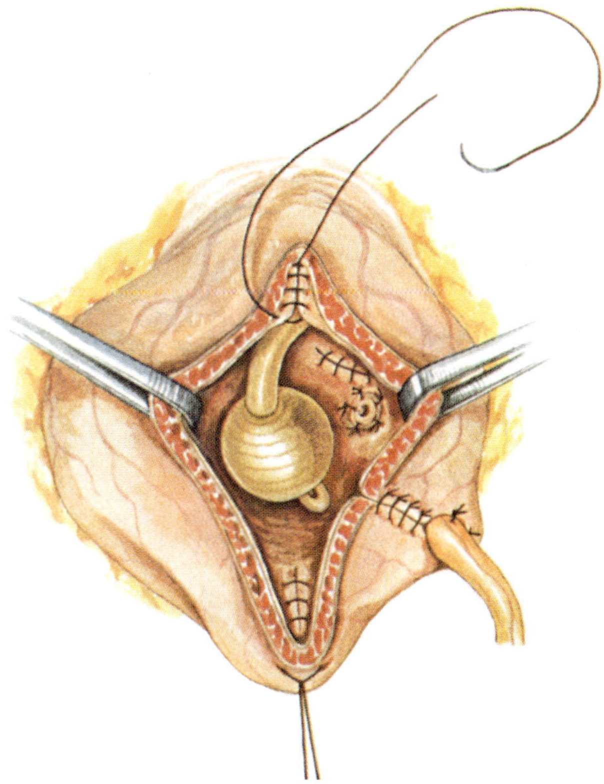

49-3

50. Radical Cystectomy and Lymph Node Dissection

This procedure is indicated when evidence for bladder carcinoma of moderate grade (II or III) invading bladder muscle has been confirmed by pathologic study after previous TUR of a bladder tumor. The tumor may also be multifocal. An intravenous urogram may confirm muscular infiltration near the ureteral orifice if obstruction is demonstrated by x-ray. We believe that CT scans of the bladder and bony pelvis may ultimately provide the best means of staging infiltrative bladder carcinoma.

We use the supine position for radical cystectomy and prostatectomy. If the bladder tumor has migrated to the prostate, then a total urethrectomy is indicated; in this in-

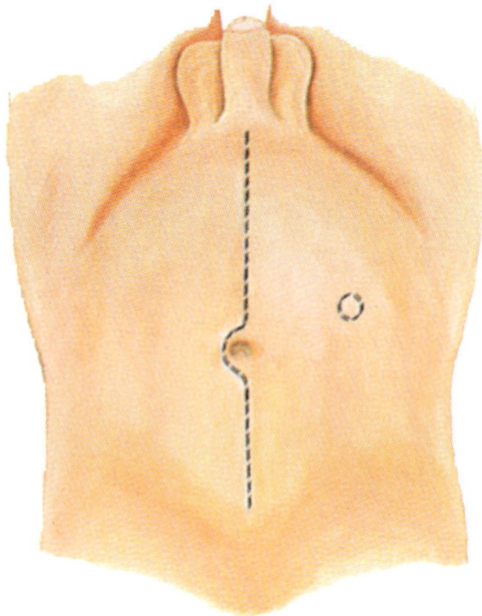

50-1

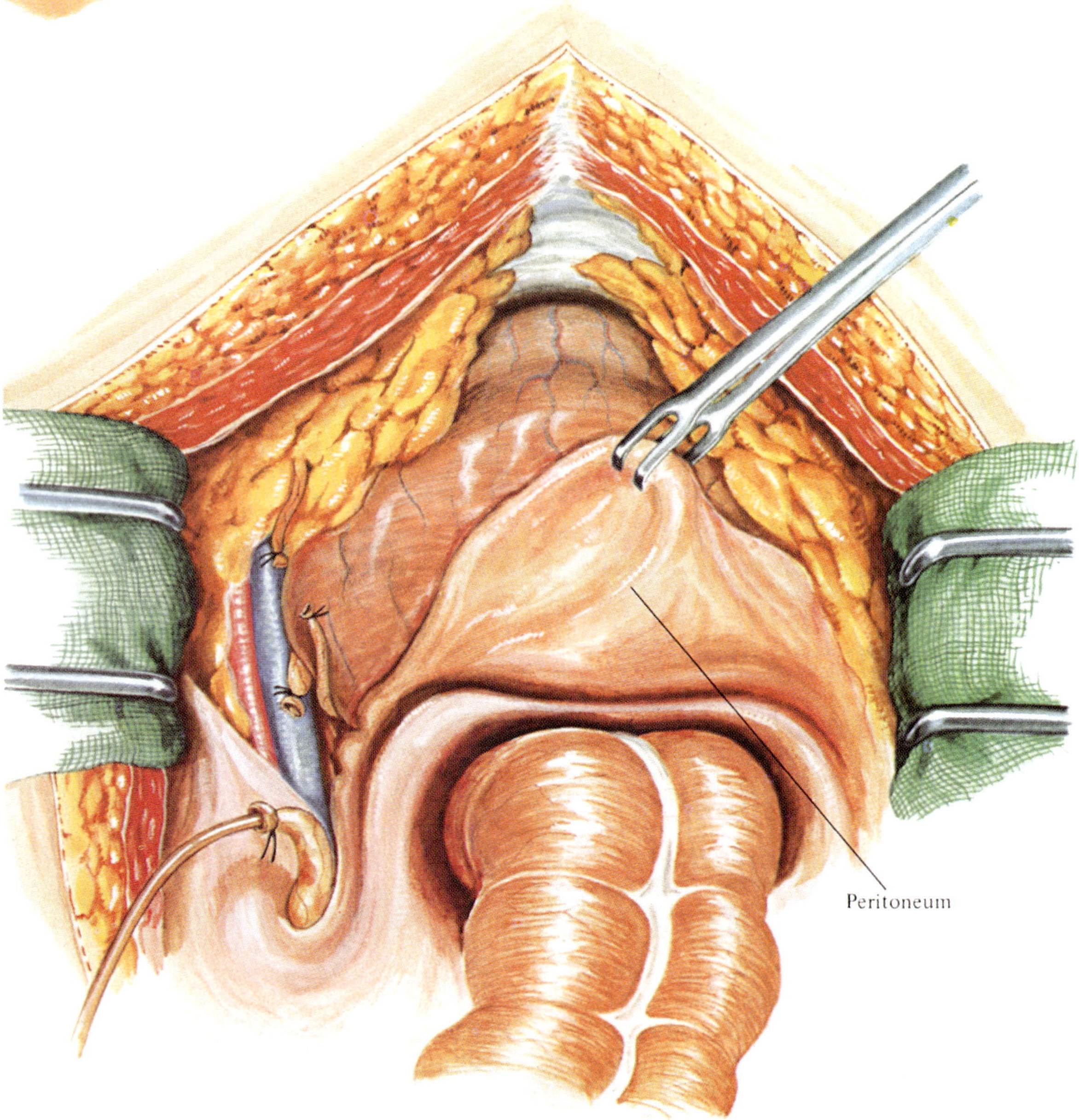

50-2

stance we use a modification of the lithotomy position. The legs, with only a slight bend in the knees, are abducted and placed on surgical protective pads. Standard leg braces are used as in the abdominal-perineal procedure. Separation of the lower extremities also allows positioning of the second assistant between the thighs.

50-1. *The future site of the ileal conduit is marked* (broken circle). A midline, vertical incision 5 cm above the umbilicus, curving around the umbilicus, and extending to the symphysis pubis is used. If a urinary diversion is also planned at this operation, then the incision may be extended superiorly for another 4–6 cm. After entering the peritoneal cavity, the bladder and pelvic area are inspected and palpated. Inspection and palpation of the liver and gastrointestinal tract are also carried out.

After placing the patient into a slight Trendelenburg position, the small bowel is carefully packed superiorly and out of the bony pelvis. A Brunswig self-retaining retractor or a Smith ring with self-retaining retractors are carefully inserted and positioned. Only the sigmoid lies posteriorly and courses inferiorly.

Dissection begins lateral to the bladder neck area on each side to free the bladder from surrounding tissue.

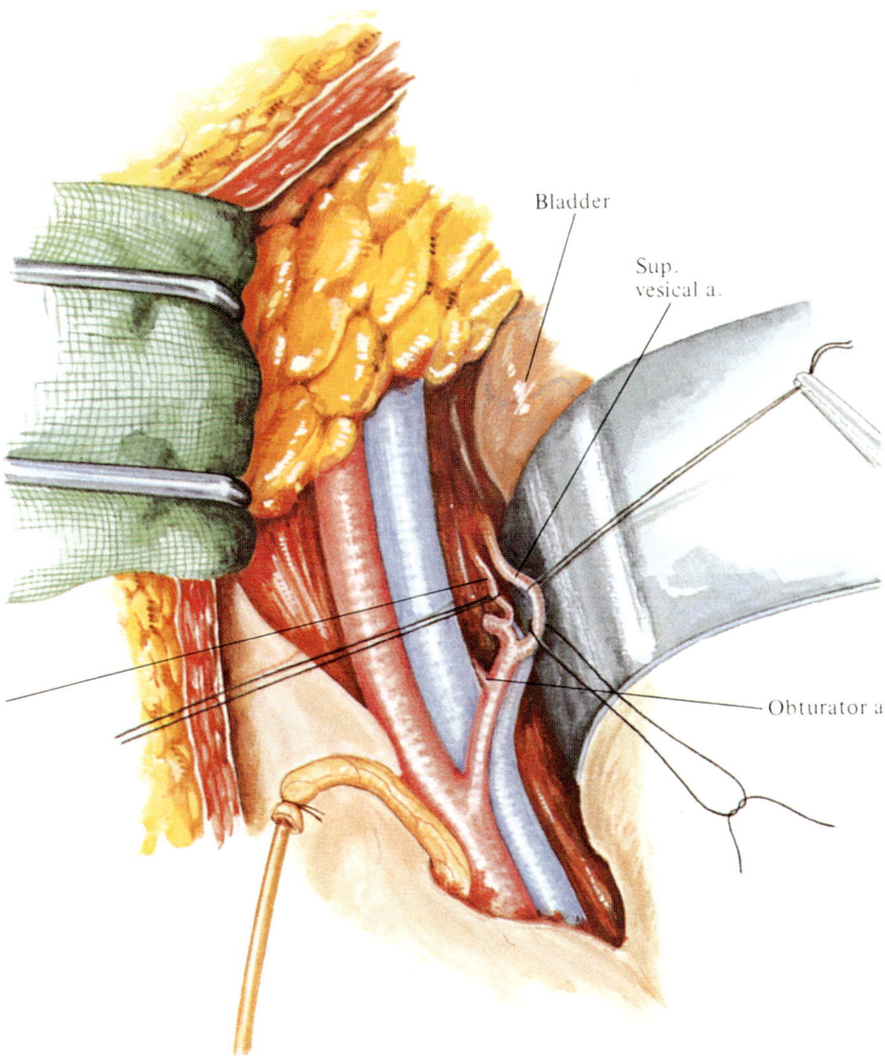

50-3

50-2. *The left ureter is isolated by incising the posterior peritoneum.* The ureter is freed and divided. A distal portion of ureter is sent to pathology for frozen section. The proximal ureter is catheterized. Lymph node dissection is begun at the bifurcation of the common iliac arteries. Areolar and connective tissue are removed on the left side between common iliac artery and iliac vein where the dissection continues laterally and inferiorly. The obturator nerve is freed and retracted laterally in the obturator bundle, allowing excision of areolar and lymphatic tissue. The obturator artery can be identified as the dissection continues to the femoral canal.

50-3. The obturator artery and middle hemorrhoidal artery are also doubly ligated and transected on the left.

The dissection proceeds inferior and lateral to the iliac vein on the right side. The common iliac artery is freed by dissecting between the vessels. The hypogastric artery is isolated and the right ureter is carefully retracted. The ureter may be divided at this point. The distal tip of the ureter is separately divided and sent to pathology for a frozen

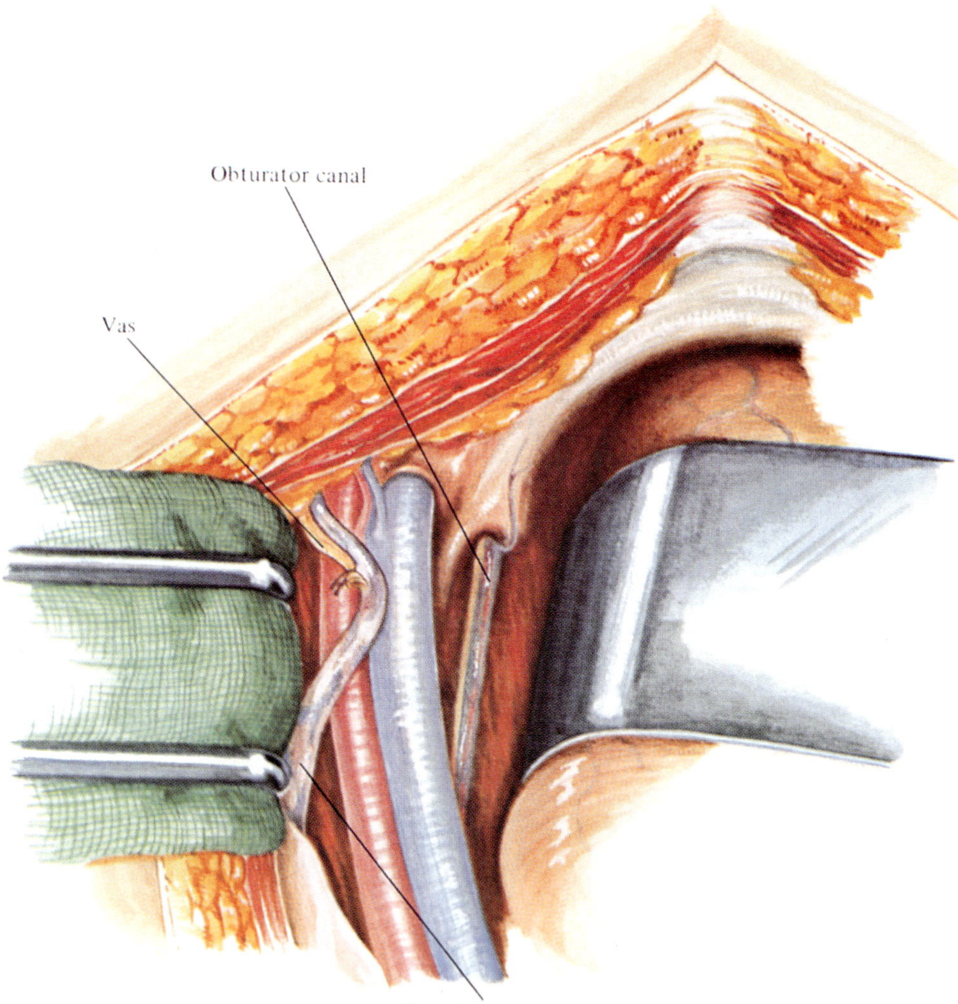

50-4

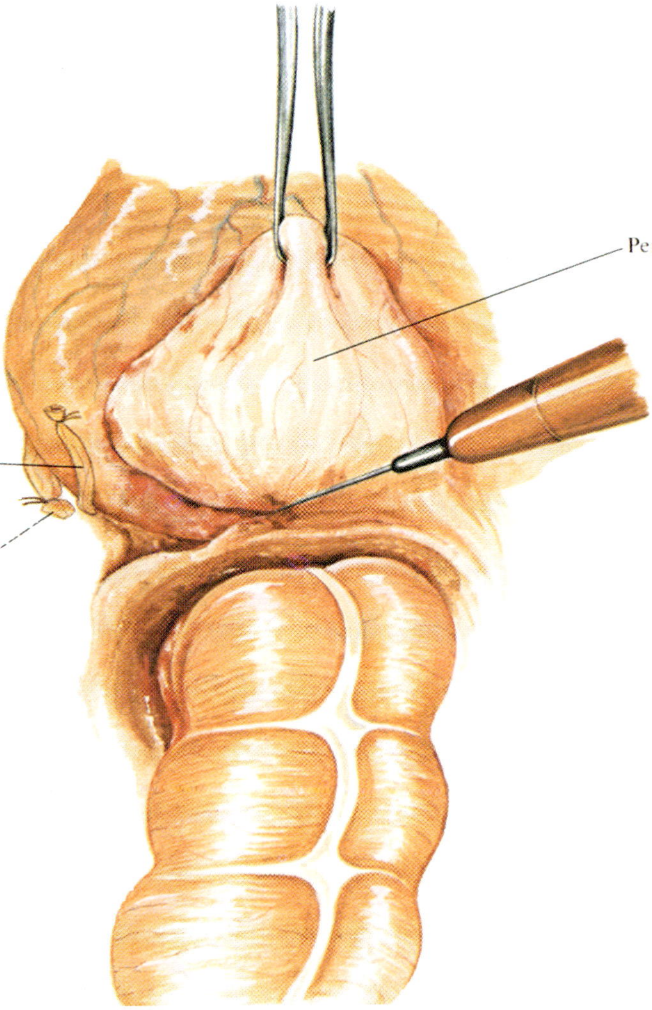

50-5

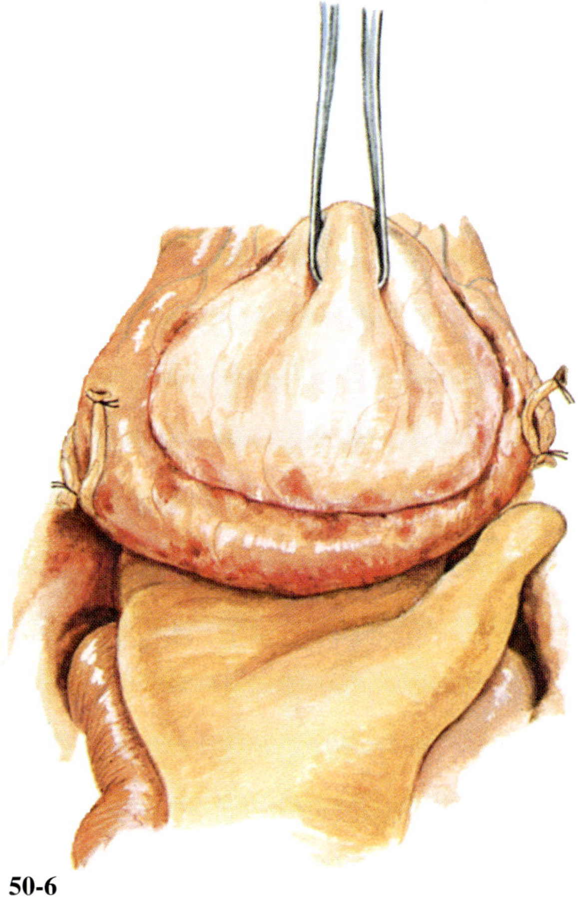

50-6

section. The proximal ureter is cannulated with a soft ureteral catheter (6 Fr) and allowed to drain outside the patient.

Dissection is continued along the right obturator bundle to the femoral canal. The hypogastric artery is carefully dissected distally, allowing double ligation and transection of the right superior vesical artery, obturator artery, and middle hemorrhoidal artery.

50-4. The circumflex vein is located at the inferior border of dissection on the left. The lateral border of dissection is the genitofemoral nerve. After dissecting and isolating the left hypogastric artery, the left superior vesical artery is freed, doubly ligated, and transected.

50-5. Removal of the bladder is now facilitated by *incising the peritoneal reflection close to the rectum and proceeding inferiorly.* The assistant lifts the bladder as the surgeon frees the posterior bladder wall. The inferior vesical arteries can now be isolated.

50-6. The plane between prostate and rectum can also be initiated.

50-7. Both inferior vesical arteries are doubly ligated and transected.

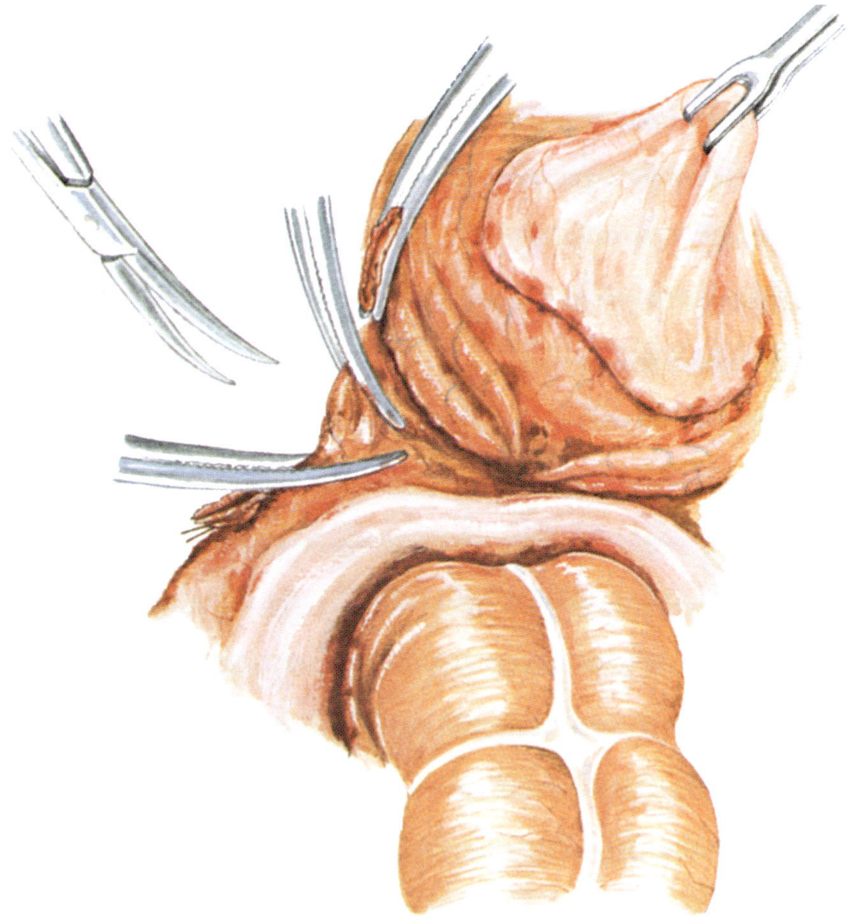

50-7

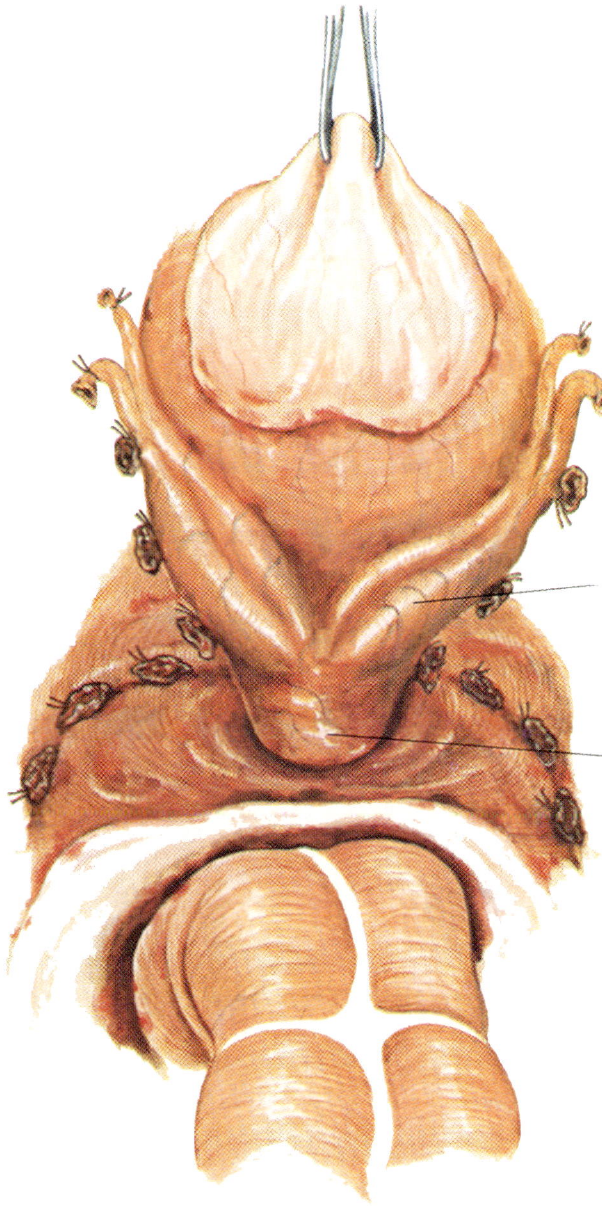

50-8

50-8. The bladder is elevated with a tenaculum. The prostate and seminal vesicles are seen along with the ligated vessels supplying the bladder and prostate. The urethral-indwelling catheter is now brought into the field. Formalin is introduced into the bladder (120 mL) for 5–10 minutes. The solution is then allowed to drain out.

50-9. Removal of Adjoining Prostate. The fatty tissue overlying the superior and anterior prostate surface is superficially removed with sharp dissection, exposing the endopelvic fascia. After using blunt dissection, the endopelvic fascia is incised in a semicircular fashion. The puboprostatic ligaments are identified and interrupted sharply. Blunt dissection is continued, allowing palpation of the apex; the membranous urethra with catheter in place and the anterior surface of the prostate are freed.

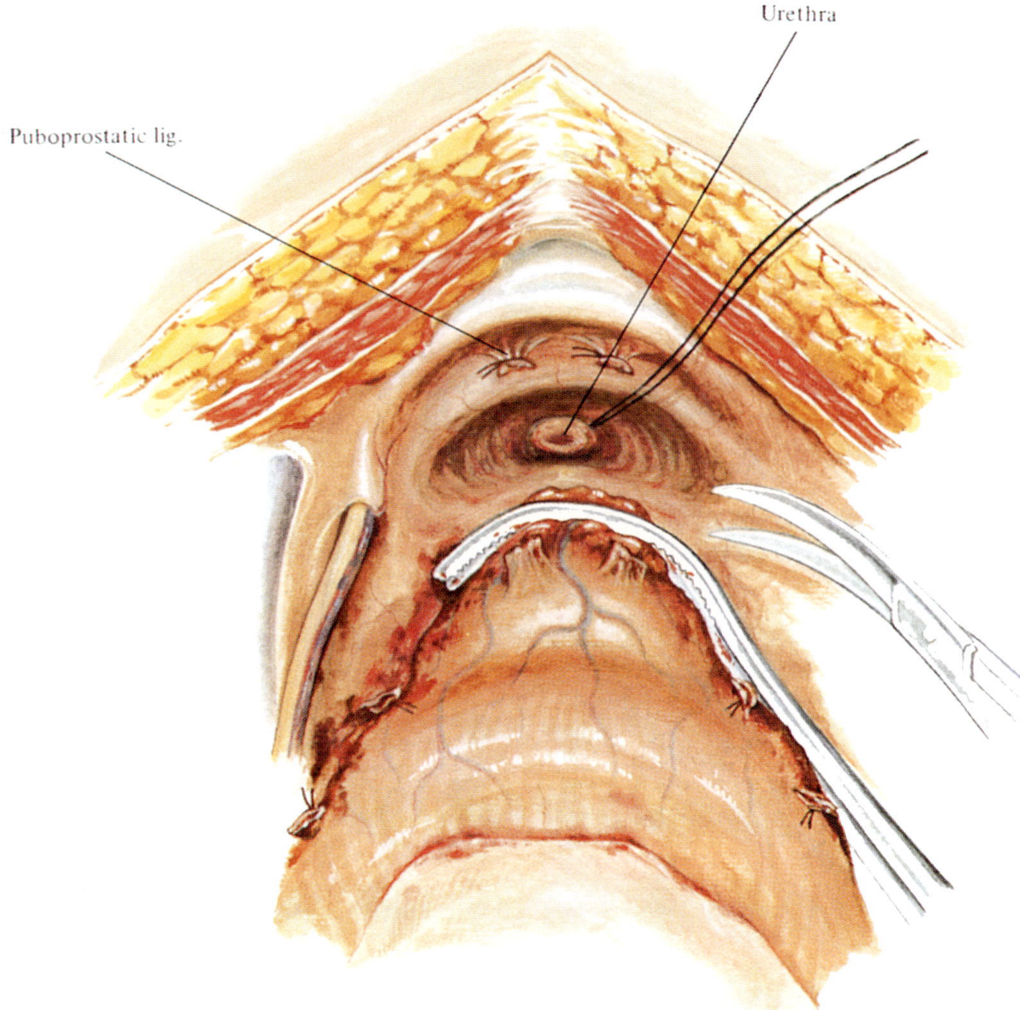

50-9

51. Urethrectomy Following Total Cystectomy and Prostatectomy

The supine patient is now repositioned (lithotomy) to allow access to the perineum. Resterilization of the perineum may be necessary, with new drapes.

51-1. *A vertical midline perineal incision is made.* The proximal urethra with its ligature is isolated and dissected. A urethral catheter or curved metal sound assists in the location of the urethra. A flat tubular drain is helpful.

51-2. *A second longitudinal incision is made along the ventrum of the penis.* The distal urethra is isolated and freed, allowing the proximal urethra to be pulled out of the surgical opening. The distal urethra is transected and ligated at the corona. The epithelium is squamous at the urethral meatus.

51-3. *Two flat tubular drains are secured.* Skin closure of both wounds is made with interrupted sutures.

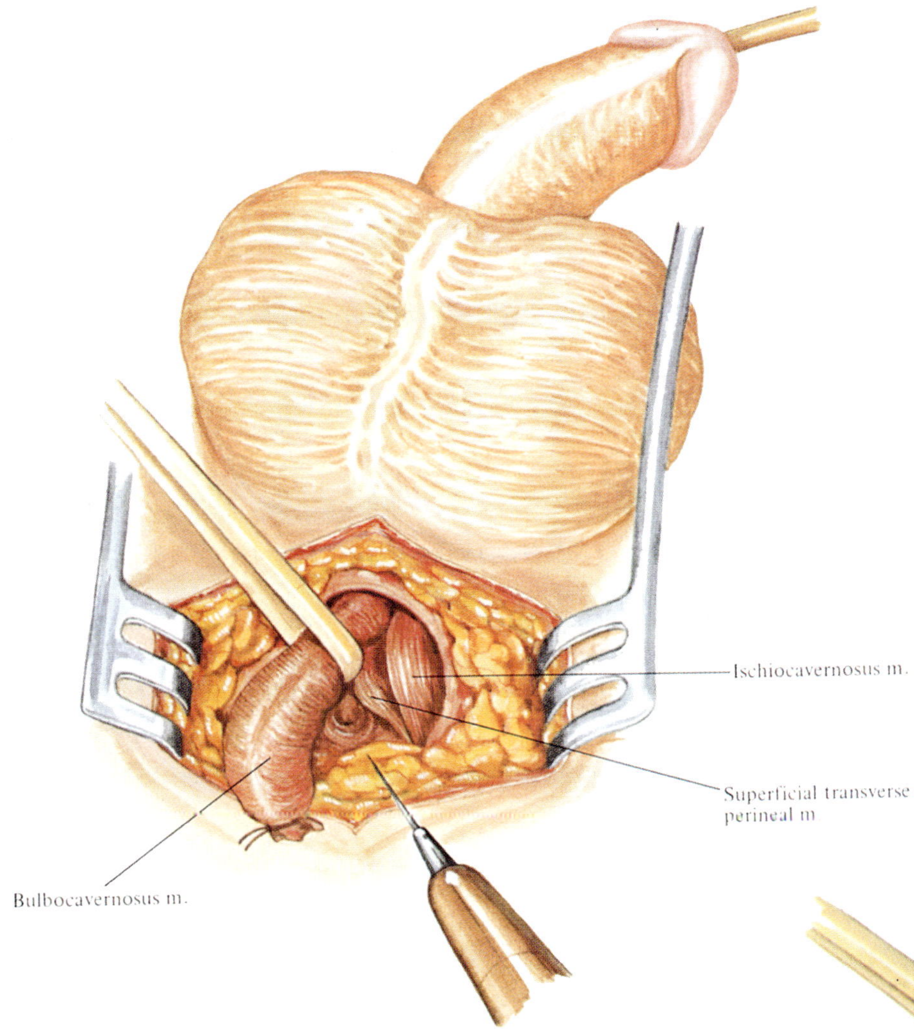
Ischiocavernosus m.
Superficial transverse perineal m
Bulbocavernosus m.

51-1

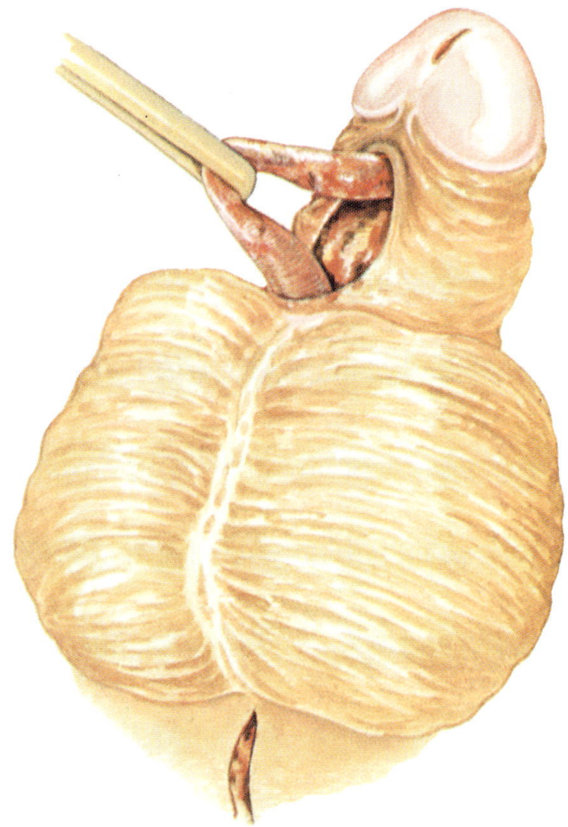

51-2

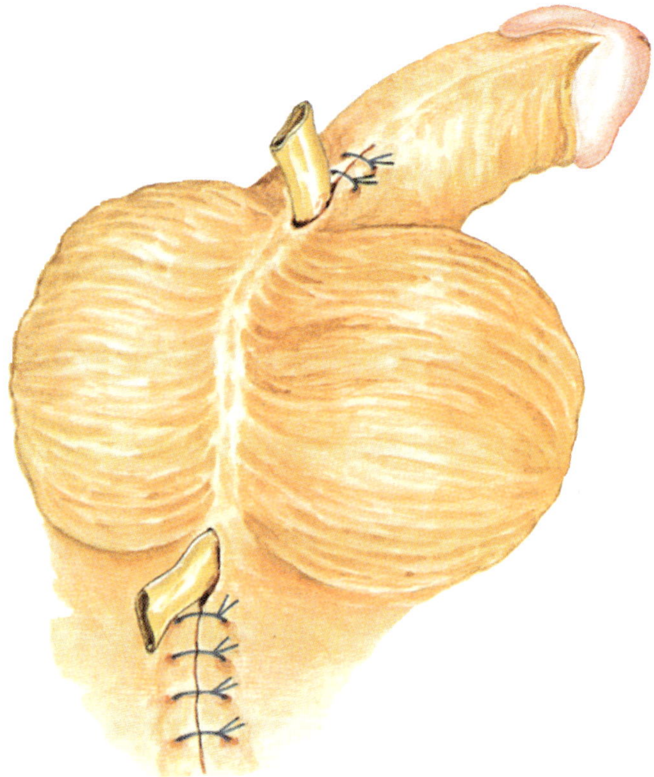

51-3

Bladder Enlargement

Candidates for the bladder-enlarging operation include patients with tuberculous cystitis, interstitial cystitis, or chemical cystitis. A bowel preparation, including the use of antibiotics, is indicated as follows:

For large bowel surgery the patient is hospitalized 24 hours prior to surgery. In selected well-motivated patients the preparation can be started at home.

For small bowel surgery the patient is hospitalized on the day of surgery. A bowel cleansing procedure can be started at home the afternoon and evening before surgery.

Our standard regimen consists of 4 liters of Colyte (Reed and Carnrick, Jersey City, NJ), a polyethylene glycol which is not absorbed. Refrigerating the solution is helpful prior to drinking it. The antibiotic regimen is as follows: neomycin 1 gm × 3 (taken orally at 1 PM, 2 PM, and 11 PM) and erythromycin base × 3 (taken orally at 1 PM, 2 PM, and 11 PM). If bowel contents are not clear, a tap water enema may be administered.

52. Goodwin Cup Patch Technique

52-1. *A segment of ileum is isolated.*

52-2. *The ileum is opened along its antimesenteric border.*

52-3 and 52-4. *A cup patch is formed.*

52-5 and 52-6. *The ileum is anastomosed to the open bladder.*

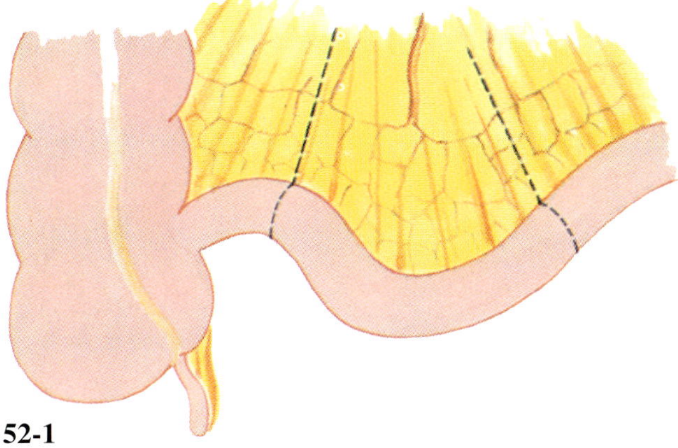

52-1

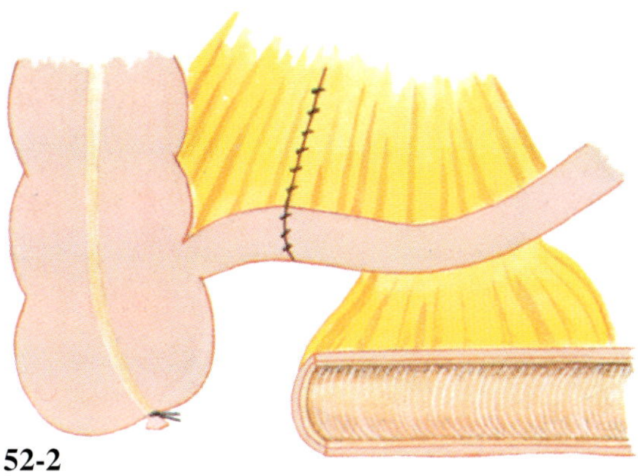

52-2

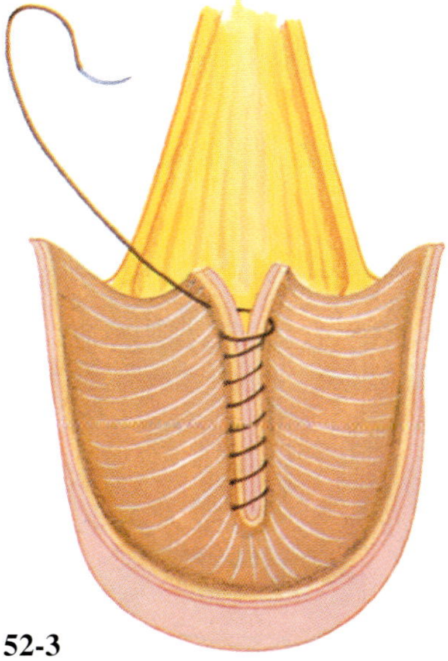

52-3

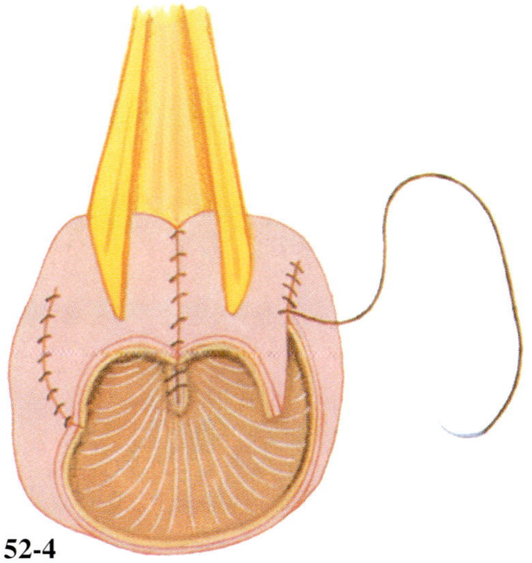

52-4

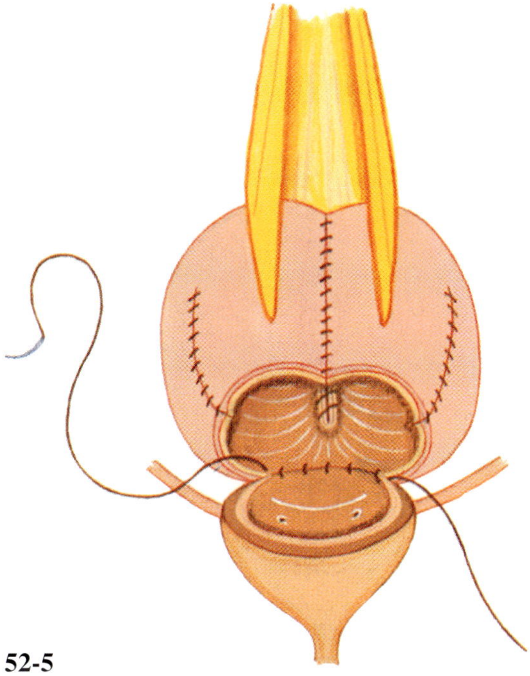

52-5

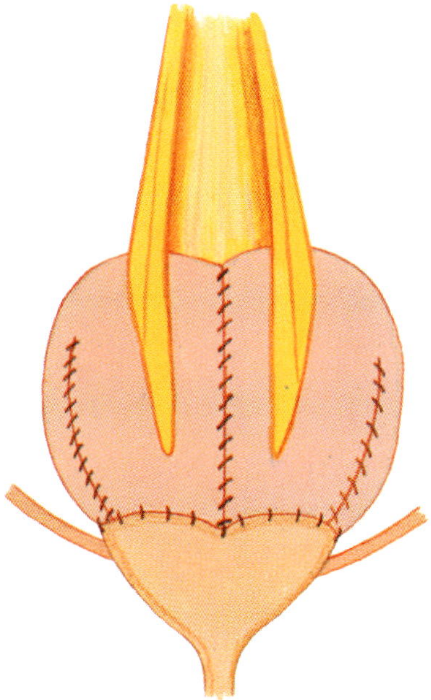

52-6

53. Sigmoid Cystoplasty

A subtotal cystectomy is performed.

53-1. *A segment of sigmoid colon is isolated* after bowel preparation.

53-2. The sigmoid is positioned, and *both ends are closed with 3–0 chromic catgut and an opening to fit the bladder is made* on the antimesenteric border.

53-3. *The sigmoid segment is attached to the bladder.*

53-4. Because of bladder irritability and urinary incontinence, *the ureters are implanted into the sigmoid* (antireflux procedure). The trigone and lower ends of the ureter are removed. The ureters lie posteriorly.

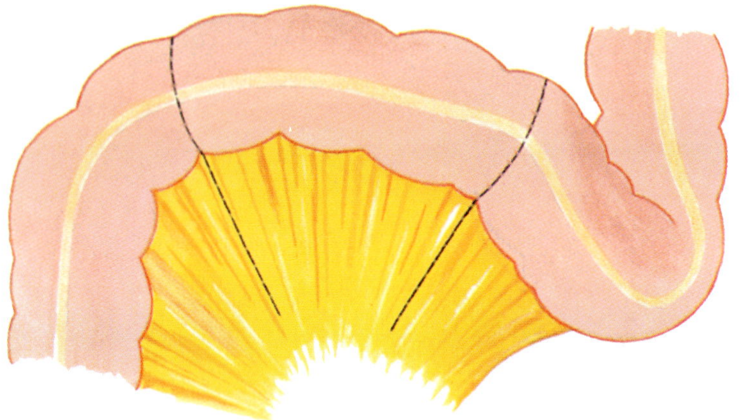

53-1

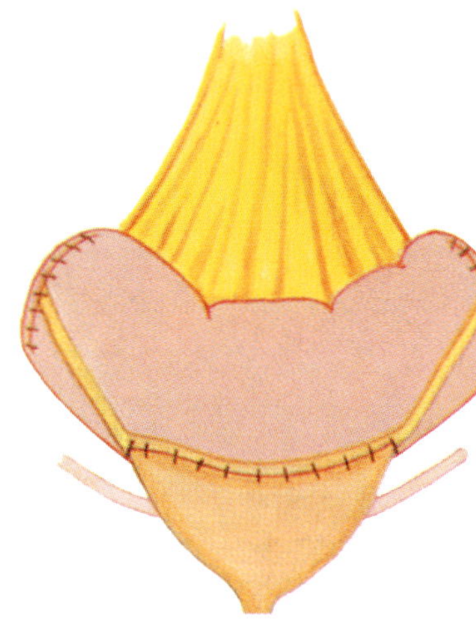

53-3

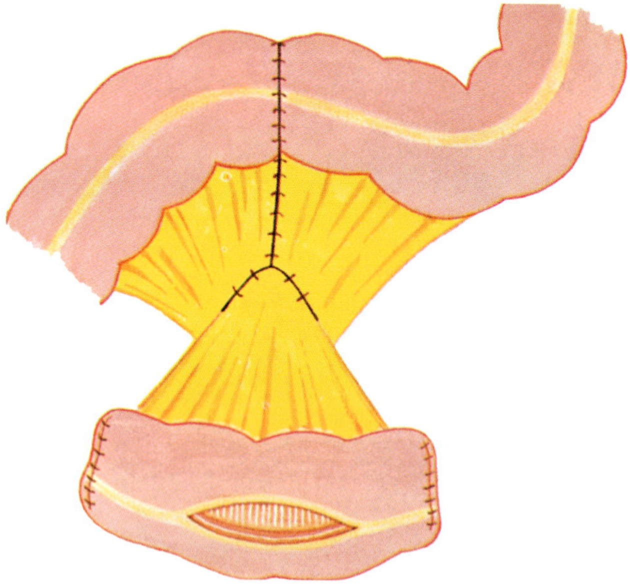

53-2

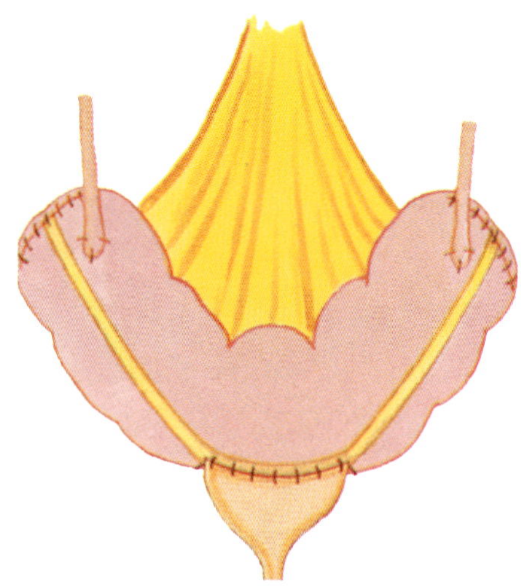

53-4

54. Cecal Bladder Construction

54-1. *The cecum and the terminal segment of the ileum are isolated surgically* prior to an appendectomy.

54-2. Reestablishment of *bowel continuity is accomplished by end-to-end anastomosis, cecum to ileum.* A 180° counterclockwise rotation is made of the isolated cecum for anastomosis to the bladder.

54-3. In selected instances *the ureters can be anastomosed to a slightly longer segment of ileum.* Urinary reflux is prevented by the ileocecal valve.

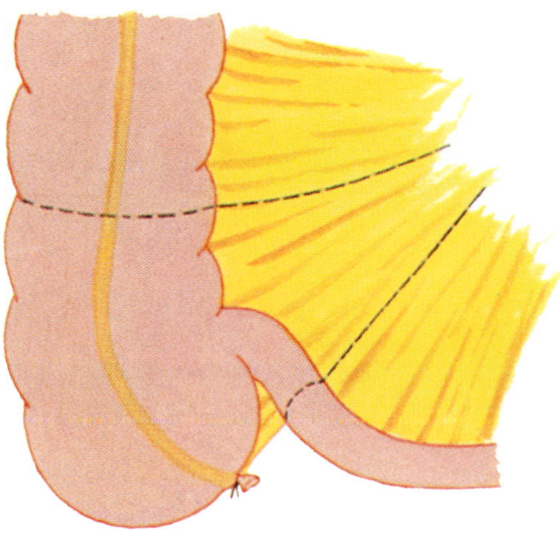

54-1

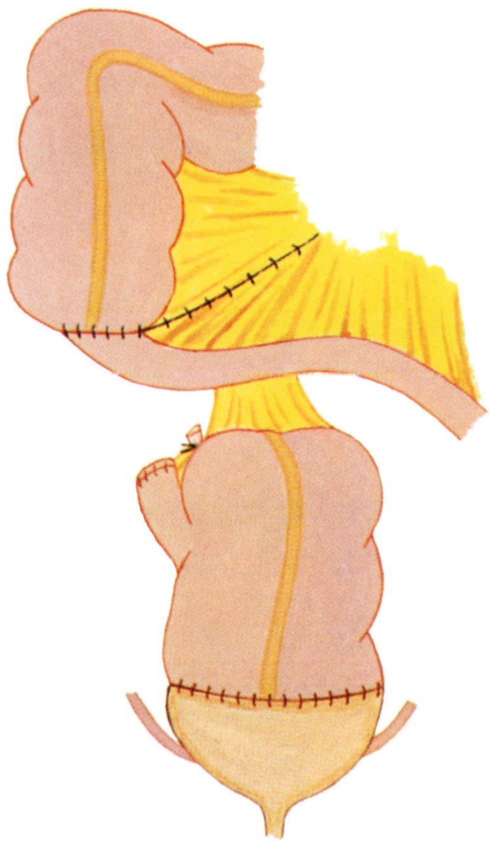

54-2

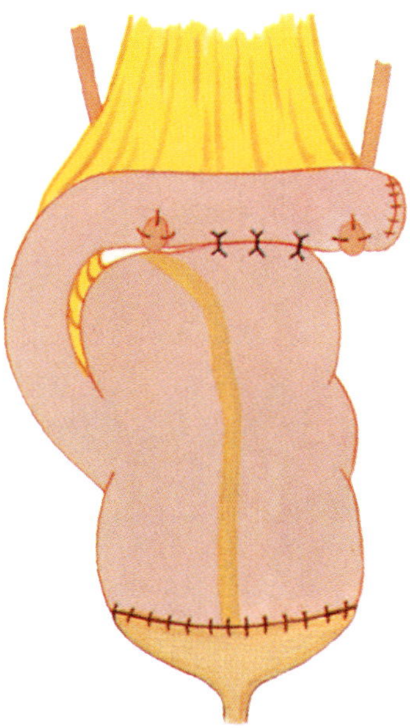

54-3

Repair of Vesicovaginal Fistula

Previous reconstructive or gynecologic surgery involving the roof of the vagina and adjacent bladder can lead to development of a urinary fistula. The added factor of infection may complicate matters. We believe that edema and infection must subside before healthy tissue can be used to surgically cover the defect. This healing period may last 2–3 months in some instances.

Careful workup of each patient is mandatory. An intravenous urogram should be performed. One should be certain that the patient does not have a ureterovaginal fistula. Cystoscopy should be performed. One can usually find the bladder opening and its proximity to the ureteral orifices.

55. Vaginal Approach

55-1. The patient is in the lithotomy position. *The vesicovaginal fistula is exposed after* a weighted vaginal speculum is inserted and stay sutures are placed for tension.

55-2. *A urethral indwelling catheter is inserted into the bladder* through the fistula. The bag is inflated and placed under tension. The broken line indicates the contour for incision.

55-3. *The fistula, with a ring of normal tissue, is excised.*

55-4. *The fistulous plug can be easily withdrawn* from the operative site. Indigo-carmine dye is injected intravenously at this point to help in visualizing the ureteral orifices.

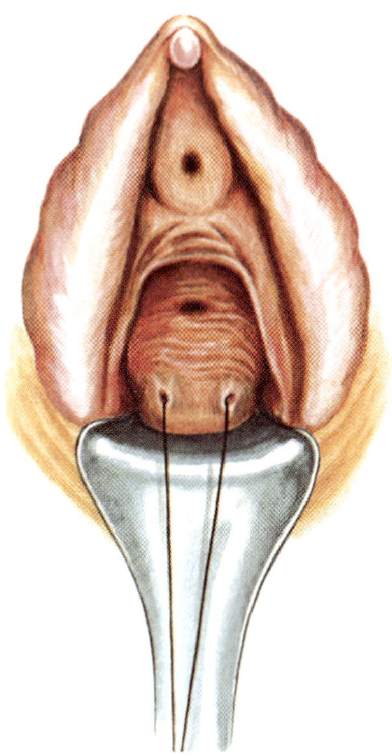

55-1

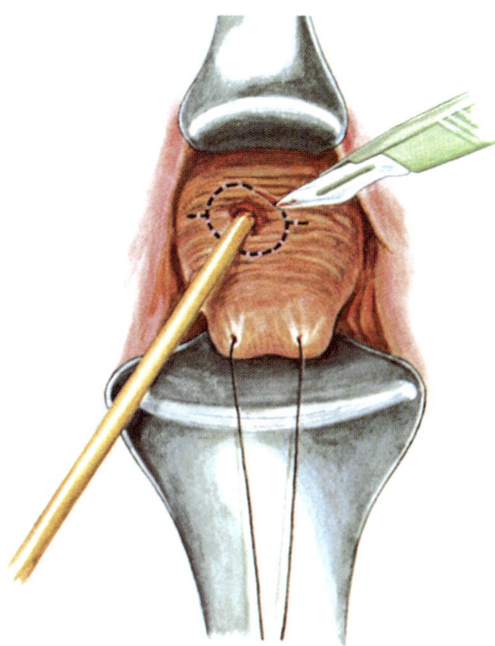

55-2

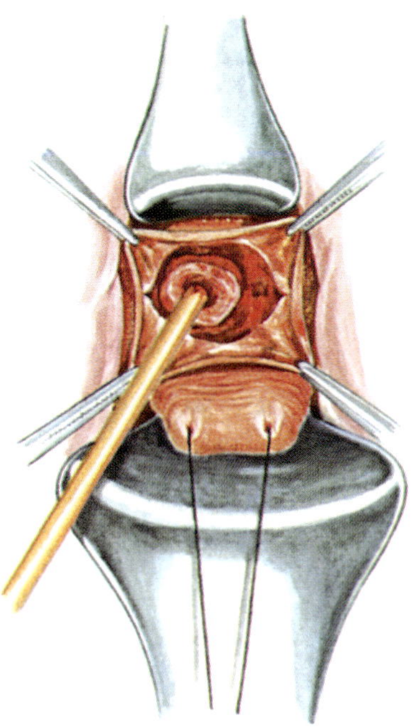

55-3

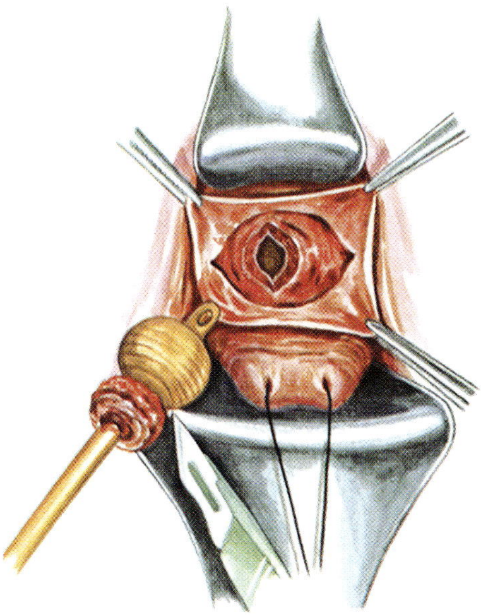

55-4

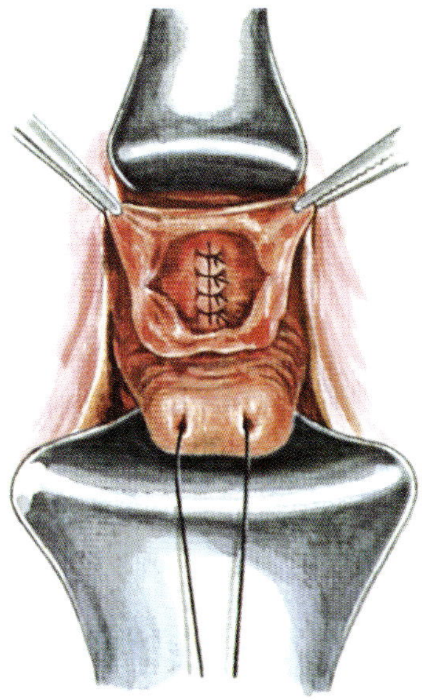

55-5

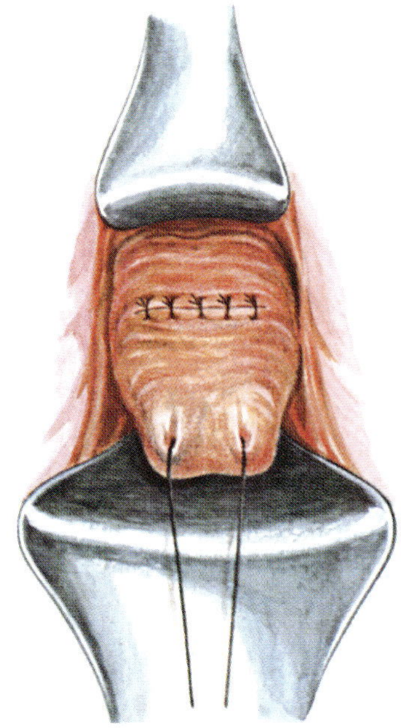

55-6

55-5. The bladder wall, muscular septum, and vaginal wall are closed in separate layers. The inner layer is closed transversely. *The middle layer is closed longitudinally.*

55-6. *The outer layer is closed transversely.* The stay sutures are removed. A urethral indwelling catheter is left in place (18–20 Fr) for 5–8 days.

56. Vesicovaginal Fistula: Transperitoneal Approach

The typical patient is a 35- to 45-year-old white female who underwent an abdominal hysterectomy 3 to 6 months earlier. The major indication for surgery was endometriosis and/or a cystocele. Since surgery, she has been totally incontinent of urine. On careful workup, the bladder incontinence has been verified. Cystoscopy and vaginoscopy reveal a large vesicovaginal fistula. Worth mentioning in any workup of similar cases is the fact that a small fistula, between the bladder and vagina, can sometimes be confirmed by placing a tampon into the vagina; the bladder is then catheterized with a 16 Fr catheter, and methylene blue dye diluted in saline is gently placed into the bladder. Seventy-five to 150 mL of blue-tinged dye may be needed to verify the diagnosis. The tampon may be only lightly stained in the case of a small fistula.

A ureterovaginal fistula can be seen by injecting intravenously 5 mL of indigo carmine with a vaginal tampon sponge in place. It is important that this procedure be performed separately on another day. Cystoscopy is useful. An intravenous pyelogram (IVP) is also helpful in finding the presence of a ureterovaginal fistula.

We prefer general anesthesia for the patient with an endotracheal tube. Spinal or epidural anesthesia is also a good option. The lithotomy position is used with stirrups lifting the thighs outward. The lower abdominal wall, vagina, and perineum are carefully prepared using povidone solution (Betadine) or other similar cleansing solutions. The vagina is particularly cleansed along with the vaginal surface and area. The modified "lithotomy position" allows excellent access to the perineum and perineal area which is elevated.

56-1. A cystoscope (21 Fr cystoscopy) with the obturator in place is carefully inserted and urine is obtained for culture and antibiotic sensitivities. The patient receives replacement intravenous (IV) fluids throughout the surgical procedure. The ureteral orifices are identified. On the posterior bladder wall, or floor of the bladder, usually slightly to the left of the midline, but away from the left ureteral orifice, a moderate fistula can be seen. (The same fistula may be located to the right for a right-sided fistula.) In our patient the fistula was approximately 2 cm in size. It connected freely with the vagina. In our opinion this is the usual location, and it is near or *at the vaginal cuff.*

Five French ureteral catheters are passed individually up each ureter and advanced to the renal pelvis. The cystoscope and the catheterizing element are carefully removed, leaving the ureteral catheters in place. A 20 Fr Foley catheter is inserted, and 8 cc of saline are used to inflate the balloon. The ureteral catheters are secured to the Foley indwelling catheter and marked separately (left and right). Maintaining the bladder and the ureteral catheters is important. Both ureteral catheters are secured to the shaft of the indwelling Foley catheter with 3–0 silk ties.

The patient is now repositioned on the operating table, being careful to protect the catheters. The patient's upper body is placed in the supine position, and the middle upper abdomen and lower chest wall are similarly cleansed with appropriate cleansing solutions. The patient is draped in a way that the surgeon has access to the vagina. This is accomplished by placing lifts between both knees, and "frog-legging" the knees and the legs, thus exposing the introitus.

A midline incision is made from the symphysis pubis anteriorly and above the umbilicus curving to the left side. A transverse incision may be used in a younger female patient. The incision is carried through subcutaneous tissue, the fascia-external oblique aponeurosis, and abdominal rectus sheath. The peritoneal cavity is entered sharply

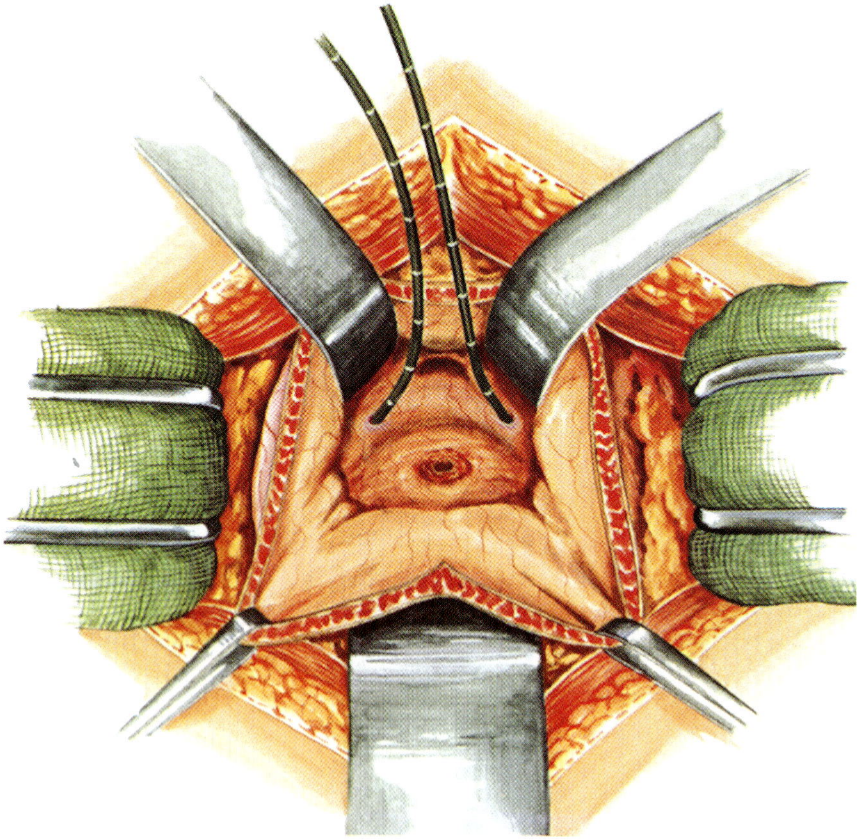

56-1

avoiding bowel. The patient is placed into the Trendelenburg position. Examination of the organs within the abdominal cavity and the retroperitoneum is carefully carried out.

56-2. Bivalving of the posterior wall to expose the fistula.

A significant amount of omentum is next mobilized from the greater curvature of the stomach. The pelvic cavity is now examined. The ureters are located by palpating the ureteral catheters. The dome of the bladder is grasped with Allis clamps and entered surgically. Exposure is obtained initially with Allis clamps: subsequently, stay sutures, 2–0 silk sutures, are used to maintain exposure along with a Balfour self-retaining retractor.

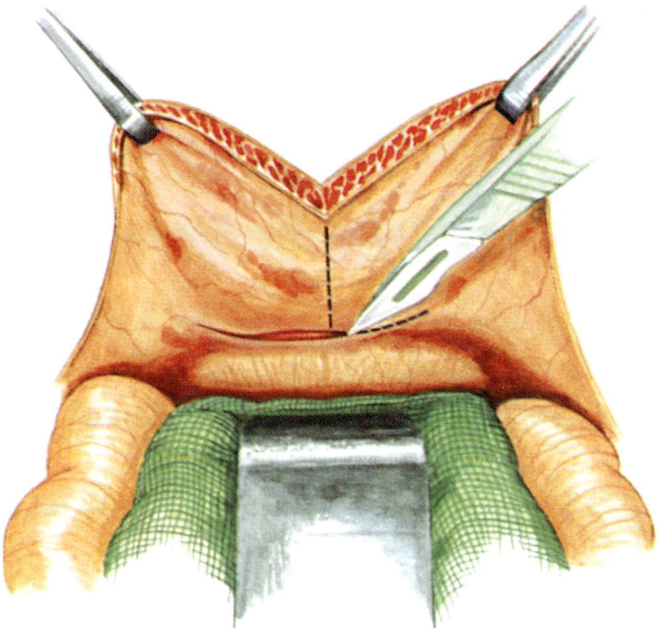

56-2

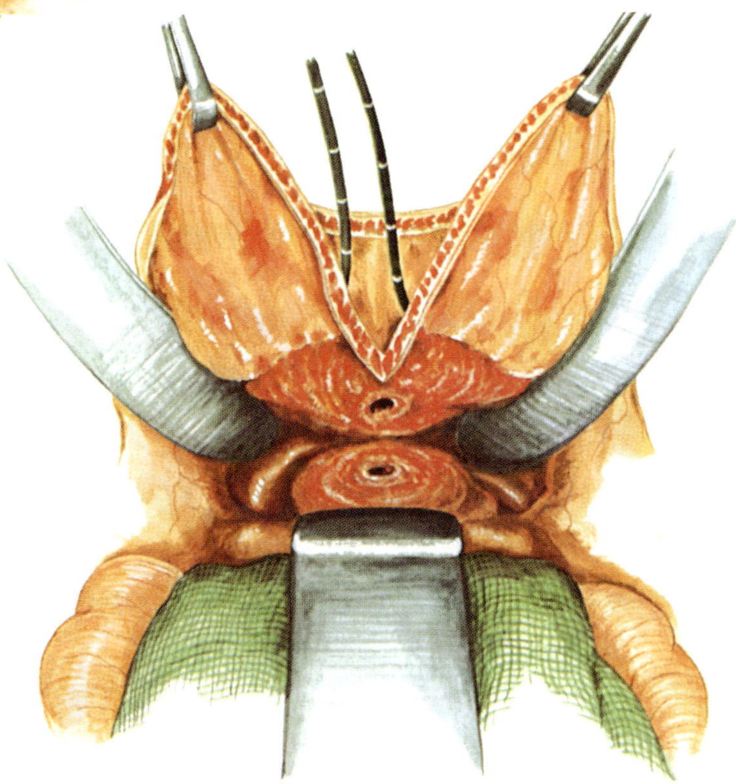

56-3

56-3. The large fistulous tract to the vagina in the vaginal cuff area is identified along the posterior bladder wall.

The incision at the midline of the open bladder wall is next extended superiorly and more posteriorly along the midbladder wall to the fistulous tract (bivalving the bladder).

56-4. The fistulous tract is then excised circumferentially using a scalpel. The tract includes a rim of posterior bladder and anterior vaginal wall. The ureters are protected. Careful attention is then directed to freeing the bladder from the anterior and lateral walls of the vagina until the vaginal wall is freely mobile.

56-5. After adequate mobilization of the bladder is accomplished, the anterior vaginal

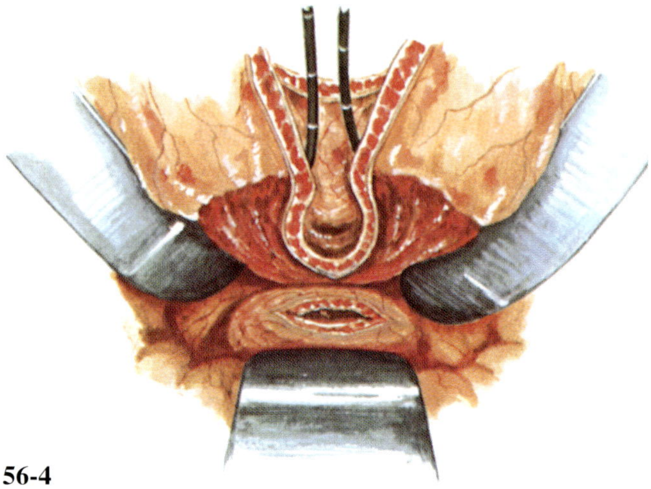

56-4

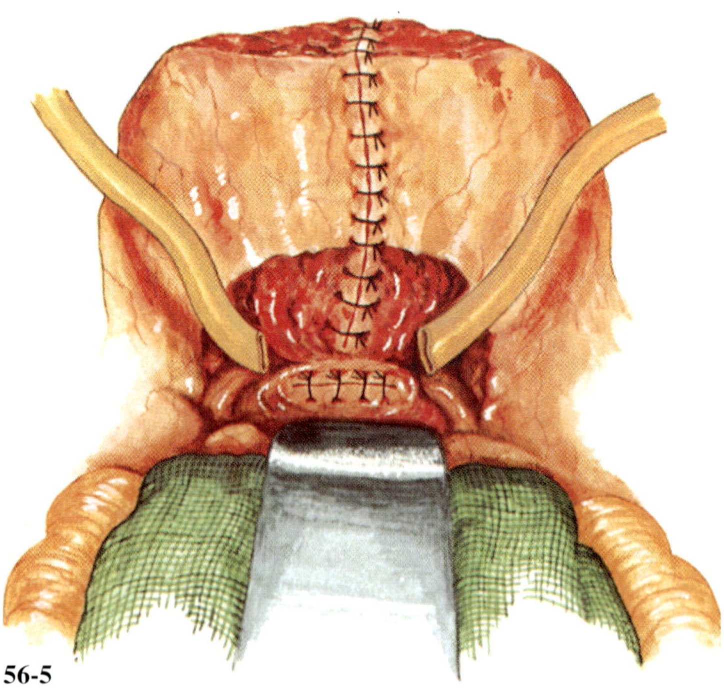

56-5

wall opening is reapproximated by using a running 2–0 chromic catgut suture, thus inverting the superficial cut edges of the vaginal opening. Interrupted reinforcing sutures are used (2–0 chromic catgut) in a second layer.

The left and right posterior walls of the bladder are mobilized, reapproximated, and closed using two layers of interrupted 2–0 chromic catgut sutures.

The ureteral catheters are kept out of the surgical field so adequate bladder closure of the posterior area is accomplished. Again, two rows of 2–0 chromic catgut suture are used. Hemostasis is accomplished with suture ligatures of 3–0 chromic catgut and electrocautery coagulation.

With the posterior bladder wall intact, a segment or "flap" of omentum, previously mobilized, is interposed between the anterior vaginal wall and posterior bladder. The omental flap is secured to the anterior vagina with 3–0 chromic catgut sutures.

A mushroom tip suprapubic catheter (26 Fr) is inserted through a separate anterior bladder incision and it is secured. The bladder is then closed superiorly and anteriorly using two suture layers of 2–0 chromic catgut. (The inner layer may be a continuous suture layer.) Wound closure is carried out using 1–0 interrupted Vicryl sutures on the peritoneum and posterior rectus sheath. The anterior rectus sheath is reapproximated with interrupted 1–0 Vicryl sutures.

The ureteral catheters are removed at the end. A nasogastric tube may be considered but is generally not necessary during the procedure. Antibiotic coverage is mandatory and is used perioperatively and postoperatively.

57. Peritoneal Flap Technique

57-1. *A peritoneal flap is made.*

57-2. *The flap is interposed between the bladder and vagina* at the site of the previous fistula and is secured.

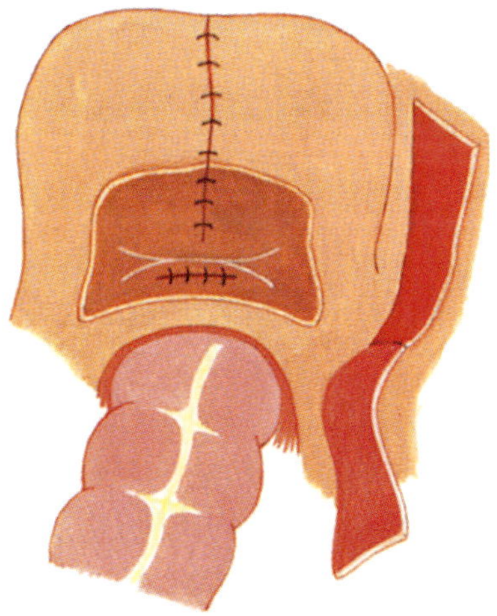

57-1

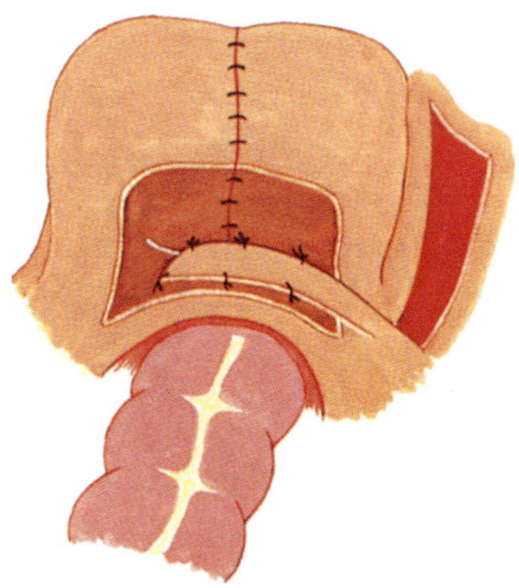

57-2

58. Omental Flap Technique

58-1. *An omental flap is prepared* if the lower omentum cannot be brought to the bladder with ease.

58-2. *The omentum is brought inferiorly and appropriately secured* along the lateral aspect of the descending colon. The blood supply is maintained by placement of sutures.

In **58–3** and **58–4** the view is from a surgical vantage point towards the symphysis pubis.

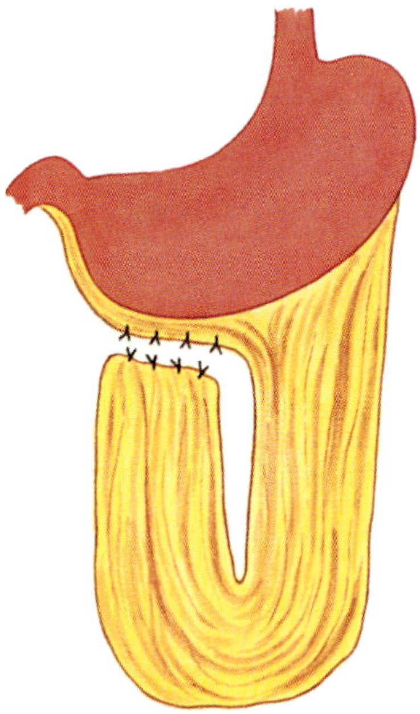

58-1

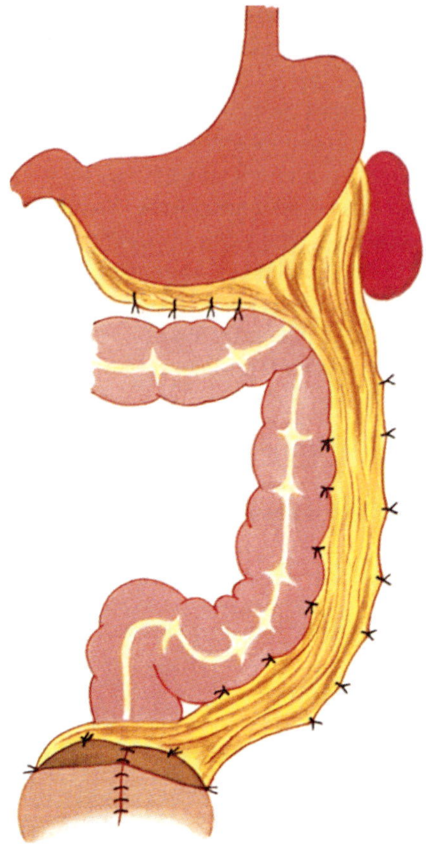

58-2

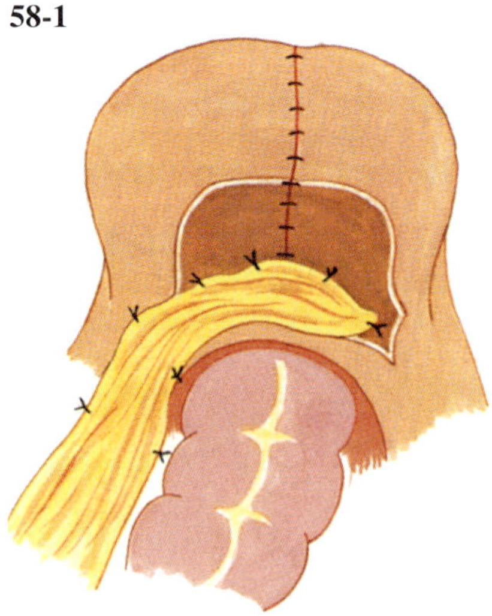

58-3

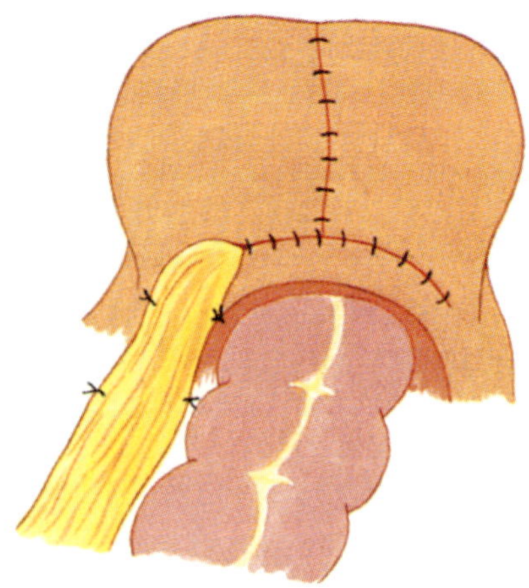

58-4

58-3. *Omentum is positioned and secured.*

58-4. *Final closure of posterior peritoneum to secure the omentum.*

Anti-Incontinence Operation for Female

59. Stamey Urinary Continence Procedure to Alleviate Stress Incontinence

Middle-aged women after the childbearing years can develop urinary stress incontinence. With time, incontinence worsens and urologic assistance is sought. A history and physical examination are performed. Urinalysis is included to rule out infection or any other organic causes of incontinence. If the patient has a pattern of uncontrolled urinary leakages or a history of urgency prior to voiding, a formal urodynamic study with cystometrogram and electromyogram recorders should be performed.

Urgency incontinence or wetting when recumbent would suggest the need for urodynamic evaluation. A moderate cystocele, if present, can usually be corrected at the time of the surgical procedure.

Cystoscopy, with the patient in the lithotomy position, is helpful in diagnosing the type of urinary incontinence. Our own workup usually does not include formal urody-

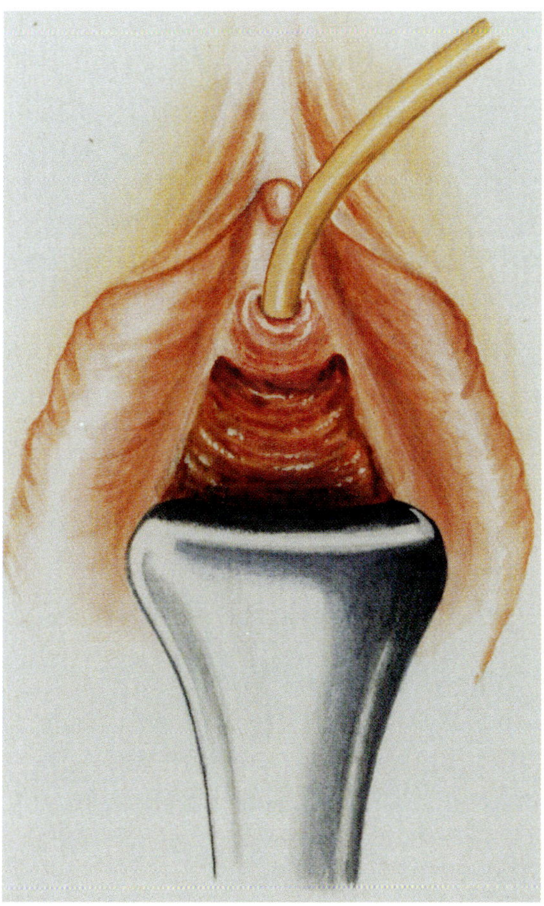

59-1

namic studies. If the patient has a neurogenic bladder with signs and symptoms of multiple sclerosis, then a careful history and urodynamic studies are included.

The Marshall test is initiated with the cystoscope in the bladder. The bladder is filled to a minimal volume of 250–300 mL. If the bladder is noncompliant, or the capacity is much larger, then a 500 mL volume may be inserted during cystoscopy. The cystoscope is removed and the patient is asked to stand upright on an elevated step. She is then asked to cough or strain. The amount of leakage is estimated after the patient coughs several times with 10 second intervals in between. The Marshall test is completed by placing the gloved index and middle finger against the bladder neck towards the pelvis through the vaginal introitus. She is asked to cough several times again. If no leakage is seen on the floor or the patient is obviously dry with this maneuver, then she has the major indication for surgery, and the procedure will correct the stress incontinence.

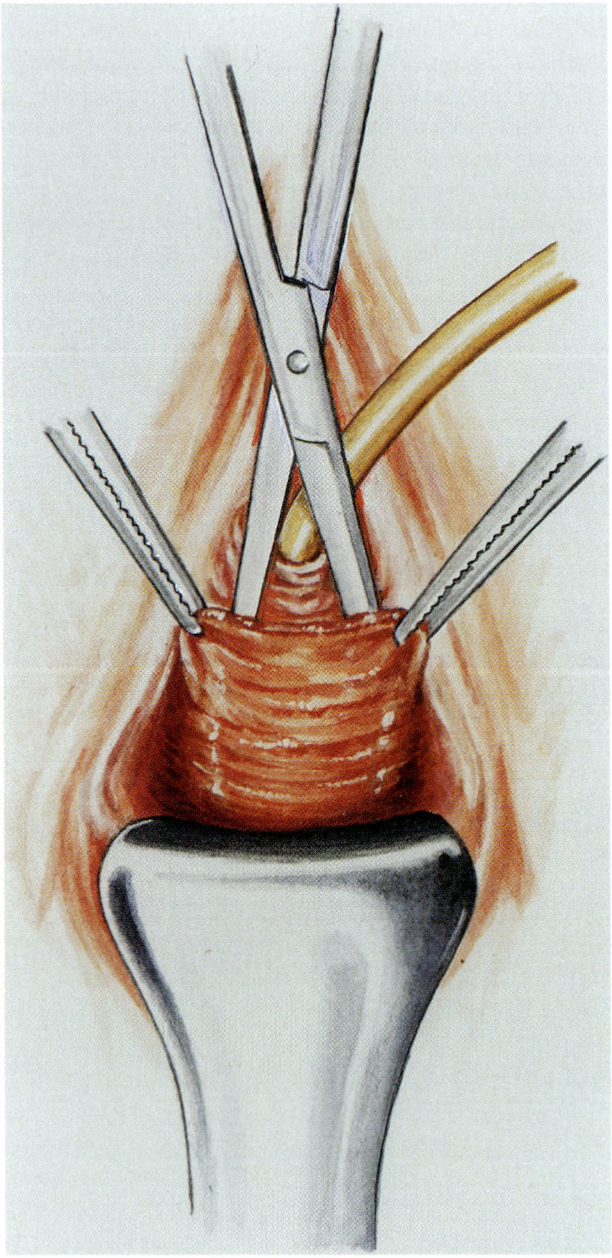

59-2

The patient receives general or regional anesthesia. She is placed into the lithotomy position and the perineal and vaginal areas are prepared (sterilized) and draped. We find it useful to sew a sterile towel above the anal region at the perineum so that the area above is sterile. The suprapubic area is also prepped and draped for the remainder of the surgical procedure.

59-1. With a vaginal speculum in place, the patient's urethral length is obtained by means of the urethral catheter with 10 cc of saline inflated into the balloon. The normal female urethra is approximately 4.5 to 5 cm in length (1-3/4 to 2 inches). This measurement is important in assisting in the operation.

59-2. With the urethral indwelling catheter in position, a transverse incision is made in the roof of the vagina with the catheter still in place. This incision extends through the vaginal epithelial layer. Careful dissection will expose the suburethral area on each side.

59-3. An improvement in the exposure by suturing the labia majora laterally in four places is shown. Skin hooks assist in the subsequent exposure. Narrow Deaver retractors can also expose the distal urethra.

59-4. The suprapubic skin incisions, 5 cm on each side, have been made and exposure is carried down to the fascia. The bladder is now emptied. The bladder must be emptied

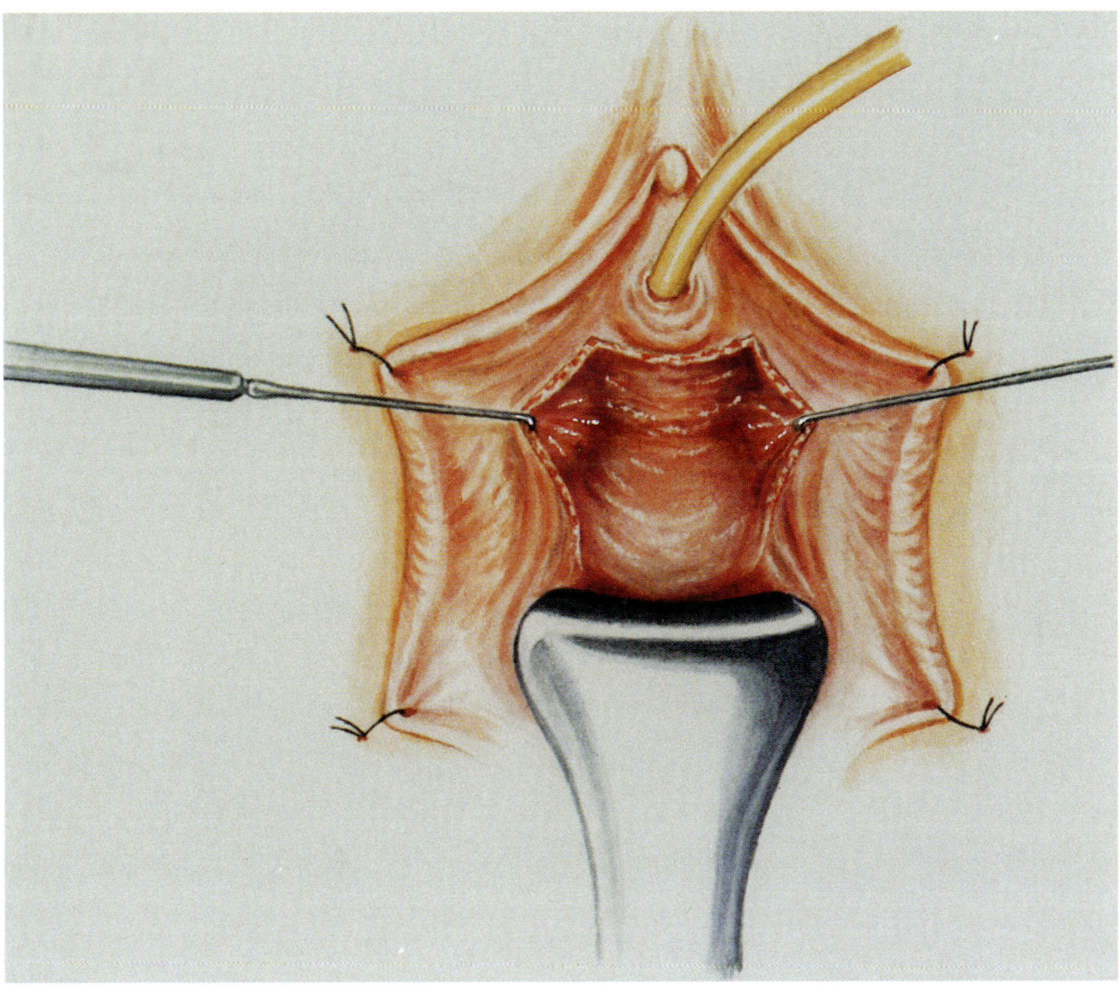

59-3

to avoid having the needle tip enter the anterior bladder lumen. The curved Stamey needles are introduced first on one side and later on the other side. The curved tip points inferiorly and toward the catheter and anterior tissue adjacent to the urethral opening on one side of the catheter. Care must be taken to avoid the urethra. After the needle tip makes a proper exit, first on one side of the urethra at the bladder neck (note the surgeon's fingers), the urethral catheter is removed and cystoscopy is performed to be sure that the needle shaft has not traversed the anterior bladder wall or bladder lumen. The 1–0 Prolene suture is attached through the eye of the Stamey needle.

59-5. A bolster has been placed as shown and the bolster is threaded over the suture. The bolster is placed longitudinally, and the end of the suture is allowed to return to the fascial site suprapubically.

The same maneuver is repeated on the opposite side of the urethra at the bladder neck urethral junction. Having the urethral catheter in place is useful in directing the needle and finding the correct pathway with the Stamey needle. Cystoscopy is performed to rule out the absence of needle encroachment into anterior bladder wall. The bolster is threaded over the Prolene suture and the needle is retracted to the anterior incisional site.

59-6. A midsagittal view demonstrates the final result. Cystoscopy can assist in judging the new bladder neck with both sutures lifted anteriorly.

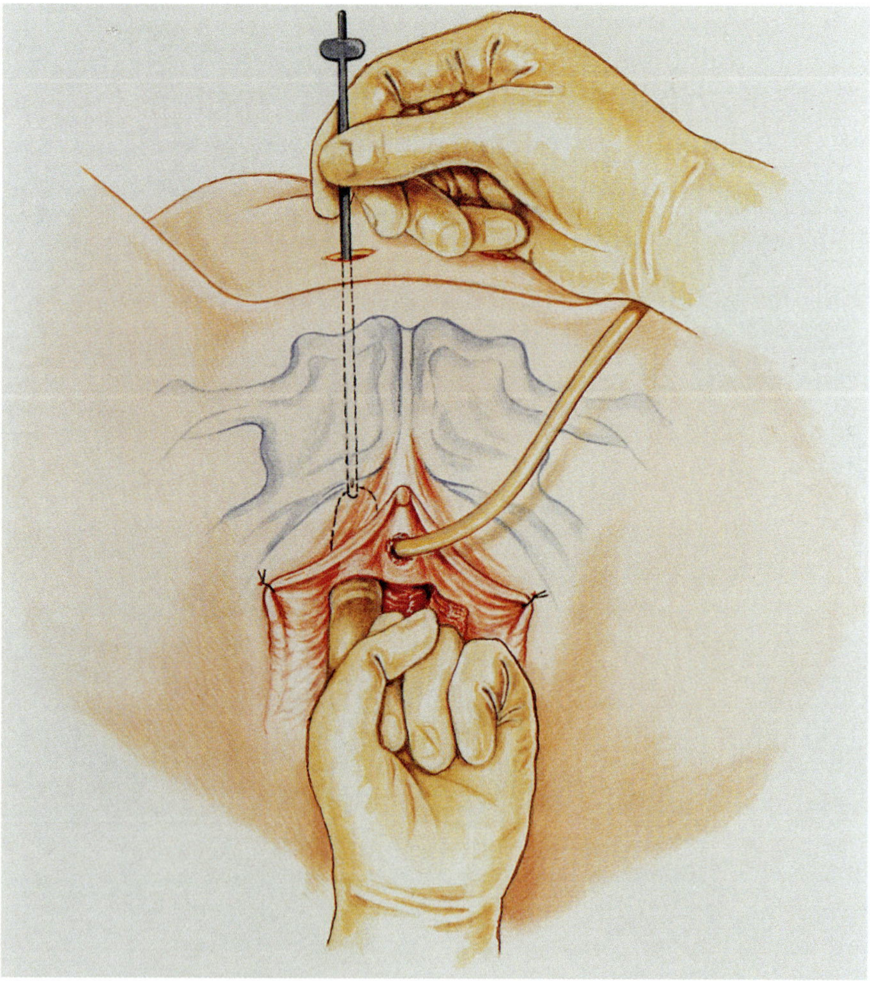

59-4

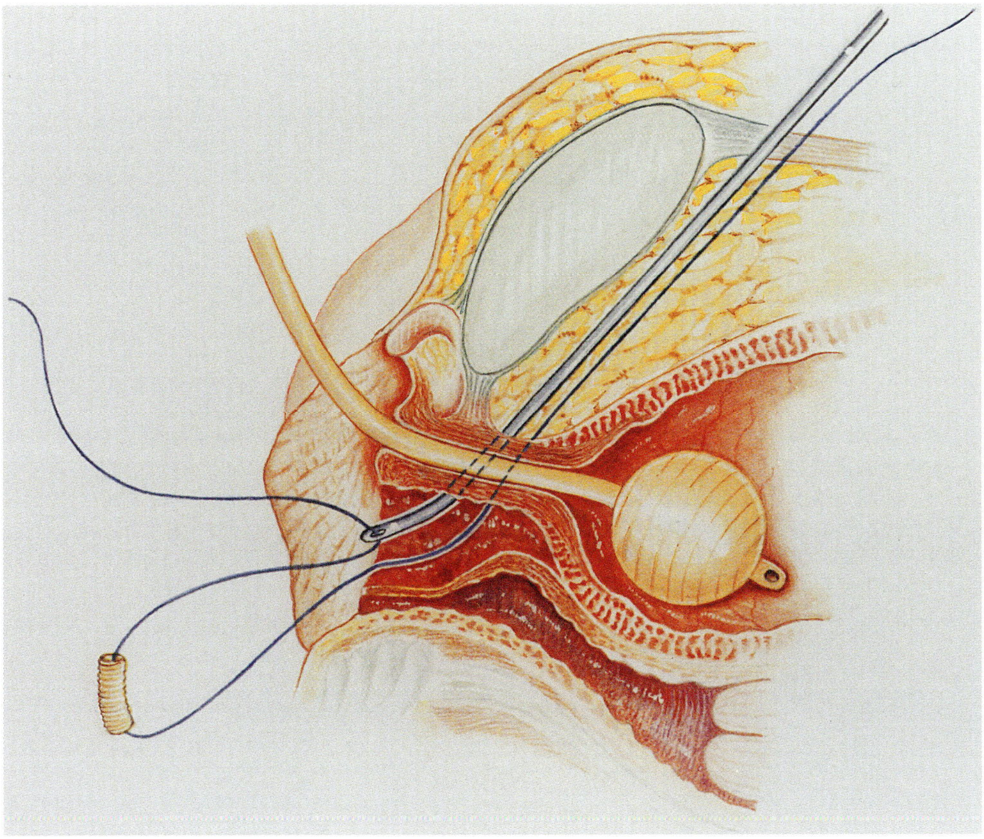

59-5

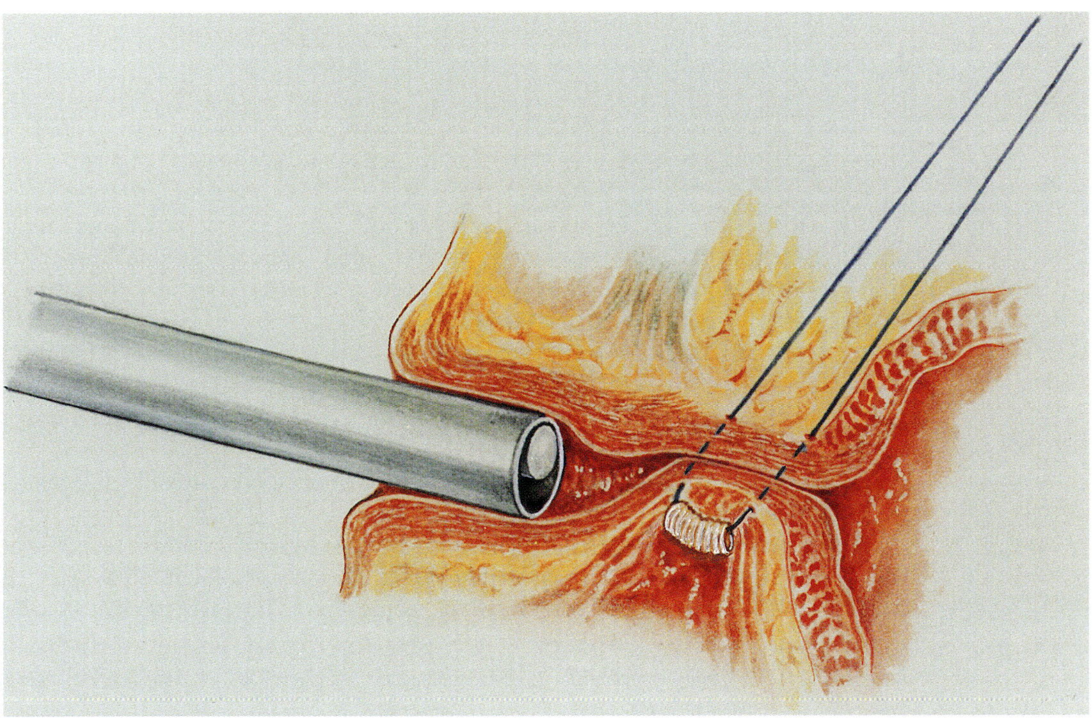

59-6

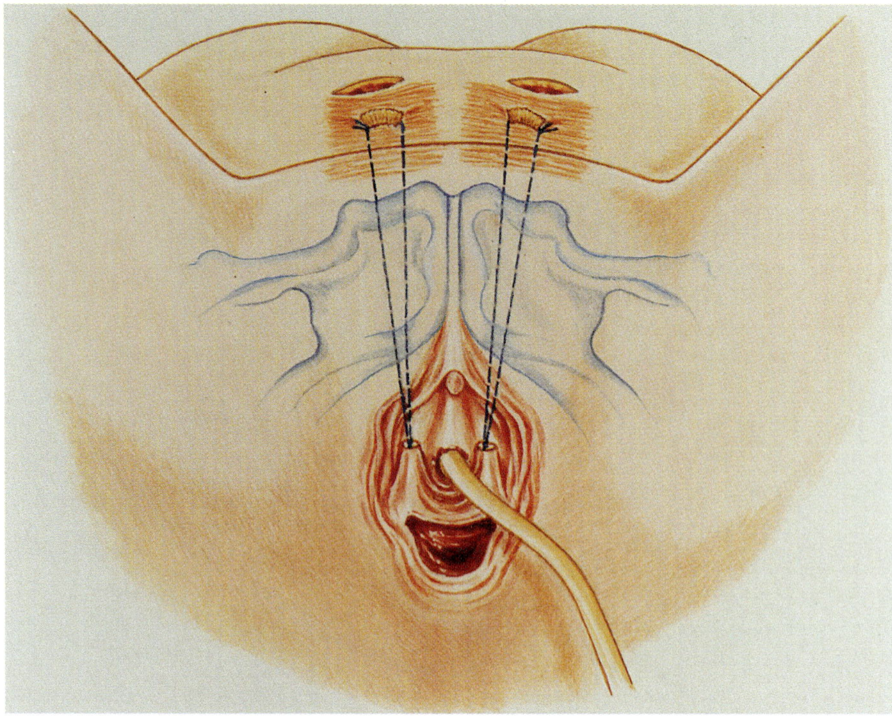

59-7

59-7. The sutures are tied over a bolster and above the anterior rectus fascia. The bolsters lie on the rectus abdominis and external oblique fascia. A Stamey suprapubic type catheter is inserted with 200 mL of saline in the bladder. A urethral catheter is usually not necessary overnight. As a rule, antibiotics are given perioperatively and continued after discharge.

60. Gittes Technique

Gittes has modified the Stamey procedure for the surgical treatment of urinary stress incontinence. His technique obviates the need for incisions. We believe a spinal or general anesthesia is necessary. We generally inject IV cephalosporin prior to anesthesia.

The patient is put in the lithotomy position, and she is prepared with appropriate cleansing solutions including povidone-iodine solution. The anus is draped out of the field. The initial exposure after draping is enhanced by using a weighted speculum to depress the posterior vaginal wall and the introitus.

A urinary catheter is inserted to empty the patient's bladder. Initial cystoscopy is not necessary because cystoscopy was performed during the initial workup. The Marshall's test had clearly demonstrated correction of the leaking bladder-urethral urinary stream after previously filling the bladder.

The Stamey needles are used and a 1–0 monofilament nylon suture is inserted into the eye of the needle.

The procedure begins with a small puncture into the suprapubic area—fat pad—just about 2 to 3 cm above the symphysis pubis but 5 cm lateral to the midline. The long Stamey needle is carefully pushed through the rectus fascia. The tip of the needle, aimed inferiorly, is advanced down the pubic bone laterally. At the same time the surgeon's other free hand is placed into the vagina and it elevates the anterior vaginal wall lateral to the catheter and the bladder neck.

60-1. Before pushing the needle through, the surgeon examines the elevated—tented up—vaginal wall to be sure of proper placement. The needle is then "popped" through the wall and then aimed forward through the introitus.

The second needle is passed through a separate rectus fascial opening (2 cm apart). Now the free tip of the needle is carefully advanced until it reaches the gloved fingers of the surgeon. If placement has been appropriate, the free end of the Prolene suture is threaded through the eye of the half-circle Mayo needle, and a distinct full bite of the vaginal wall will be taken as shown. Several circular sutures can be taken.

The second arm of the Stamey needle is attached to the vaginal end of the long suture and can be threaded. Both ends of the suture can now be lifted, and the uplift should be clearly demonstrated.

We generally perform cystoscopy after removing the urethral indwelling catheter. Generally the Stamey needle has not entered the bladder wall.

With the long arm of a second Stamey needle, the opposite side is manipulated following the opposite pubic bone. The exact maneuvers, described on one side previously, are repeated again. With the urethral catheter in place the Stamey needle with the Prolene suture enters the roof of the opposite vaginal wall.

Care is taken again to suture the vaginal wall anteriorly as seen. Cystoscopy is repeated after the indwelling catheter has been removed. When both sutures are lifted anteriorly, the angulation in the urethral wall can be observed. Care is taken to not injure the urethral wall.

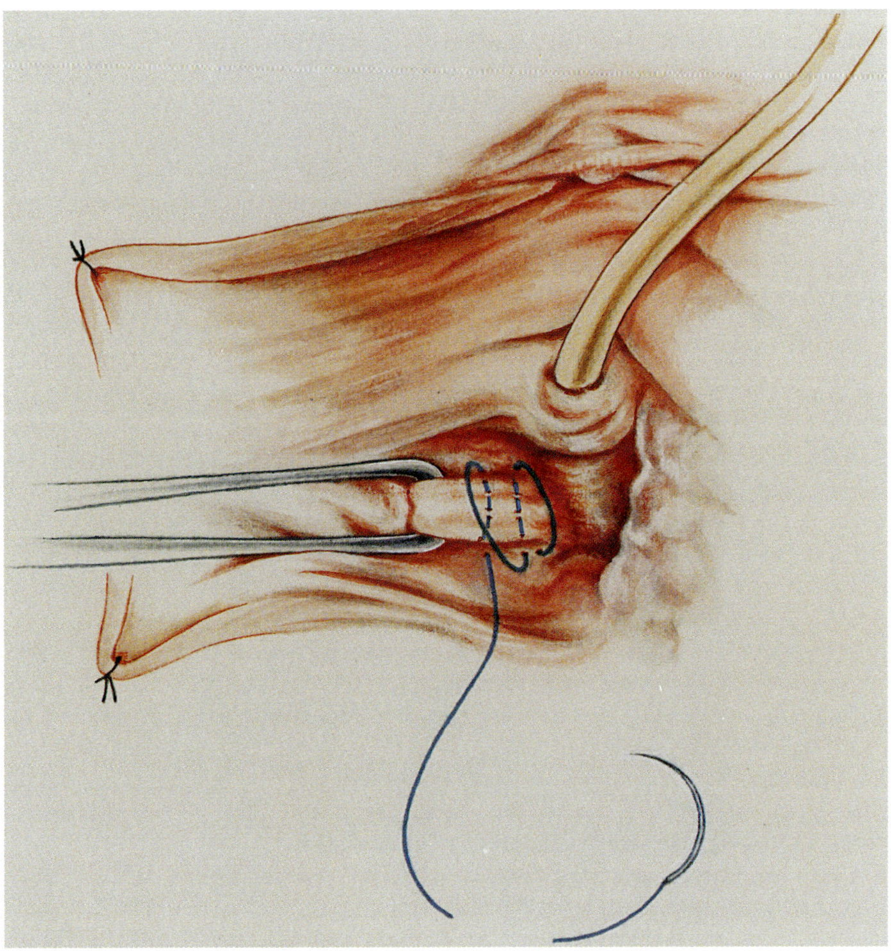

60-1

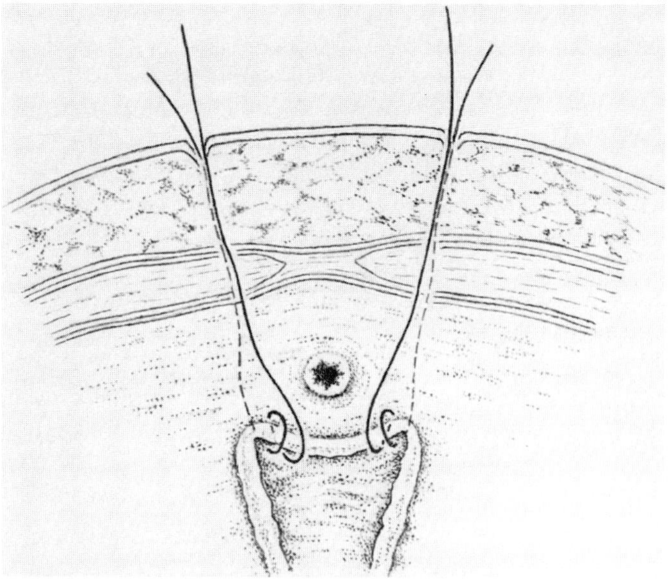

60-2

60-2. The position of the two Prolene sutures is revealed. The angulation and uplift of the urethra can be adjusted to provide urinary continence. This maneuver can be demonstrated by filling the bladder with 250–300 mL of saline. When the stress incontinence has been corrected, no leakage will appear even after pressing downward on the bladder wall.

The patient must keep the indwelling catheter in place for 2 to 4 days. She can be discharged after an overnight stay if she has traveled a long distance for this surgical correction.

61. Raz Technique: 4-Point Suspension

Prolapse of the anterior vaginal wall is a common outcome particularly after the childbearing years. Fortunately, selected procedures can correct the moderate cystocele.

According to Raz, there are three anatomic structures that are involved in the prolapse: the bladder base, the bladder neck, and the urethra. Usually all three structures can be seen and palpated in the female with stress incontinence.

On some occasions, one may see a urethral prolapse alone or in combination with a bladder cystocele. The signs and symptoms which are anatomically presented by the female include urinary incontinence, a vaginal mass or prolapse, urinary obstruction, and recurrent infections due to incomplete bladder emptying.

It is important to document that the patient has incontinence particularly after coughing or lifting a moderately heavy package. Cystoscopy and the demonstration of incontinence in the standing position are important diagnostic steps. A urodynamic study may be indicated.

We prefer spinal or general anesthesia. The patient is in the lithotomy position. A weighted vaginal speculum is used in the vagina. The labia folds are sewn laterally for exposure. We usually inject cephalosporin IV before surgery.

Unlike other incontinence procedures which focus on fixing the lax structures from below, Raz et al. insist that lifting up the bladder and resuspending it are the key steps. Permanent sutures support the bladder base by lifting it up and resuspending it. We believe that female patients with moderate cystoceles can benefit from this procedure.

61-1. A U-shaped incision is made as shown. The apex of the incision is midway between the urethral meatus and bladder neck. The base of the inverted U incision is extended further posteriorly beyond the bladder neck to the bladder base where the anterior extension of the cardinal ligaments is located. If the uterus is present, the incision is extended laterally to the cervix. Do not extend beyond this location.

61-2. The retropubic space is entered and adhesions are freed. The urethropelvic fascia is detached sharply from its attachment to the pelvic wall on both sides.

61-3. Blunt dissection of the retropubic space is used with the use of the index finger to mobilize the urethra and bladder neck.

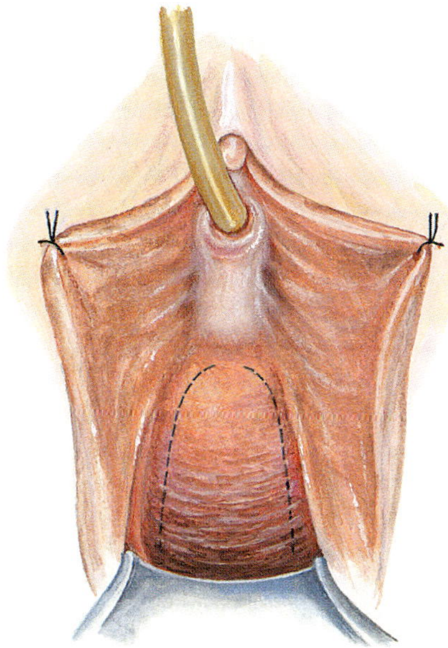

61-1

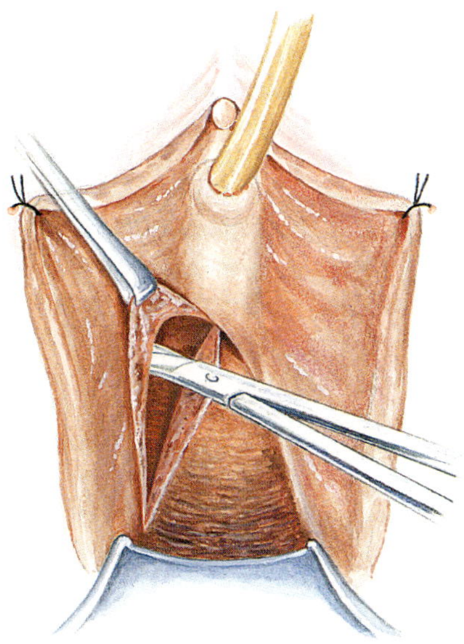

61-2

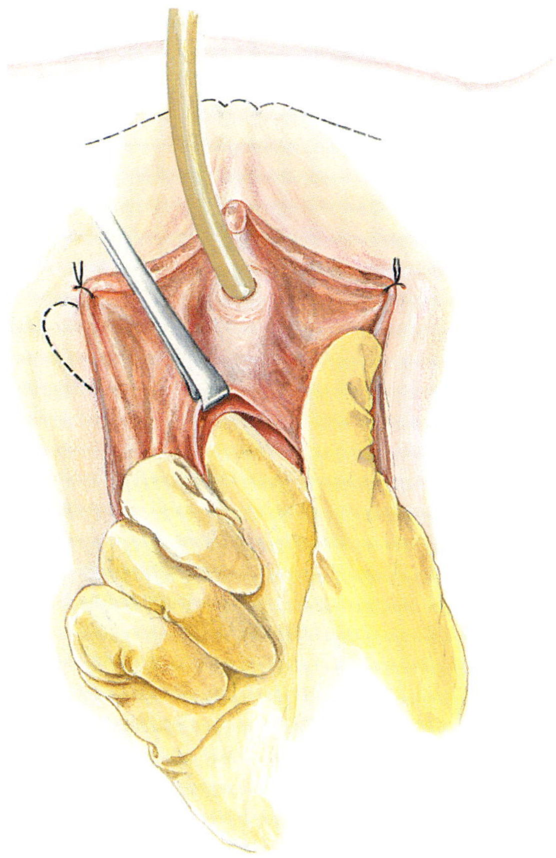

61-3

61-4. Placement of two pairs of nonabsorbable sutures is carried out including vaginal wall minus epithelium, pubocervical fascia, and medial edge of urethropelvic fascia at the level of bladder neck and the cystocele base.

61-5. Using the guidance of the index finger—left hand as shown—the Raz double pronged needles are passed from the suprapubic incision to the vaginal incision. Two sets of Prolene sutures are placed, one on each side. These sutures include vaginal wall (no epithelium), pubocervical fascia, and medial edge of the urethropelvic fascia. These sutures are near the bladder neck and include the cystocele base.

61-6. The four sets of suspending sutures are transferred to the suprapubic incision. Closure of the incision in the suprapubic area may be necessary. A suprapubic catheter is inserted. Vaginal packing is left in place until the following morning. Suprapubic tube may be removed at postoperative day 1 or 2.

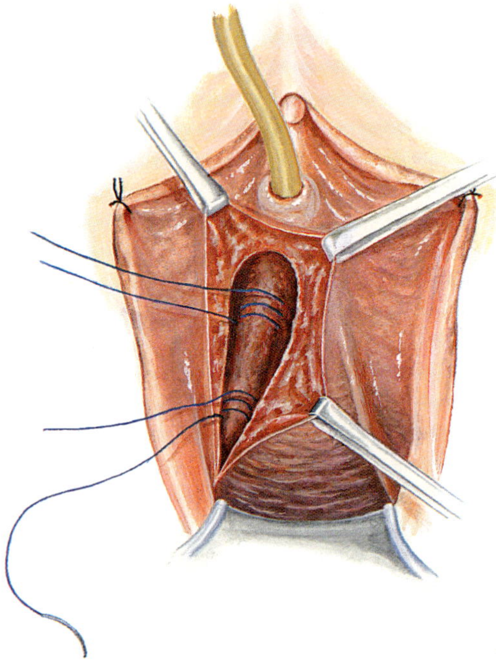

61-4

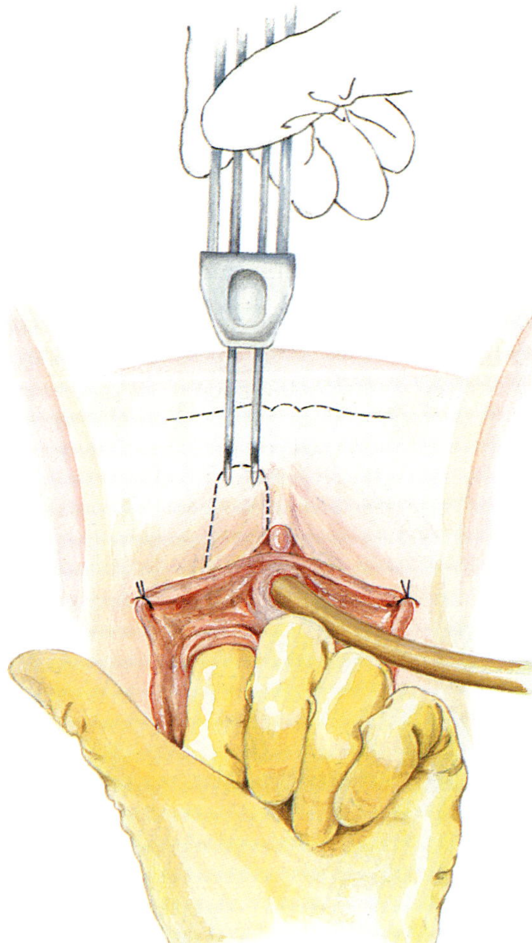

61-5

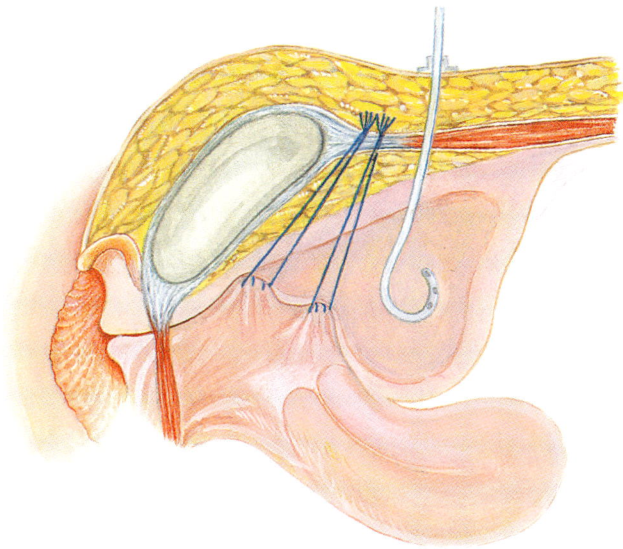

61-6

62. Marshall-Marchetti-Krantz Procedure

When a middle-aged female presents with stress incontinence, care must be taken to rule out other causes of urinary incontinence. Infection will cause an urgency incontinence coupled with frequency. Overflow incontinence must be excluded. Every attempt must be made to rule out the presence of a neurogenic bladder.

We routinely schedule each patient for urologic evaluation, obtaining a history and performing a physical examination. The presence of a cystocele and/or urethrocele is noted. Urinalysis will assist in ruling out urinary infection. If infection is present, then an intravenous pyelogram may be indicated.

We usually obtain a cystometrogram at the second office visit. In addition, we perform cystoscopy. If bladder capacity is normal, and stress incontinence is present, then we perform the Marshall test by refilling the bladder with 300 mL saline. We have been pleased with the voiding phase of the test performed in the upright position. The patient with a full bladder sits on the edge of the cystoscopy table with her lower extremities in the dependent sitting position. While the gloved hand raises the superior vesicourethral angle, the patient is urged to cough. This exercise is repeated after the pressure on the bladder neck is released. Selected patients who respond and become continent when the bladder neck is elevated are excellent candidates for the procedure.

If the middle-aged female patient has a cystocele, urethrocele, and a rectocele, then we refer her to the gynecologist for an anterior and posterior colporrhaphy.

The patient is placed in the lithotomy position and her lower legs are placed into stirrups. An alternative position can also be used. The knees are separated and the thighs are elevated on several long rolls; access to the vagina is important during this procedure.

The skin in the suprapubic area is prepared in the usual manner. The vagina and introitus are also carefully prepared and cleansed with povidone-iodine (Betadine). After the wound has been draped, the bladder is filled with approximately 250 mL saline. The 18 Fr Foley catheter is left indwelling.

In an older patient, a vertical midline incision may be used. We prefer a transverse skin incision in the younger or middle-aged patient.

The incision is made. Fascia is incised. Rectus abdominis muscles are separated from the vertical midline. The prevesical fat is removed from the anterior bladder and urethra.

62-1. *Four parallel pairs of 0-0 chromic catgut sutures elevate and reform the posterior vesicourethral angle.* The sutures are placed into the anterior vaginal wall lateral to urethra and left untied. The indwelling catheter assists in demarcating the location of the urethra and bladder neck. The first pair of sutures is placed approximately 1 cm inferior to the bladder neck and attached to the inferior periosteum covering the symphysis pubis. The second set of sutures is placed lateral to the bladder neck and into the periosteum, located more anteriorly and superiorly than the first set. These sutures also are not tied at this point. The third set of sutures is placed 1 cm superior to the bladder neck, and the sutures then enter the outer two-thirds of the bladder wall. The same sutures enter the periosteum still more anteriorly and superiorly. A fourth set of sutures is placed 2 cm superior to the bladder neck and inserted into the rectus fascia on each side.

An assistant now places his index and middle finger into the vagina and elevates the bladder neck. The four pairs of sutures are tied and secured during this maneuver.

62-2. *A midsagittal view through the midbladder, symphysis pubis, and urethra.* The sutures have been placed and tied.

The catheter is left indwelling for 7 days. We close the wound in the usual fashion. If hemostasis is maintained, a flat tubular drain is not needed. We usually place a vaginal pack deep into the vagina to assist in maintaining the proper bladder neck angle. The pack is removed after 36 to 48 hours. The patient should avoid lifting or increased activity for 7 to 10 days.

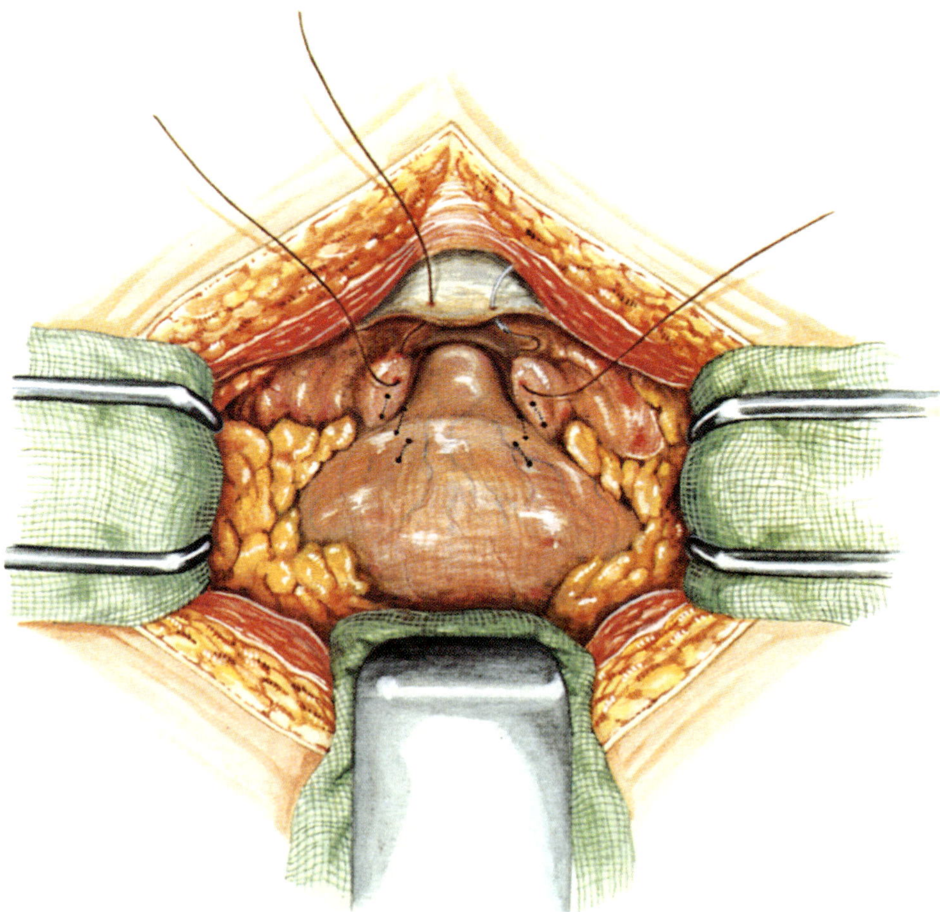

62-1

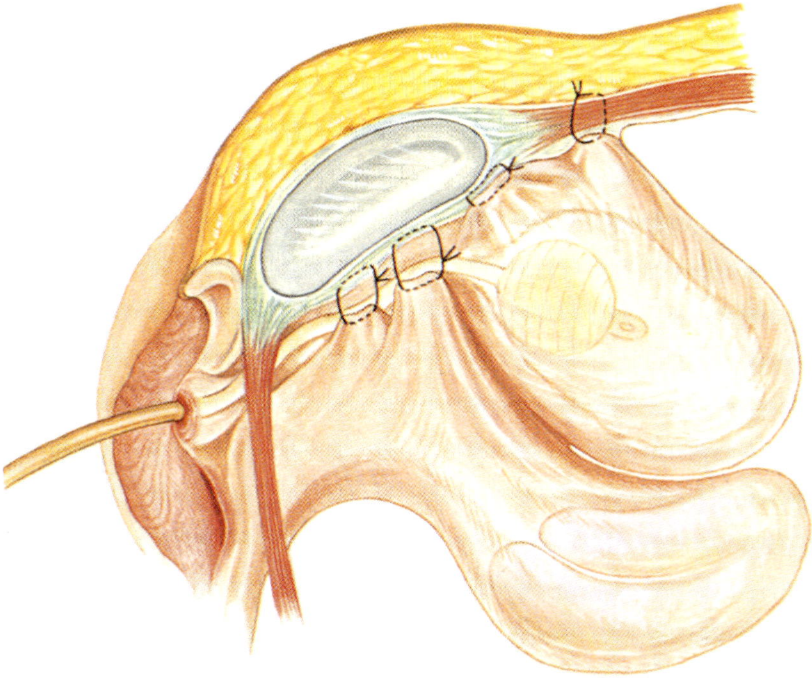

62-2

INTRAOPERATIVE AND POSTOPERATIVE ANTIBIOTIC TREATMENT

Ceftriaxone is a broad spectrum cephalosporin which can be given intravenously or intramuscularly. Depending on the size of the patient, the initial dose can be 1 g in an average adult or 1.5 to 2 g in a large adult. Twelve hours following intramuscular administration the blood levels are in the 50% range from the initial dose of 1 g.

Suggested Readings

Bischoff PF. Operative treatment of megaureter. J Urol 85:268, 1961.

Bricker EM. Bladder substitution after pelvic evisceration. Surg Clin North Am 30:1511, 1950.

Cockett ATK, Davis RS, Cos LR, Wheeless LL, Jr. Bacillus Calmette-Guérin and interleukin-2 for treatment of superficial bladder cancer. J Urol 146:766–770, 1990.

Cockett ATK, di Sant'Agnese PA, Hamlin DJ, Keys HM. Porcine sensitized lymph node cells (immunotherapy) and attenuated irradiation for infiltrative transitional cell carcinoma of bladder. Urology 19:593–598, 1982.

Gittes RF, Loughlin KR. No incision pubovaginal suspension for stress incontinence. J Urol 138:568–570, 1987.

Goodwin WE. Ileocystoplasty. Surg Gynecol Obstet 108:240, 1959.

Hamlin DJ, Cockett ATK. Computed tomography of bladder: staging of bladder cancer using low density opacification technique. Urology 13:331–334, 1979.

Jewett HJ, Strong GH. Infiltrating carcinoma of the bladder: Relation of depth of penetration of the baldder wall to incidence of local extension and metastases. J Urol 55:366, 1946.

Marshall VF. The relation of the preoperative estimate to the pathologic demonstration of the extent of vesicle neoplasms. J Urol 68:714, 1952.

Ockerblad NF. Reimplantation of the ureter into the bladder by a flap method. J Urol 57:845, 1947.

Raz S, Klutke CG, Golomb J. Four-corner bladder and urethral suspension for moderate cystocele. J Urol 142:712–715, 1989.

4 Urinary Diversion

Operative Techniques

63. Unilateral and Bilateral Cutaneous Ureterostomy

This procedure can be useful for patients suffering from renal insufficiency or for palliation in patients with carcinoma. For long-term urinary diversion, the procedure is contraindicated because of infection and progressive narrowing of the stomas.

63-1. *Potential sites for placement of ureteral stomas* (circles on left and right sides). In the midline inferior to the umbilicus, both ureteral ends can be joined and brought out as a single stoma.

After potential sites on the skin are marked, a vertical midline transabdominal incision is made to allow access and to conveniently locate both upper ureters. The peritoneum and fascial lining lateral to the ascending and descending colon are incised longitudinally, allowing medial retraction of the large bowel for full exposure of the ureters. The ureters are severed at the most inferior point to allow optimum placement without tension. The lower ureteral ends are ligated, using 2–0 chromic catgut.

63-2. The ureter is freed. *A clamp is used to initiate the new ureteral pathway* to a previously selected stomal site. A small skin incision is made and carried through the fascia to allow the clamp free access to the skin opening. A rubber ureteral catheter (6 French) can be grasped and drawn into the peritoneal space, where it is introduced into the ureter and appropriately tied.

63-3. *The catheter is grasped and gently withdrawn* through the newly created tunnel. Two 3–0 chronic catgut sutures are used to secure the ureter (periadventitial ureter to fascia) at the stomal site.

63-4. The *catheter is withdrawn.* Excessive ureter is excised and the ureteral stoma is widened.

63-5. The flat tubular drain is seen. We now use a Jackson-Pratt closed drainage tube

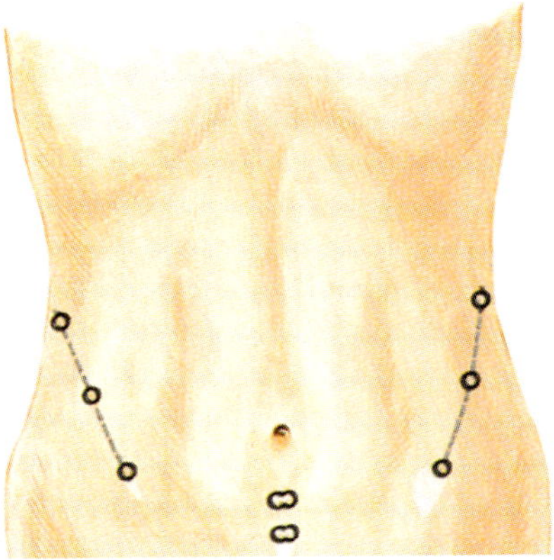

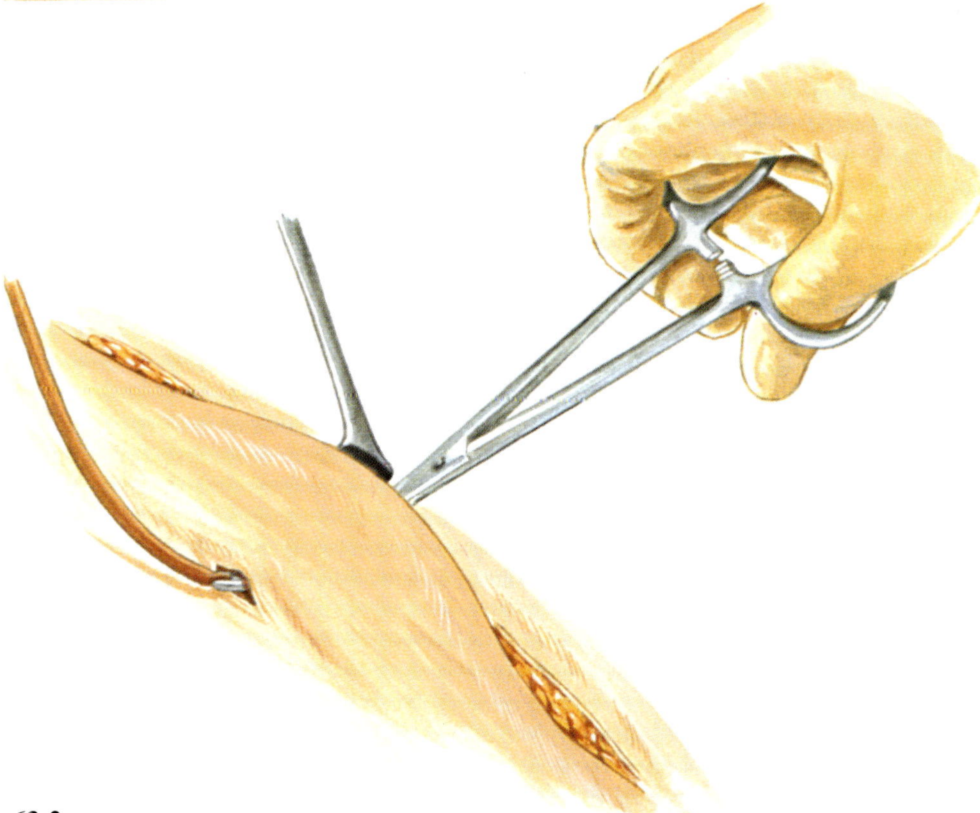

63-2

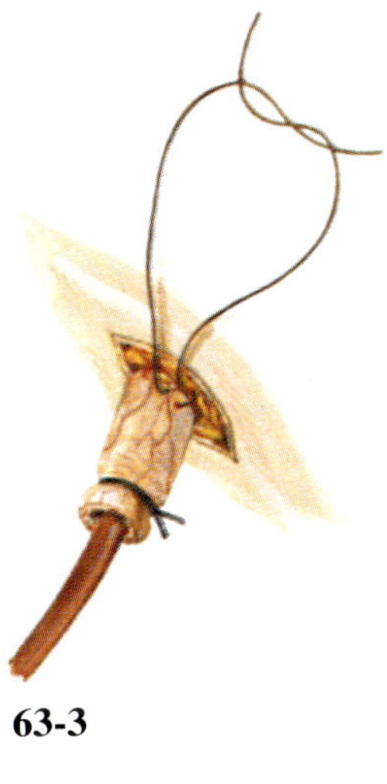

63-3

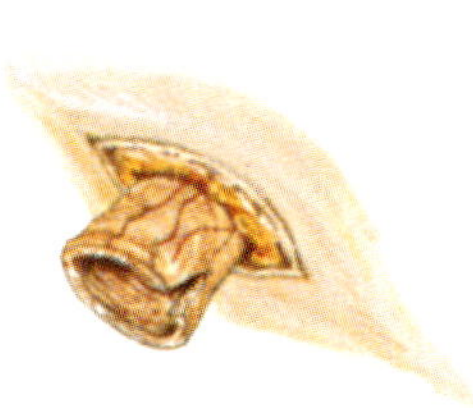

63-4

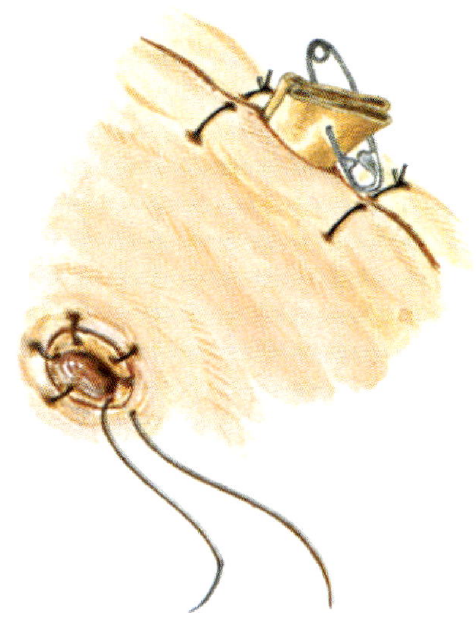

63-5

to discourage infection. The compressible bulb on the distal end provides a negative pressure, thus allowing the tissue fluid to collect in the lumen of the bulb or the closed drainage bag.

64. Creation of Stomal Nipple

The advantages of this approach over the foregoing method include the extraperitoneal exposure of the ureter and formation of a skin nipple for more convenient stomal management.

64-1. The *incisions are made for ureteral access and creation of a skin flap.* The ureter is brought out through the peritoneum and is freed and severed. The inferior end is ligated. A ureteral catheter (6 Fr) is introduced, secured, lifted, and withdrawn to the mid-incision site.

64-2. *The ureter is in place for creation of the stomal nipple.* Note the presence of a Penrose drain. A Jackson-Pratt closed drainage tube has replaced this drain.

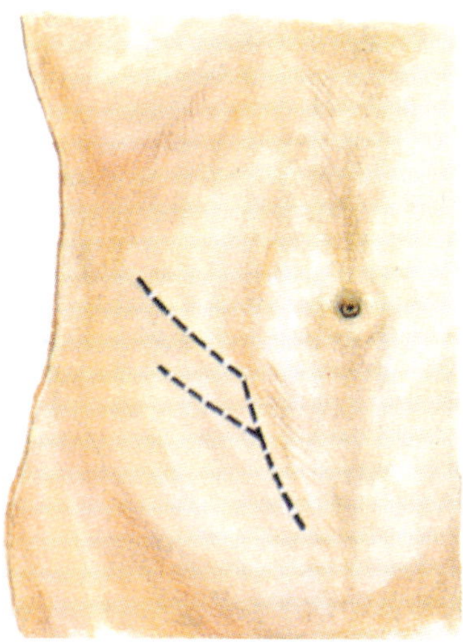

64-1

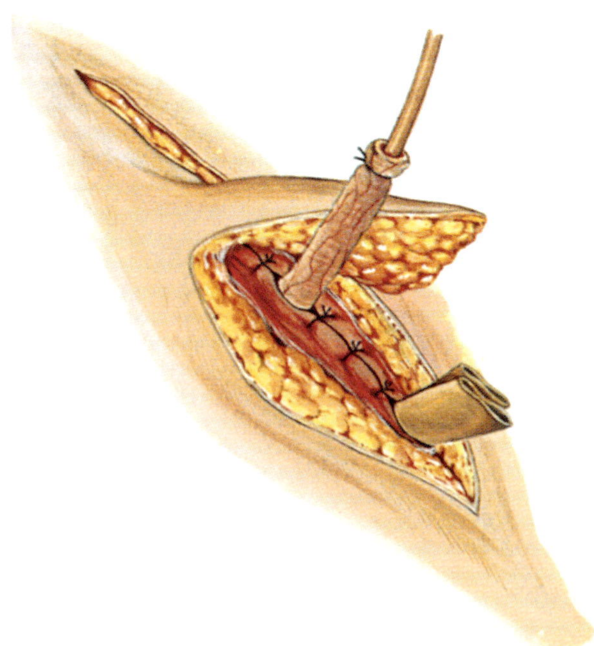

64-2

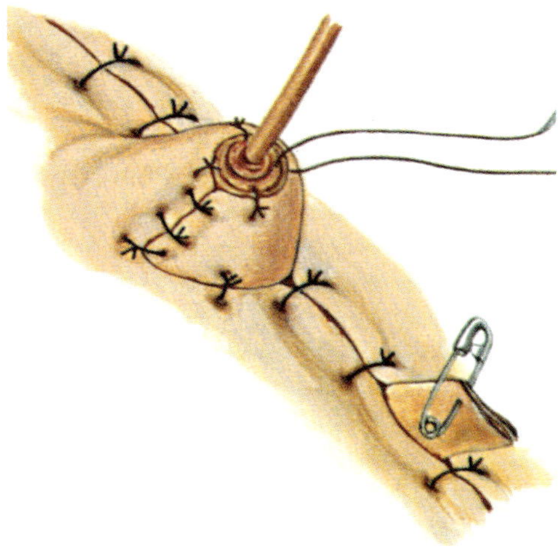

64-3

64-3. *The nipple has been formed* and the stomal site has been secured with interrupted sutures (4–0 chromic catgut).

65. Bilateral Cutaneous Ureterostomy with Combined Stoma

See **37–1** for the potential site of midline ureteral stomal placement. A vertical midline transabdominal incision is made from the midepigastrium to the umbilicus.

65-1. The schematic demonstrates the selected *location of the combined stomal site* and the approximations of the lower freed ends of the ureter. The development of the stomal tunnel is facilitated by intraperitoneal access to this region. An incision is made as indicated by the dotted line. The ureters are brought through the opening. This maneuver is facilitated by the use of stay sutures.

65-2. Each ureter is incised longitudinally for 2 cm in a line facing each other. The *newly created common posterior stomal wall* is reapproximated and sutured as shown.

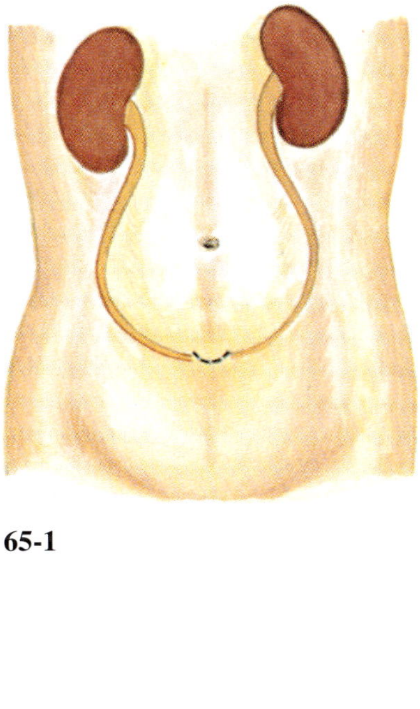

65-1

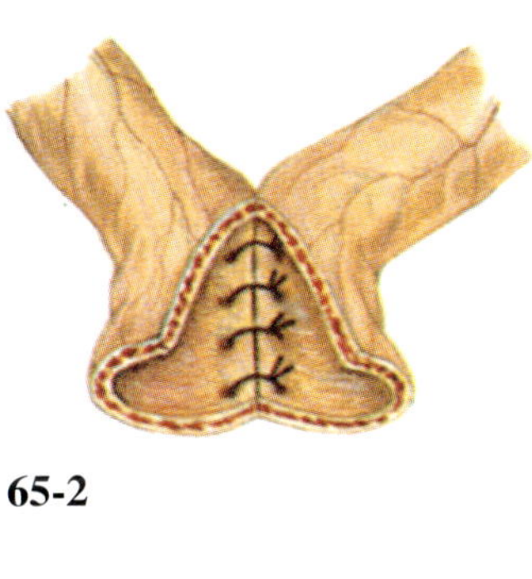

65-2

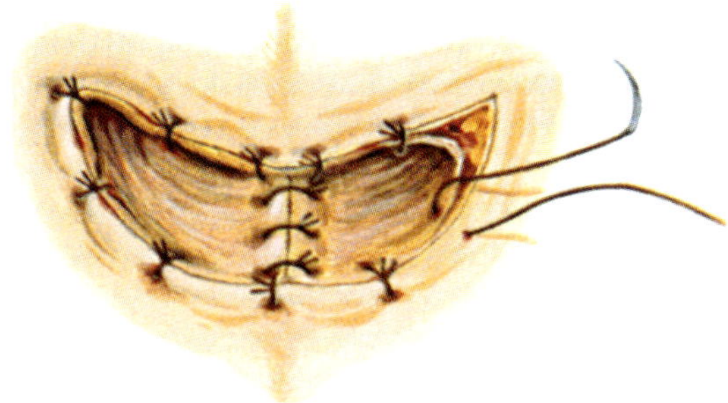

65-3

65-3. *The stoma is large and broad* enough to be secured directly to the skin margin and appropriately sutured.

A urinary collection bag (ileostomy bag) can easily be placed over the new stoma.

Sterilization of Large Intestine Prior to Surgery

Our standard regimen consists of 4 liters of Colyte (Reed and Carnrick, Jersey City, NJ), a polyethylene glycol mixture that is not absorbed. Refrigerating the solution prior to drinking it is helpful.

The antibiotic regimen is as follows: neomycin 1 g × 3 (taken orally at 1 PM, 2 PM, and 11 PM) and erythromycin base × 3 (taken orally at 1 PM, 2 PM, and 11 PM). If bowel contents are not clear, a tap water enema may be administered.

66. Bilateral Ureterosigmoidostomy (Goodwin Procedure[1])

Goodwin stated that this operation "is due for a renascence."[2] We agree.

Patient selection is important in this procedure. The ureters must be of normal caliber. Total renal function should be close to normal levels. A competent anal sphincter must be present. This can be determined by introducing a fluid load of 5 to 7 ounces through the anal sphincter. Any fluid leakage would preclude use of the procedure. If megavoltage irradiation is contemplated to the pelvic bed, e.g., in infiltrative bladder carcinoma, then this operation is contraindicated. However, a modified alternative can be substituted. A sigmoid segment of the colon can be fashioned and isolated to serve as a urinary conduit. The distal end is brought to the skin. The ureters are implanted through a submucosal tunnel, preventing urinary regurgitation.

The obvious advantages of this procedure are 1) no external urinary collecting device is needed and 2) the ureteral antireflux procedure discourages reflux and prevents pyelonephritis.

Preoperative Considerations. Adequate bowel sterilization procedures are mandatory. An antibiotic—neomycin—for 48 hours before surgery is mandatory. The generous use of enemas is necessary. A low-residue diet is helpful.

Incision. A vertical midline transabdominal incision is extended from the mid-epigastrium, curving around the umbilicus, and continuing inferiorly for 10 cm. The peritoneal cavity is entered, and routine inspection and palpation of the abdominal contents are carried out.

The small bowel is placed in a moist plastic bag, the noose in the bag is tightened at the base of the small bowel mesentery. The small intestine and bag are lifted out of the abdominal cavity and placed on the right anterior abdominal wall.

The posterior peritoneum is incised longitudinally over each mid-ureter. The ureters are found as they cross the bifurcation of the common iliac arteries. The ureters are freed inferiorly, clamped, transected, and ligated inferiorly. The free ureteral ends are secured with stay sutures and passed into the peritoneal cavity.

66-1. *The contiguous sigmoid colon at the promontory of the sacrum is elevated* by means of a rubber-shod intestinal clamp. The freed left ureter is seen.

66-2. *The right ureter* is seen.

66-3. *The sigmoid colon is incised anteriorly* along the taenia. Stay sutures are strategically placed. The bowel lumen is readily visible.

66–4. *The sigmoid mucosa has been incised posteriorly* in two areas to accommodate the ureters. A right-angle or curved cystic-duct clamp can be used to dissect through the bowel wall and adjacent posterior serosa. The stay suture is grasped, and the ureter is gently drawn through the posterior wall. A similar maneuver is used for the contralateral ureter. It is important to prevent kinking, tension, or twisting of the ureters as each courses through the mesosigmoid and posterior sigmoid segment of the bowel.

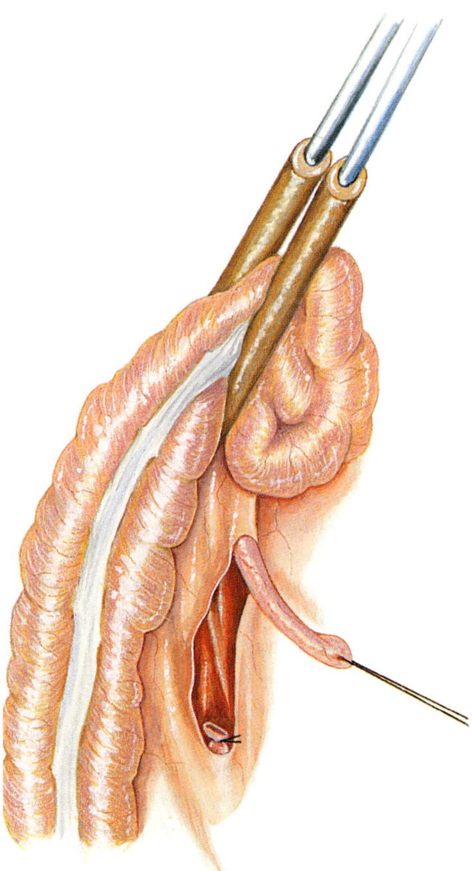

66-1

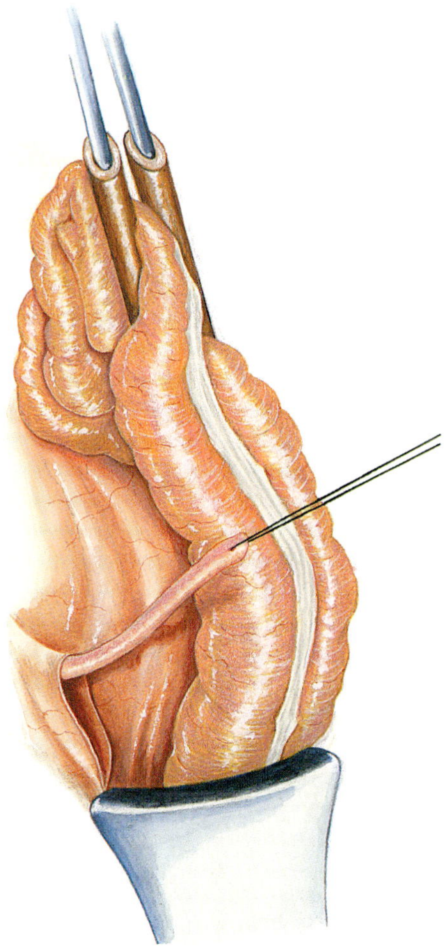

66-2

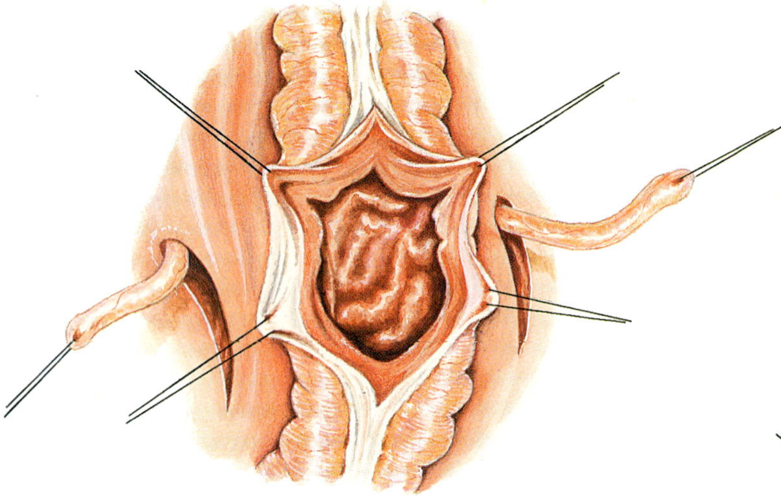

66-3

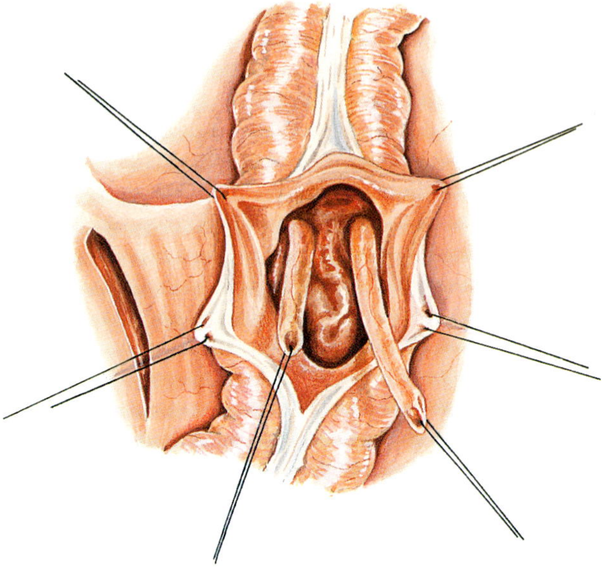

66-4

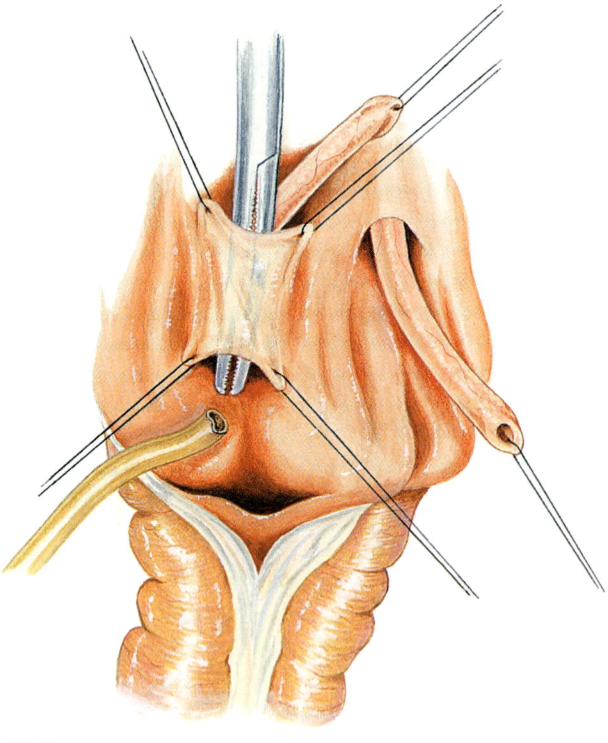

66-5

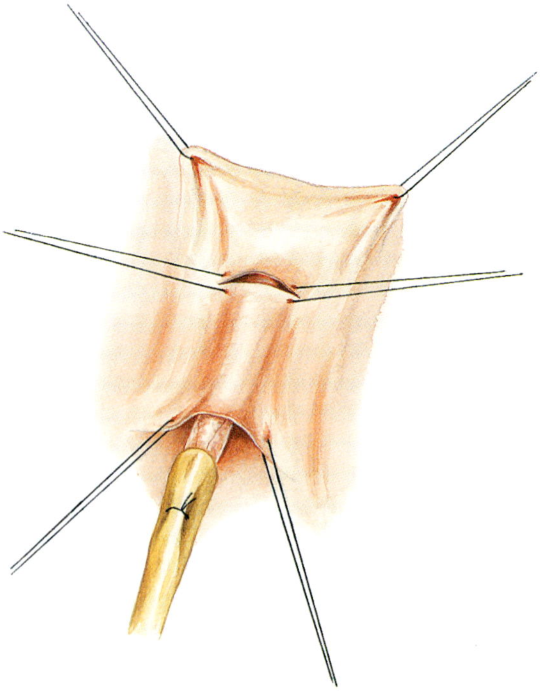

66-6

66-5. *A submucosal tunnel is created inferior to the point of ureteral insertion.* Four stay sutures assist in marking the length of the tunnel (tunnel length should be six times the diameter of the ureter). A small flat tubular drain is grasped.

66-6. *The flat tubular drain is pulled through the tunnel superiorly* and positioned so that the open end caps the end of the ureter. A single suture is used to secure the junction.

66-7. *The flat tubular drain is grasped and slowly pulled back out of the tunnel,* bringing the secured ureter along with it. Note that stay sutures placed superiorly help flatten redundant mucosa.

66-8. *The superior opening in the mucosa is sutured* (4–0 chromic catgut). The terminal point of the ureter in the sigmoid lumen is fixed by interrupted 4–0 chromic catgut sutures as shown. A ureteral stent (5 Fr pediatric feeding tube) is introduced into the ureter to rule out obstruction. The contralateral ureterosigmoid anastomosis is carried out in the same manner.

66-9. *The ureterointestinal anastomosis is completed on both sides.* The superior ends of the ureteral stents reside in the renal pelvis.

To accommodate the inferior position of the stents, a sterile rectal tube is passed to the open sigmoid. The stents are tucked within the lumen, and the rectal tube is withdrawn. Ureteral stents remain in place for 3 to 4 days.

66-10. The sigmoid and peritoneal opening are closed. Closure of the sigmoid is performed in two layers. The inner mucosal lining is reapproximated and sutured with running 3–0 chromic catgut. The taenia is reapproximated with interrupted 3–0 silk sutures. The peritoneal openings are sutured with 4–0 chromic catgut.

Closure of the abdominal wound is performed in the standard manner. A Jackson-Pratt closed drainage tube, placed extraperitoneally, may be used for 1 to 2 days.

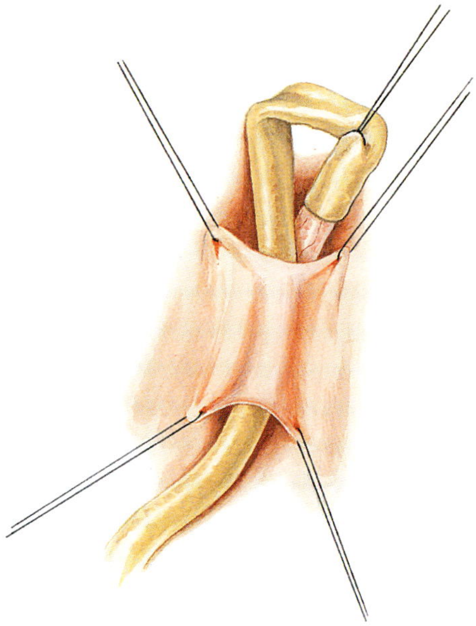

66-7

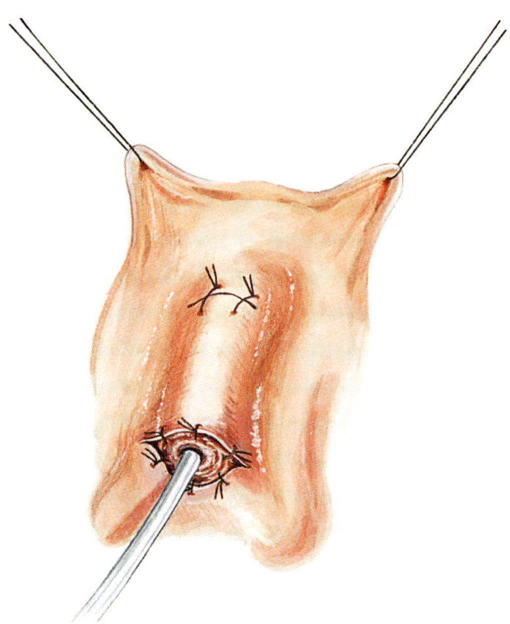

66-8

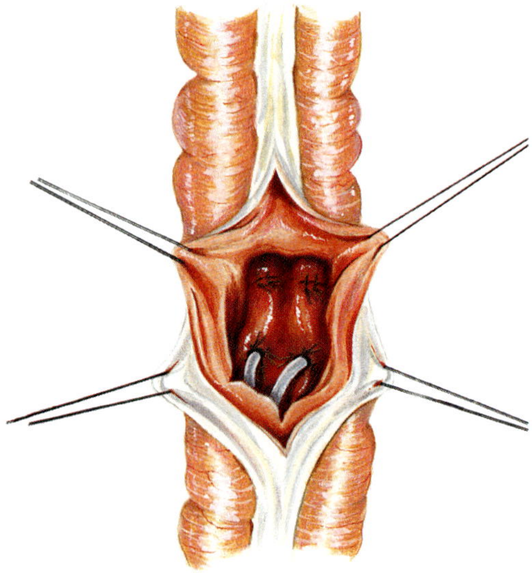

66-9

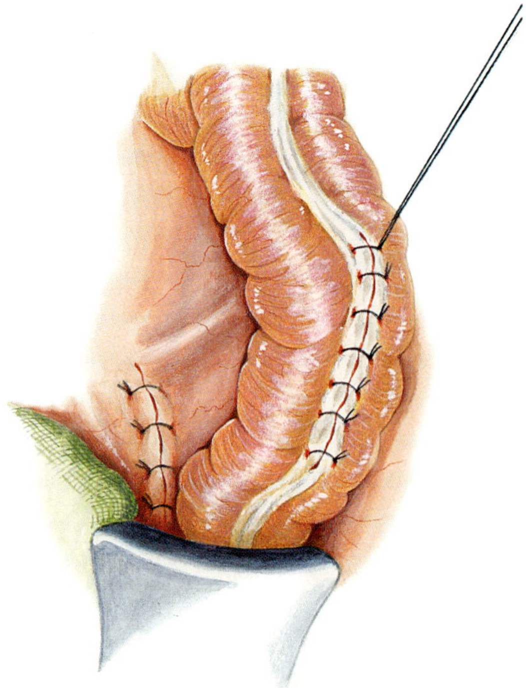

66-10

67. Ureterosigmoid Anastomosis from Outside the Sigmoid

67-1. Schematic of an *anastomosis through the posterolateral sigmoid.* The ureter is being sutured to bowel mucosa (at left). After the anastomosis is completed, the adjoining ureter is laid in the trough between submucosa and longitudinal muscle layers and the trough is closed (at right).

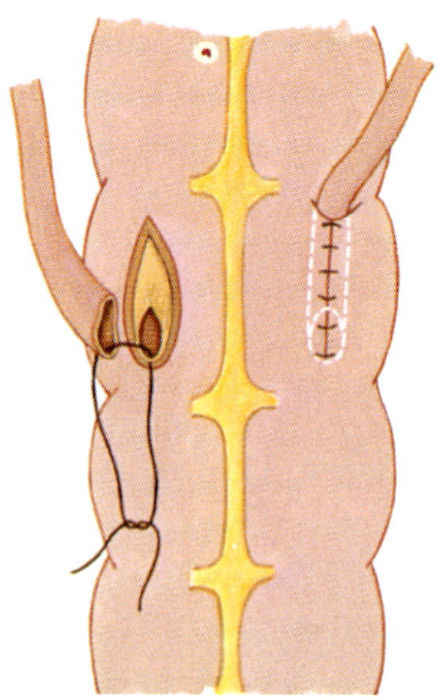

67-1

68. Other Ureterointestinal Anastomotic Procedures

A ureteral substitute may be formed from a segment of ileum.

68-1. Schematic of *ureterointestinal anastomosis to an isolated segment of ileum.* Urine is transported in isoperistaltic fashion. The distal tip of ileum is anastomosed to the posterior bladder wall.

68-2. *In this ipsilateral ureteral anastomosis,* a segment of ileum serves as a ureteral substitute.

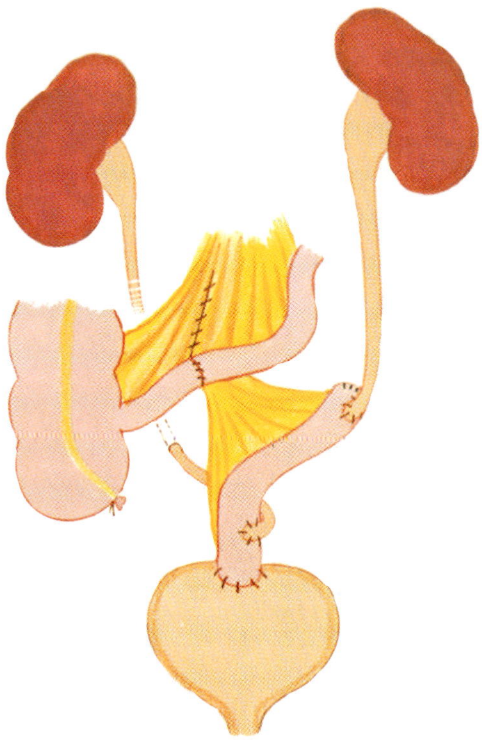

68-1

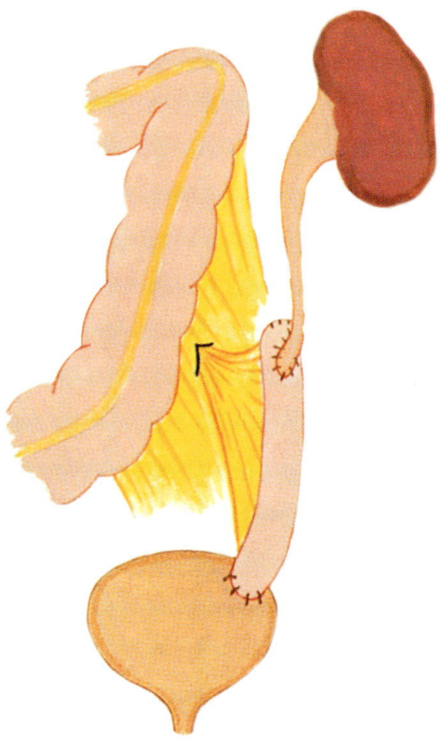

68-2

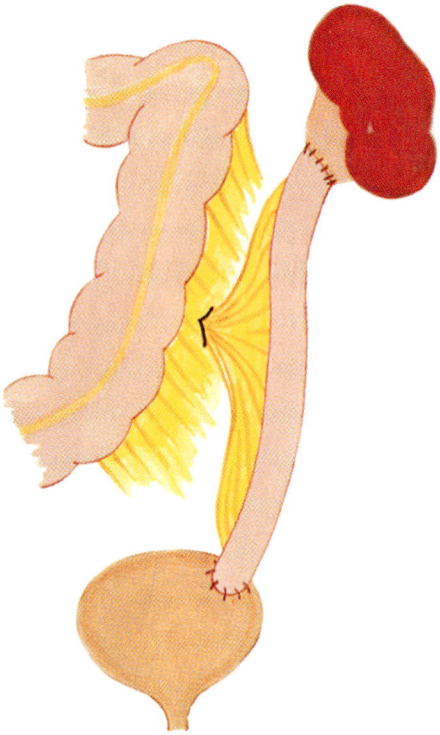

68-3

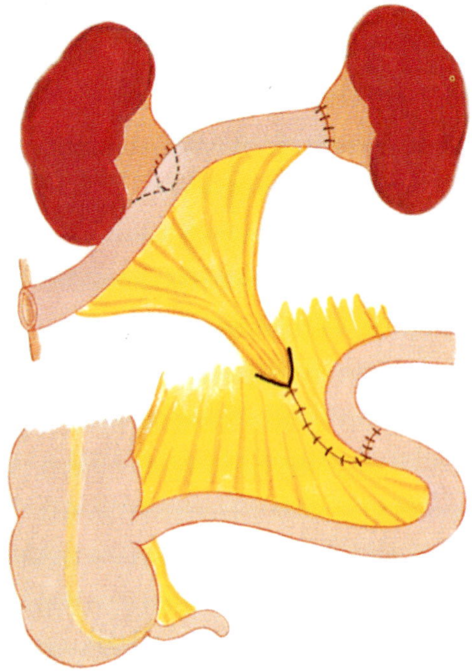

68-4

68-3. *Total ureteral substitution* is accomplished by an isoperistaltic segment of ileum.

68-4. *A segment of ileum serves as a common ureter for both kidneys.* The left renal pelvis is sutured end to end; the right renal pelvis is end to side, and the tip of the ileum is fashioned into a cutaneous stoma. The ileal segment transports urine from left to right in isoperistaltic fashion.

69. Ileal Conduit (Bricker Loop[3])

69-1. This procedure is sometimes staged and performed independently prior to cystectomy. *The segment of ileum with its blood supply is prepared.* Bowel continuity is reestablished. The proximal end of the isolated ileum is closed with two layers of 3–0 chromic catgut sutures. An appendectomy is performed. The distal opening of the ileum is catheterized to flush out residual mucoid material.

69-2. *The upper segment of the left ureter must now be carefully guided behind the mesosigmoid to a new location in a more medial position.* Care must be taken to prevent kinking in the upper left ureter.

Each ureter is brought through the posterior peritoneum and cut on a bias. An opening in the antimesenteric border of the ileum is made to accommodate the exact diameter of each ureter. Redundant mucosa is usually included in the small button of ileal wall removed. The ureteral anastomoses are made using 4–0 chromic catgut. The size of the intestinal conduit is noted so that an appropriate incision can be made at the previously determined skin site (see 69–1). A circumferential button of skin is excised. A similar size circle of fascia is removed. The abdominal muscles are separated by blunt dissection. A button of anterior peritoneum is removed. The opening in the abdominal wall is ready to accommodate the distal isolated segment of ileum.

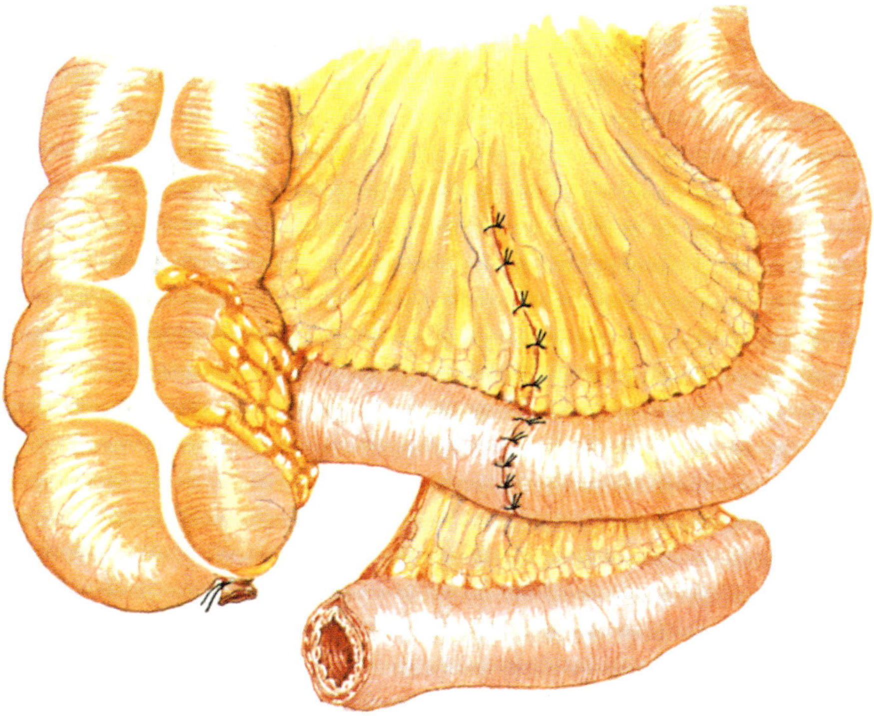

69-1

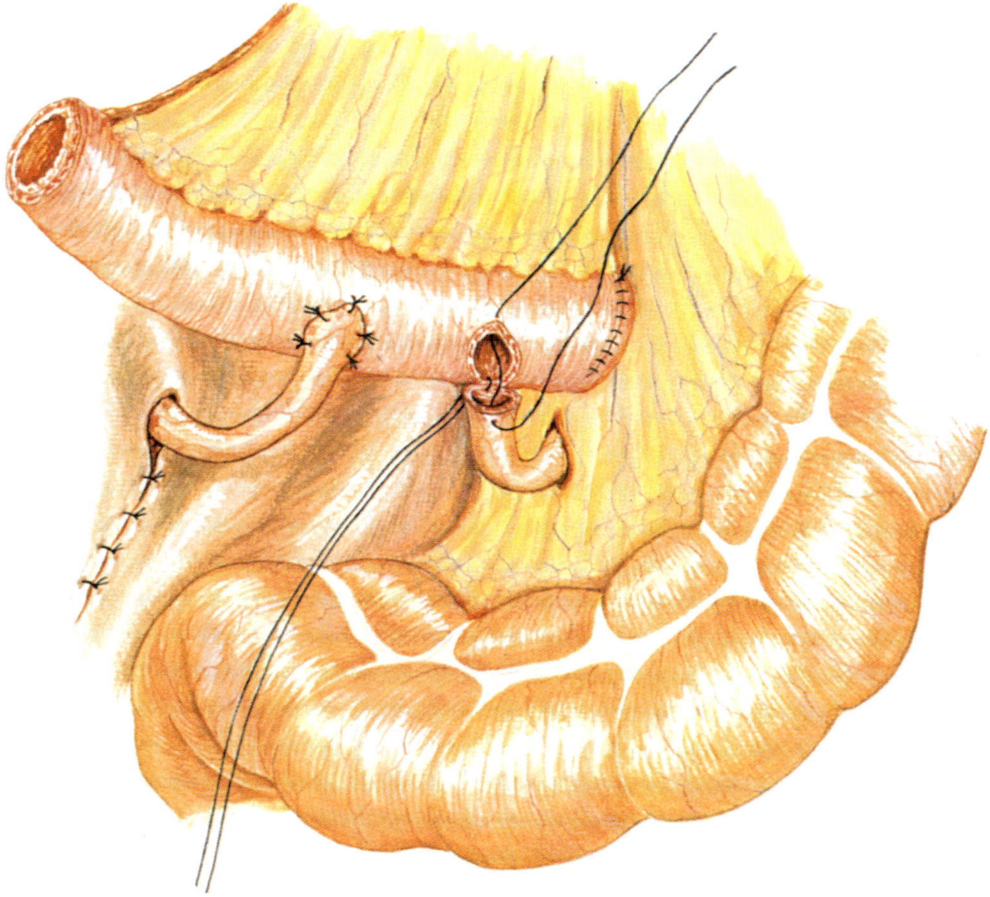

69-2

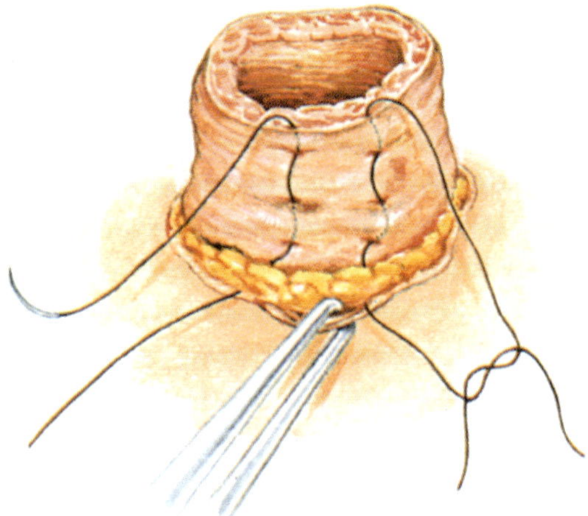

69-3

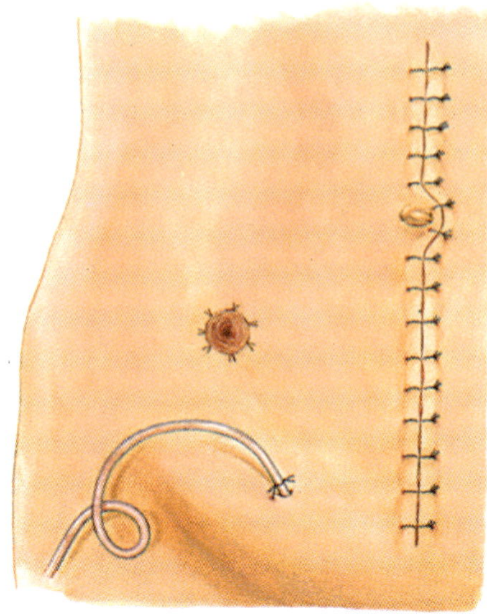

69-4

69-3. *The distal ileum is grasped and gently pulled through the stoma* with Allis clamps. The ileum is secured to the anterior peritoneum to prevent potential herniation. The ileum is then sutured to the fascia. Chromic catgut (3–0) stitches are placed circumferentially prior to eversion.

69-4. *The ileum is everted into a cuff.* The interrupted sutures are tied. A hemovac tube is positioned as shown to drain the pelvic cavity and is secured to the skin for 4 to 6 days. The muscles are reapproximated. The fascia is closed with interrupted nylon sutures (1–0). The abdominal skin is closed with interrupted sutures.

70. Variation of a Technique for Ileal Loop Urinary Diversion

70-1 and 70-2. The David Wallace technique. In this procedure the left ureter is cut longitudinally along one side as shown and the ureter is used to cap the proximal end of the ileal segment (70–1). The advantage of this technique is that the ureteral cap allows good healing (70–2) and there is less likelihood of stenosis developing. We have found that prior to completing the anastomosis, we pass a double J stent, 6 or 7 Fr in size, up the left ureter allowing the one J to curl inside the pelvis of the left kidney. After completing both ureteral anastomoses and creating the ileal stoma through the body wall, both double J stents are brought out through the stoma. A suture is placed around each stent to maintain its position for at least 7 days. The excessive distal J is cut and discarded. We mark the left stent by cutting the distal end without the J in a biased or oblique position representing the left side. The right single ureteral J stent has a right angle cut at the ileal stomal margin. Both stents are carefully sutured to the ileal stoma initially.

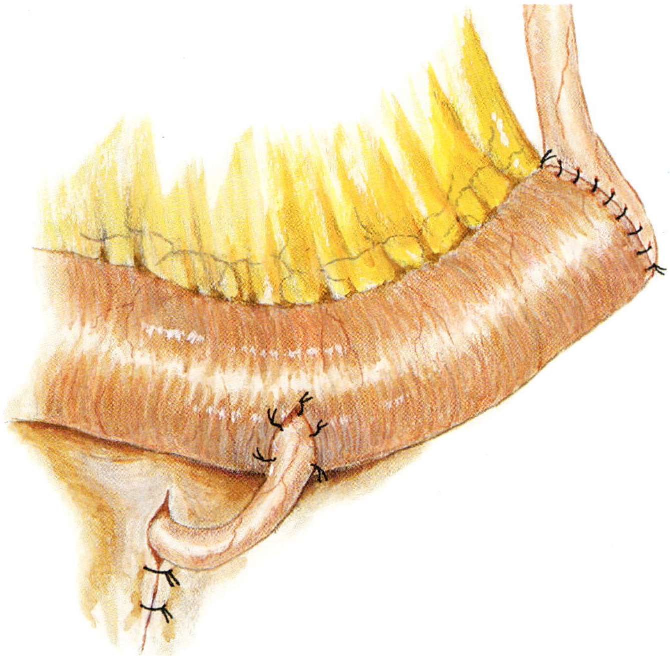

70-1

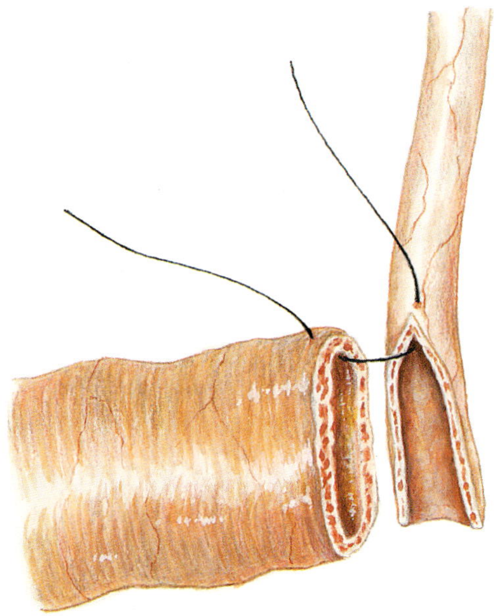

70-2

71. Use of a Transverse Colon Conduit for Urinary Diversion

The technique of fashioning a transverse colon conduit and bringing the distal stoma to the lower left abdominal quadrant near the umbilicus has gained some popularity.

Prior to the procedure the large bowel is cleansed and rendered aseptic using Colyte and the appropriate nonabsorbable antibiotics. The stoma site is marked in the left lower quadrant. An incision is made starting in the midline approximately 6 cm above the umbilicus. The incision curves to the right at the umbilicus and is extended to the symphysis pubis. The pelvic lymph node dissection bilaterally and the cystectomy are performed first. In males a total prostatectomy is also performed.

71-1. The transverse colon conduit is isolated as shown. The large bowel clamps have been removed. The greater omentum and mesocolon have been freed and the segment of transverse colon has been isolated. A major portion of the middle colic artery supplying the transverse colon segment for diversion must be preserved as shown. Reanastomosis of the remaining colon is accomplished in the usual fashion using two layers. The outer layer is closed with interrupted sutures. Both upper ureters are freed from the transected lower ureteral boundaries. Care is taken to preserve the ureteral blood supply which is on the medial borders of the ureters.

71-2. We like to implant the ureters next. We usually cut the distal ureter on a bias so that a direct anastomosis can be performed. The subserosal muscle layers are carefully exposed and the tunnel length is extended about 5 cm. The actual length of the submucosal tunnel is dependent on the size of the ureter. A chronically obstructed ureter is thicker and needs a longer tunnel. We use four chromic catgut interrupted mucosal-ureteral sutures; five to six may be needed if the ureter is enlarged. The serosa and overlying muscle layer is reapproximated taking care not to bend the ureter excessively as it exits from the submucosal layer. A single J stent may be used for each ureter, and the

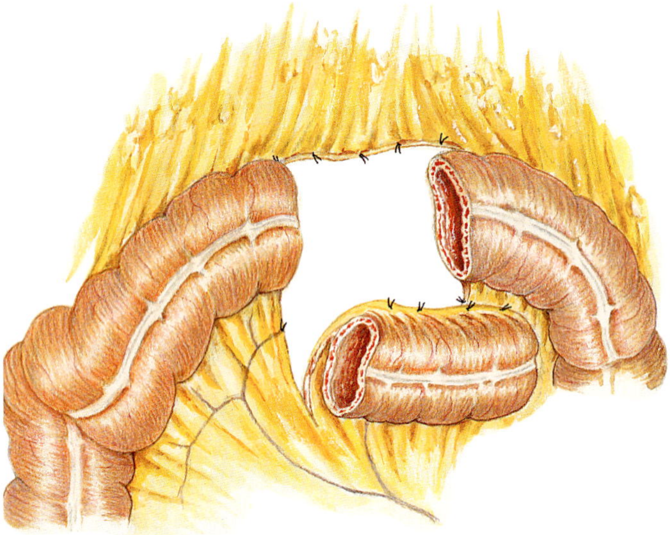

71-1

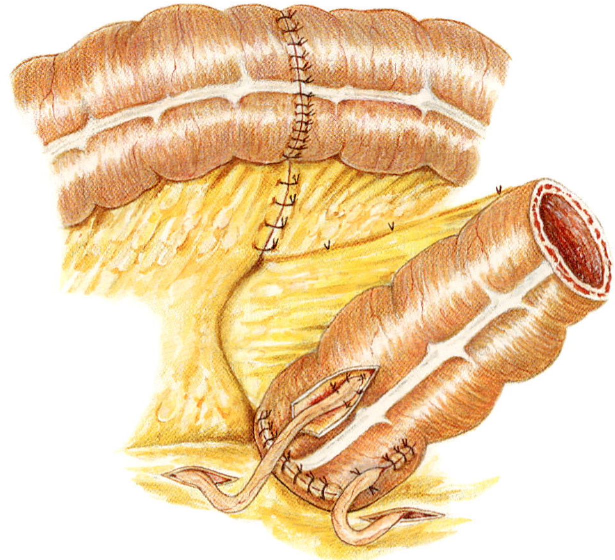

71-2

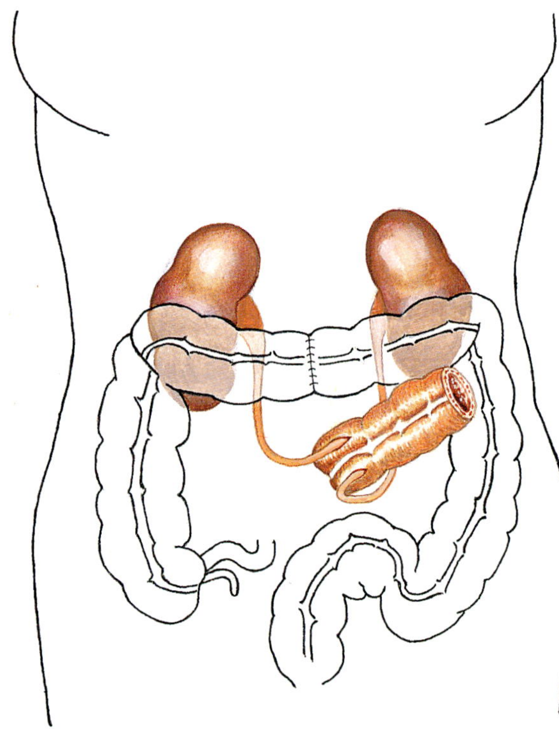

71-3

long straight end will exit out the stoma. We mark the ureters by cutting the distal stent on a bias to mark the left ureter.

71-3. The stoma is fashioned in the usual way . A normal disk of skin is again identified. It has been previously marked with the sharp end of a needle. A circular segment of anterior fascia is removed in the proper location. The muscles are separated. The fascial layer and peritoneum are identified with Kocher or Allis clamps and a disc of tissue is removed. The single J stent is separately shortened and sutured to the skin surrounding the stoma. A urinary conduit bag and attachment are fixed over the stoma. We leave J stents in place for 7 days.

72. Sigmoid Colon Conduit

72-1. *Urinary diversion using a segment of sigmoid colon.*

Although depicted anteriorly by the following schematics, the operative technique includes placement of the distal ureters in a posterior location. An antireflux procedure can be performed, as described in 66-6 to 66-9.

73. Rectal Bladder and Concomitant Colostomy

73-1. The rectal baldder lies vertically in the pelvic cavity. The ureters are implanted separately. The rectal bladder can accommodate the uterus anteriorly or slightly posteriorly. The choice is made depending on the more normal anatomic position of the ureters. The ureters should lie flat.

74. Rectal Bladder

74-1. A rectal bladder is formed. The sigmoid colon is brought inferiorly but anterior to the rectum, and it is also brought through the anal sphincter.

74-2. In this instance the sigmoid colon is brought posterior to the rectum.

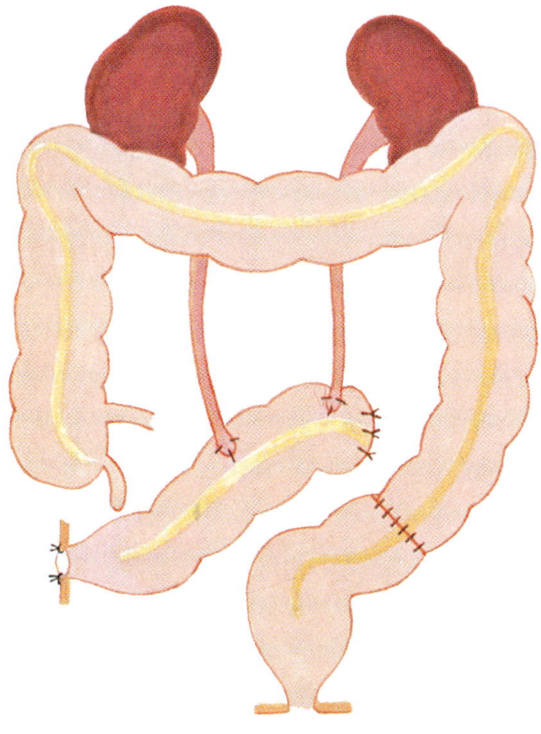

72-1

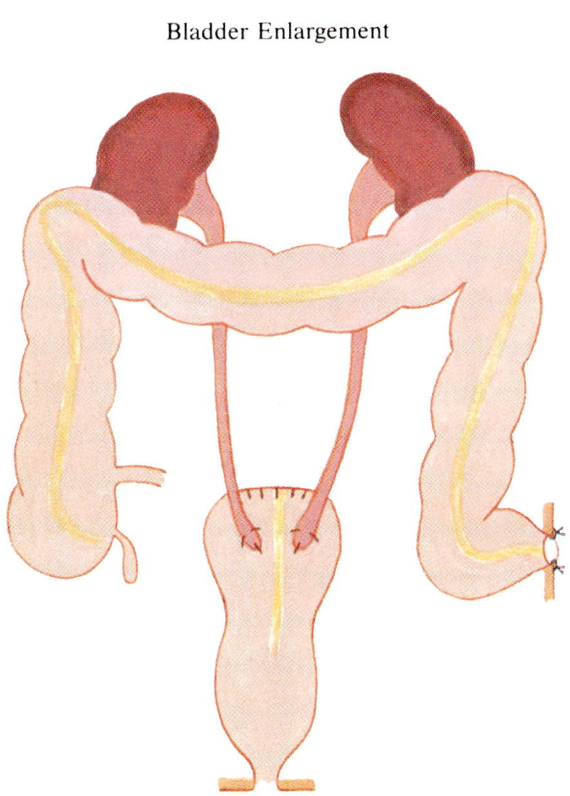

73-1

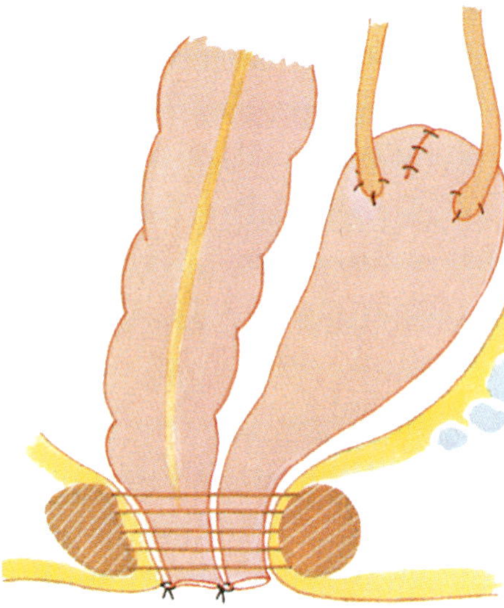

74-1

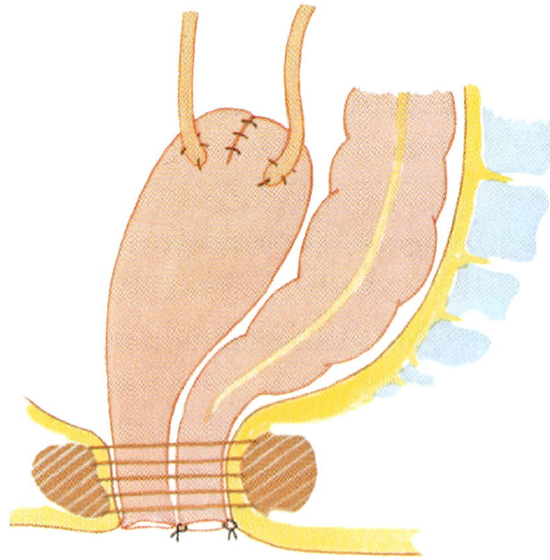

74-2

75. The Modified Kock Pouch: A Continent Ileal Reservoir and an Alternative to Ileal Cutaneous Urinary Diversion

As previously conceived by Kock et al.,[4] the continent ileal reservoir has been used to produce a low pressure system, and also serve as a storage pouch for urine. The Kock pouch is a continent, high-capacity reservoir with nonrefluxing valves and is constructed from ileum to hold approximately 500 to 800 cc of urine. Pressure in the pouch rarely exceeds 15 to 20 cm of water; whereas ileum or cecum elicit pressures above 60 cm of water.

Skinner and associates have published their results of a large series of patients. More than 350 patients have had the Kock pouch fashioned by these authors—300 patients from Aug 1982 to 1987. More than 200 have undergone simultaneous radical cystectomy for bladder cancer.[5]

In an earlier report by Skinner et al., about two-thirds of the patients underwent a radical cystectomy. Another 60 patients underwent a different type of urinary diversion and now a Kock pouch was constructed to rectify the problems. At least one-third of the patients had also undergone irradiation therapy before a Kock pouch was fashioned surgically.

75-1. The surgical technique with modifications by Dr. Skinner are described. A longer segment of ileum is used. The afferent and efferent limbs are 17 cm long.

75-2. The pouch is constructed from two 22 cm segments. A new modification by Skinner et al. makes good sense.

75-3. A 4 to 6 cm segment of ileum proximal to the measured segments are discarded with its mesentery divided next to serosa. The purpose of this modification is to provide a better arterial blood supply to the pouch. This modification also increases the mobility of the afferent limb.

Prior to preparation of the ileum to create the pouch, 8 cm of mesentery are stripped off the serosa of the ileum from the afferent and efferent limbs adjacent to the pouch.

75-4. Then a 2-cm wide strip of polyglycolic acid mesh is passed through the next window as shown by the Dever.

75-5. Skinner has demonstrated that now the ileal intussusception can be fashioned without incorporating the mesentery. The illustration shows the formation of a Marlex (or fascial) collar around each nipple base.

75-6. Experience has shown that during the intussusception process, the polyglycolic acid mesh will move adjacent to the pouch wall where it can be fixed with 2–0 chromic catgut sutures. This illustration shows the formation of the continent-proving and reflux-proving nipples.

The intussuscepted segment should be fashioned without crushing the bowel. Four rows of 4.8 mm stainless steel staples, non-hemostatic type, are applied to the intussuscepted segment (75–7). The acid mesh (polyglycolic) must not be incorporated into the staples. If one inadvertently incorporates the staples, the increased thickness can prevent proper closure of the segment.

The importance of using the pin of the stapler to avoid misaligned staples is worth underscoring. The pinhole created must be closed with 3–0 polyglycolic sutures to prevent urinary leakage bypassing the intussuscepted nipple.

Skinner mentions initially using three rows of staples which are placed evenly around the anterior 180° of the intussusception. A new stapler, PI-55 automatic stapler

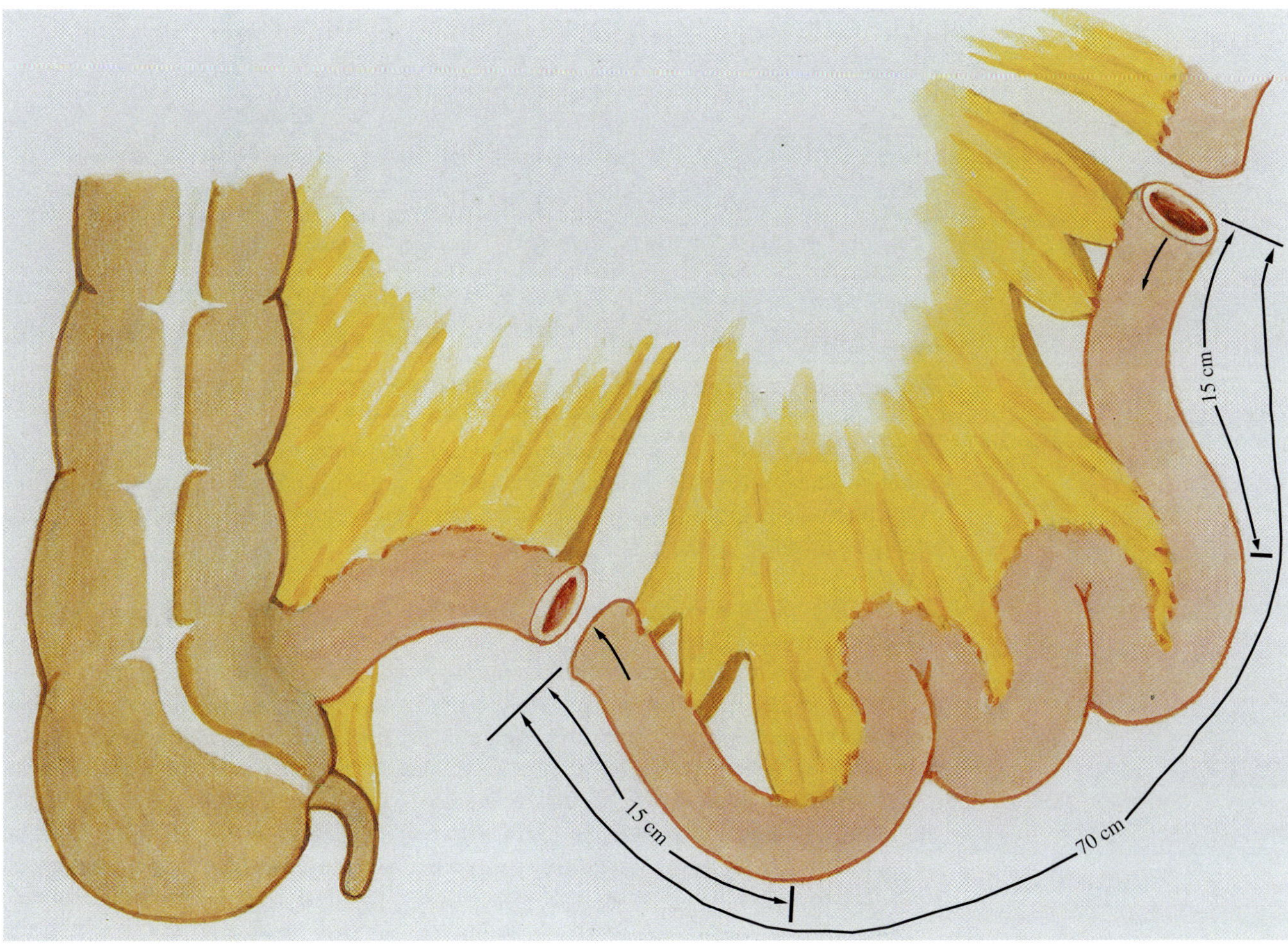

75-1

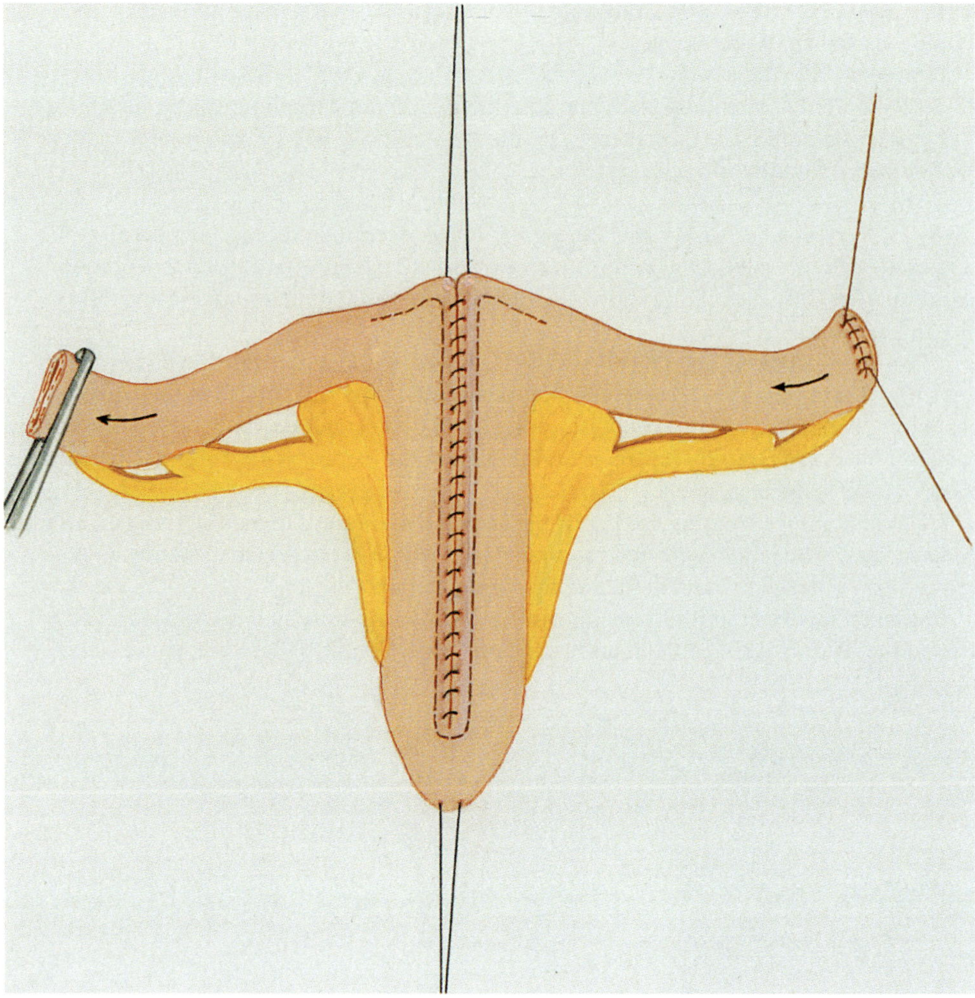

75-2

with custom staples provided by the manufacturer, is advocated. The A.V. Mueller company has manufactured a stapler in which six staples from the proximal portion of the cartridge have been removed prior to shipment. The staples at the end of the nipple do not contribute to the maintenance of the intussusception, and remain exposed to urine. The creation of a nidus for stone formation can occur. The staples are removed from the stapling cartridge.

75-7. The fourth row of staples fixes the intussuscepted nipple to the back wall of the pouch and also provides fixation of the pouch. Now the anvil stapling device is passed into the inside of the nipple from outside the pouch, initiating the procedure at the mesentery at the base of the nipple. These modifications fix the two layers of bowel; the back wall of the pouch is one layer of the nipple valve. A full cartridge with all staples must be used, because the more important staples are those at the nipple base. The pin hole must be closed; however, a small hole may be made just beyond the point at which the intussuscepted nipple will lie. Skinner advocates that the anvil of the stapler be brought through this hole from outside the pouch. The intussuscepted nipple is advanced over the anvil, which allows slippage up the ileum beyond the intussusception, as the illustration demonstrates. Skinner's modification staples three thicknesses of ileum: the back wall, and two layers in the intussusception. A special custom cartridge is used with

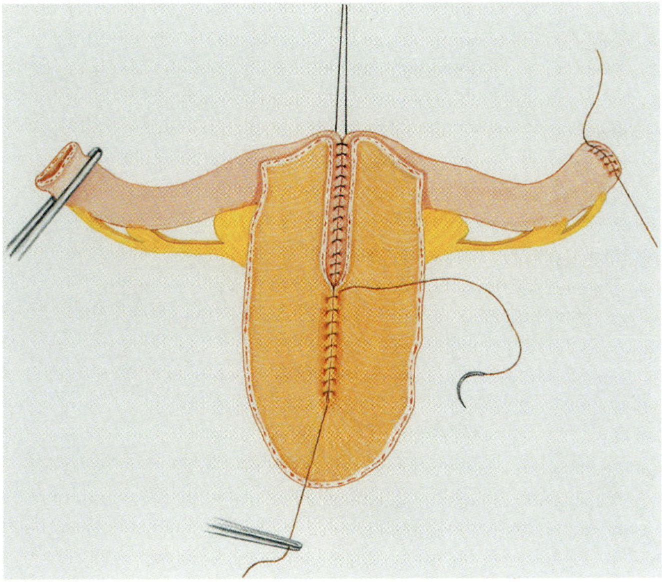

75-3

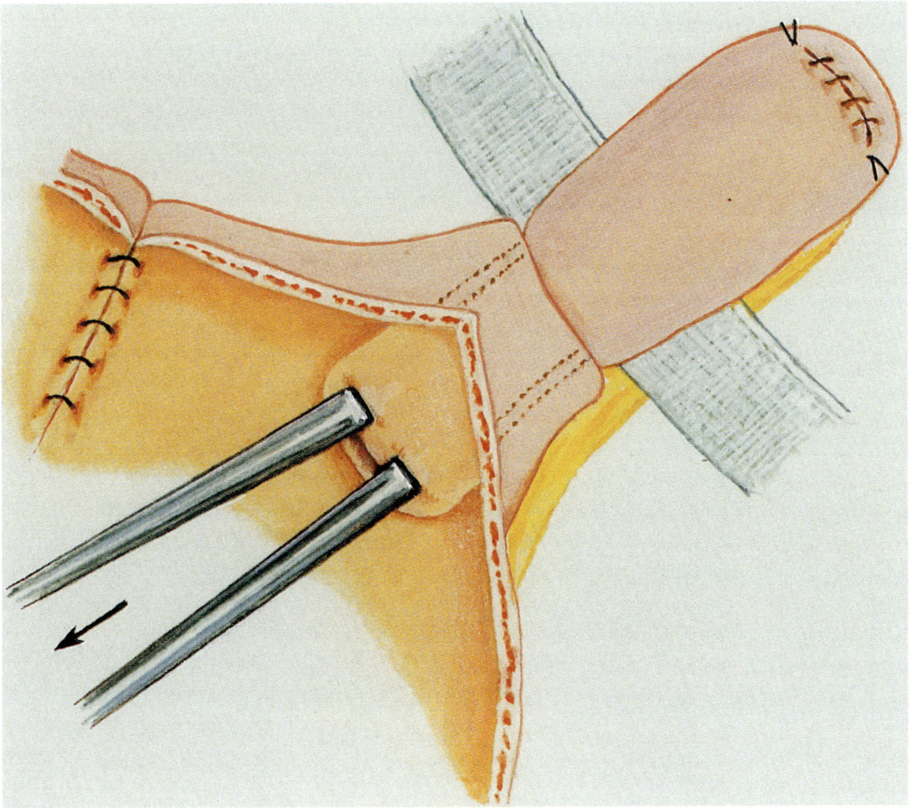

75-4

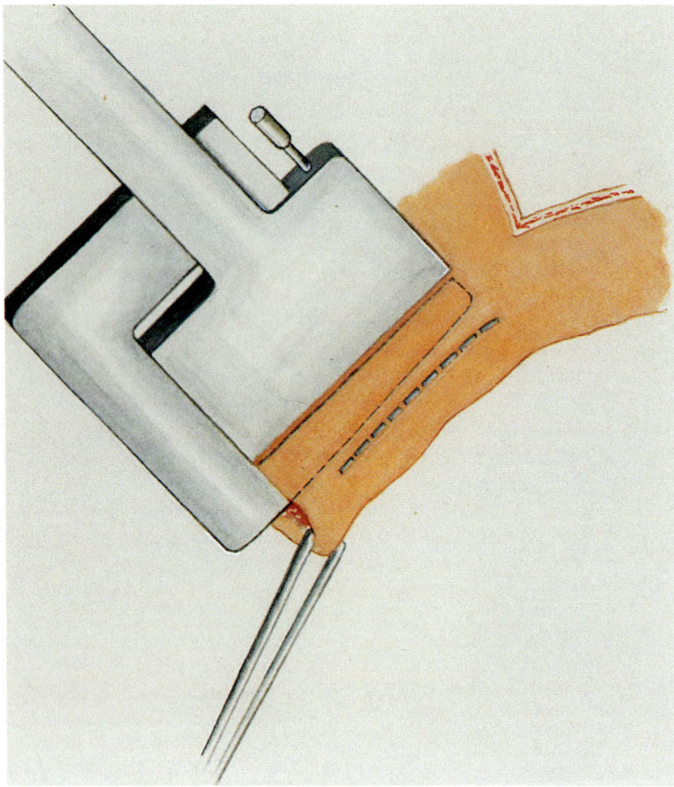

75-5

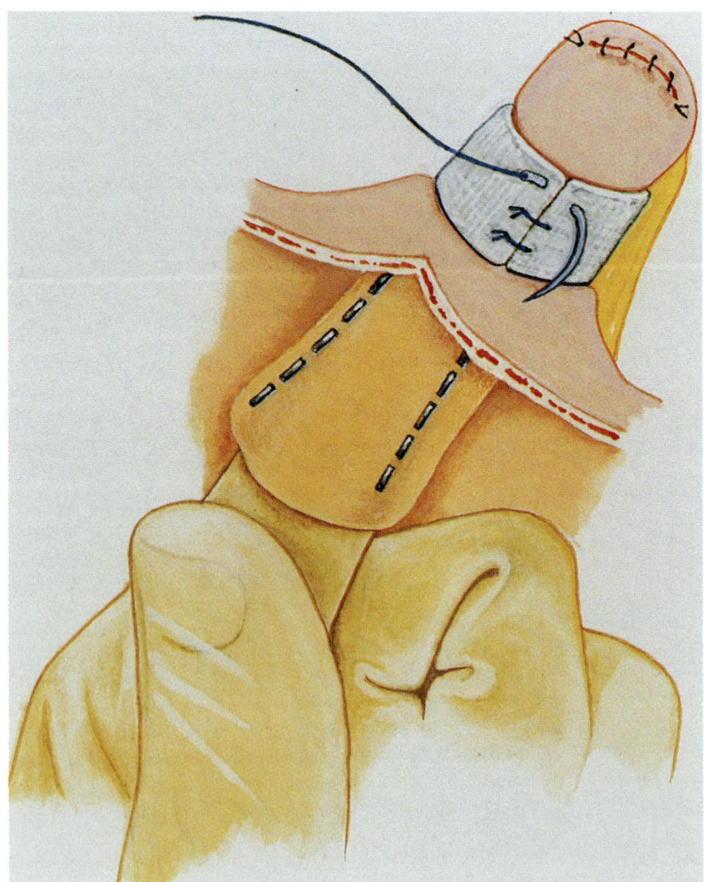

75-6

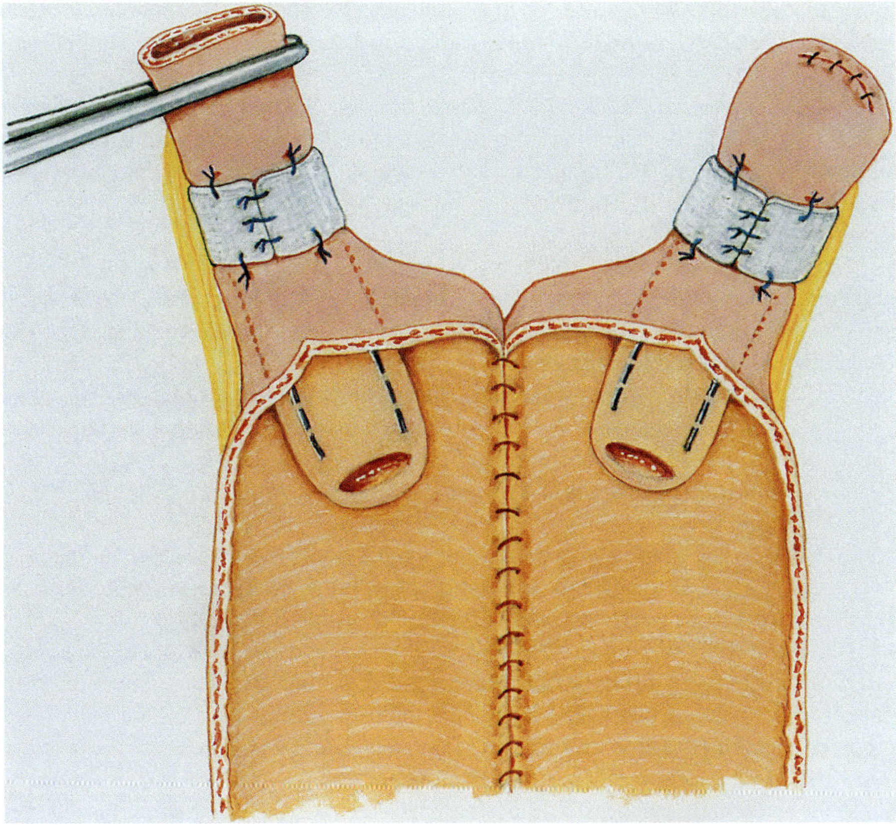

75-7

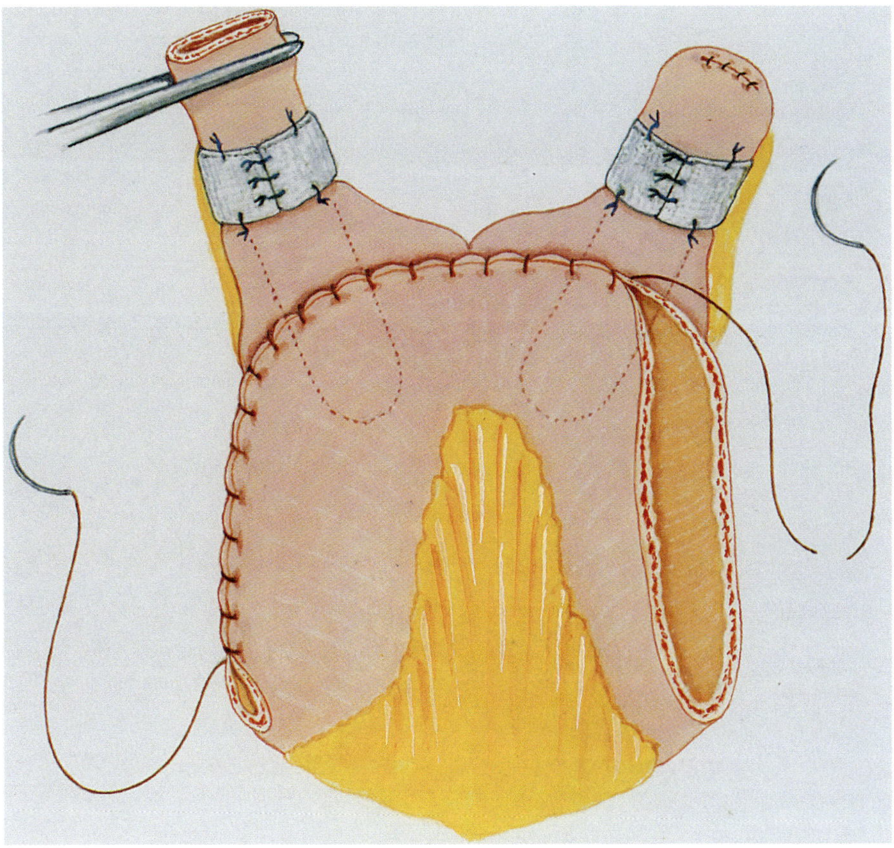

75-8

this modification. Finally, the ends of both nipples are sutured to the pouch wall with 3–0 polyglycolic acid sutures. The hole in the pouch wall must now be sutured and closed.

The next step is passing a 30–0 Medina tube through the nipple and the polyglycolic acid mesh strip is secured circumferentially around the ileal segment with 2–0 chromic catgut interrupted sutures. This allows further attachment and fixation at the mesh to the pouch and ileal segment.

75-8. Next, the pouch is closed, placing two mattress sutures of 1–0 nylon from the anterior rectus fascia to the medial and lateral aspects of the efferent Marlex (or fascial) collar. A second suture line of interrupted catgut can be used to reinforce the pouch. The ureters are then implanted into the pouch.

A more recent modification by Skinner adds a 2 cm wide strip of Marlex. The mesh is fixed with a 1–0 nylon suture to the anterior peritoneum and abdominal wall fascia, at a location lateral and slightly cephalad to the opening in the abdominal wall through which the efferent limb of ileum will exit.

75-9 and **75-10.** The Marlex strip then is brought out the window of Dever at the ileal mesentery at the base of the efferent intussusception adjacent to the polyglycolic acid mesh collar. Two 1–0 polyglycolic acid sutures are placed as horizontal mattress sutures entering through the abdominal wall fascia. One is lateral and one is medial to the pouch. The efferent limb is now brought out through the abdominal wall and any redundant ileum is excised. The purpose of the horizontal mattress sutures is to fix the bowel and help provide a continent valve mechanism to the abdominal wall fascia.

Now the Marlex strip is sewn to the peritoneum and posterior rectus fascia that is medial to the pouch. This Marlex strip does not cause erosion and it is important in preventing a parastomal herniation. It also fixes the continent valve mechanism and still allows self catheterization.

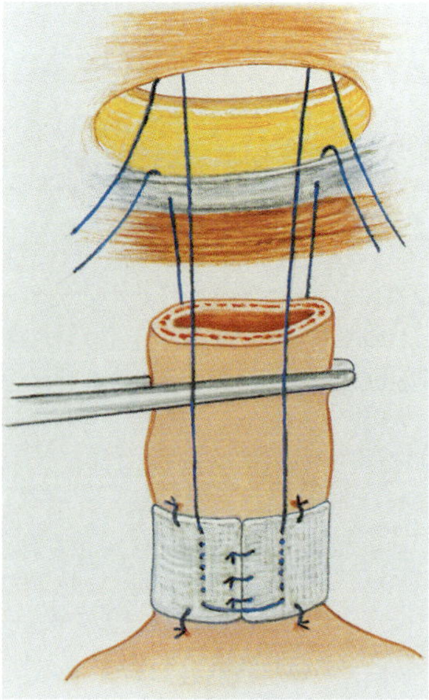

75-9

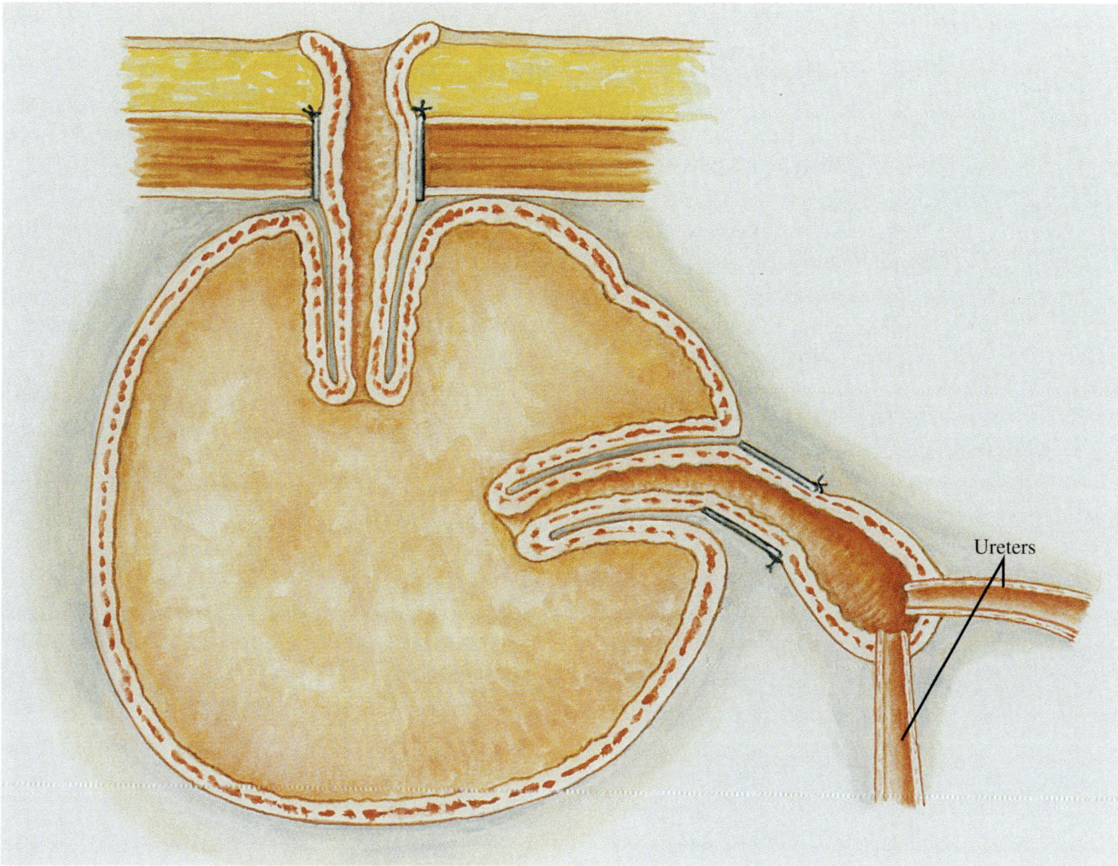

75-10

76. The Mainz Pouch: A Complete Bladder Substitution After Radical Cystectoprostatectomy

The above procedure was previously described for use in patients who underwent radical cystectoprostatectomy for bladder cancer. More recently the indications for the Mainz Pouch have been extended to include bladder augmentation and/or continent urinary diversion.

The Mainz group headed by Prof. Hohenfellner have had a very large experience with the "Mainz Pouch." The first 100 cases were reported recently in 1988. Twenty of the 100 cases included children.

The surgical technique described by Hohenfellner and colleagues remains the same. Three similar segments of bowel are employed.

76-1. 10–15 cm of cecum, 10–15 cm of distal ileum and 10–15 cm of ileum extending from the distal segment for 10–15 cm.

76-2. End-to-end anastomosis of ileum 6 to ascending colon.

76-3. The anastomosis is completed

76-4. Mechanical end-to-side anastomosis using the EEA stapler.

76-5. Blind closure of ascending colon by TA55 stapler.

76-6. Antimesenteric splitting of intestine.

76-7. Side-to-side anastomosis of ascending colon and terminal ileal segment. Then, the second anastomosis is between the two ileal segments.

76-8. Anastomosis of the posterior wall of the pouch to the subtotally resected bladder and antireflux implantation of ureters without rotation of intestine.

76-9. After 180° counter-clockwise rotation of intestine for tension-free anastomosis with short mesentery.

76-10. After complete closure of bladder augmentation without rotation of the pouch.

76-11. Operative situation after complete closure of bladder augmentation after 180° rotation of the pouch.

It is clear that on occasion the completed pouch cannot be easily placed into the bony pelvic cavity following a radial cystectomy. Lampel and Hohenfellner[6] recommend that increased mobilization of the pouch can be achieved by mobilizing the right colon up to the right colon–flexure. This will provide appropriate mobilization so that the pouch can be placed into the bony pelvic cavity.

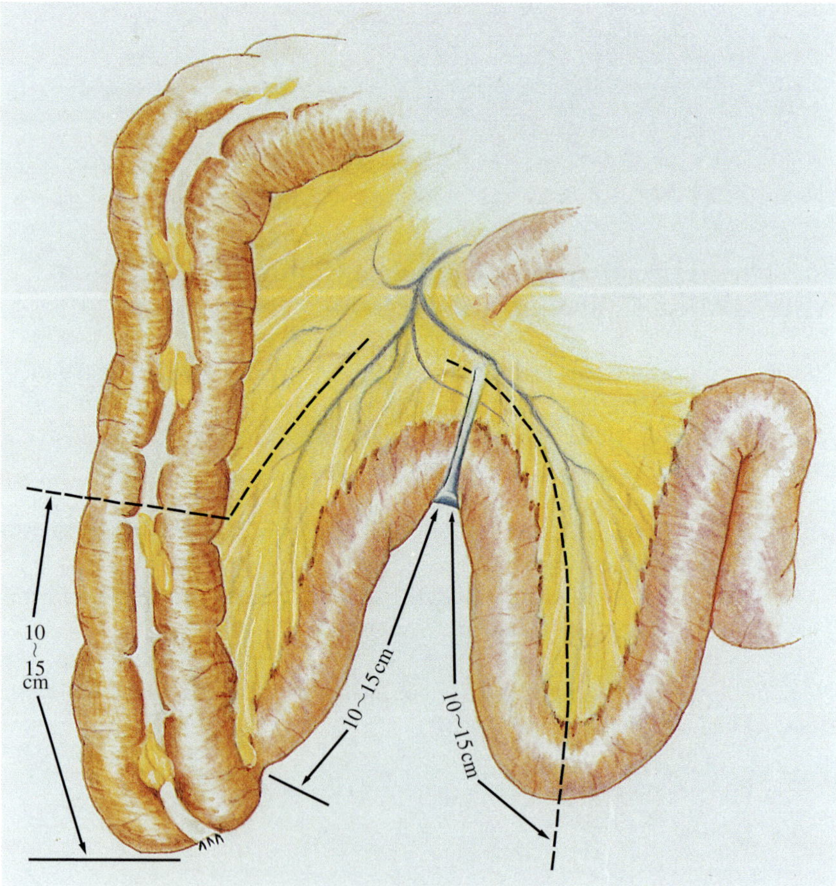

76-1

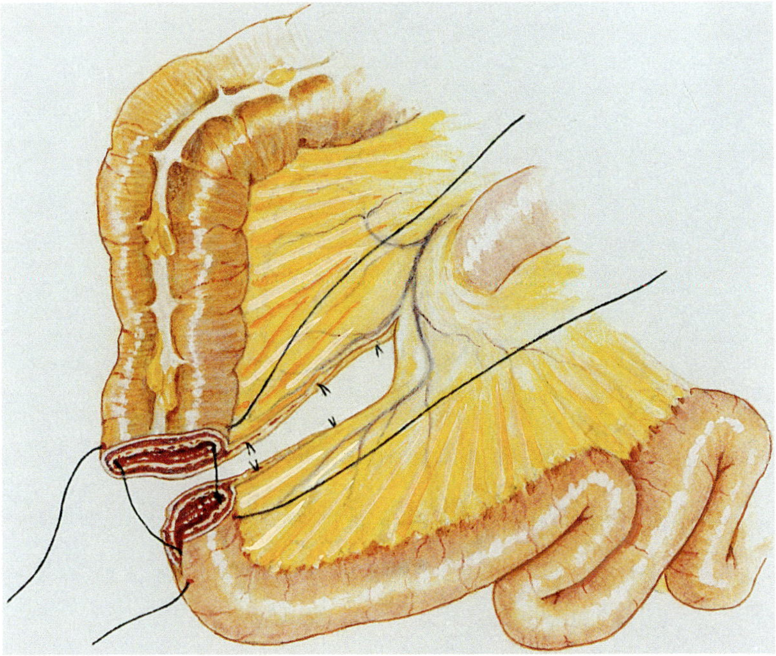

76-2

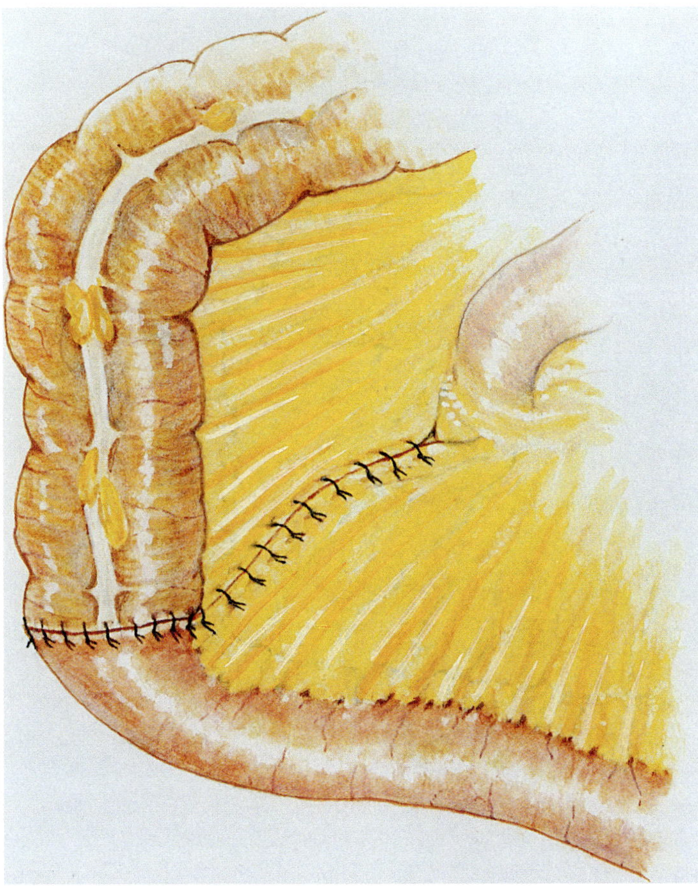

76-3

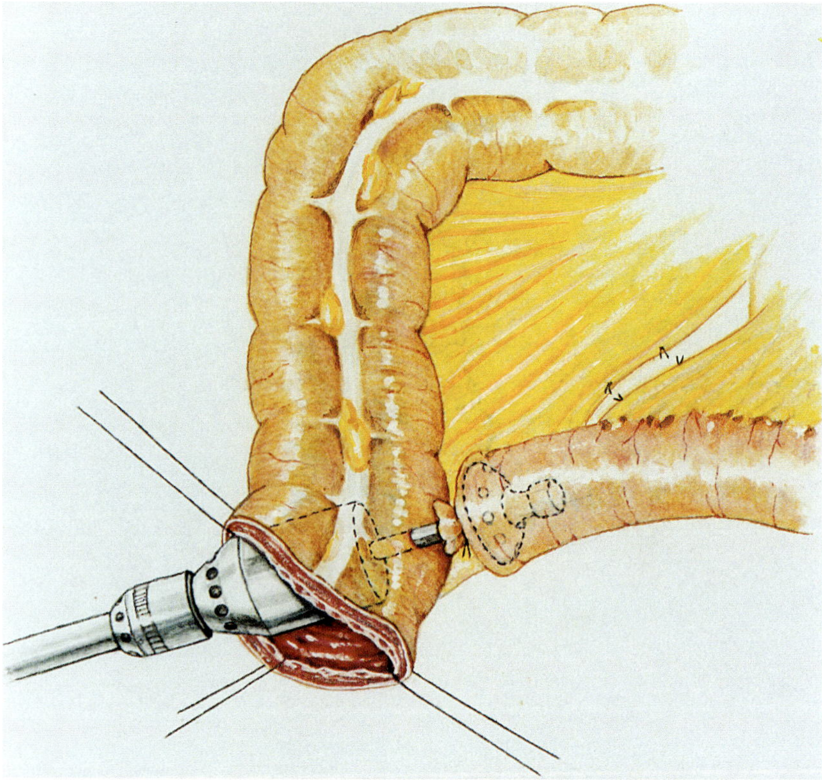

76-4

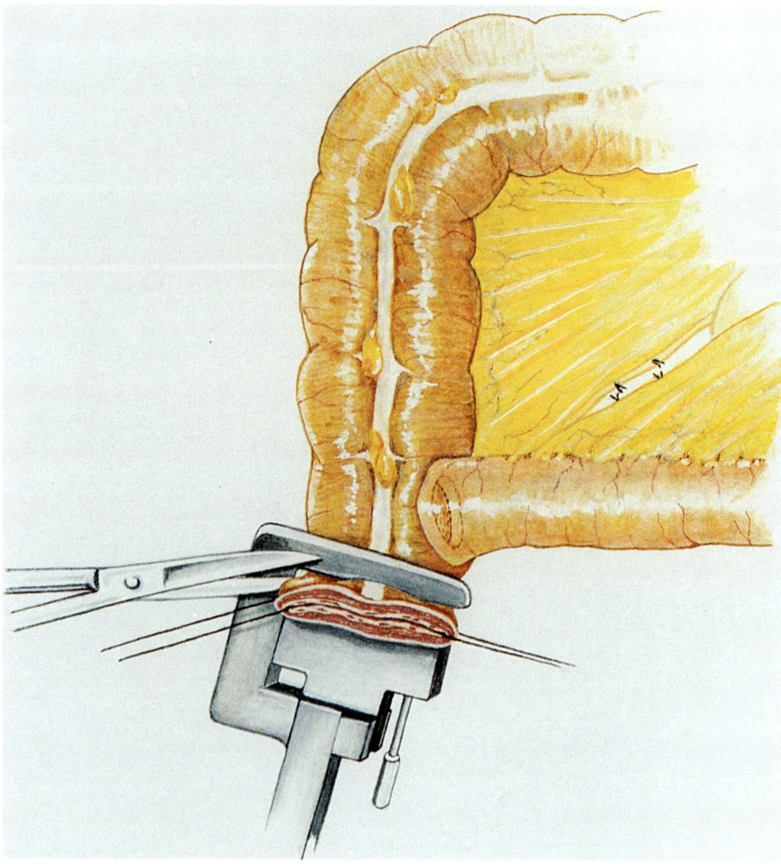

76-5

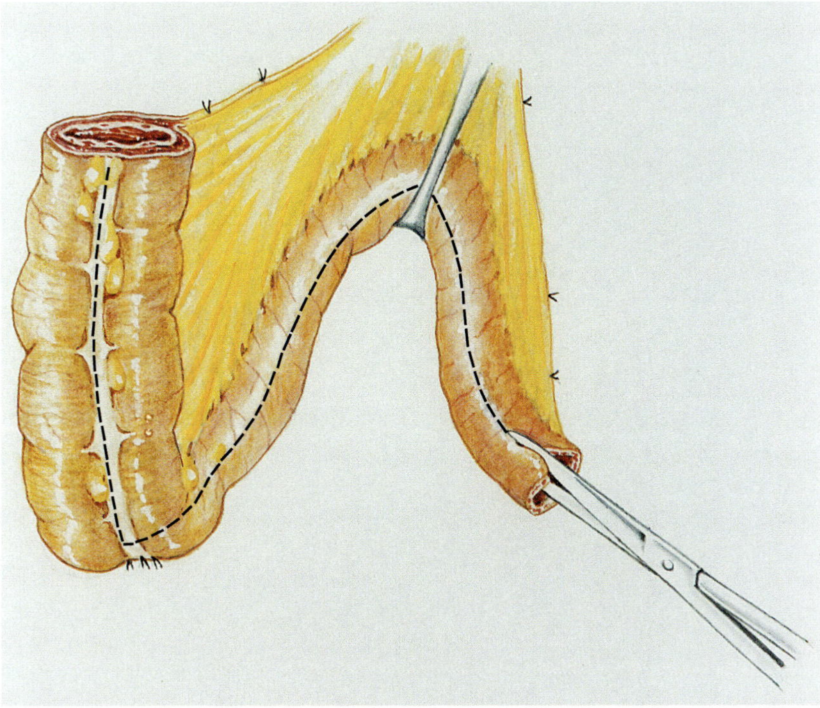

76-6

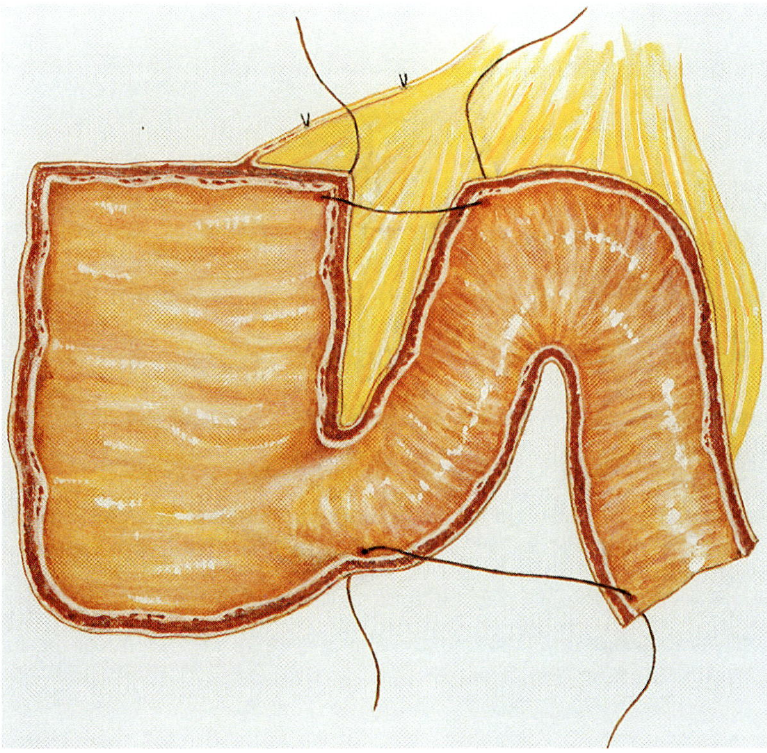

76-7

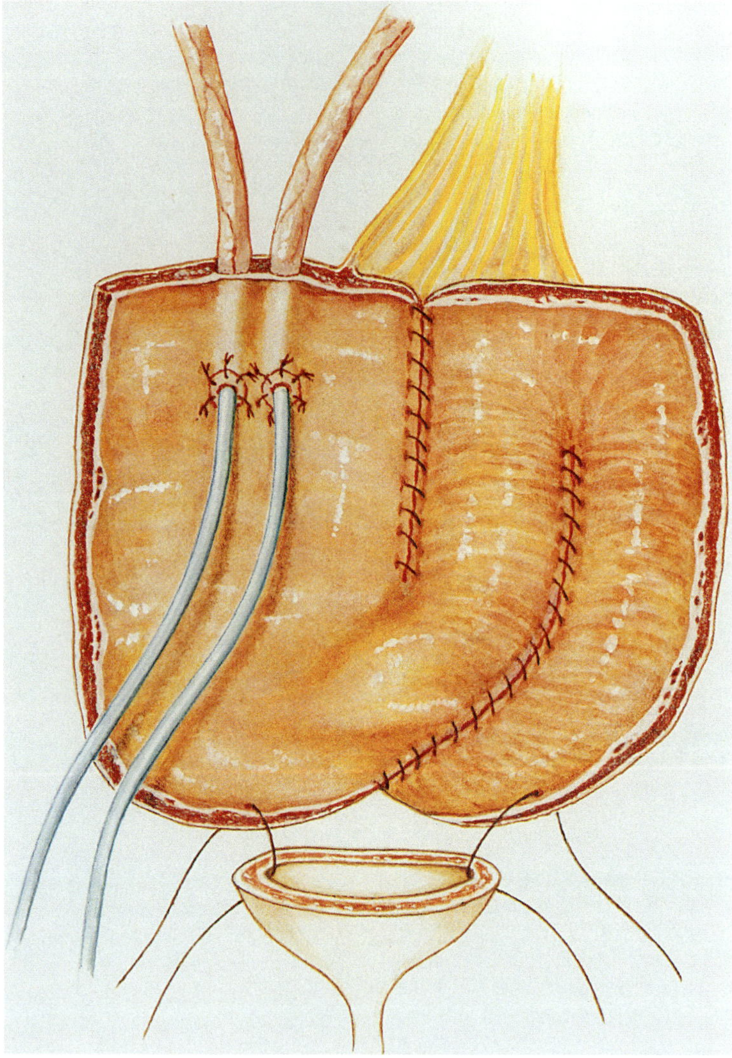

76-8

Mainz Pouch Continent Urinary Diversion Technique

76-12. Intestinal segment to be isolated for Mainz pouch continent urinary diversion.

76-13. Antimesenteric splitting of the intestine for continent pouch.

76-14. Anastomosis of ascending colon and terminal ileal segment, and of the latter with the next proximal loop.

76-15. Mainz pouch urinary diversion with antireflux implantation of ureters into ascending colon. The proximal ileal loop remains intact for the ileo-ileal invagination valve.

76-16. Ileo-ileal invagination on technique division of 6 cm of mesentery for mesenteric exclusion from the invagination valve.

76-17. Completed invagination secured by several rows of interrupted seromuscular sutures and a fascial strip around the base of the invagination.

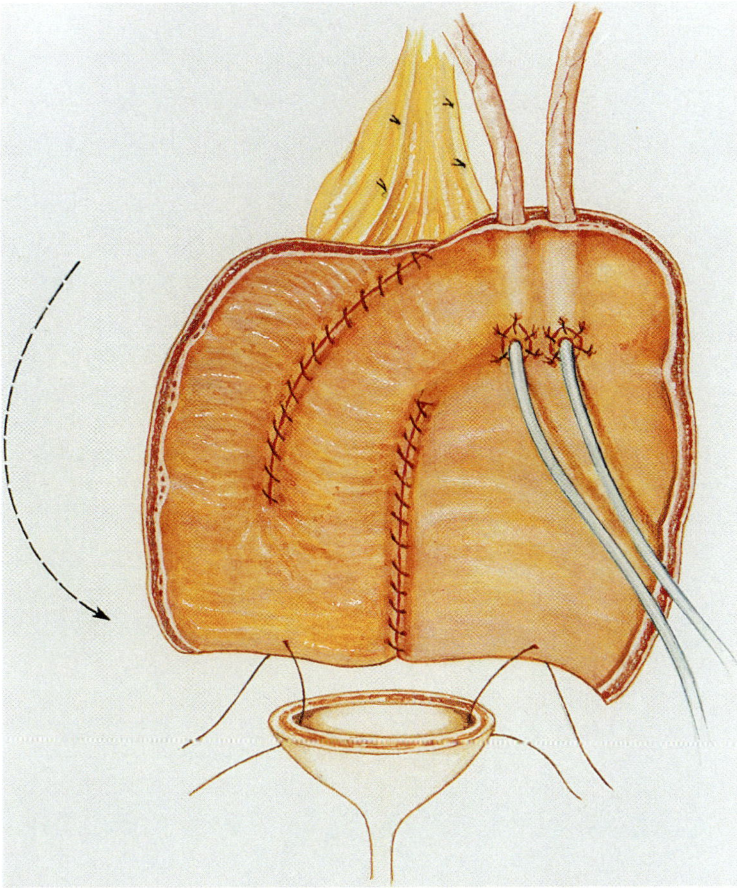

76-9

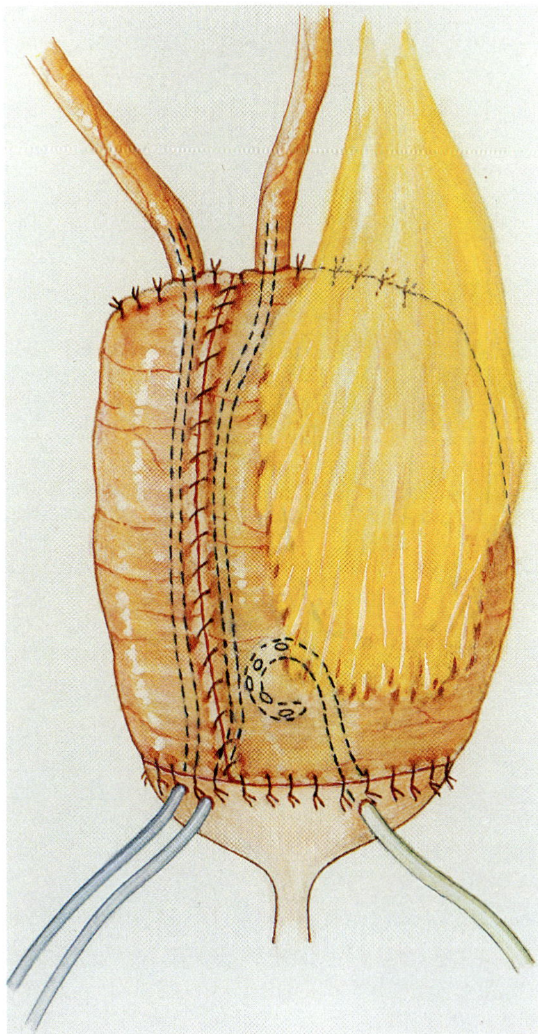

76-10

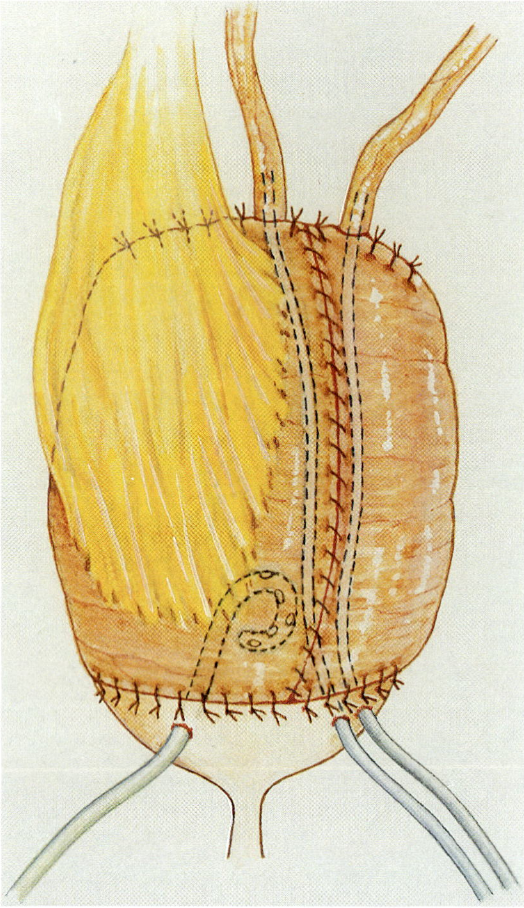

76-11

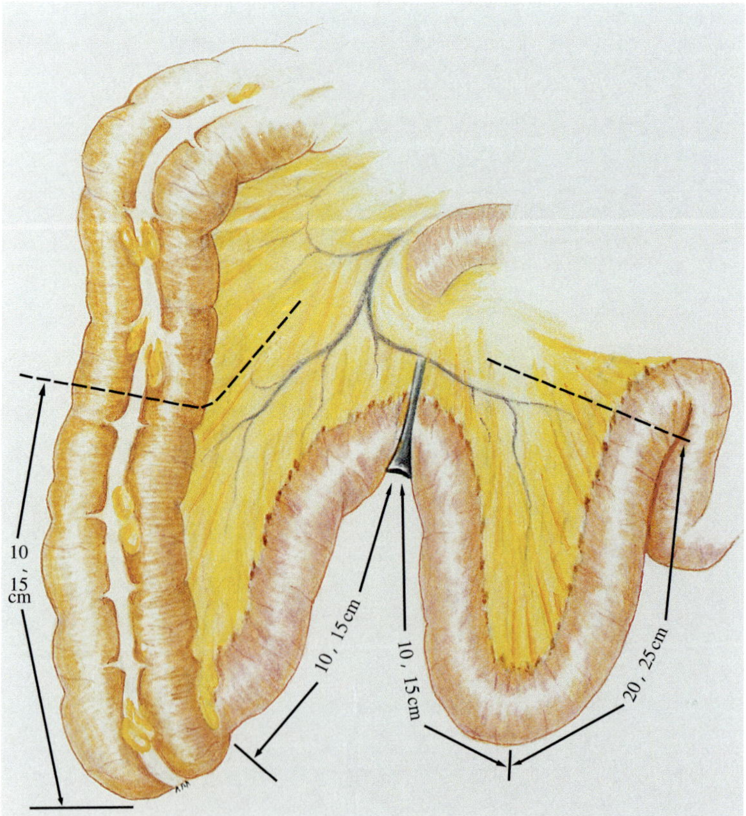

76-12

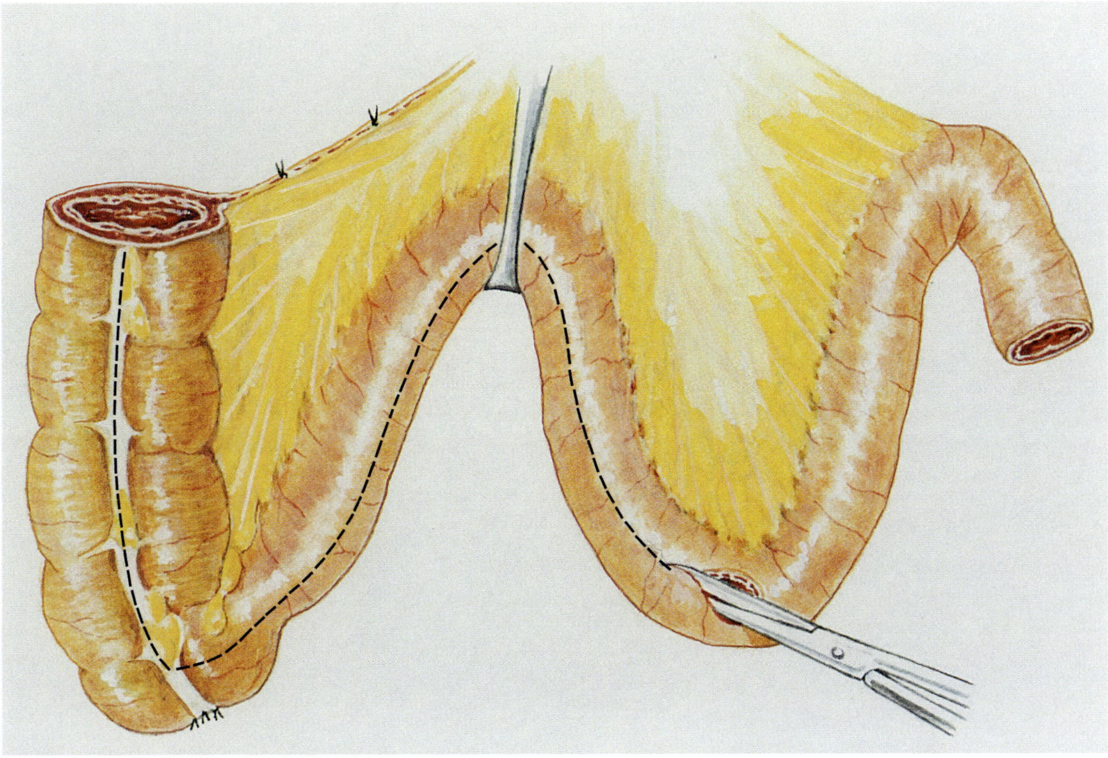

76-13

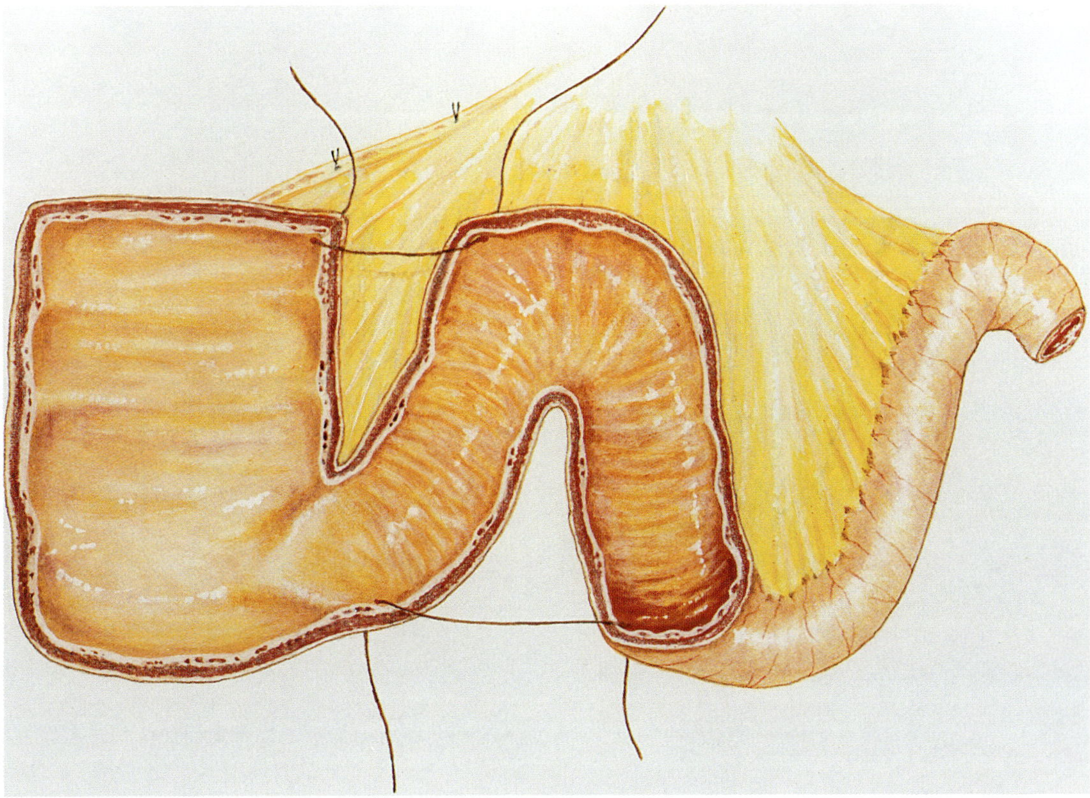

76-14

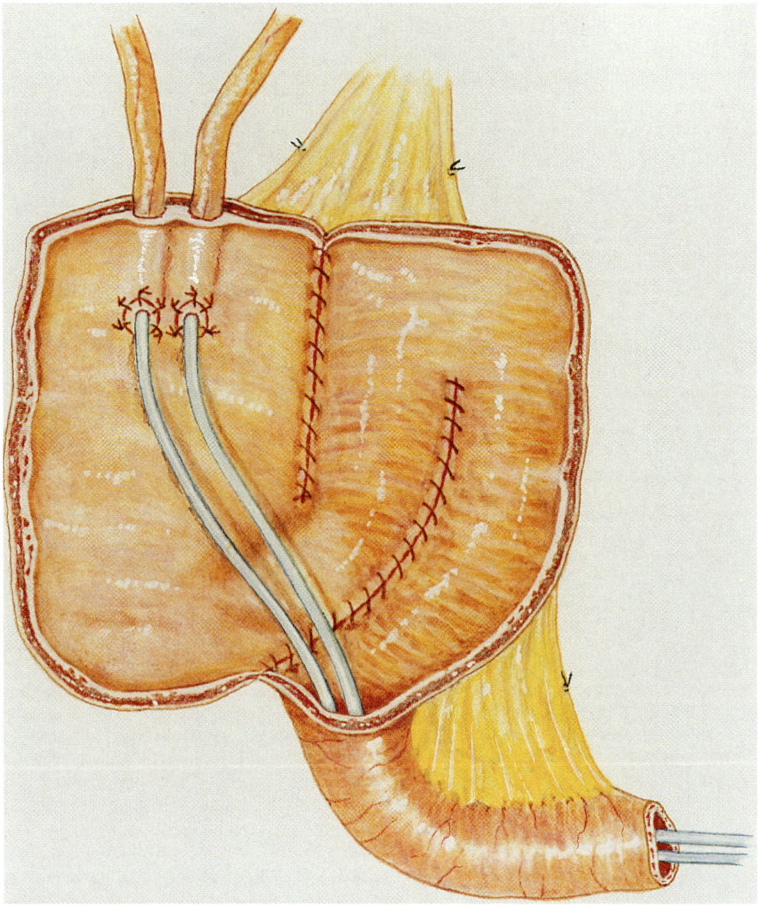

76-15

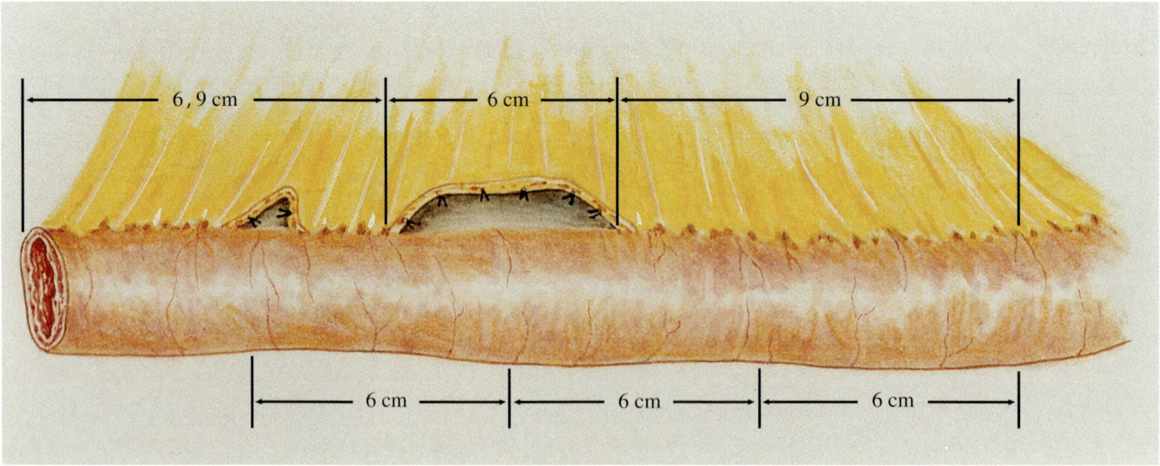

76-16

76-18. Alternative fixation of the invagination valve to the intussuscepting ileal wall with 4 rows of staples.

76-19. Completed continent stoma: The fascial strip around the base of the invagination is sutured to the abdominal fascia for anchoring the base of invagination within the abdominal wall.

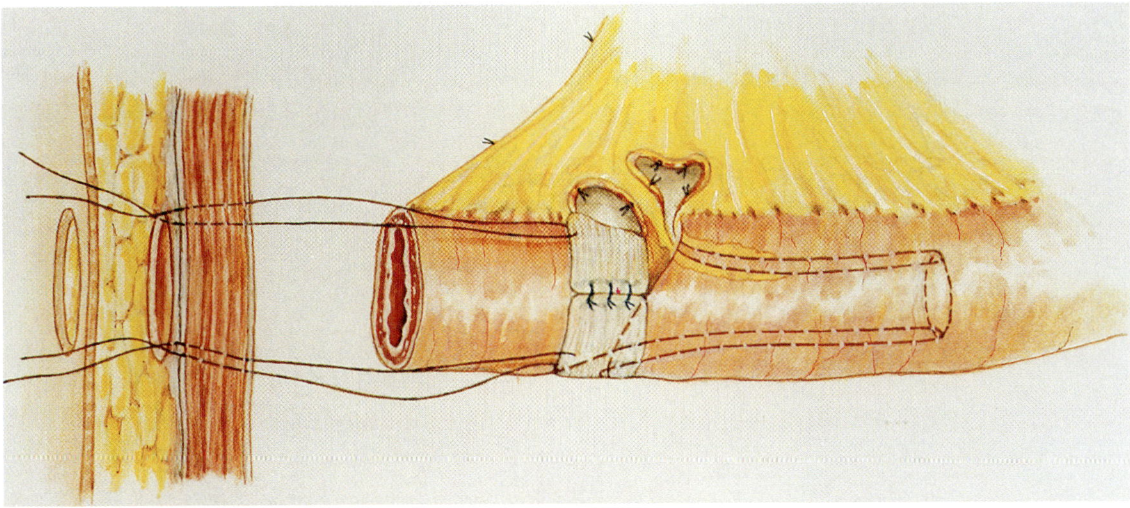

76-17

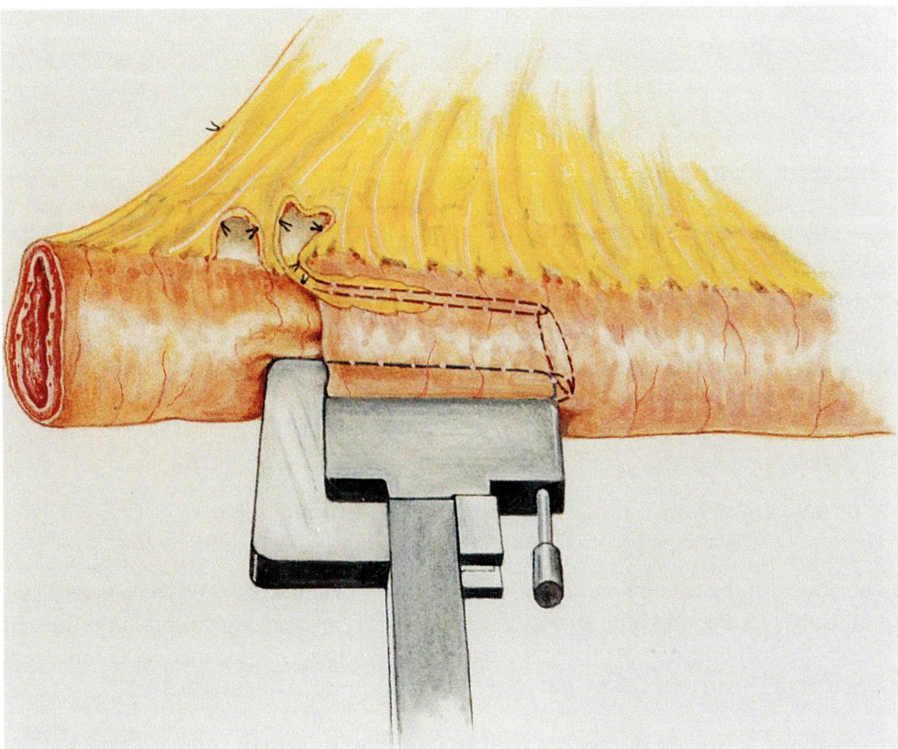

76-18

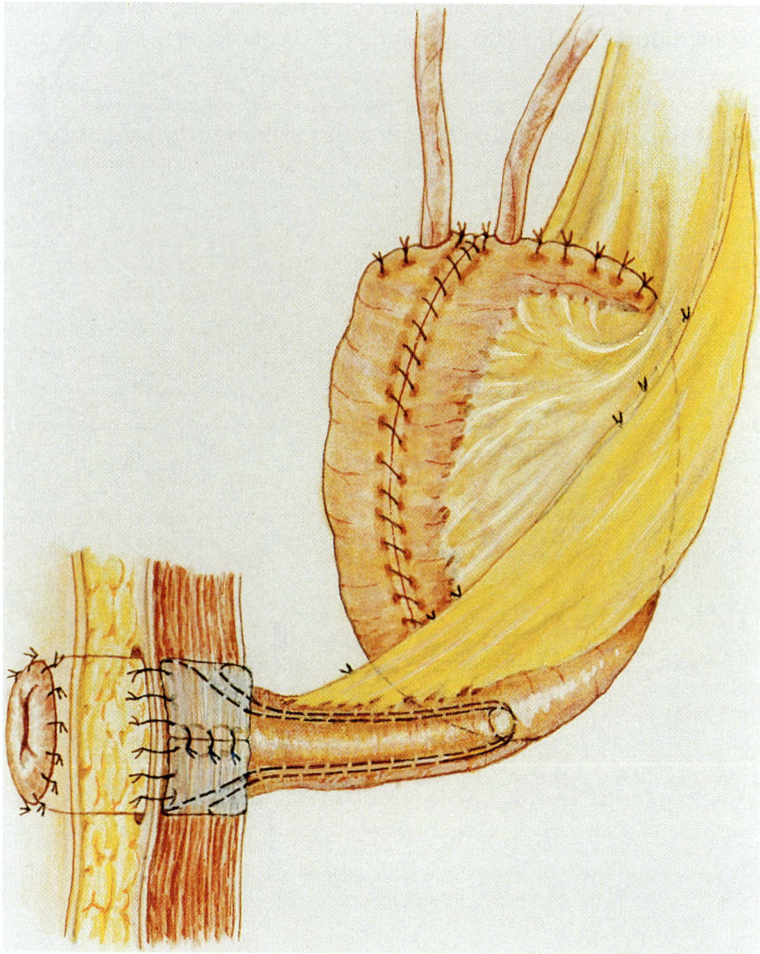

76-19

77. Indiana Pouch

The Indiana Pouch for continent urinary diversion has been described by Rowland, Mitchell, and others.[7] Preoperative care includes mechanical cleansing and antibiotic bowel preparation. Hydration of the patient is important preoperatively.

The incision on the skin to be used depends on the location of the stoma. After laparotomy the cystectomy and prostatectomy in men are performed and completed. The right colon is mobilized to the proximal transverse colon.

77-1. Appropriate lengths of bowel are measured as follows:

1. The continent segment of ileum is 8 to 12 cm of terminal ileum.
2. The reservoir is formed from a 26 to 30 cm segment of ascending colon.

The pouch of the ascending colon is opened with cautery between the anterior taeniae coli down to the appendix that is circumscribed. An appendectomy is performed and completed by clamping the mesoappendix and ligating it. The appendix is removed. The segment of ileum that is isolated is opened on its antimesenteric border.

77-2. Both lower ureters have been previously isolated and catheterized following the cystectomy. The ureterocolic anastomosis on each side is started after a tunnel has been made between the muscle layer of the colon and the mucosal margin. In the right colon it is not difficult to find the appropriate layer posteriorly between muscularis and mucosa for the ureteral tunnels. The left ureter is brought under the inferior mesenteric artery. The location of both ureters is at the midportion of the pouch. The ureteral anastomoses lie posteriorly. To prevent partial obstruction, one must not angulate the left ureter. Care must be taken to avoid kinking or twisting the ureter. We usually spatulate the ureter and use 5 to 6 sutures of 4–0 polyglycolic acid sutures to the mucosal and adjacent muscle layer of the bowel. The created tunnel is closed over the ureter with 4–0 interrupted polyglycolic acid sutures. A 6 Fr single J stent is used for each ureter. The J stent is in the kidney pelvis. We secure the stent up each ureter with 4–0 plain catgut suture to the mucosa of the colon distal to the stomal opening where the ureteral orifices are stented.

The pouch is closed in a transverse (Heineke-Mikulicz) fashion with 2 layers of 3–0 and 4–0 polyglycolic acid sutures. After final closure of the reservoir-pouch, the pouch is secured to the abdominal wall by tacking it with absorbable sutures. The terminal ileum—the continence mechanism—can be led to the right or left lower quadrant depending on the anatomy. A left handed patient may request a left-sided stoma. The stents are fixed with a 3–0 chromic pursestring sutures. The ileal segment that is isolated is opened on its antimesenteric border.

The open ileal segment will be used to cap the segment of colon which has been reconfigured to form a cecal pouch. This enlargement is necessary if the pouch is small.

77-3. In some instances where a larger pouch is warranted, a sigmoid segment can be used. The isolated sigmoid segment is opened on its antimesenteric border. The large bowel segment is used to cap the reconfigured cecal segment.

The distal ileal segment to the cecum as shown is preserved and will serve as a continent ileal conduit after imbrication sutures are placed. The more proximal ileal segment still attached to the ileum in continuity must be anastomosed to the ascending colon as shown to reestablish bowel continuity.

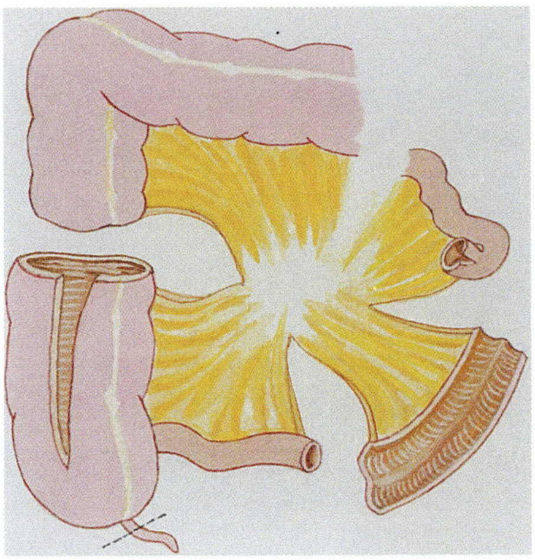

77-1

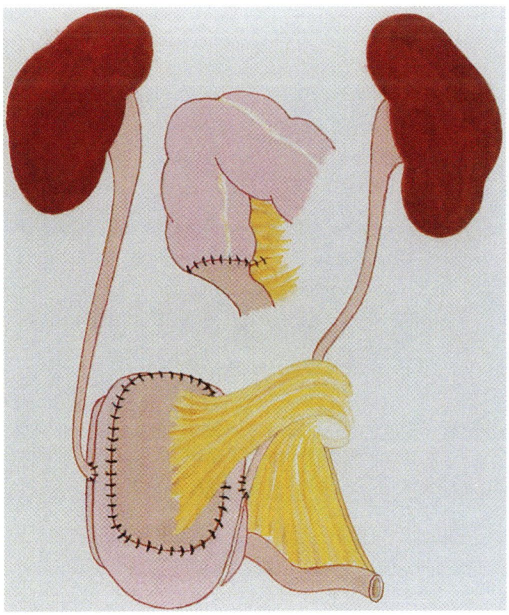

77-2

77-4. The cecum of the ileocecal segment is opened on its antimesenteric border. A segment of sigmoid has been isolated, irrigated free of mucus, and finally opened on its antimesenteric border as shown. The sigmoid cap will enlarge the new cecal bladder reservoir. In this illustration the isolated sigmoid is opened and it can serve as a cap for the cecal segment. The sigmoid in continuity and the descending colon must be reanastomosed using a two-layer closure.

The outer layer can be 3–0 silk or interrupted Vicryl sutures.

77-5, 77-6, and 77-7. A third option is illustrated. A longer segment of cecum and its attached distal ileum are isolated. Using a Heineke-Mikulicz infolding maneuver as shown in 77–6, the cecum is folded over and used to cap the pouch. Sutures are used to maintain the pouch first at the "corners." A double layer closure is appropriate using interrupted sutures to secure the infolded cecum. 77–7 demonstrates the final cecal pouch. The ileum still in continuity must now be attached to the ascending colon to reestablish bowel continuity. If needed, the ileum at the distal tip can be incised for 2 cm on the antimesenteric end and enlarged. This wider opening is for the anastomosis to the ascending colon. Two layers of sutures are used. The outer layer has interrupted sutures.

77-8, 77-9, and 77-10. The formation of a plicated terminal ileum using Lembert sutures. This configuration provides continence. 77–10 is a schematic. It is important to use a Robinson catheter (12 Fr) to maintain a non-constricting lumen at the distal stoma of the ileum.

77-11, 77-12, 77-13, and 77-14. These depict the distal ureteral-cecal anastomosis performed from the exterior of the cecum. A muscular submucosal tunnel is easily made posteriorly with blunt and sharp dissection along the taenia of the cecum. In our opinion the length of the tunnel should be 2.5 times the width of the ureteral lumen. When the anastomoses are completed, the ureteral mucosal–cecal anastomoses can be tested with a ureteral catheter through the open end of the cecal pouch. Single J ureteral stents can

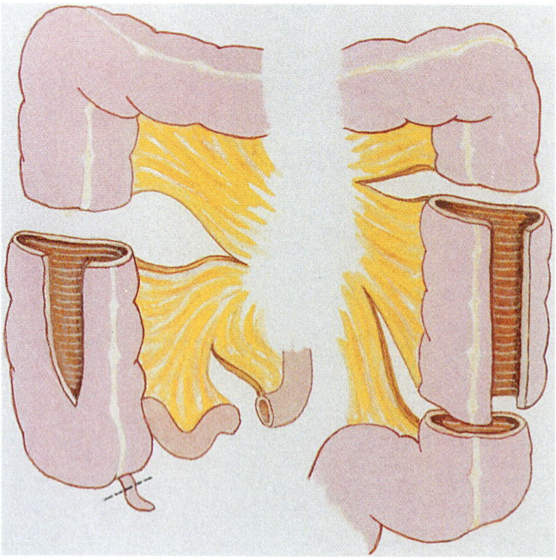

77-3

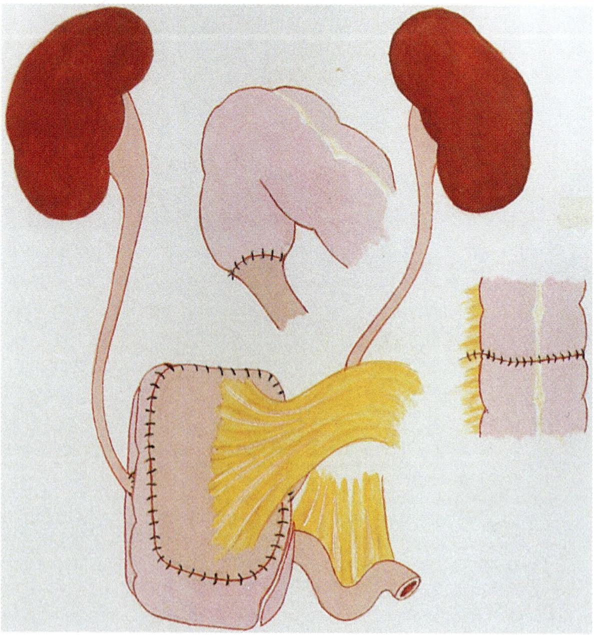

77-4

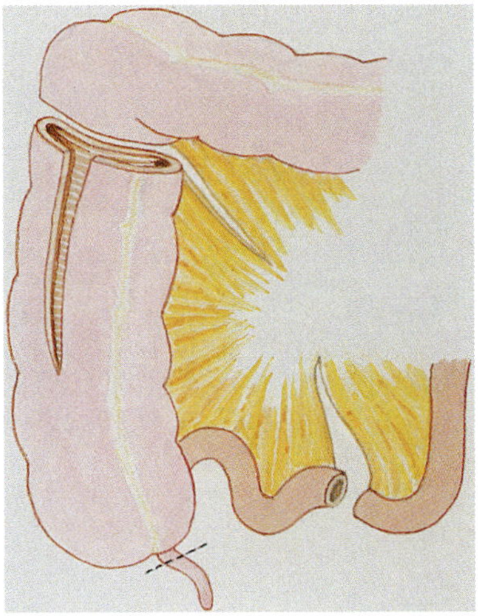

77-5

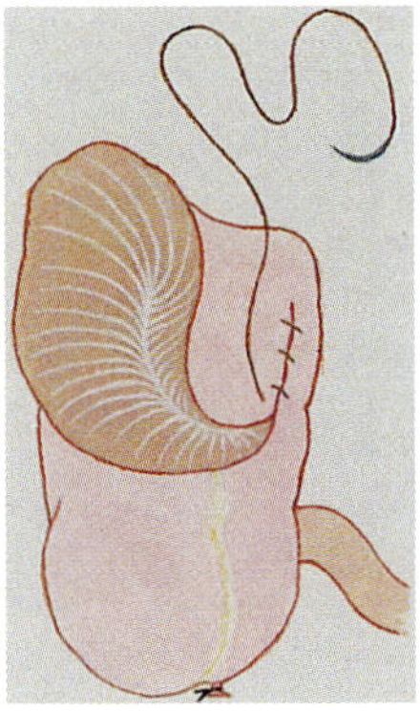

77-6

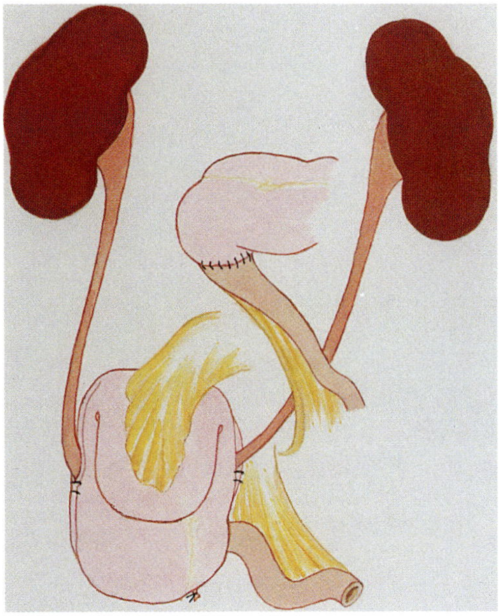

77-7

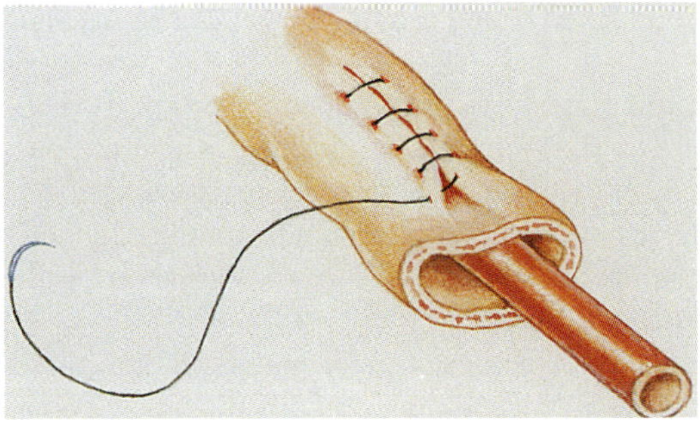

77-8

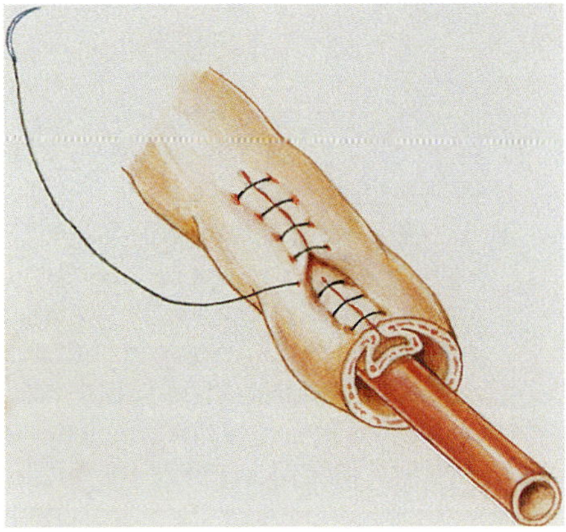

77-9

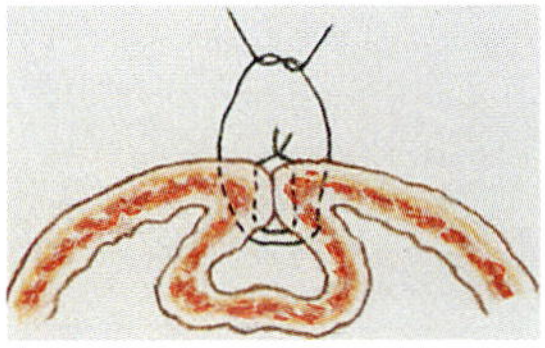

77-10

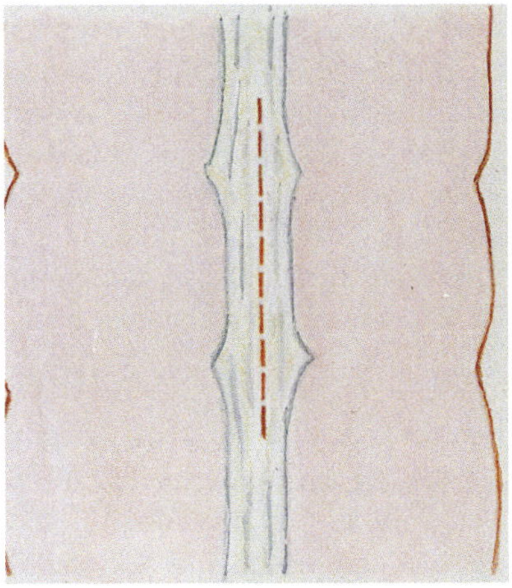

77-11

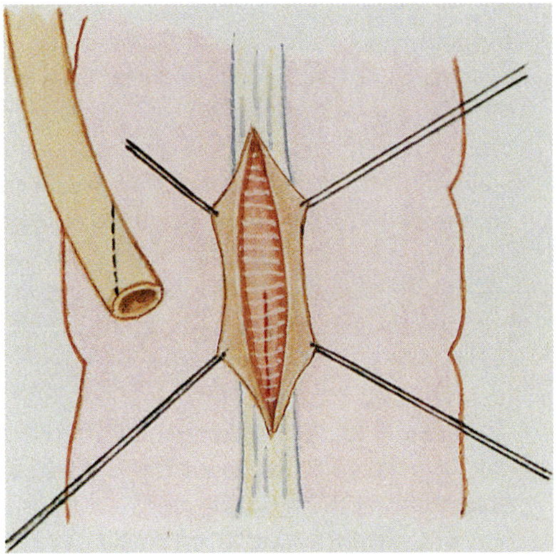

77-12

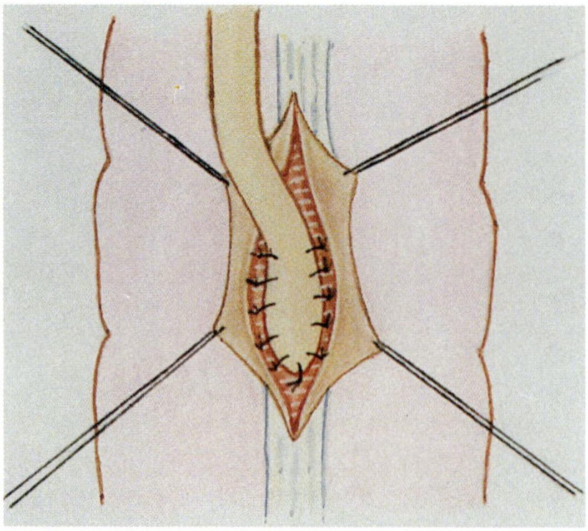

77-13

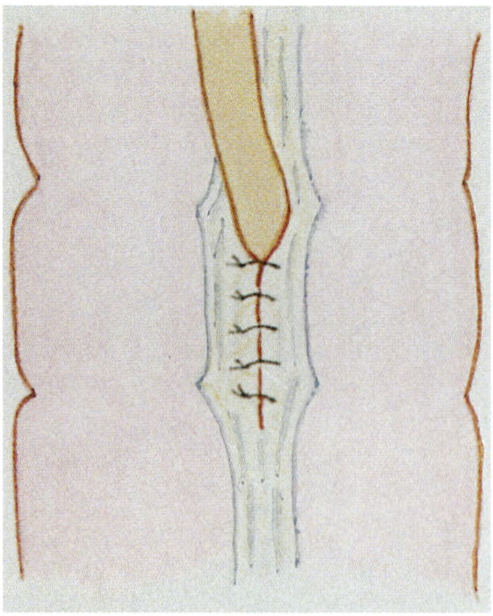

77-14

be brought out through the ileal conduit attached to the cecum. Bowel continuity must be reestablished.

Attention is now directed to the continent ileal limb attached to the pouch. It is best to pass a 12 Fr or a 14 Fr Robinson catheter through the ileal segment which has been tapered with interrupted 3–0 silk Lembert imbricating sutures on the antimesenteric border. A 12 Fr red Robinson catheter provides guidance in creating the continence mechanism in children. The sutures should be spaced about 8 mm apart. One uses sutures about 5–6 mm apart as one nears the ileocecal valve.

In a modification of the Indiana Pouch, one may use tighter spacing of interrupted sutures as you near the ileocecal valve. At the ileocecal junction one places 3 Lembert sutures on the anterior, posterior, and antimesenteric surfaces to tighten the continence mechanism. Note the schematic. Continence is tested by filling the new pouch with 250 mL of saline. If leakage occurs, further plication of the ileocecal valve junction is performed.

Next, a 24 Malecot catheter with its proximal tip within the pouch is placed through the anterior colonic pouch and is secured with a pursestring suture of 2–0 chromic catgut. The Malecot tip catheter and pouch are carefully secured to the anterior abdominal wall. The ureteral stents are brought out through the distal ileal conduit wound and secured with 2–0 or 3–0 silk sutures adjacent to the ileal stoma or at the stomal entrance.

The stoma is positioned inferior to the cecostomy tube in an area marked preoperatively. The efferent limb is brought out through the abdominal wall and an excessive or particularly long limb can be trimmed or shortened. Closure of the abdominal wall is performed in the usual fashion. Retaining sutures may be necessary in an older or undernourished patient.

Postoperatively the insertion of contrast medium by gravity into the pouch can be performed 7 days postoperatively. If no extravasation is seen, we remove both stents on separate days (8th and 9th days).

The patient is taught to catheterize his pouch every 3 hours during the day and every 3 to 4 hours at night. Volumes are recorded.

References

1. Goodwin WE, Harris AP, Kaufman JJ. Open transcolonic ureterointestinal anastomoses. A new approach. Surg Gynecol Obstet 97:295, 1953.
2. Goodwin WE, Scardino PT. Ureterosigmoidostomy. J Urol 118:169, 1977.
3. Bricker EM. Bladder substitution after pelvic evisceration. Surg Clin North Am 30:1511, 1950.
4. Kock NG, Nilson AE, Nilson LO, Norlen LJ, Philipson BM. Urinary diversion via a continent ileal reservoir clinical results in 12 patients. J Urol 128:469, 1982.
5. Skinner DG, Lieskousky G, Boyd SD. Continuing experience with the continent ileal reservoir (Kock Pouch) as an alternative to cutaneous urinary diversion An update after 250 cases. J Urol 137:1141, 1987.
6. Lampel A, Hohenfellner M, Schultz-Lampel D, Thuroff JW. In situ tunneled bowel flap tubes: 2 new techniques of a continent outlet for Mainz pouch cutaneous diversion. J Urol 153: 308–315, 1995.
7. Rowland RG, Mitchell ME, Bihrle R, Kahnoski RJ, Piser JE. Indiana continent urinary reservoir. J Urol 137:1136–1139, 1987.

5 The Prostate

The prostate in men aged 20 to 40 years is a small, walnut-shaped organ located deep in the bony pelvic region. It is less than 12 g in weight in adolescents. It increases in size from 15 to 20 g in middle adulthood (30 to 40 years). After age 50 to 65 the gland may increase in size from 25 to 60 g or more in most men. Large volumes of prostate, more than 100 g, have been reported. In the enlarged prostate, the configuration of the prostate may resemble a "croissant." Exceptions in volumetric size are probably due to neuroendocrine, paracrine-type hormonal influences that act in an independent fashion. These cells do not directly affect the conversion of testosterone to dihydrotestosterone (DHT). Neuroendocrine cells, staining positive for Chromogranin A, serotonin, and calcitonin have been identified in the prostate. These cells are located in the basal cell layer next to the prostatic glandular epithelial cells. In the older male, approximately 60 to 65 years of age or more, these neuroendocrine cells seem to stimulate the smaller, active hyperplastic adenomas (<1 cm) which are undergoing active growth and enlargement.

Recently, finasteride has been shown to reduce prostatic growth. A male who is approximately 60 years of age and has a prostate approximately 40 g in size will experience a 20% reduction in prostatic volume after taking 5 mg of finasteride on a daily basis for 1 year. Five mg of finasteride for 1 year will reduce the glandular epithelial cells of the prostate, particularly in the transitional zone, due to blockage of 5 alpha-reductase activity. Testosterone is not converted to DHT by the enzyme. Overall, urinary flow rates have been slightly disappointing after taking 5 mg on a daily basis for 1 year. A slightly increased (1.9 to 2.1 mL/sec) improvement in flow rates after 1 year of therapy have been reported.

DHT has a biochemical and physiologic impact in the prostate. Recently, it has been mentioned that finasteride masks the rise of prostate-specific antigen (PSA), a blood test used to detect early prostatic cancer. More research is needed to determine how PSA is influenced in men with early prostatic cancer and early benign prostatic hyperplasia (BPH). Early data show that epithelial cells in the small prostatic glands undergoing growth also manufacture PSA. Finasteride treatment for 1 year can reduce PSA levels by 50% in the BPH patient.

New studies would indicate that cancer of the prostate is the second most common cancer in the aging male. In the United States, more than 45,000 deaths will occur in 1995 as a result of prostate cancer. Approximately 319,000 new prostate cancers will arise in 1996. The American Cancer Society estimates that prostate cancer will occur in

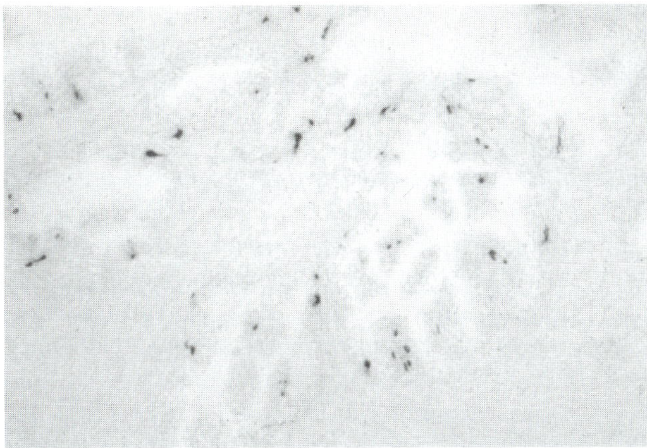

FIG. 1.
Immunohistochemical stain demonstrating neuroendocrine cells.

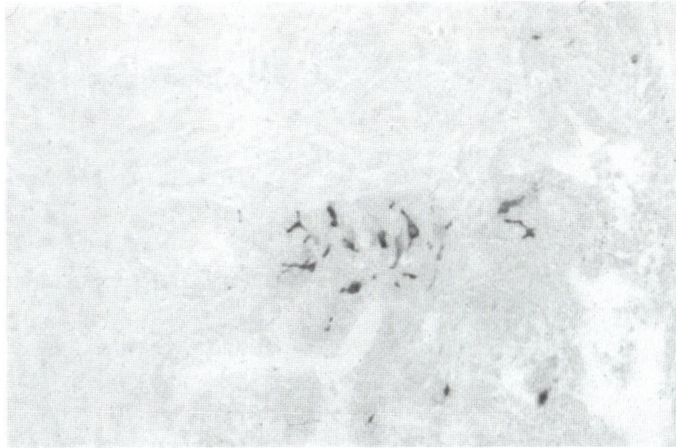

FIG. 2.
Neuroendocrine cells stained positive for serotonin.

one out of four men over 55 years of age. Cancer of the prostate is the most proliferative abnormality found in any human organ. We have preliminary evidence that neuroendocrine cells in the prostate provide a stimulus for early growth of prostate cancer in most cases.

We also have evidence that neuroendocrine cells provide the stimulus for BPH. Figure 1 is an immunohistochemical stain demonstrating Chromogranin A stained neuroendocrine cells around a small hyperplastic nodule from BPH. The proliferation cell nuclear antigen (PCNA) revealed a loci of cellular hyperplasia in a nodule < 1 cm. Figure 2 shows numerous serotonin-stained neuroendocrine cells in a focal area at the periphery of a BPH nodule.

Urologists are familiar with the inflammatory lesions found in the prostate. Subacute prostatitis, when incompletely or inadequately treated, may lead to chronic prostatitis and calculus formation in the prostate. It is not within the scope of this atlas to discuss the diagnosis and treatment of inflammatory disorders of the prostate. Nor is it within the scope of this book to discuss the constituents of the seminal plasma that can be altered by disease, including prostatitis, BPH, or prostate cancer.

Studies by di Sant'Agnese[2] and others in our group have clearly demonstrated that the prostate gland functions as a paracrine-endocrine organ. Di Sant'Agnese and our colleagues worldwide have demonstrated serotonin, calcitonin, bombesin, and somatostatin secreting cells—neuroendocrine cells—in the prostate. Calcitonin and serotonin secretory cells appear to be more abundant in many prostate cancers. We believe that the calcitonin cells may be important in altering prostatic secretions in the ejaculum, and perhaps reducing fertility depending on their specific intraprostatic hormonal-like secretions. For example, calcitonin gene-related peptides can change the concentrations of ionized calcium in the prostate, and affect sperm motility when the ejaculum is collected and evaluated.

Benign Prostatic Hyperplasia (BPH)

In the United States during the years 1975 to 1986 the surgical treatment of BPH was the second most common operation performed on men over 65 years of age. The only operation that exceeded transurethral prostatic resection (TURP) was cataract extraction. In 1986, over 400,000 transurethral prostatectomies were performed in the U.S. The cost of the operations throughout the U.S. in the late 1980s was approximately \$4 billion, when one includes the costs of hospital care. The prevalence of BPH among men over 60 years of age is approximately 45 to 50%. This prevalence is found in whites. The actual prevalence rate among Japanese or Chinese living in their own countries is much less. When Chinese men or Japanese men move to a new culture in western countries (e.g., the U.S.), prostate growth simulates that of men in the western world, suggesting the fact that environmental differences play a major role.

Guidelines for the treatment of BPH are now established. Use of a symptom score, or some index in which the patient's symptoms can be carefully evaluated, appears to be advantageous. The physical examination includes a general examination and the digital rectal examination of the prostate. A routine PSA blood test is obtained in all patients over 50 years of age. When BPH becomes more obvious in terms of increased symptomatology, then more frequent PSAs (every 6–9 months) are needed. In the workup of BPH, we include a symptom evaluation sheet, which was recently summarized by one of us. The symptomatology can be listed as obstructive or irritative (see Table 5.1).

As men grow older, BPH becomes a major clinical problem. The symptoms related to prostatic hyperplasia have all been described. The AUA Symptom Score clearly validates the severity of the major symptoms, and the increasing score denotes a more symptomatic BPH due to a restrictive urinary flow.

Seven symptoms are described in Table 5.1, and they can be judged on their own by determining the severity of the symptom. The symptoms are a feeling of incompletely emptying the bladder; two different frequencies of urination; urinary intermittency; urgency (or postponing urination); a weak urinary stream; and, finally, straining to urinate at the beginning or during urination. An additional question—quality of life due to urinary symptoms—was also added.

It is now clear that significant BPH (symptom score over 12 points) needs to be treated either with medication or removal of the enlarged BPH tissue. In the workup of the older patient, a uroflow study—peak urinary flow and average urinary flow—should be obtained. An ultrasound bladder scan is also obtained to measure postvoiding residual urine after urination. We believe that the symptomatic male needs to void 140–150 mL of urine to be able to document the extent of prostatic glandular blockage. Some investigators believe that a voiding volume of 125 mL is satisfactory.

What seems to complicate the symptomatology are irritative symptoms. They include urgency, a sensation of incomplete voiding, and some incontinence that is slightly uncontrollable.

The collection of objective data includes uroflowmetry (minimal volume of 150 mL) with maximal flow and average flow. Residual urine is obtained from the bladder after voiding based on ultrasonography using an anterior bladder scanner. Cystoscopy and urethroscopy are exceedingly important. Urethroscopy will rule out a stricture. Cystoscopy will provide some evaluation of the obstructive prostate. By measuring urethral length, one can also determine what the various options for treatment might include. The bladder neck is carefully evaluated. It is important to be sure that if a fairly thin posterior bladder neck is present, then several therapeutic options may be available. One option is transurethral incision of the prostate (TUIP), or incision of the bladder neck and posterior prostate tissue from bladder neck to near the verumontanum. At this time, one cannot find data based on randomized studies that support the effectiveness of balloon dilation 1 year after the procedure. We no longer use balloon dilatation. To complete the cystoscopy evaluation, the bladder is carefully examined. The presence or absence of calculi is noted. The degree of trabeculations is documented. In addition, the presence of cellules or diverticula is documented.

While still somewhat debatable, we believe that the patient develops indications for prostatic treatment based on symptom score; uroflowmetry data, including residual urine; and cystoscopic findings. Regarding urine flow studies, the patient is asked to void at least 150 mL of urine. In some studies, a voiding volume of 125 mL is acceptable. The maximal peak flow is noted. Normally, this maximal peak flow in a 40 year old would be more than 25 mL/sec. With beginning prostatic hyperplasia, the peak flow

Table 5.1 International Prostate Symptom Score (I–PSS)

	Not at all	Less than 1 time in 5	Less than half the time	About half the time	More than half the time	Almost always	
1. Over the past month, how often have you had a sensation of not emptying your bladder completely after you finished urinating?	0	1	2	3	4	5	PVR
2. Over the past month, how often have you had to urinate again less than 2 hours after you finished urinating?	0	1	2	3	4	5	FREQ
3. Over the past month, how often have you found you stopped and started again several times when you urinated?	0	1	2	3	4	5	INTER-MITT
4. Over the past month, how often have you found it difficult to postpone urination?	0	1	2	3	4	5	URGE
5. Over the past month, how often have you had a weak urinary stream?	0	1	2	3	4	5	↓ FLOW
6. Over the past month, how often have you had to push or strain to begin urination?	0	1	2	3	4	5	STRAIN
	None	1 time	2 times	3 times	4 times	5 or more times	
7. Over the past month, how many times did you most typically get up to urinate from the time you went to bed at night until the time you got up in the morning?	0	1	2	3	4	5	NOCT

Quality of Life Due to Urinary Symptoms

	Delighted	Pleased	Mostly satisfied	Mixed about equally satisfied and dissatisfied	Mostly dissatisfied	Unhappy	Terrible
1. If you were to spend the rest of your life with your urinary condition just the way it is now, how would you feel about that?	0	1	2	3	4	5	6

Quality of Life Assessment Index L=

Increased dribbling at end of voiding has 2 components
- ↓ urethral muscle tone
- BPH & obstruction

will be reduced to the level of 15 mL/sec. When that maximal peak flow is in the 10 mL/sec range or less, then moderately significant BPH has developed. The average flow in the person who is obstructed is somewhere in the range of 5–8 mL/sec. At this reduced level the older male may have a residual urine volume of approximately 100 mL or more.

Urodynamic studies are indicated in some patients who have urge incontinence and prostatic obstruction. These pressure flow studies provide excellent information and assist the urologist in the decision-making process.

Previously, a study was conducted by the American Urological Association and selected urological centers. The purpose of the study was to reexamine the mortality rate of TURP. It has now been demonstrated that the increased mortality rate may be unrelated to the operation itself. Significant co-morbidities, including heart disease or hypertension, may be a better explanation. The final study, which has recently been published, suggests that an increased mortality is not seen after TURP in the United States.

At the present time there are a number of studies which have been structured so that randomized data are being collected. These studies, including ours, are carefully evaluating BPH. When the older men are symptomatic and objective parameters reveal significant obstruction, then the patient is randomized into three non-operative categories and one operative category (TURP).

To date, approximately 150 patients have been randomized, and clinical data are accumulating. In 1996 it is anticipated that a number of publications will appear, including our own, and the value of nonoperative medical therapies (an alpha blocker such as terazosin or doxazosin) will appear. In addition, studies that will have randomized data may show longer term results using finasteride 5 mg, or 4 to 8 mg of doxazosin per day, for BPH.

It would appear that, over the long term, treatment of BPH will allow the older patient a whole array of therapeutic options. Although the nonoperative selection of finasteride may not be ideal, since there may be some masking of the PSA blood test particularly in older patients who select finasteride, newer therapies may become available. Urologists will need to be aware of what these options are and if the studies are randomized. The selection of options for treatment of BPH should be based on randomized data clearly demonstrating the efficacy of drugs or the effectiveness of urological-surgical procedures employing laser or other new devices.

Surgical Anatomy

STRUCTURE AND LOCATION

The prostate is a multilobar glandular and fibromuscular organ that surrounds the first part of the urethra between the bladder and the urogenital diaphragm: it is covered by a fibrous capsule.

It is roughly truncated in shape, with its base contiguous with the bladder and its apex pointing toward the urogenital diaphragm (Fig. 3).

The prostate consists of five lobes: anterior, posterior, median, left, and right lateral lobes (Fig. 4). The anterior lobe has fewer glandular elements and adenoma rarely occurs in this location. The posterior lobe lies behind the median lobe, forming the entire posterior surface of the gland, and is the lobe palpated during rectal examination. Primary adenocarcinoma may occur in this lobe as a palpable nodule.

The median lobe is, clinically, an important lobe. It lies in front of the ejaculatory ducts, below the neck of the bladder, and contains much glandular tissue. Adenomas frequently grow in this lobe and may lead to urinary obstruction.

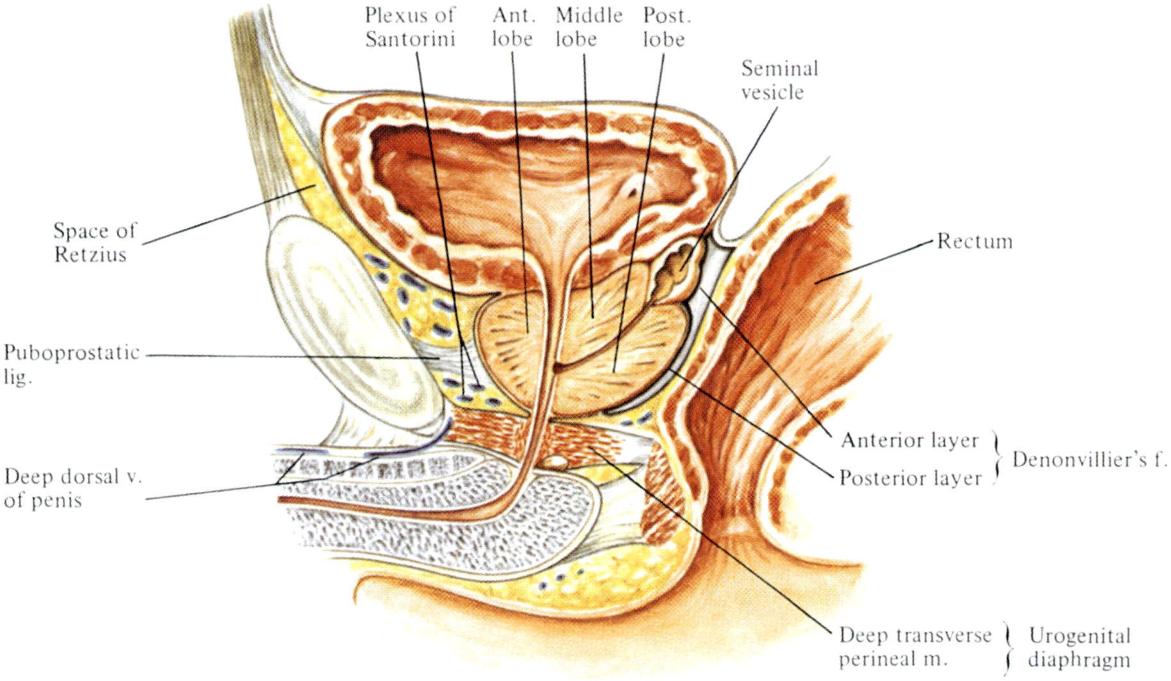

FIG. 3.
Midsagittal view emphasizing fascial relationships.

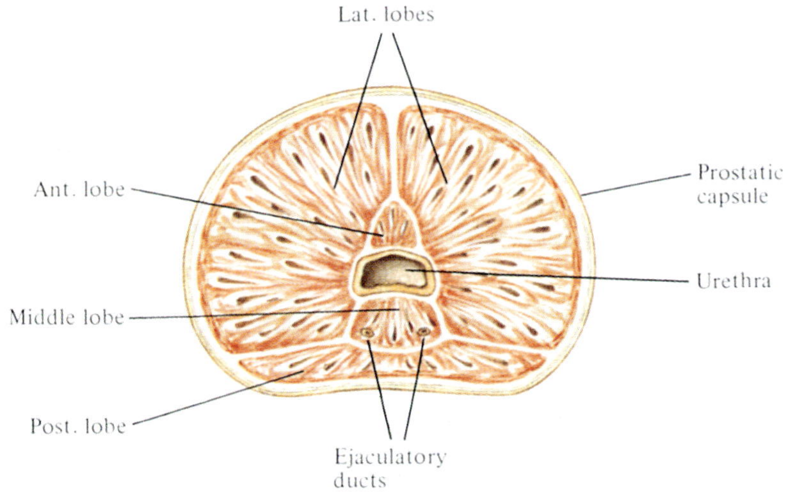

FIG. 4.
Cross-sectional view, showing lobes.

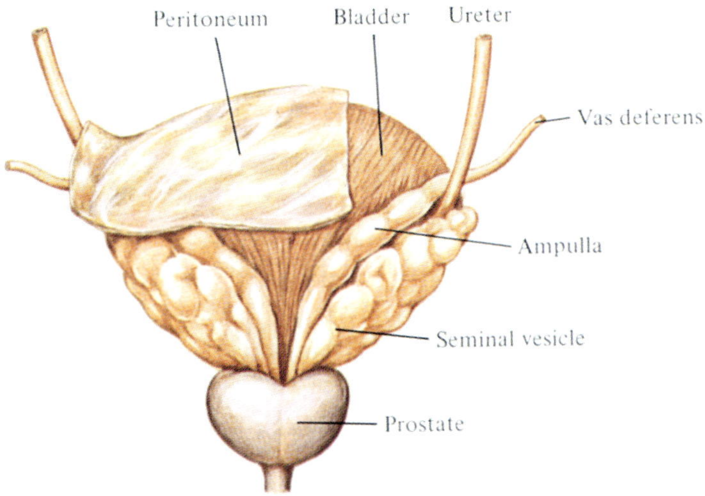

FIG. 5.
Posterior view showing seminal vesicles and ejaculatory ducts entering prostate.

Both lateral lobes contain much glandular tissue in the elderly male. Hyperplasia of the inner (periurethral) glands may form large adenomas: the outer normal prostatic tissue is displaced peripherally and compressed into a thin fibroglandular structure that is known as the "surgical capsule." Hypertrophy of these lateral lobes is the most frequent cause of urinary obstruction in the older male.

The seminal colliculus (verumontanum) is a rounded prominence on the lower posterior surface of the prostatic urethra. It has a small depression in its central surface, the prostatic utricle. The ejaculatory ducts open into the prostatic urethra on either side of the colliculus (Fig. 5).

The prostatic glands consist of a compounded tubular structure and form about 20 ducts that open into the prostatic urethra (Fig. 6).

FASCIAL RELATIONSHIPS

The prostate is surrounded by the endopelvic fascia, which lies outside the prostatic capsule. The puboprostatic ligaments anteriorly, triangular ligaments inferiorly, and rectovesical fascia of Denonvilliers posteriorly also surround the prostate (Fig. 1). A narrow area at the anterior midline toward the base of the prostate is left uncovered by the puboprostatic ligaments (width of one finger) (Fig. 7).

The anterior layer of the rectovesical fascia is firmly attached to the prostate and seminal vesicles, but the posterior layer is attached loosely to the pelvic fascia and separates these organs from the rectum. The space between these two layers is called the retroprostatic space of Proust and is an important anatomic landmark when total perineal prostatectomy is being performed.

The periprostatic plexus of veins lies between these surrounding fasciae and the true prostatic capsule. By dissecting close to the levator ani muscle, the fascia containing blood vessels and lymphatics can be removed with the prostate and seminal vesicles when radical perineal prostatectomy is being performed.

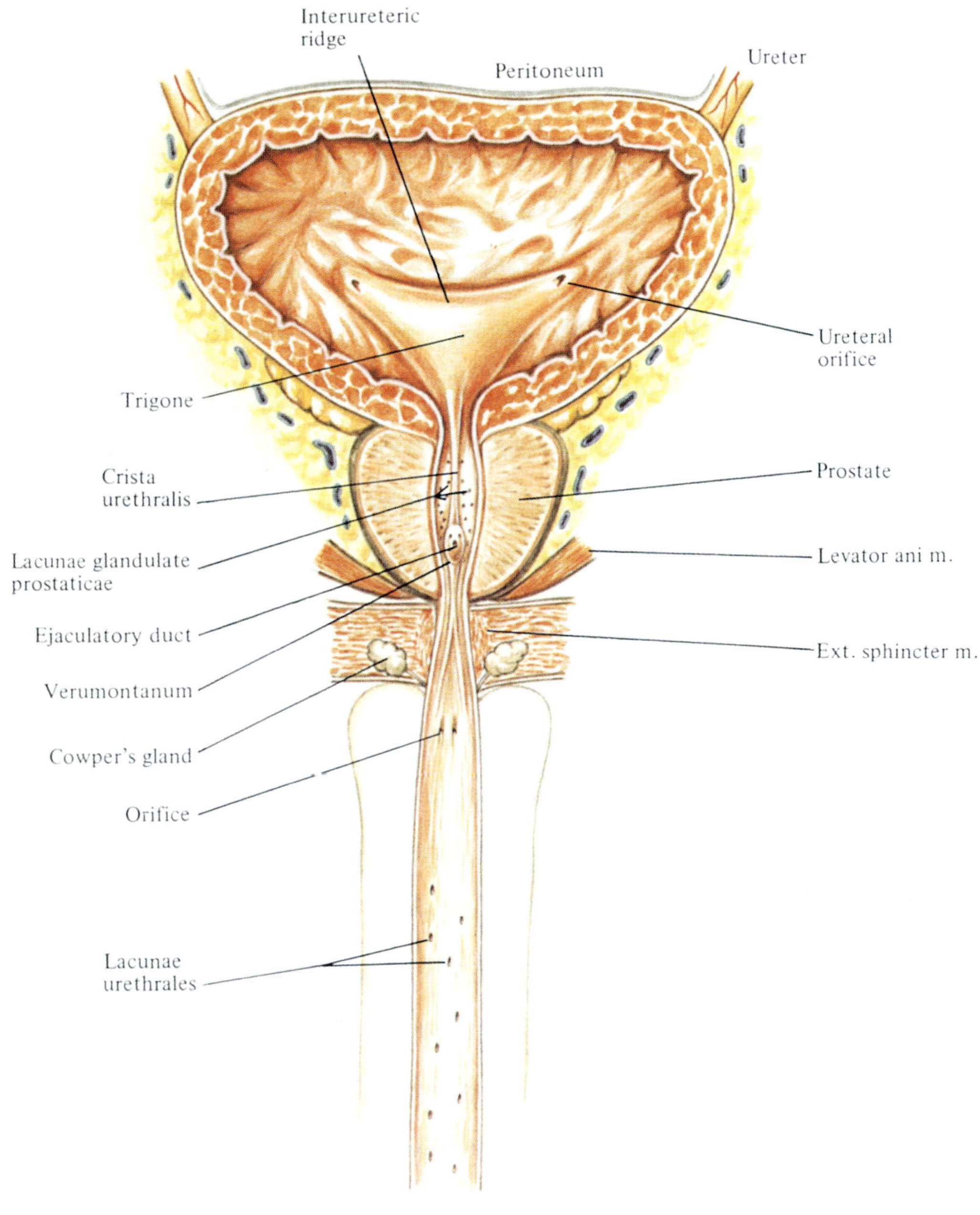

FIG. 6.
Interior of bladder, prostate, and proximal portion of urethra.

VASCULAR SUPPLY

The main arterial supply to the prostate is derived from the inferior vesical artery, which is a branch of the internal iliac artery. Additional arterial supply is frequently received from the middle hemorrhoidal and internal pudendal arteries, which enter the gland at the vesicoprostatic junction. Flocks made a comprehensive study of the intrinsic arterial distribution within the prostate and found two groups of arteries, the urethral and the cap-

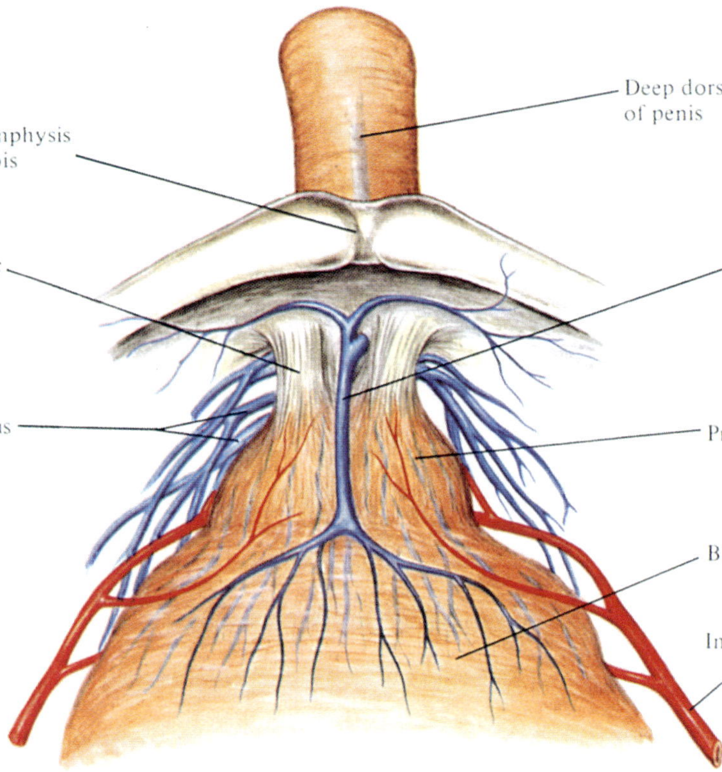

FIG. 7.
Venous supply.

sular groups. The urethral group of arteries penetrates the capsule at the posterolateral vesicoprostatic junction and supplies the vesical neck and periurethral portion of the gland. The capsular group of arteries enters the gland laterally, giving off several branches, which mainly supply the peripheral portion of the prostate (Fig. 8). This group of arteries shows little change with age or with the development of hyperplasia.

With BPH, the urethral group of arteries enlarges to supply the whole of the adenoma. It is an extremely important anatomic principle when a surgical procedure of the prostate is being considered. Regardless of the type of adenectomy, the main arterial bleeding will be from this group of arteries in the posterolateral quadrants of the vesical neck. Ligation or cautery of the vessels in the early stage of any type of operative procedure will minimize subsequent bleeding.

Veins form a plexus on the anterior and lateral aspects of the prostatic capsule, particularly around the base of the gland at the vesicoprostatic junction. The veins receive branches from the deep dorsal vein of the penis, communicate with the pudendal venous plexus and vesical plexus, and drain into the internal iliac veins. The superficial branch of the deep dorsal vein of the penis, which lies on the midline of the anterior surface of the prostatic capsule, is of considerable surgical importance in retropubic prostatectomy (Fig. 7).

The lymphatics from the prostate glands form a periprostatic network and unite to form several main channels and drain into the internal iliac, external iliac, obturator, and presacral nodes.

THE McNEAL DIAGRAM

McNeal has clearly outlined the zones or segments of the prostate. Figure 9A is a three dimensional, 3/4 frontal view of the McNeal diagram. The posterior region is the pe-

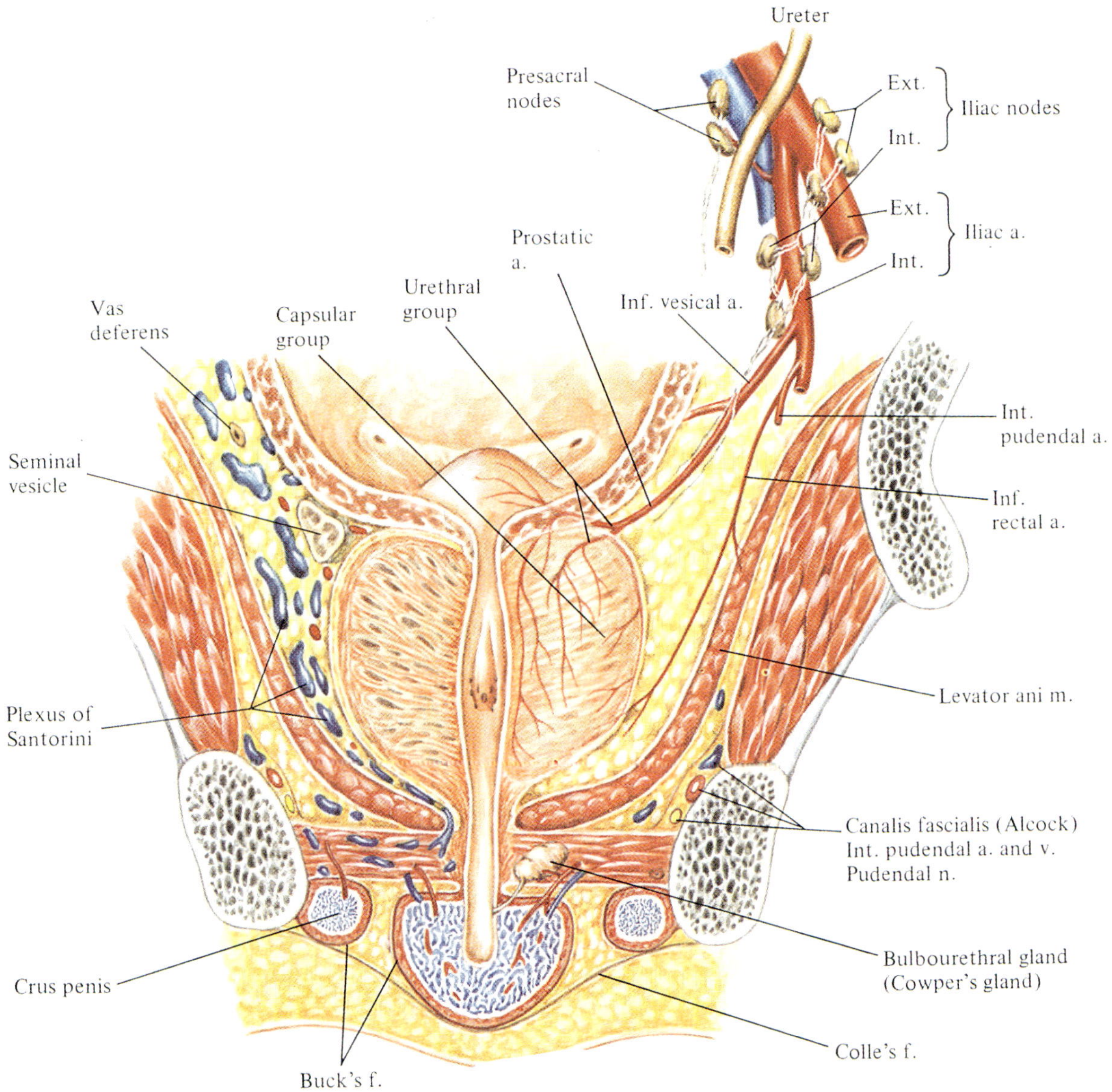

FIG. 8.
Arterial supply.

ripheral zone. From other studies we have learned that about 50% of the prostate contains stroma. When BPH occurs, the stromal portion of the prostate may increase significantly along with glandular hyperplasia.

Figures 9B–D show the sagittal diagram (Fig. 9B), coronal section diagram (Fig. 9C), and the oblique coronal section diagram (Fig. 9D), respectively, after the McNeal diagram.

In BPH, one can identify areas of nodular hyperplasia and expansion of the transitional zone. When the transitional zone expands further (Fig. 9E), the proximal urethral segment is elongated. The distal urethral segment, however, is shortened. Since the verumontanum is located just proximal to the external sphincter, care must be taken to not resect beyond, or distal to, the verumontanum. An aggressive resection (TURP) in this distal area may lead to urinary stress incontinence.

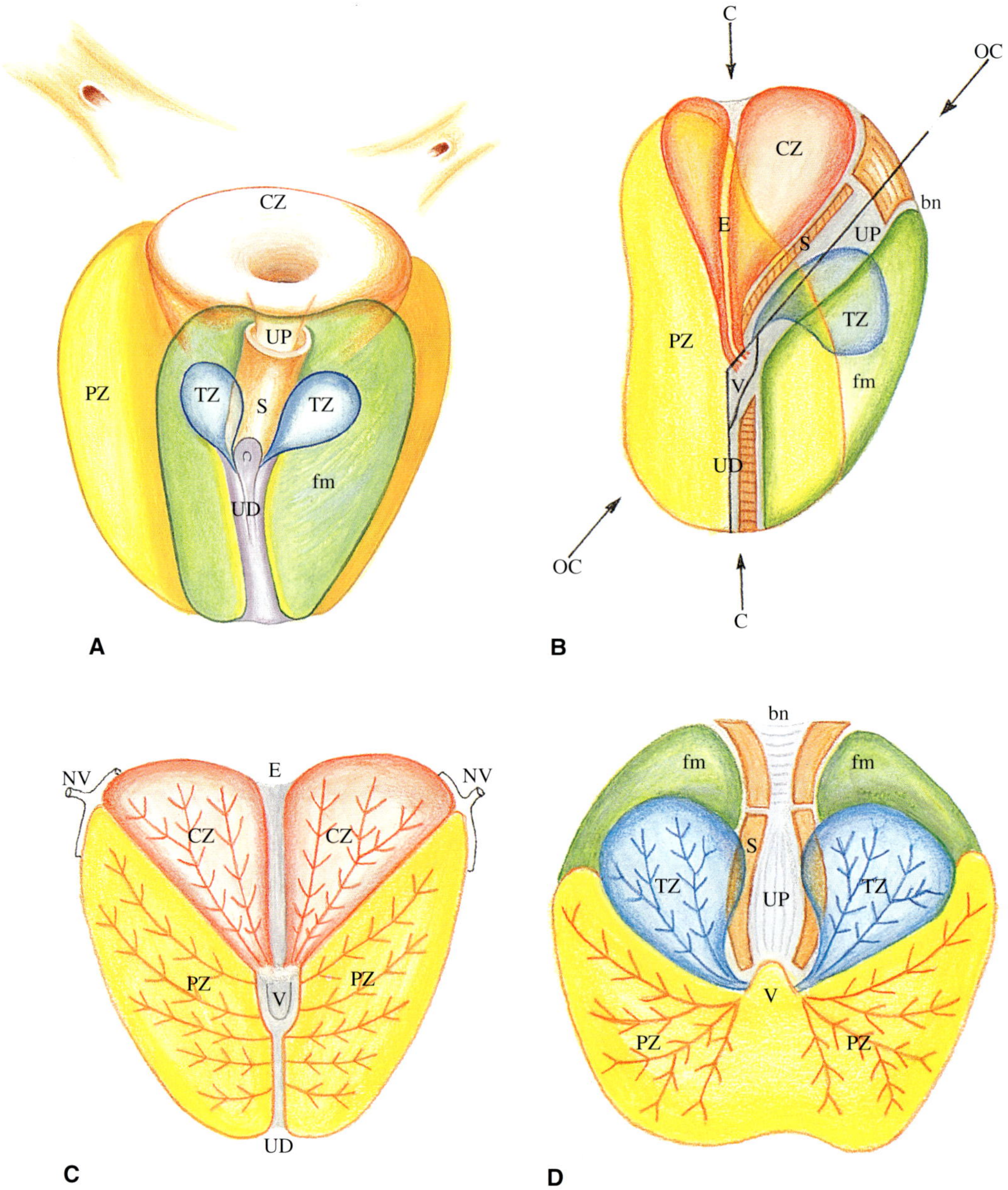

FIG. 9.
A. Three dimensional view of prostate. The prostate is turned 25% ($\frac{1}{4}$) from frontal view. **B.** Sagittal view of prostate. **C.** Coronal section of prostate. **D.** Coronal section turned slightly oblique. Bladder neck (bn) and verumontanum (V) are shown. **E.** BPH in the transitional zones. **F.** Distribution of carcinoma originating in the prostate. Legends: CZ = central zone, bn = bladder neck, TZ = transitional zone, PZ = peripheral zone, UP = proximal urethra, UD = distal urethra, fm = fibromuscular stroma, S = preprostatic sphincter, OC = oblique coronal plane, E = ejaculatory ducts, NV = neurovascular bundle, and V = verumontanum. Figures 9A to D are original illustrations, but they follow the descriptions and findings published by John E. McNeal, MD. The 1988 *Monographs in Urology.* Copyright 1988 by Thomas Stamey.

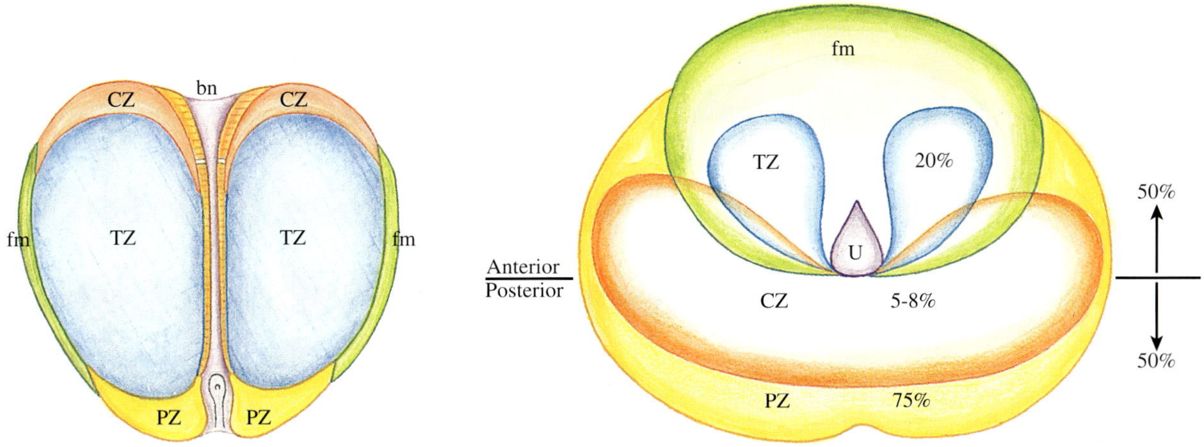

E F

FIG. 9. *(continued).*

In most cases, BPH (as shown in Fig. 9E) is almost entirely the result of bilateral nodular expansion of the transition zone. The proximal urethral segment is elongated, the distal urethral segment is relatively shortened, and the verumontanum is located just proximal to the external sphincter. Care must be taken not to resect beyond the level of verumontanum at TURP to avoid incontinence.

Operative Techniques

78. Retropubic Prostatectomy (Vesicocapsular Prostatectomy)

78-1. Position of the patient is exaggerated. *The sacrum of the patient is placed on a rectangular sandbag.* The table is flexed slightly to open the retropubic space.

78-2. *A vertical midline incision is made* and carried through skin and fascia. The rectus abdominis muscles are separated, exposing prevesical fat.

78-3. *The inferior bladder wall and prostate are carefully exposed.* The self-retaining retractor provides adequate exposure.

78-4. *The major arterial blood supply of the right prostate is ligated;* an aneurysm needle carries the ligature. A sponge on a ring forceps assists in providing appropriate traction.

78-5. *A vertical midline incision is made from the prostate to the bladder neck* by means of a Bovie type electrical cutting current. The capsular vein is ligated on each end to prevent excessive bleeding.

The classic capsular incision for retropubic prostatectomy is made in a transverse direction. If this alternative is chosen, then suture ligatures (three for the inferior plane and three for the superior plane) must be placed prior to making the horizontal incision. We have used both capsular incisions with equal success.

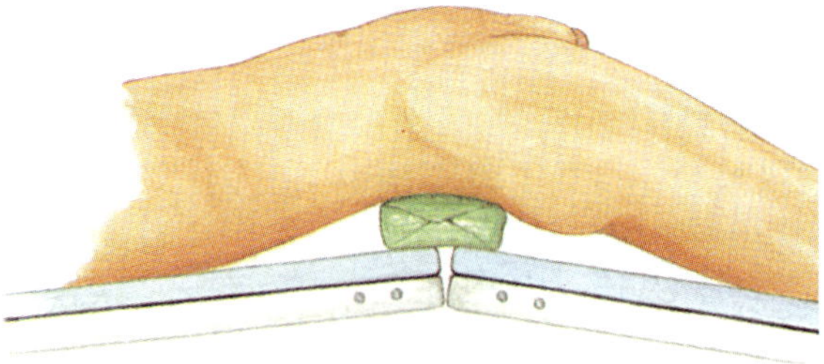

78-1

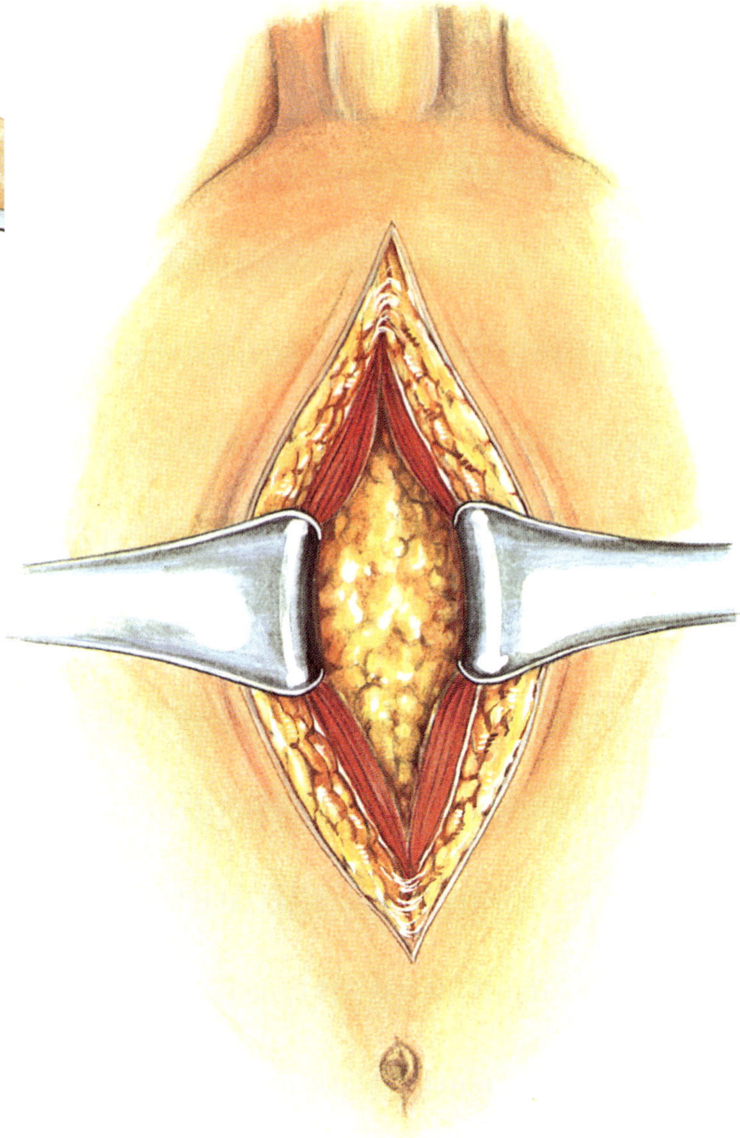

78-2

Enucleation of Prostatic Adenoma and Wedge Resection of Posterior Bladder Neck

78-6. *The cleavage plane is established* by using blunt and sharp dissection. The adenoma is freed.

78-7. *The adenoma is detached from the prostatic fossa* near the external sphincter. Care must be taken not to injure the sphincter, either by sharp dissection or by vigorous dissection with the finger in an inferior direction.

78-8. *The posterior bladder neck is grasped at 6 o'clock by an Allis clamp.* The right posterior neck is cut as shown.

78-9. *The posterior bladder neck has been excised.* Figure-of-eight sutures (2–0 chromic catgut) are placed at 5 and 7 o'clock for hemostasis. The bladder mucosa is attached to the proximal prostate floor with several 3–0 chromic catgut sutures. The indwelling catheter (22 French) is placed, and the balloon is tested.

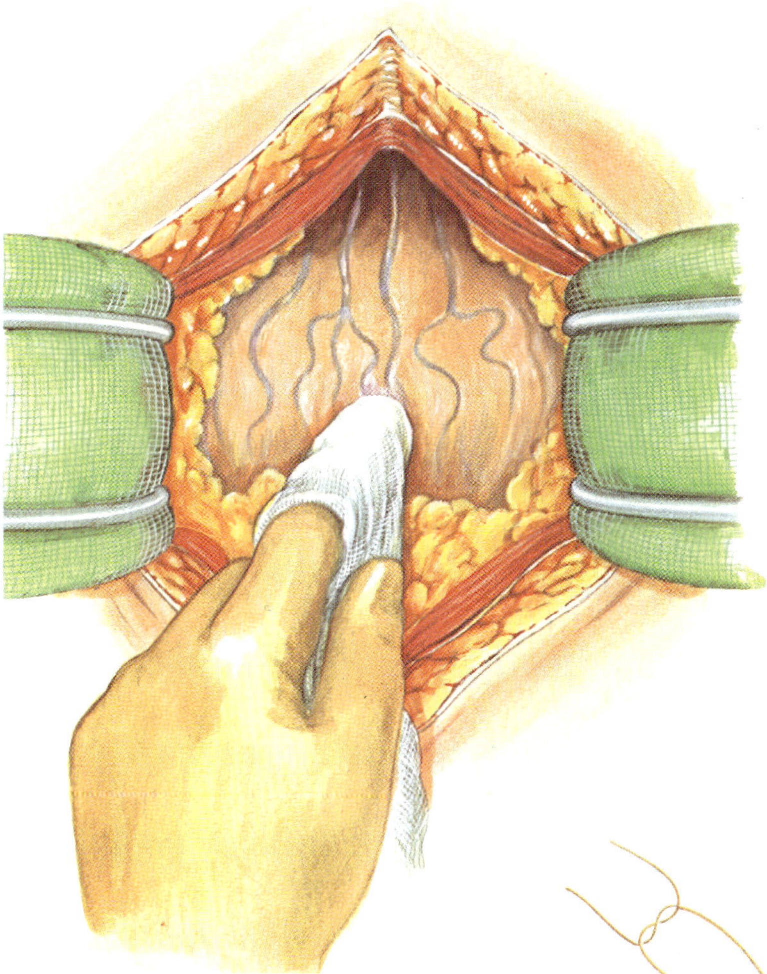

78-3

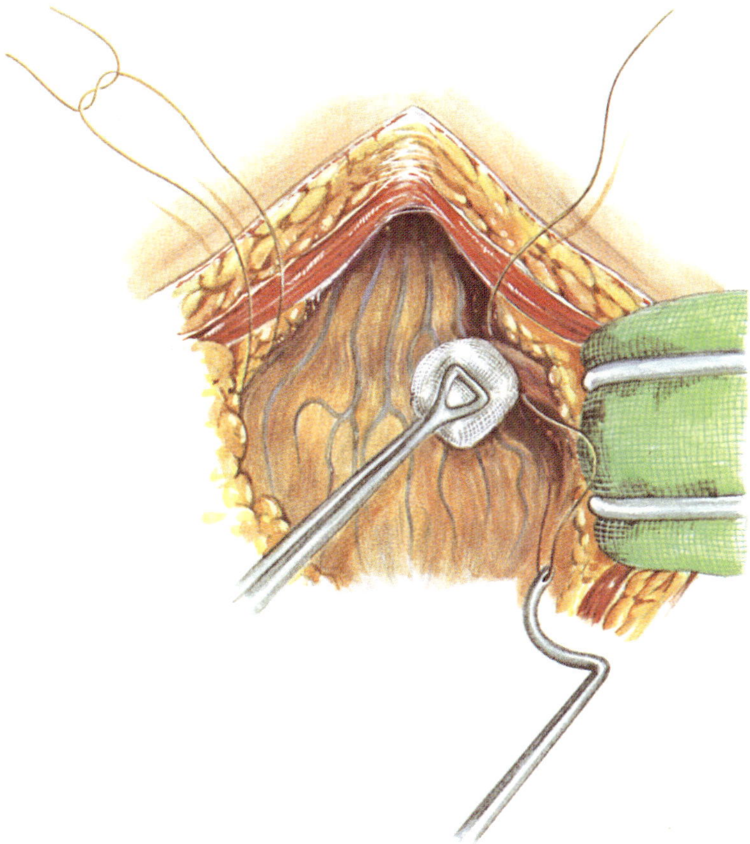

78-4

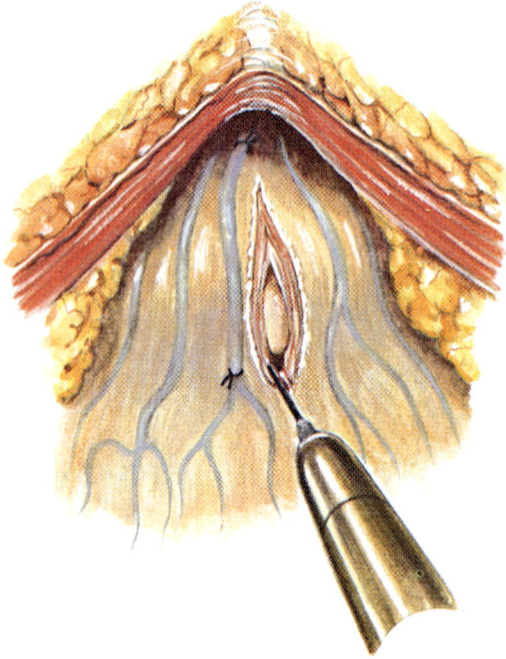

78-5

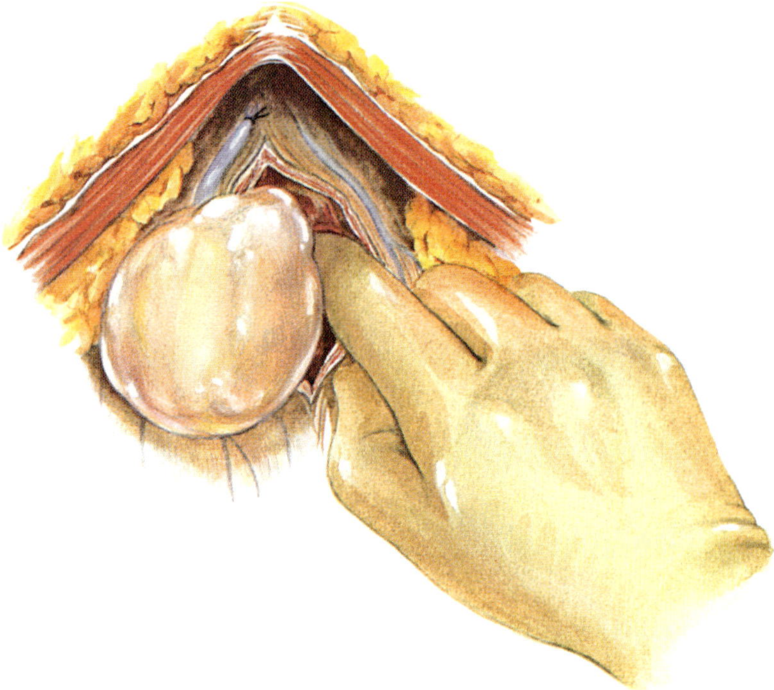

78-6

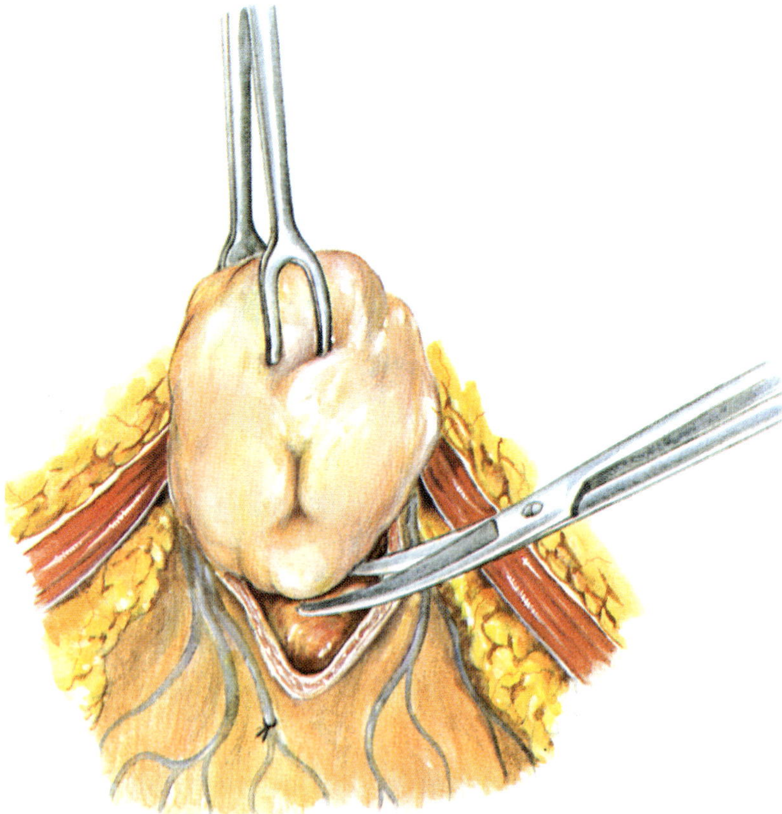

78-7

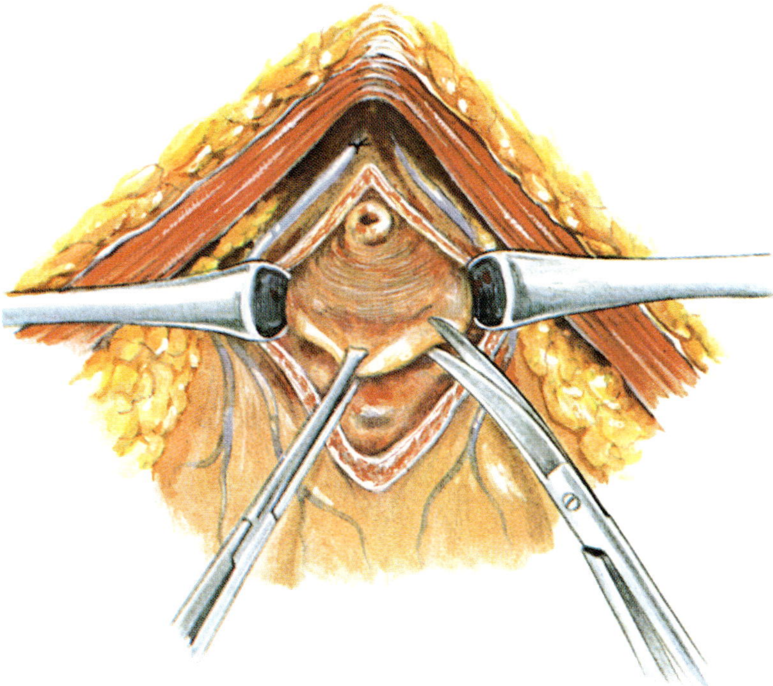

78-8

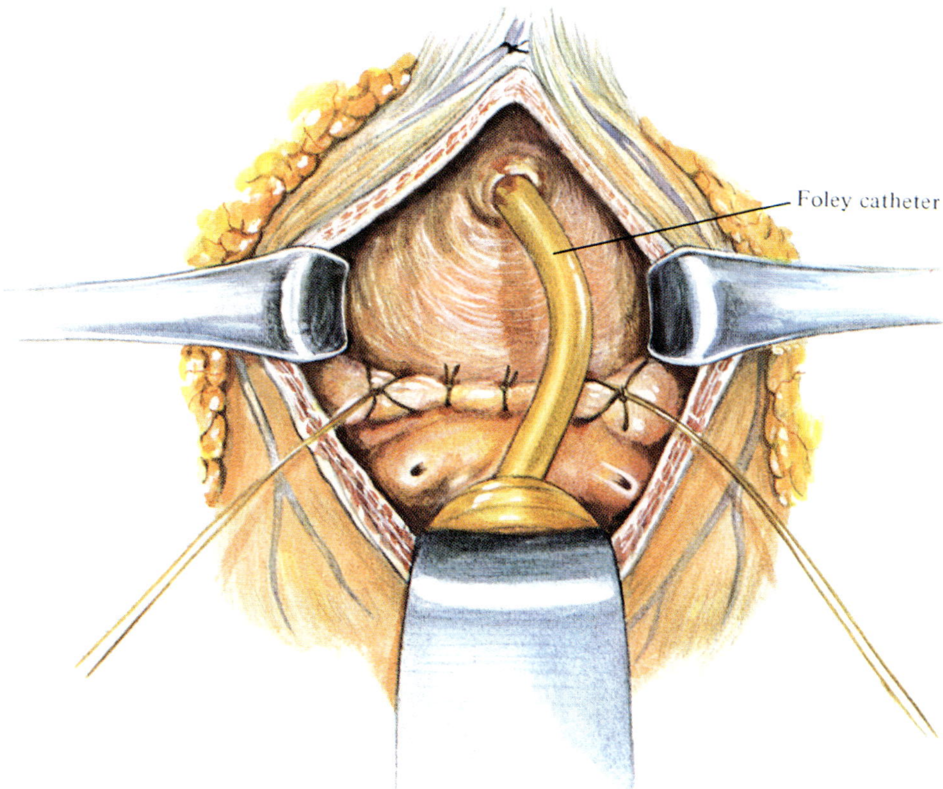

78-9

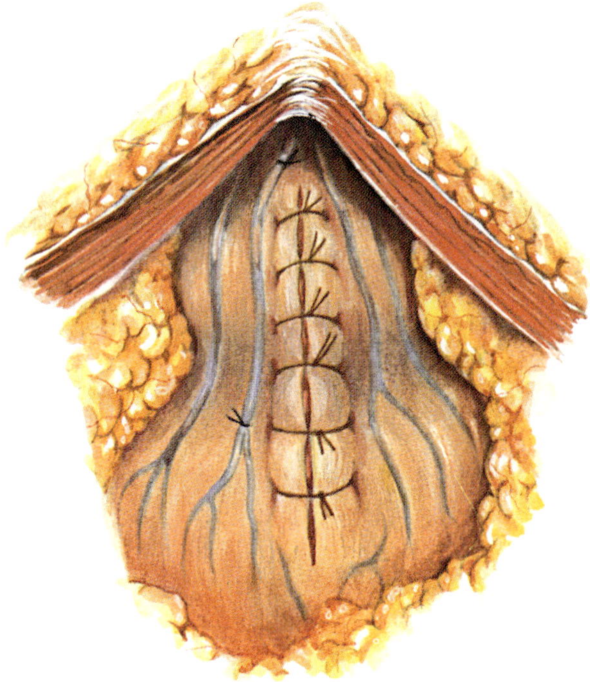

78-10

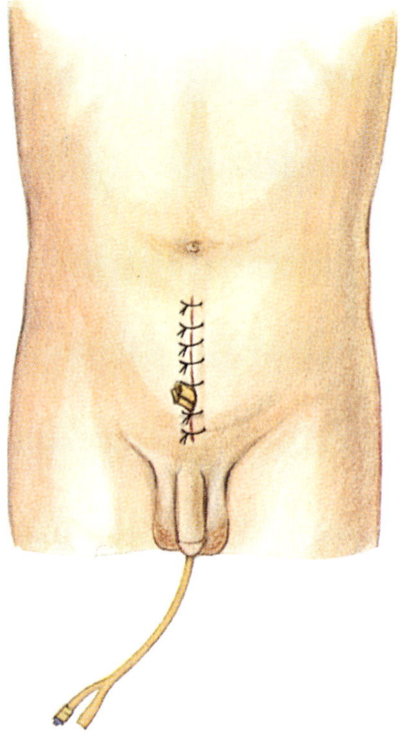

78-11

Closure

78-10. *The prostatic capsule and bladder neck are reapproximated* with 2–0 chromic catgut. One flat tubular drain is inserted on the lateral aspect of the prostate, and the tubular connection is attached to a plastic bulb which has been deflated.

78-11. The indwelling catheter (22 Fr) is tested again. Thirty mL of saline is used to inflate the balloon. The fascia is reapproximated with interrupted sutures (0–0 chromic catgut). The skin is closed with 4–0 nylon sutures. Although *the flat tubular drain emerges from the inferior portion of the incision,* we now make a separate skin stab for the tubular drain that lies near the capsular incision.

79. The Walsh Technique: Radical Retropubic Prostatectomy for Prostatic Adenocarcinoma

Overview of Organization and Perspectives

Prostate cancer is a major health problem in older men. In 1996 approximately 317,000 new cases of prostate cancer will be detected, and approximately 45,000 deaths from prostate cancer will be reported. Areas of controversy and disagreement exist with regard to the best treatment for these patients.

The latest data on prostate cancer, as we have it and interpret it today, needs some clarification. This introduction will include a critical discussion regarding the detection and treatment of early stage prostate cancer. The best reference for a thorough discussion of prostate cancer is the *Journal of Urology*, supplement issue, November 1994. Partner organizations participating included the American Urological Association, American Cancer Society, American College of Surgeons' Commission on Cancer, and the cooperation of the National Cancer Institute.

Several major issues require clarification. What is meant by screening and early detection? We need to separate screening programs from those on early detection of prostate cancer. Screening for prostate cancer, by definition, focuses on asymptomatic men. Early detection focuses on men with symptoms similar to those for BPH. Men who are 50 years old or older have mild to moderate BPH with an incidence of 60 to 70%. They should undergo testing with PSA and digital rectal examination to ensure early detection of abnormalities at least once a year according to recommendations of the American Urological Association and The American Cancer Society. Black men and those with a strong positive family history of prostate cancer should begin evaluation starting at age 40 years, including a PSA test and a digital rectal examination initially. If both tests are normal, PSA and digital rectal examination should be repeated 6 months to 1 year later, and continued each year.

What is the role of digital rectal examination and PSA? How should they be used in an early detection program? Digital rectal examination for cancer detection, unfortunately, underestimates cancer volume. The use of the available tests and transrectal ultrasonography, including when to perform biopsy will be discussed later. These modalities are related to important confirmatory steps in an early detection program of cancer. Should the 8 to 9 million older men ages 76 to 80 years with latent cancer (Gleason grade 2 to 4 of 10) be followed expectantly? How can we separate latent cancer from cancer with a Gleason grade of 5 to 7? We agree that men in the former group may be watched expectantly; the patient with moderate undifferentiation (Gleason 5 to 7) probably requires radical prostatectomy given the heterogeneity that occurs in prostate tissue and the fact that 6 to 8 biopsies may not be fully representative of the highest prostate cancer Gleason grade.

What is the appropriate age limitation for radical prostatectomy? What important co-morbidities should limit the procedure or increase the chronological age for surgery? Can urologists agree to an upper age limit for radical surgery of 70 to 74 years?

What are the long-term results of irradiation therapy if patient characteristics are adjusted for Gleason grade, age, and stage? What are some of the problems that arise when radical prostatectomy is performed in smaller cities and communities? Are these operations resulting in excessive impotence rates and high urinary incontinence rates? The *Journal of Urology*, November 1994, addresses most of these controversies.

Urodynamic changes in the bladder occur with the progression of BPH. Our Scandinavian colleagues tell us that symptoms of urge incontinence can occur in probably a third of older men with BPH. Do these tendencies influence our interpretation of prostate cancer study results? Are men with latent cancer (75 to 80 years old or older) undergoing a radical operation? Guidelines are clearly needed to deal with this tendency.

Diagnosis and Treatment of Prostate Cancer

Worth emphasizing is the important role of radical prostatectomy for cure of significant stages of prostate cancer. The indications for surgery include stages A_1, A_2, B_1, and B_2 (Gleason score of 5 to 7 out of 10, or moderate undifferentiated cancer). One of the major problems with accurate staging of prostate cancer is the heterogeneity of the prostate. The biopsy needle may uncover a well differentiated cancer (Gleason 2 to 4) while a lesion with a higher Gleason grade nearby has not been biopsied. A rising PSA, e.g., 4.1 ng/mL at the initial stage that is elevated 6 months later to 4.7, and, subsequently, after another 6 months has risen to 5.3 ng/mL is suspicious for early cancer. The patient needs to be re-biopsied. He probably has early prostate cancer, a Gleason score of 5 to 6, or moderate undifferentiation. Some C lesions have been included for surgery by a few investigators; however, this indication is controversial. The final decision for removal of the involved neurovascular bundle is made at surgery. We do not believe that a radical retropubic prostatectomy is indicated for Stage D_1 adenocarcinoma. By definition, Stage

D_1 means that the pelvic lymph nodes—obturator nodes—are involved with cancer (two or more nodes). Prostate Cancer Awareness Week over the past 5 years (1990–1995), lasting for 2 weeks, has allowed 2000 urologic centers to screen about a million men (ages 50 or more). In the case of Blacks, they are encouraged to undergo a digital rectal exam and a PSA blood test after age 40 years because of a higher incidence of cancer.

The location of most early prostatic carcinoma is assisted by transrectal ultrasound imaging. Hypoechoic lesions can usually be detected. The ultrasonic guided needle biopsies can identify the cancer. The usual patient, age 58 to 65 years of age, will present with an elevated PSA (4.1 to 8 ng/mL). The prostatic specific antigen serum test has been effective in the early detection of prostate cancer. Based on the Symposium Issue (*J Urol*, November 1994, No. 2) we strongly believe that monitoring the blood PSA levels, particularly at 6-month intervals, is useful. An initial PSA rise in a 60 year old with early BPH may reveal a PSA of 4.1 ng/mL to 4.8 ng/mL. The transrectal ultrasound scan (TRUS-P) may not reveal hypoechoic areas particularly in the peripheral zone (PZ). Digital rectal examination reveals a mild to moderate enlargement of the prostate. The TRUS-P Scanner will provide the size of the prostate and the BPH diagnosis is recorded. A third PSA should be obtained in about 4 to 6 months. A rise in the PSA to 4.8 (more than 0.5 ng/mL) is suspicious for cancer because BPH is slow growing. The digital examination is negative for cancer. BPH is still the "working" diagnosis. After another 6 months, if the PSA now has risen to 5.4 ng/mL, we become suspicious of cancer. This elevation of PSA may be due to prostatic cancer (moderate undifferentiation, Gleason sum [Gleason score] 5 to 7). Transrectal ultrasound scanning of the prostate is repeated. If small, hypoechoic lesions are seen, they are biopsied. In addition, 6 to 8 random biopsies are obtained from other zones, including the transitional zones. In our view, the rise in the PSA (more than 0.5 ng/mL) over each subsequent 6-month study interval is very important. We agree with Dr. William Catalona that it is important for the urologist to re-biopsy the prostate even if the digital rectal exam is negative for cancer but suggestive of early BPH.

Lilja, Gershagen, and our group in Rochester believe the new PSA test evaluating ACT, alpha-1 antichymotrypsin, is probably a better diagnostic test for separating BPH from prostate cancer. A higher ratio of free PSA over the complex form (PSA attached to alpha 1 antichymotrypsin) is seen in BPH. In early prostatic cancer, the complex form of ACT predominates. It behooves the urologist to perform more biopsies as the PSA levels rise over two 4- to 6-month intervals.

Digital rectal examination is also helpful in about 20% of patients depending on the level of PSA. In our view, a PSA in the range of 4–10 ng/mL is useful in diagnosing cancer of the prostate in about 20–30% of patients. A PSA elevated between 10–20 ng/mL is also useful in diagnosing prostate cancer in approximately 35–50% of patients. PSA values more than 10–20 ng/mL may actually suggest cancer spread beyond the prostatic capsule in 50% of cases.

If hypoechoic areas are localized by transrectal ultrasonography, these sites are usually the foci for cancer. If the PSA is 10–20 ng/mL and digital rectal examination is negative, we perform random biopsies of the prostate taking cores from at least eight sites. The sites include the posterior peripheral zones, the anterior quadrants, and the transitional zones.

A magnetic resonance imaging (MRI) coil developed by Pollack et al. has been evaluated by our group in staging intracapsular or local extracapsular extension of prostate cancer. The higher stage cancers infiltrating the capsule, for example, on one side or at the apical prostate can be visualized by the MRI coil. Overall, a single coil MRI device is not beneficial for the early detection of most prostate cancers (Gleason 5 to 7). Today, we do not suggest that MRI examination be performed for early detection of prostate cancer localized within the prostatic capsule.

Pollack has recently developed a double coil magnetic resonance imaging (MRI) apparatus. Early reports suggest that the double coils can focus on prostate cancer within and at the capsular margin. Cancer infiltrating the prostatic capsule and extending outward for 3 to 4 mm can apparently be detected.

We believe that new future prostatic markers in the seminal plasma may provide useful approaches for early detection of cancer. Mirror imaging studies with prostate cancer may be useful using new antibodies (immunohistochemical staining). These new tests may prove useful in ascertaining the potential degree of infiltrating prostatic cancer. Chromogranin A and parathyroid hormone-related protein (PTHrP) are two new tissue markers undergoing evaluation and localization in neuroendocrine cells. The more useful marker may be PTHrP. We believe that these markers may be able to characterize the degree of differentiation in prostatic carcinomas. Early reports suggest that an increasing degree of neuroendocrine differentiation correlates with aggressive tumor behavior. New specific immunohistochemical stains of prostatic cancer, e.g., prostatic intraepithelial neoplasia (PIN), have the potential to become useful in detecting some cases of early prostate cancer. The importance of this finding is that if prostatic cancer is detected early, and the new markers are moderately elevated, aggressive surgical therapy can be initiated with an outcome of cure.

Preparation of the Patient

A bone scan is performed prior to deciding whether the candidate should undergo radical prostatectomy. Evidence of bone spread is a contraindication for radical surgery.

About 2–3 weeks prior to surgery, the patient visits the hospital or an experienced Red Cross Blood Bank to provide two units of autologous blood for his planned future surgery (usually two units of blood will suffice). Use of the Chu-Holtgrewe retractor has been useful in exposing the dorsal vein and its branches. This maneuver has significantly lessened the need for autologous blood.

The patient may be admitted 24 hours prior to surgery if he lives outside the region. A large bowel preparation using a standard routine, including Colyte (Reed and Carnrick, Jersey City, NJ), to encourage cleansing of the large bowel, enemas, and antibiotics are beneficial. This preparation may be started at home and the patient can be admitted the next morning, ready for surgery.

On the morning, 2 hours prior to surgery, the patient may receive a single dose (4000–5000 units) of heparin subcutaneously. This is optional and we do not routinely use heparin. In the operating room automatic inflatable leg and thigh cuffs are applied to both lower extremities to promote the return of venous blood. The patient is in the operating room at this time. An antibiotic, a cephalosporin, is injected prior to induction with anesthesia.

Operative Procedure

Our routine is to use epidural anesthesia for most patients. The anesthetized patient has his legs separated slightly in abduction. His anterior abdomen from above the umbilicus is carefully and surgically cleansed. The scrotum and adjacent perineum, along with the penis, are also surgically cleansed using at least two disinfectants. Surgical drapes expose the penile shaft and anterior abdomen up to and at least 4–5 inches above the umbilicus.

79-1. A vertical midline incision is made from the symphysis pubis superiorly to the left of the umbilicus and returns to the midline, particularly in obese patients. After incising the anterior fascia, the rectus abdominis muscles are separated in the midline. A new urinary catheter, 22 Fr with a deflated balloon, is inserted and the bladder is emptied. At the time of insertion an aliquot of urine is obtained for culture and sensitivities. The bladder is partially filled with saline to permit easier dissection of the space of Retzius. The bladder is then emptied. The peritoneal reflection is freed and sharply dissected off the bladder surface to assist with bladder mobilization and exposure of the pelvic lymph nodes. The peritoneum is not entered. Bilateral partial vasectomy may be performed in the pelvic cavity where the vas deferens turns medially.

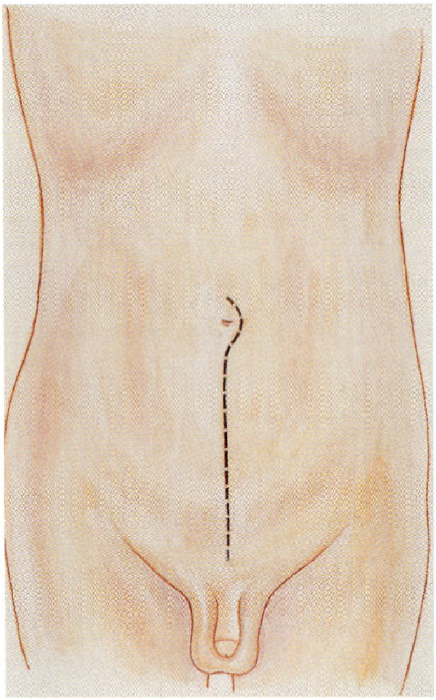

79-1

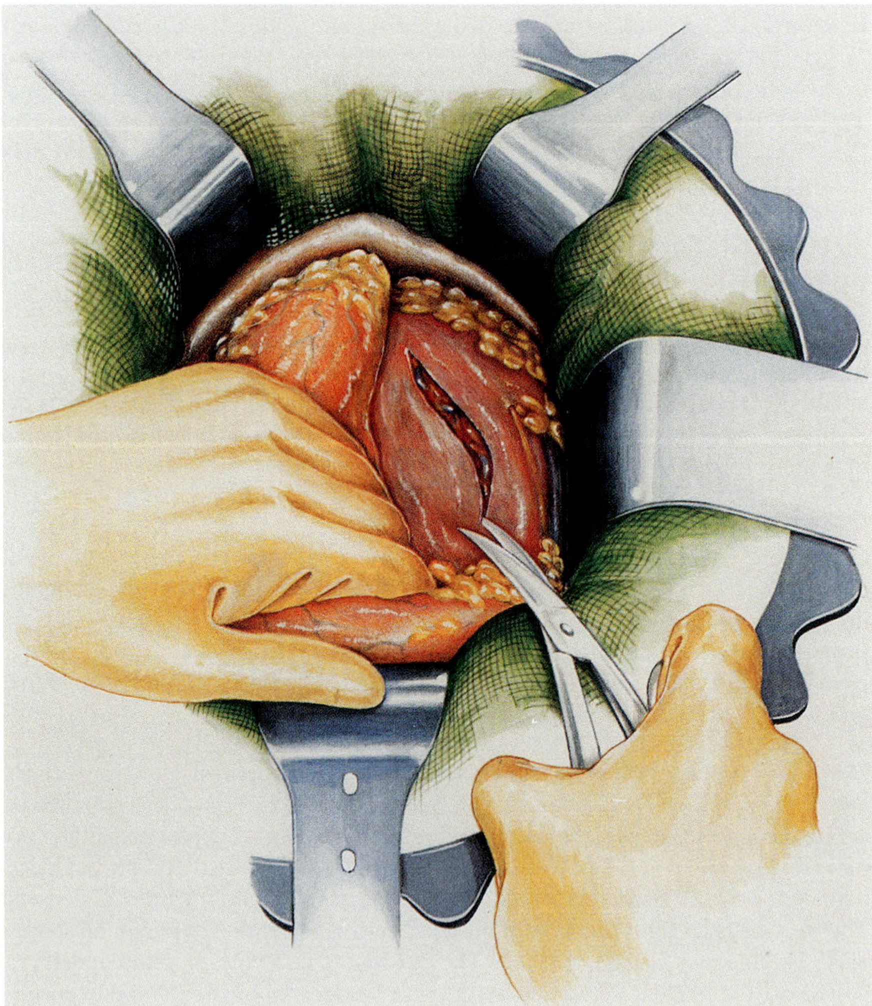

79-2

79-2. With careful exposure, using a self-retaining Balfour retractor and a padded Deaver retractor, the right obturator lymph node chain is exposed. All areola tissue and lymph nodes from the right circumflex veins are dissected from and removed up to and superior to the junction of the bifurcation of the external and internal iliac arteries and veins. A vein retractor is useful in protecting the iliac vein. Electrocautery is used to maintain hemostasis, the posterior margins for dissection include all nodes and areola tissue surrounding the obturator nerve and the obturator artery. The obturator artery and nerve are carefully protected and preserved. The tissue is submitted for frozen section. While we are waiting for the pathologist's report, exactly the same procedure is performed on the left side. If the reports reveal that all the nodes are negative, then the operation is continued with the goal of removing the prostate and seminal vesicles.

The fatty tissue overlying the superior and anterior prostate surface is superficially removed with sharp dissection, exposing the endopelvic fascia. After using blunt dissection, the endopelvic fascia is incised in a semicircular fashion.

79-3. The puboprostatic ligaments are identified and interrupted sharply. Blunt dissection is continued, allowing finger palpation of the apex, the membranous urethra with catheter in place, and the anterior surface of the prostate.

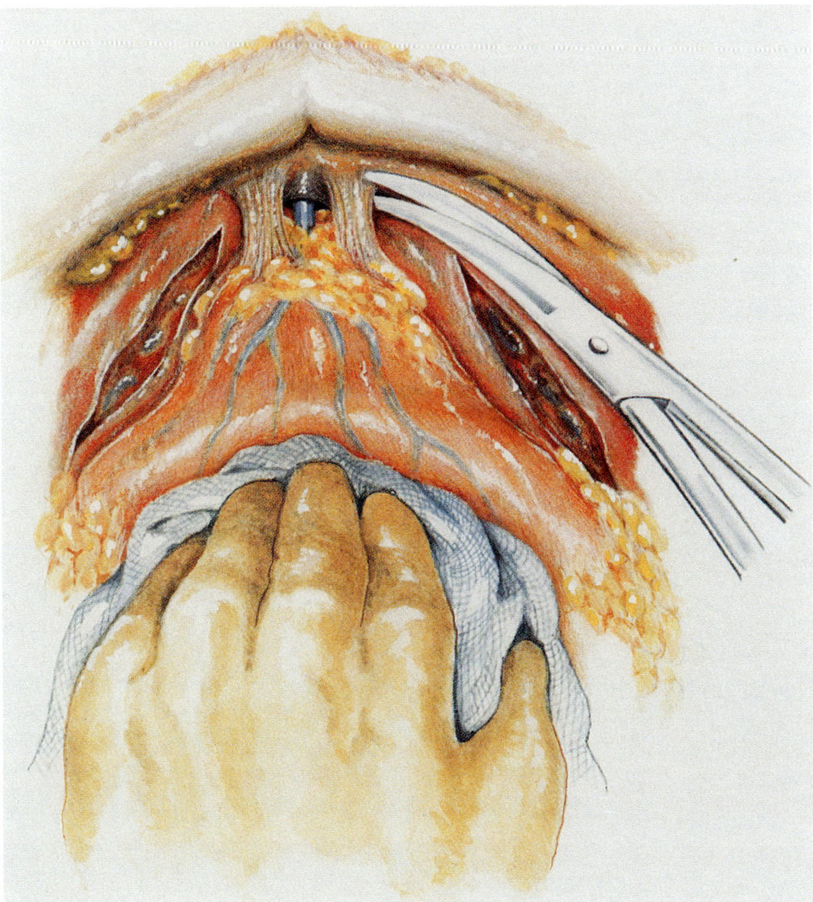

79-3

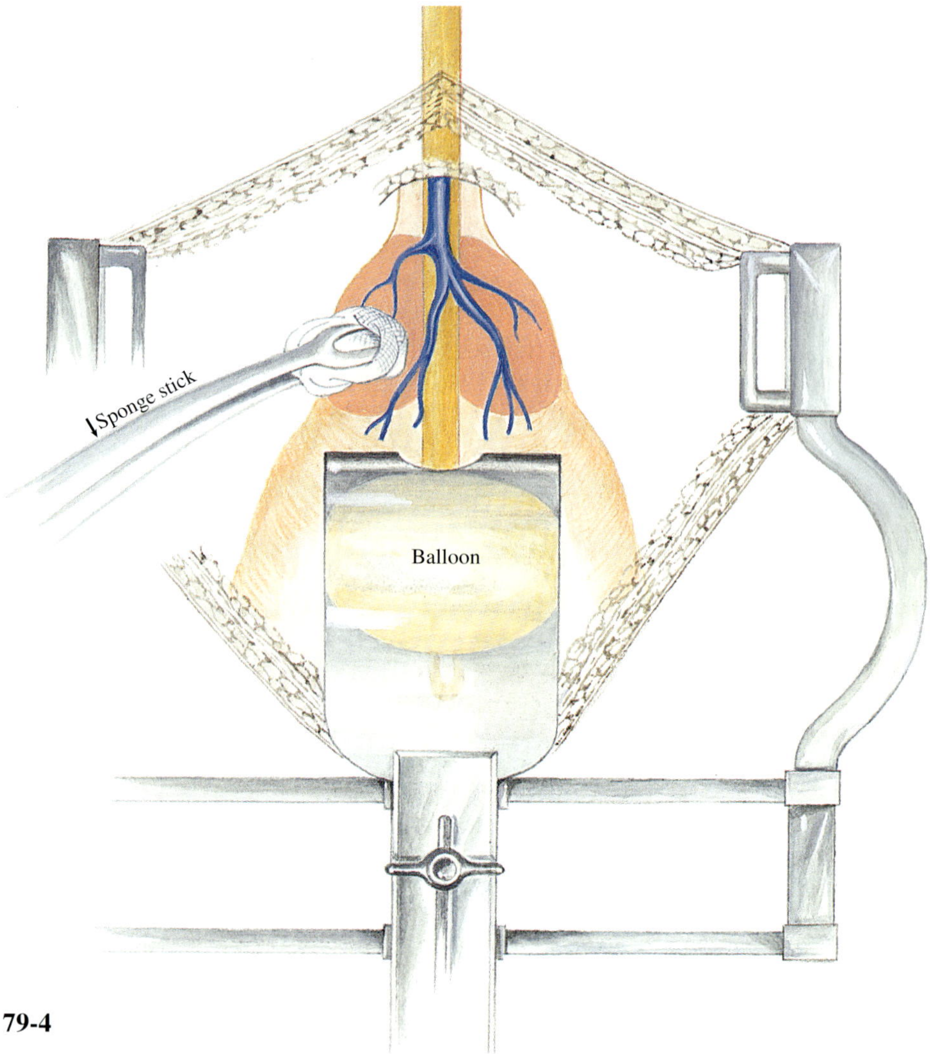

79-4

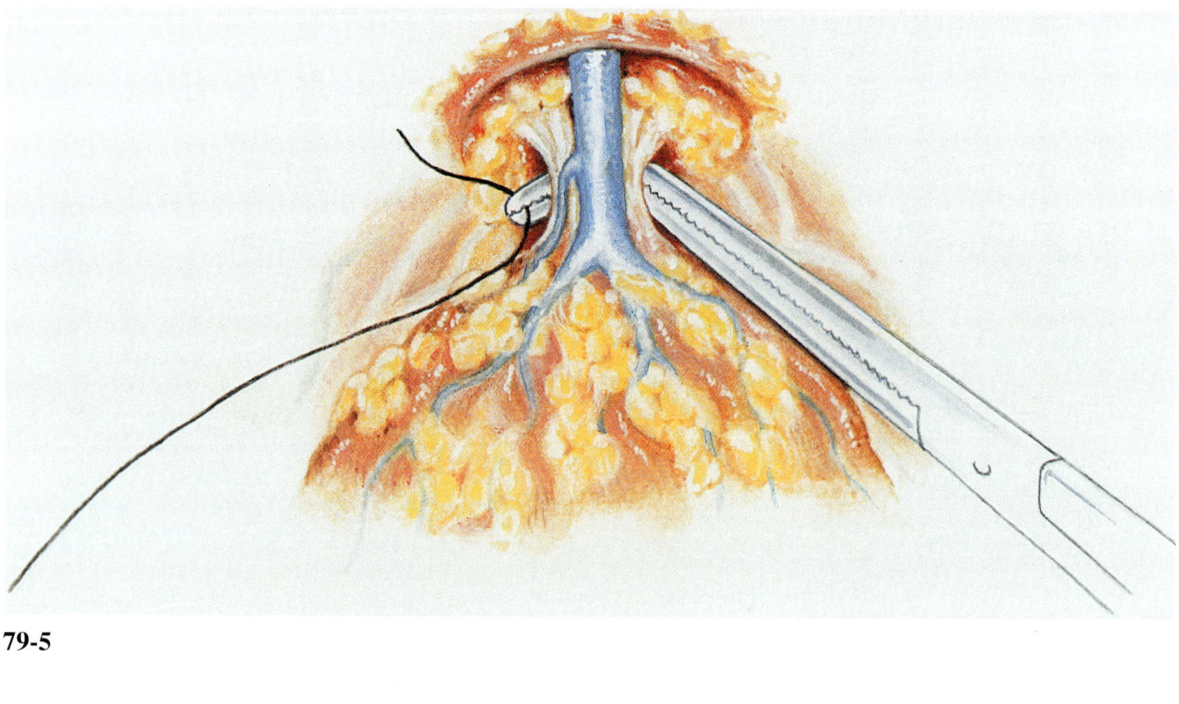

79-5

79-4. Since exposure is difficult because of the anatomy and the fact that the patient is short and obese, we use a modification. The Chu-Holtgrewe retractor is readied. Forty mL of saline is then placed into the balloon of the Foley catheter. The balloon is moved superiorly away from the bladder neck (3 cm superiorly), and the new retractor with the U-shaped slot is placed below the balloon about 3 cm superior to bladder neck. Gentle but firm downward and superior directional pressure is applied over the U shape of the special retractor and increased to expose the prostatic fossa.

A ring forceps with a sponge in place is used to direct downward posterior pressure, thus allowing the prostate to be pushed superiorly and posteriorly exposing the dorsal venous complex, particularly at the apex of the prostate.

79-5. Now a curved clamp can be passed around the dorsal venous complex distally and the dorsal vein including adjacent tributaries can be encompassed by the clamp. 1–0 silk sutures are used for ligation. After ligating the distal dorsal veins, the proximal veins are similarly encompassed, ligated and tied. The veins in between are divided.

79-6. If the venous complex has an aberrant pattern, the dorsal venous complex can be separately ligated inferiorly. Suture ligatures can be used to ligate the dorsal venous complex near the proximal prostatic margins. The prostatic branch of the inferior vesicle arteries provides the major blood supply to the prostate. It is well to remember that the prostate is shaped like a "croissant" in most instances.

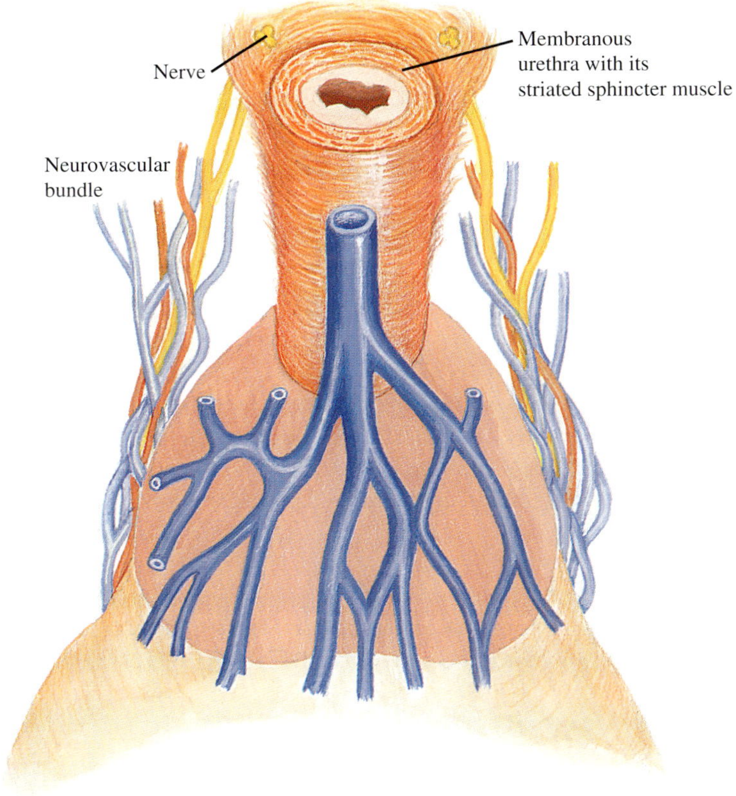

79-6

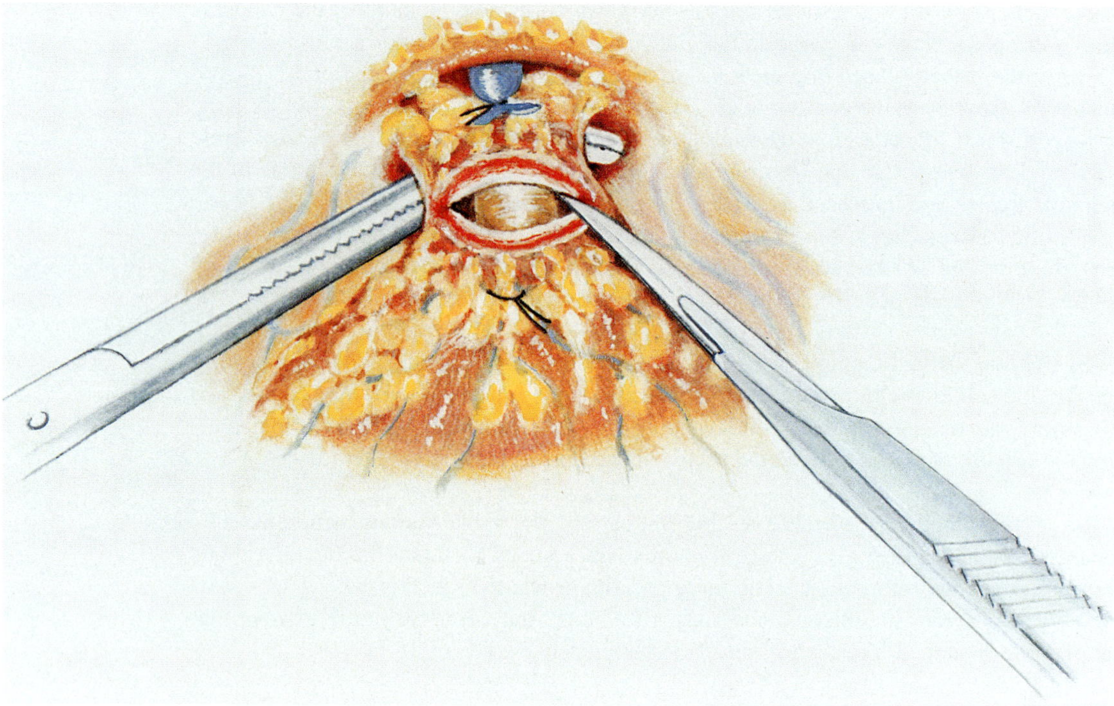

79-7

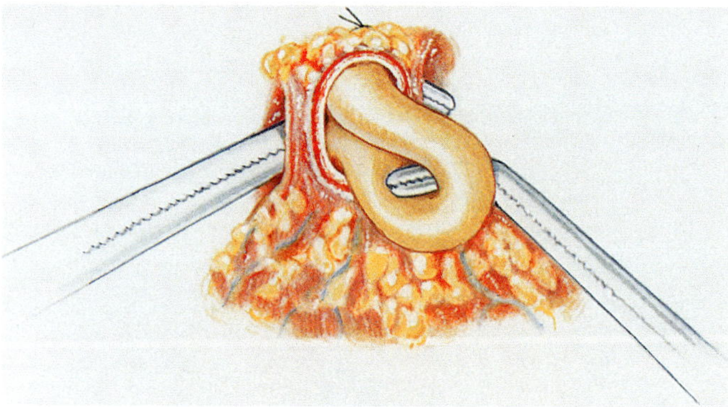

79-8

Next, the plane between rectum posteriorly and urethra anteriorly and posteriorly is developed at the apex of the prostate. Care is taken to dissect close to the urethral wall at the apex of prostate and catheter to avoid injuring the neurovascular bundles on each side. We dissect the plane between prostatic capsule and levator fascia to expose the neurovascular bundle on one side. The dissection includes apex of the prostate. A right angle clamp is used to dissect closely around the lateral and posterior urethral wall at the apex.

79-7 and **79-8**. The anterior surface of urethra is incised exposing a previously placed 16 Fr. urethral catheter with a balloon inflated in the bladder. Lifting the catheter shaft allows the remaining urethra to be incised. We now place upward and lateral traction on the catheter shaft to expose the neurovascular bundle on one side. The prostatic apex can be moved to expose the opposite neurovascular bundle. By careful traction to one side the appropriate neurovascular bundle is dissected free. The same opposite catheter traction is used to expose and free the opposite neurovascular bundle. If cancer has extended through prostatic capsule on one side, that adjacent neurovascular bundle is sacrificed.

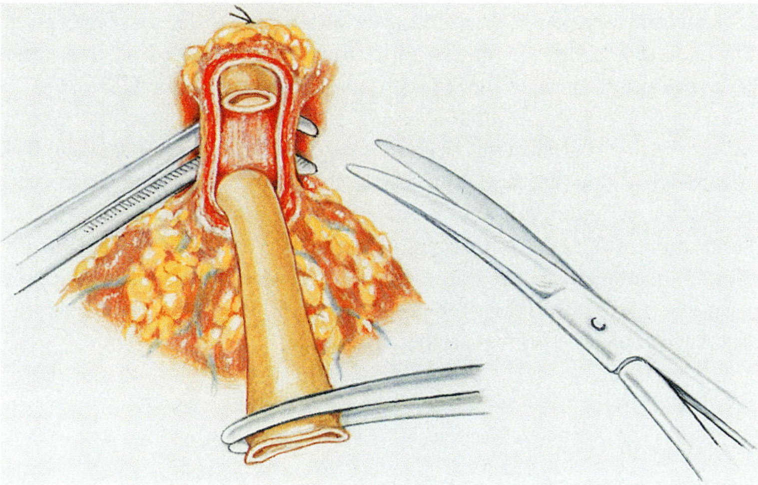

79-9

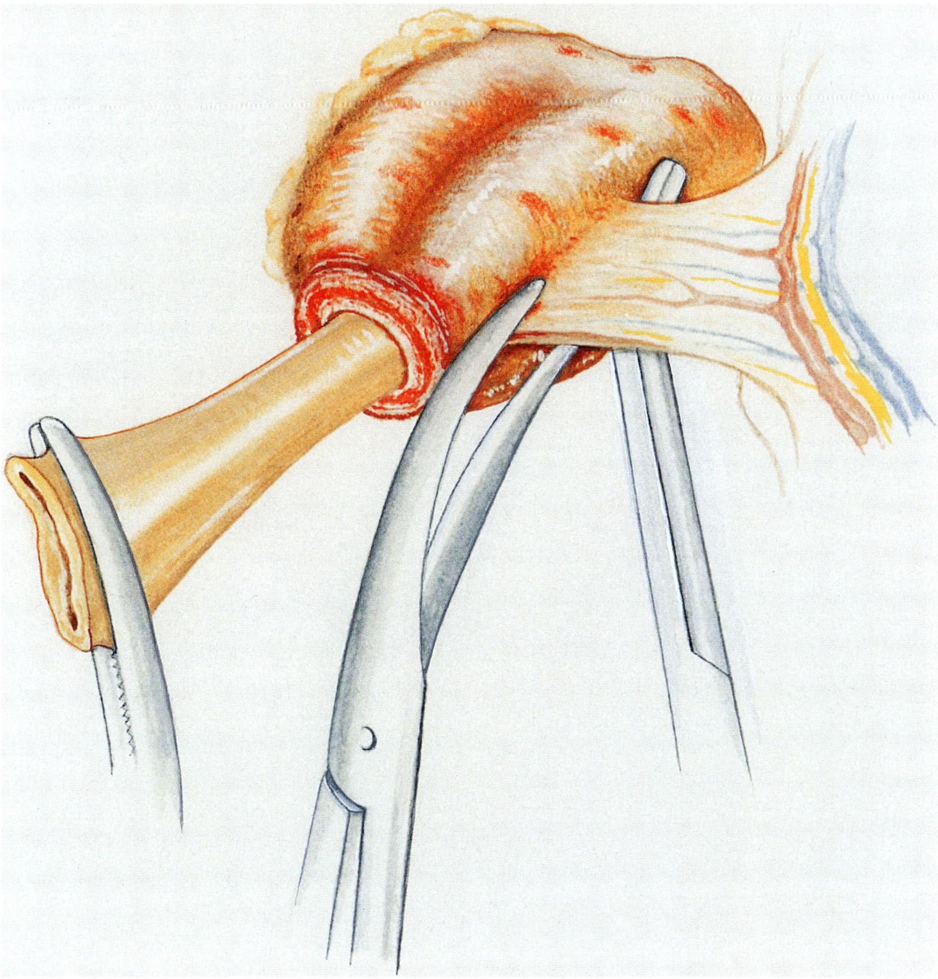

79-10

Preservation of the neurovascular bundle first on one side and then on the other allows the inferior vesicle artery (main prostatic arterial supply) to be dissected free, doubly ligated and cut between ties. Both prostatic arteries are divided after double ligation. If the exposure is poor, an alternative technique can be substituted (79-11).

79-9 and **79-10.** After the distal urethra has been incised completely two 3–0 monocryl sutures are placed through distal urethral mucosa at the 3 and 7 o'clock positions. Urethral smooth muscle is *not* included. We avoid the perineal body by not placing a 6 o'clock suture. Three more monocryl sutures are placed at 9, 3 and 12 o'clock. The sutures are now shielded, and the apical prostate can be lifted so that the posterior outer covering of the prostate can be incised near the posterior midline to expose the ejaculatory ducts and seminal vesicles. We prefer another technique.

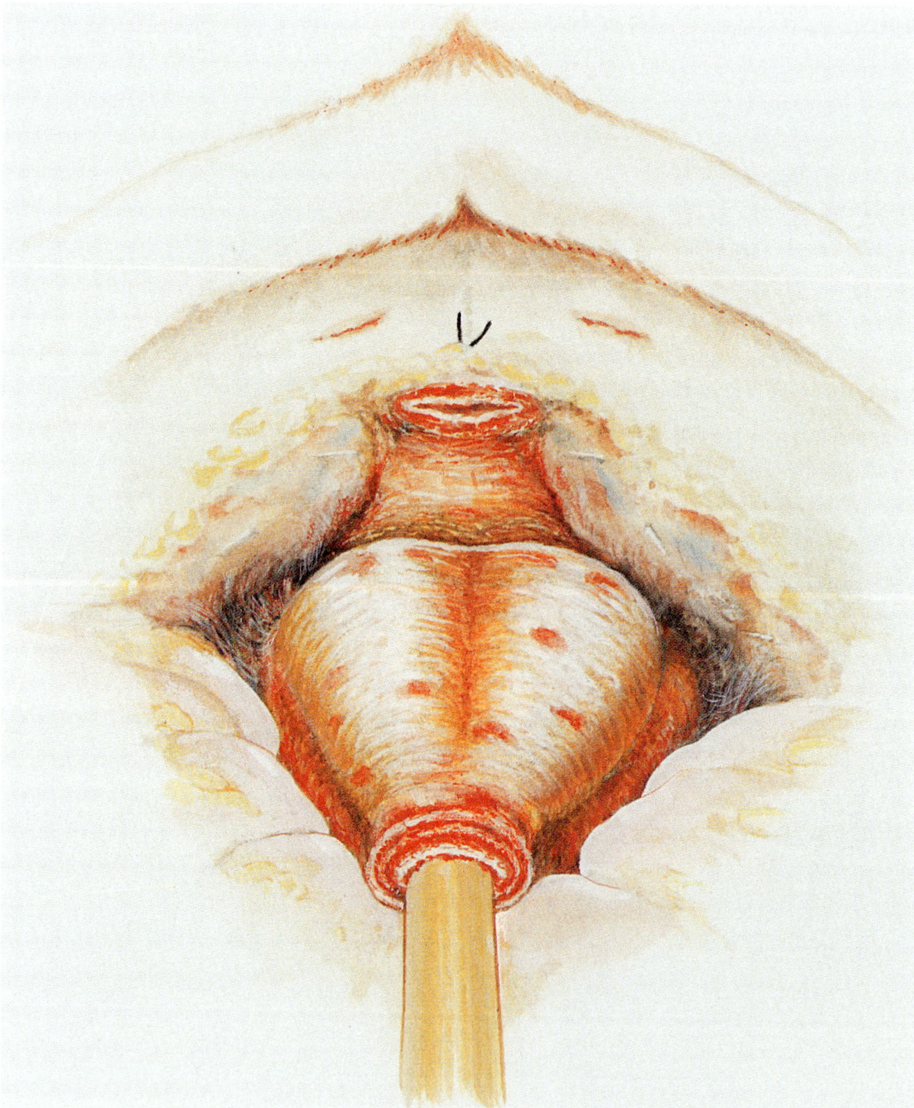

79-11

79-11. By incising the anterior bladder neck at the prostatic junction one can begin to separate bladder from proximal prostate. Continuing the incision down both sides of bladder neck, one exposes the inferior vesicle (prostatic) arteries at 5 and 7 o'clock. Indigo carmine injected by IV10 minutes earlier helps to isolate the ureteral orifices on the trigone. The prostatic arterial supply can be doubly ligated (left and right) at this time.

79-12, 79-13 and **79-14.** Allis clamps can now lift the anterior prostate and capsule so that the posterior bladder neck is incised. The bladder neck is protected. The seminal vesicles and ejeculatory ducts can now be dissected and isolated on the posterior side. The ejaculatory ducts lie more medial to the seminal vesicles. The superior and posterior end of seminal vesicles after dissecting Denonvilliers fascia extend behind the trigone and course posterolaterally.

79-15. The ejaculatory ducts are isolated and divided. The blood supply to the seminal vesicle courses in the sheath surrounding the ejaculatory duct. Both ejaculatory ducts are doubly divided and ligated.

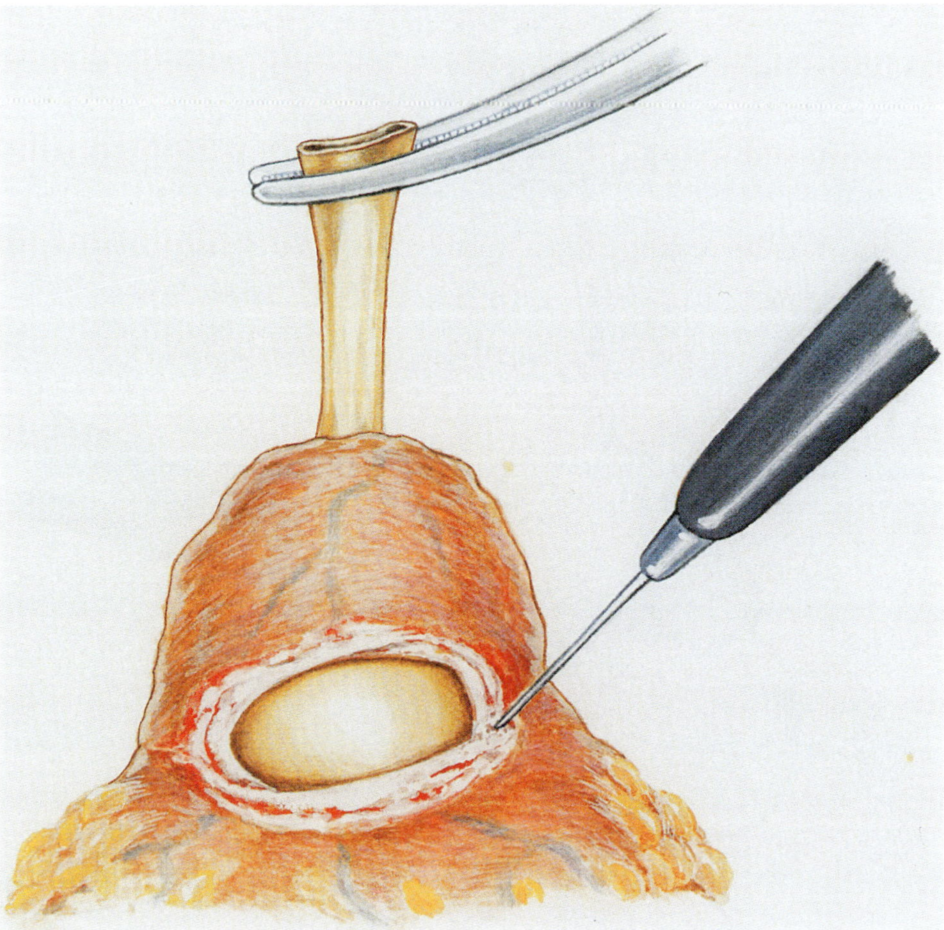

79-12

79-16. When satisfactory hemostasis is obtained, particularly in the pelvic cavity and prostatic fossa, the Foley catheter with its balloon is deflated. We use a No. 1 Prolene suture to provide a second means of anchoring the Foley catheter after the anastomosis is completed. This is useful in an obese person. A No. 1 Prolene suture with a large circular needle wedged on, is passed through the double eyes of the proximal catheter tip; this is a new 22 Fr silicone catheter. The suture is tied six times, always attempting to manipulate the knots so they lie in the part of the lumen where the two distal openings are located at the proximal tip. The needle is then blindly, but carefully, placed through the mid-right lateral anterior bladder wall so that this catheter-retaining suture is brought out through the anterior-lateral bladder wall near the bladder dome. On the opposite side will be the location of the Jackson-Pratt drainage tube which will be subsequently placed into the pelvic fossa where the prostate was removed. It is brought out through the fascia, muscle walls, and skin through a separate left lateral incision. The bladder neck and distal urethra are aligned.

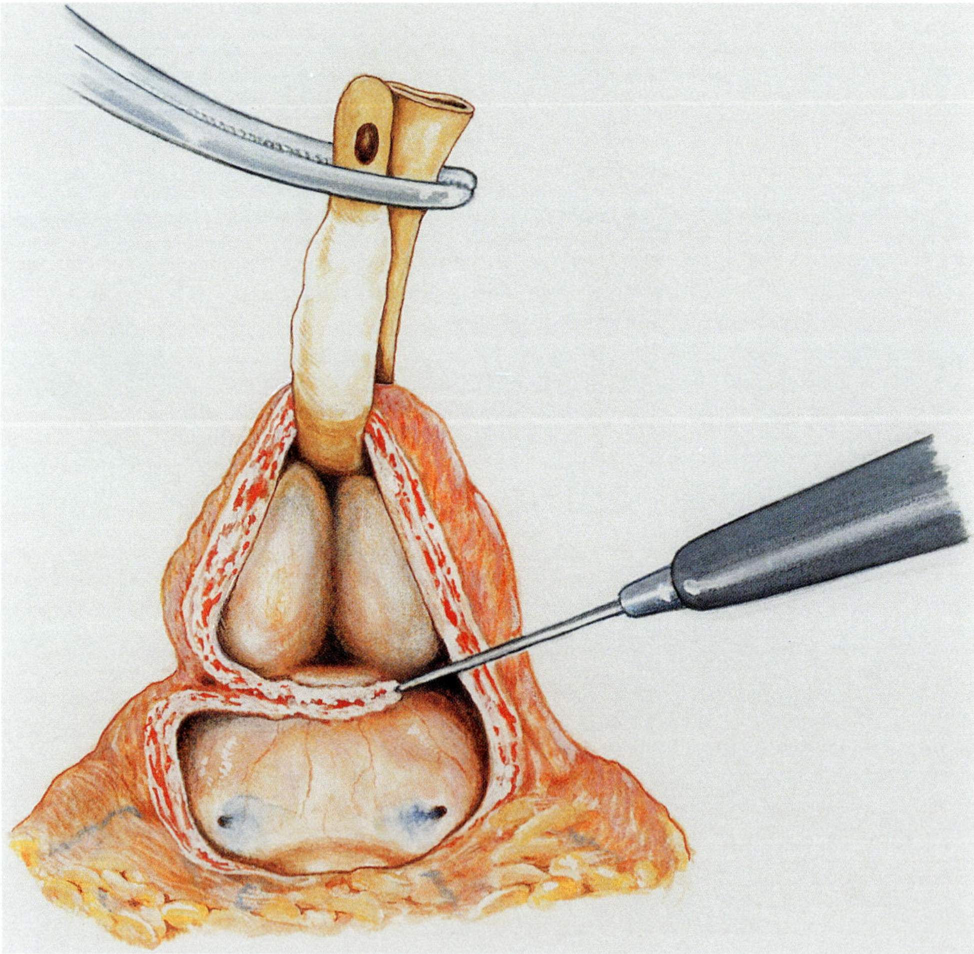

79-13

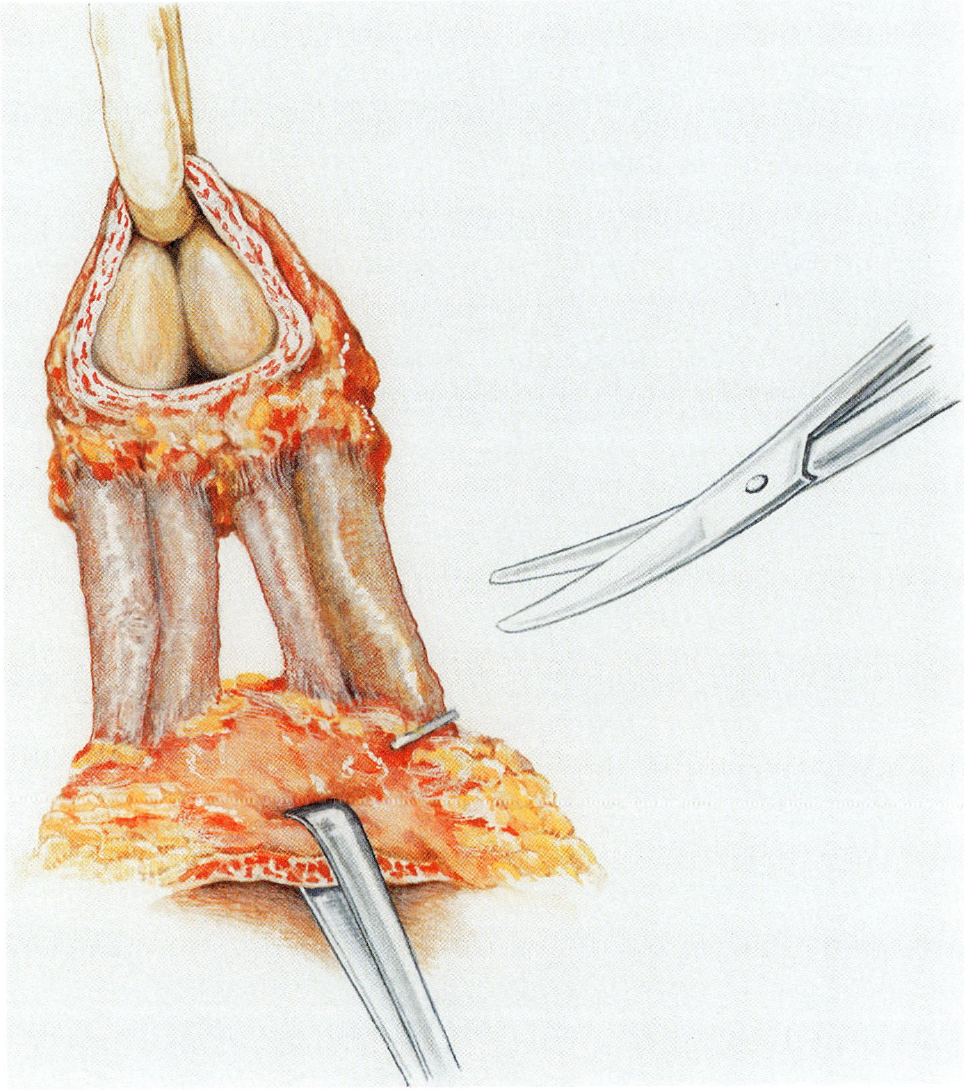

79-14

The five sutures on the distal urethra are carefully positioned on the bladder neck to correspond to the clock-like location that was described with the distal urethra. Make sure to catch circular striated muscle fibers around cut end of the distal urethra. We now place slight traction on the nylon sutures as we insert a new Foley catheter. The balloon is inflated inside the bladder cavity. This allows significant reapproximation of both distal urethra and bladder neck. We leave the curved needles on the 9, 12, and 3 o'clock sutures to remind the surgeon that he needs to thread the other end and suture the bladder neck inside out, so that all knots are eventually tied on the outside. Similarly, the 5 and 7 o'clock sutures are threaded again using a curved needle and placed appropriately through the new bladder neck so that the knots will be on the outside. The catheter, with the proximal tip now inside the bladder lumen, has the balloon inflated up to 50 mL with saline and gentle traction is now brought inferiorly to approximate the bladder neck and urethra. The 5 and 7 o'clock sutures are tied initially. The remaining anterior sutures are also tied and cut. The Foley catheter is placed on gentle traction while the pelvic wound is inspected. Hemostasis is important. The Jackson-Pratt drainage tube is adjusted if it is not properly placed. The flat end of the Jackson-Pratt drain starts transversely on the right over the prostatic urethra, then across the bladder neck. The tubular portion is brought out the left side anteriorly.

79-17. A schematic sagittal diagram exposes the right side of the prostate and bladder. The major structures on the right side are demonstrated. The striated urethral sphincter is clearly shown.

We generally leave the urethral catheter in place for 10–14 days. The patient is discharged about 3 to 5 days postoperatively depending on the co-morbidities. We reduce the Foley balloon size from 50 mL to 30 mL to reduce bladder irritability prior to discharge.

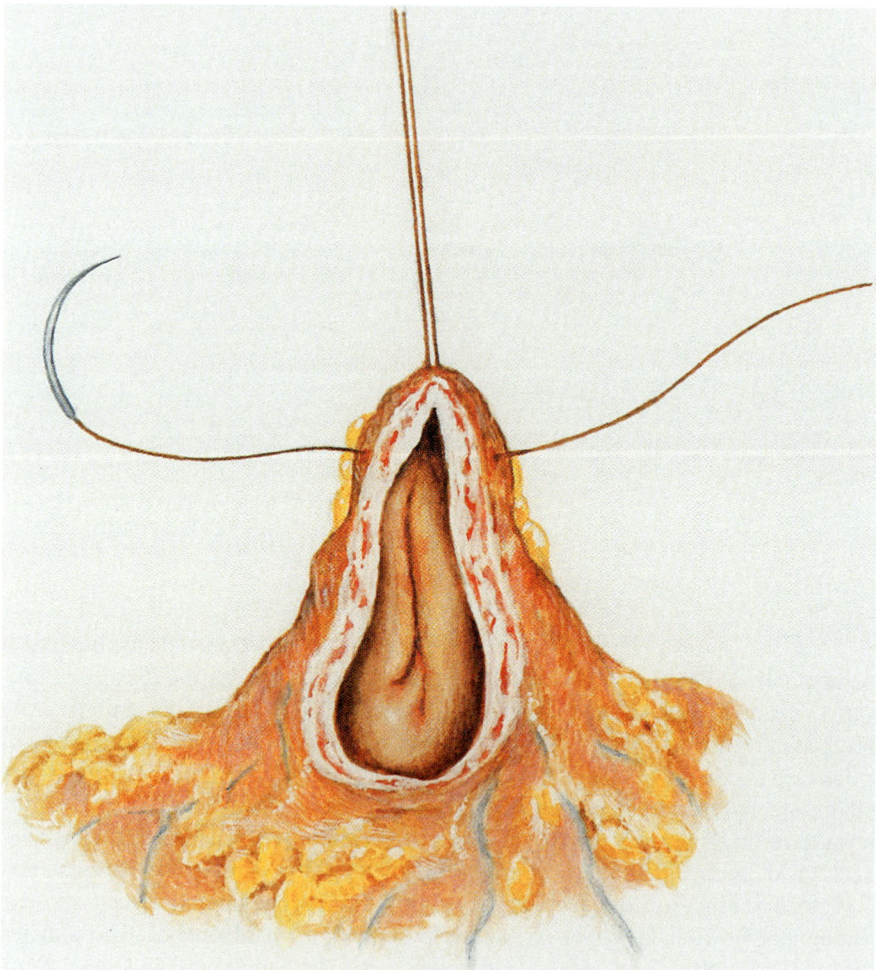

79-15

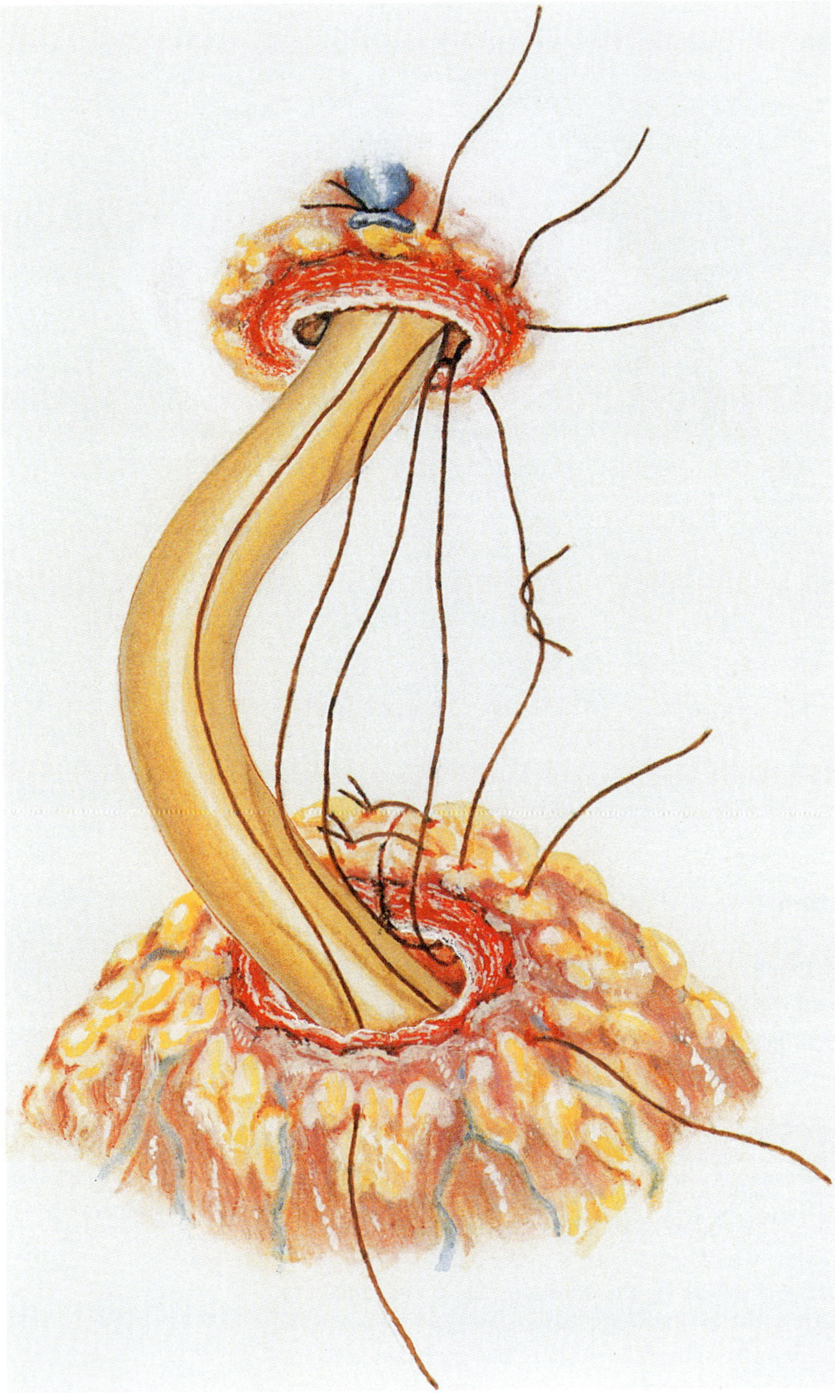

79-16

The patient is instructed in the act of performing anal external sphincter exercises well before discharge. I personally instruct the patient in this maneuver using a gloved index finger. He also begins to appreciate the "duck walk" and pelvic floor exercises over the next week and a half.

Of importance is the fact that PSA has a 2.5 day half life. Therefore, by the time the

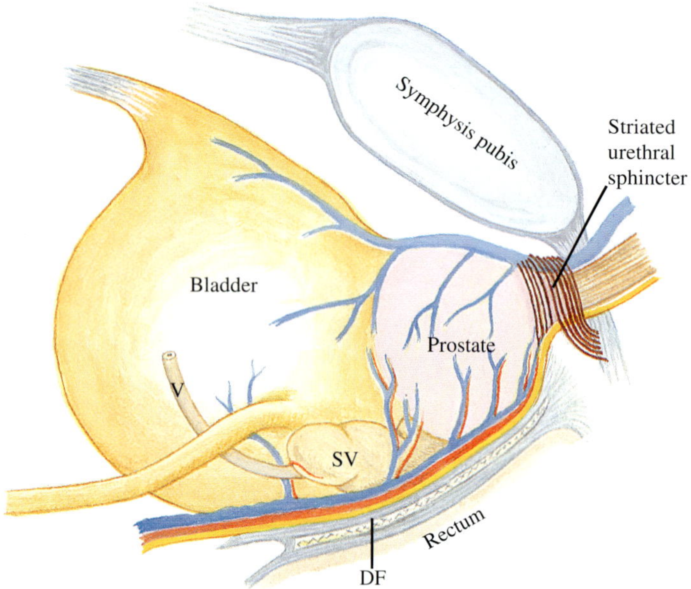

79-17

patient is seen in the office at 12–14 days postoperatively, his PSA should be less than 0.2 ng/mL.

80. Pelvic Lymph Node Dissection

Bilateral pelvic lymph node dissection should be carried out prior to removal of the prostate. This dissection, when performed early, will allow proper staging of the obturator lymph nodes. Examination of frozen sections of the lymph nodes can be made if large matted nodes are encountered.

80-1. *The lymph nodes are to be dissected free of the boundaries* in the schematic *(dotted line).* A meticulous dissection of the pelvic lymph nodes is imperative bilaterally. The dissection includes 1) the common iliac nodes overlying the proximal and distal one half of the common iliac artery and vein; 2) the nodes extending superiorly to the aorta at the bifurcation; 3) the external iliac nodes, which are adjacent to the entire course of the external iliac artery and vein; and 4) the nodes along the obturator nerve and canal. This dissection includes all fat, nodal tissue, and areolar tissue between the hypogastric artery and its ramifications medially. The pelvic side wall laterally is also included, next to the hypogastric vessels.

80-2. *The lymph node dissection is completed on the right side in the schematic.*

80-3. The *nodes along the right external iliac artery and vein,* the *right internal iliac artery, and the ureter are visible* prior to dissection.

80-4. In the nearly completed dissection on the right, *the ureter is retracted medially by a flat tubular drain.* A vein retractor lifts the iliac vein laterally. A single node remains at the obturator canal. This node is removed.

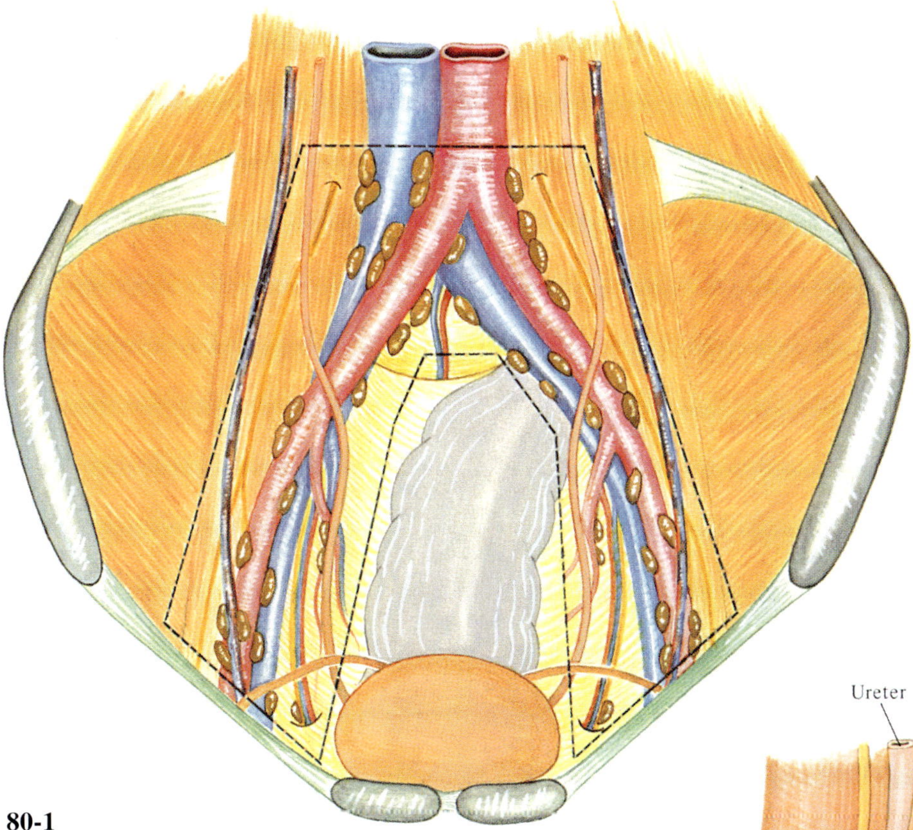

80-1

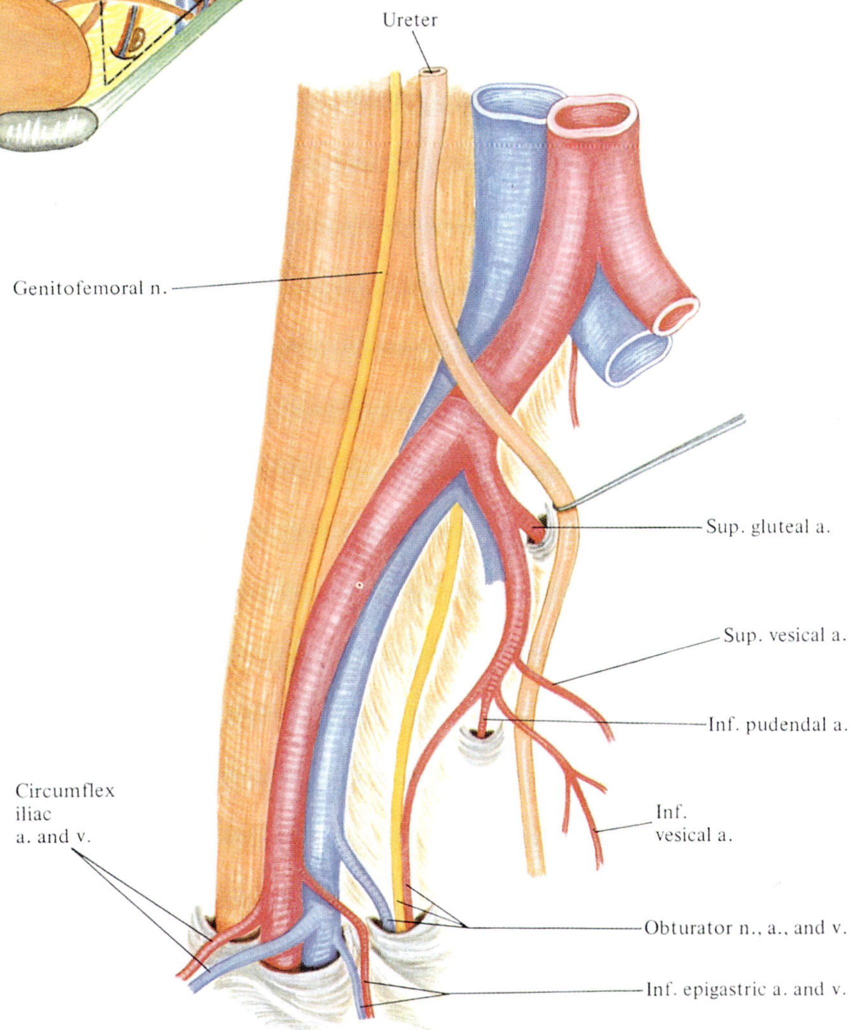
Ureter
Genitofemoral n.
Sup. gluteal a.
Sup. vesical a.
Inf. pudendal a.
Circumflex iliac a. and v.
Inf. vesical a.
Obturator n., a., and v.
Inf. epigastric a. and v.

80-2

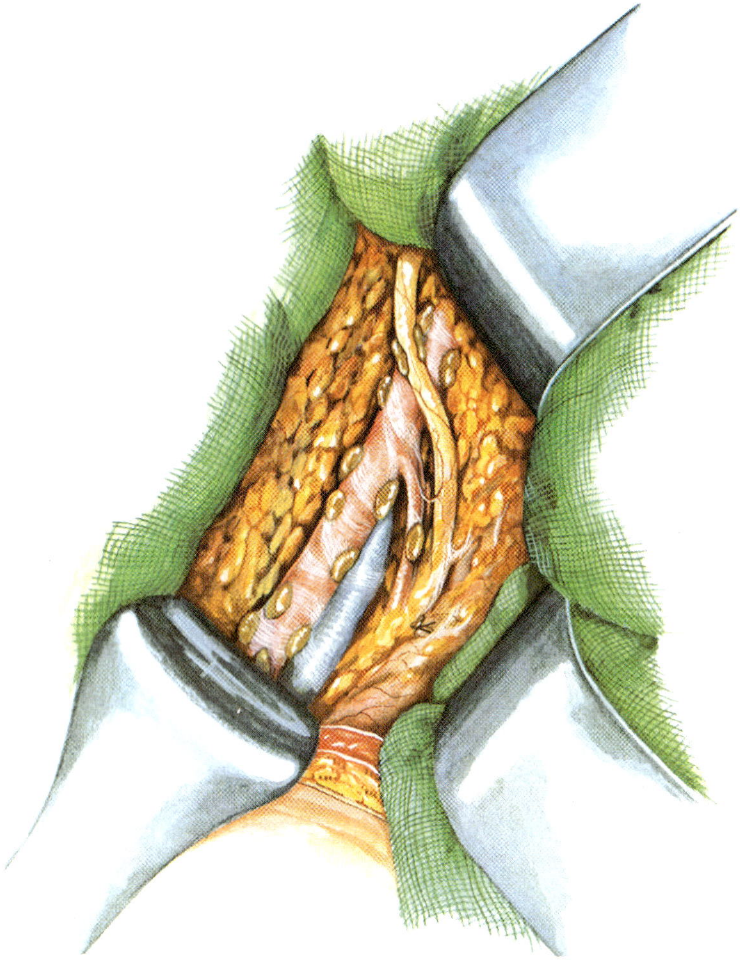

80-3

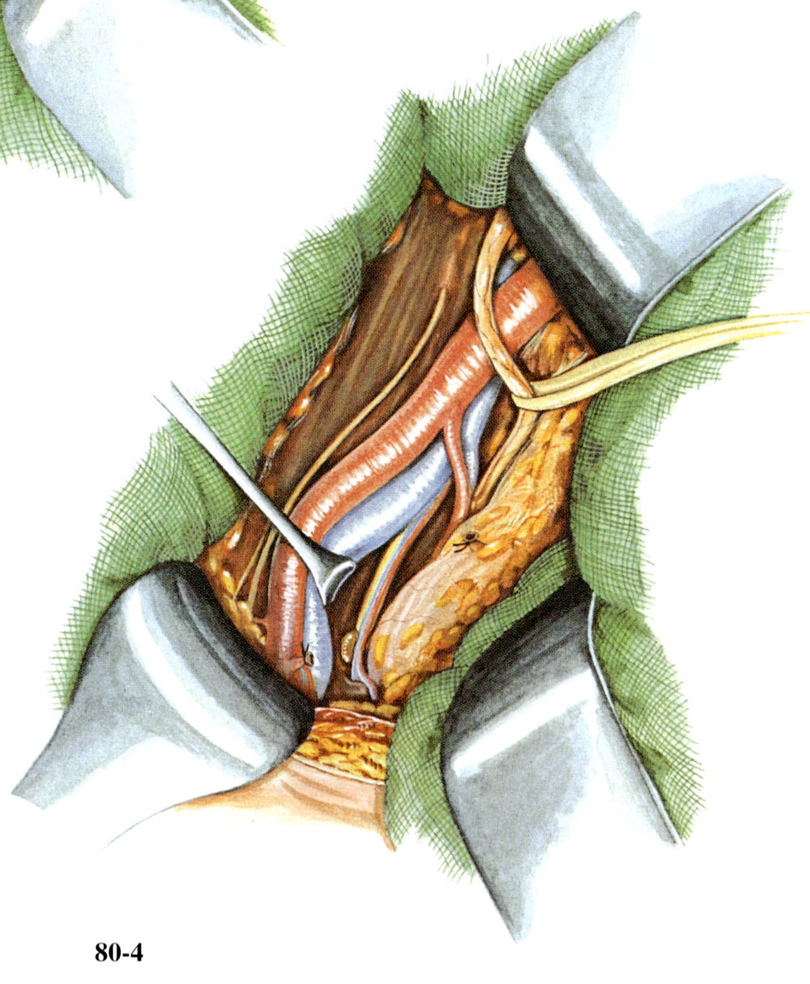

80-4

81. Radical Perineal Prostatectomy—Belt Approach

The indication for radical perineal prostatectomy is early cancer confined to the prostate gland. Subtotal prostatectomy is performed for severe prostatic stone disease associated with fibrosis. Prior to the operation, it is important to perform a biopsy on the suspicious prostatic nodule to prove the diagnosis of cancer, or to have evidence of multifocal prostatic carcinoma after transurethral resection of the prostate. We believe that a single focus of cancer found after examining all the resected fragments of glandular prostatic tissue removed transurethrally represents a "clinical cure," and no further treatment for the prostatic cancer is necessary. The PSA blood test will also confirm the absence of cancer.

When an open perineal biopsy of a suspicious area is performed, frozen section of the biopsy is indicated. If a positive diagnosis cannot be made, then the patient's incision is closed, and permanent microscopic sections are examined a few days later to confirm the diagnosis. As a secondary surgical procedure, we advocate either performing radical prostatectomy within 7 to 9 days of previous transurethral surgery, or waiting at least 3 months to allow inflammation to subside.

We suggest bowel preparation with antibiotics and mechanical cleansing procedures to sterilize the rectal area. For large-bowel surgery, the patient is hospitalized 48 hours before surgery when home care and proper cleansing is not possible. In selected, well-motivated patients, the preparation can be started at home. For small-bowel surgery, the patient is hospitalized 24 hours prior to surgery when the preoperative care in a distant suburb is marginal.

1. A low-residue diet is begun and continued during the preoperative period.
2. Enemas (tap water) are administered once daily until the day before surgery, when enemas are given twice a day.
3. As a laxative, 16 mL aqueous solution of sodium phosphate (Phospho-Soda) is given twice daily throughout the preoperative period.
4. Oral neomycin (500 mg) and tetracycline (250 mg) are administered four times a day until surgery. An alternative antibiotic protocol includes 1 g neomycin and 1 g erythromycin base, which are given three times on the day prior to surgery. Both medications are given orally at 1300, 1400, and 2300 the day before surgery.

In our experience, tumor involvement of the prostatic capsule (stage C) may be unsuspected, and the rectal wall, including Denonvilliers's fascia, may be surgically thinned inadvertently. A proctotomy can be surgically repaired because there has been previous bowel sterilization. The rectal wall is closed in three layers using 3–0 chromic catgut sutures.

We are now convinced that approximately 25% of male patients with stage B_2 adenocarcinoma of the prostate may have extension of tumor to the lymph nodes along the obturator canal. Therefore, we advocate bilateral pelvic lymphadenectomy as a staging procedure before total perineal prostatectomy is attempted.

We agree that pedal lymphangiography is optional for demonstrating metastatic lymph node areas along the hypogastric artery and external iliac nodes.

Ultrasound scans of the prostate are not helpful in BPH. However, ultrasound scans—hypoecholic areas—are indicative of adenocarcinoma.

Our experience with a single coil—an MRI—has been disappointing. A new double coil MRI apparatus would indicate that cancer can be detected up to 3 mm outside the prostate capsule.

81-1. *Positioning the patient into an extreme lithotomy posture is important* in this procedure. We like the padded straight poles for elevating the lower extremities. Wrapping both legs from the mid-thigh to the mid-calf area assists in maintaining proper position. The use of shoulder braces is important in maintaining the position. The padded brace should be placed against the bony shoulder prominence. Pressure must be avoided over the brachial plexus.

We have learned that placing several rolls of rectangular pads or plastic-covered sandbags beneath the midsacrum also assists in elevating the perineum into an optimal position. The perineum is in a horizontal position if the patient has been properly positioned.

81-2. *An inverted U-shaped incision is made,* starting medial to the ischial tuberosities and curving anteriorly about 2 cm above the mucocutaneous junction. The second dotted line, larger than the first, is the Hugh H. Young incision line. This incision at the anterior end is above the subcutaneous anal sphincter.

81-3. *The subcutaneous tissue and fat are incised sharply at the anterior margin.* The anal sphincter is avoided. Gentle downward traction, using a sponge and index finger motion, will usually reveal the proper bloodless plane of dissection beneath the sphincter. When the external anal sphincter is lifted with the knife handle in one hand, one can move superiorly toward the prostate, with the sponge and index finger of the other hand

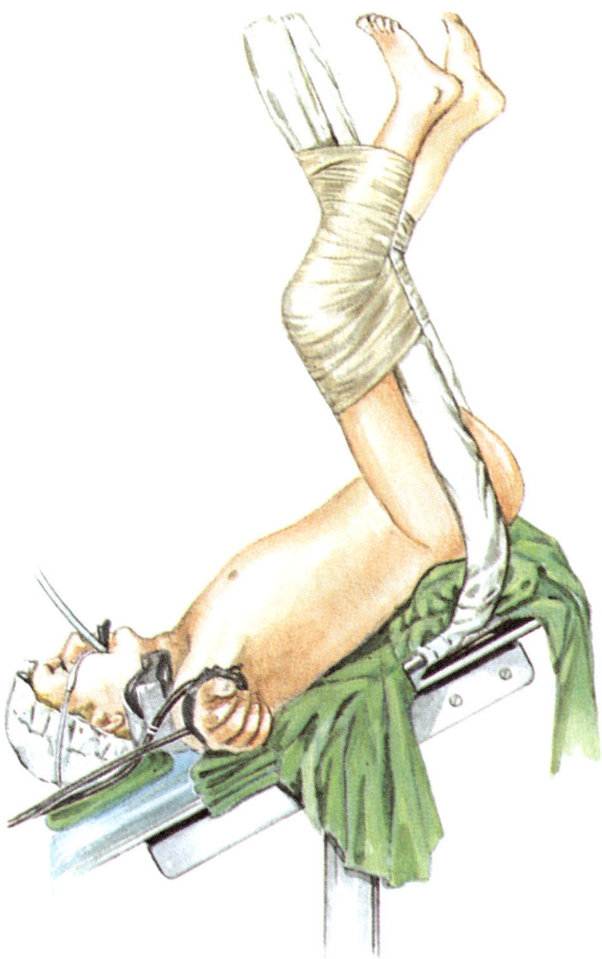

81-1

providing countertraction against the rectum; the prostate can soon be palpated deep to the levator ani muscles. Superficial lateral paired retractors assist in elevating the anal sphincter.

81-4. *The curved urethral retractor is inserted into the bladder and rotated* to be sure it is in the bladder lumen. Then the blades are opened by clockwise rotation of the knob on the handle. The levator ani muscles are seen, prior to their separation. Superficial lateral retractors are in place at 10 and 2 o'clock positions. A flat-angled posterior retractor is in place over a protective sponge and serves also to protect the rectum.

81-5. *Now the prostate can be moved to the wound edge.* Deep lateral retractors are placed in the wound at 10 and 2 o'clock positions. The levator ani muscles are now separated laterally by blunt dissection, exposing the posterior layer of Denonvilliers's fas-

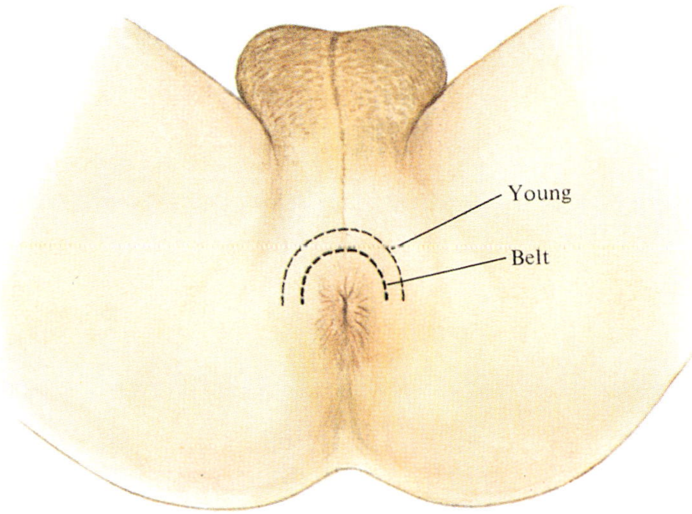

81-2

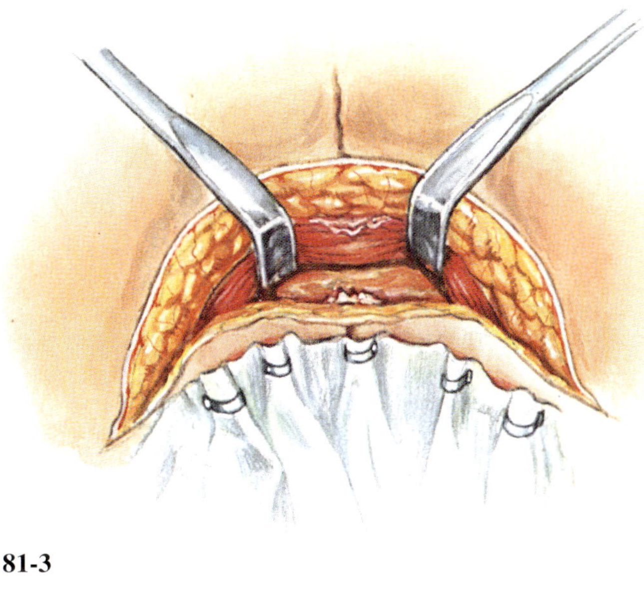

81-3

cia. The longer, posterior, perineal retractor is replaced over a sponge, which protects the outer rectal wall.

The rectal wall can be separated from the prostate if the proper cleavage plane has been achieved. The rectum and posterior layer of Denonvilliers's fascia are separated from the prostate by lifting the handle of the curved urethral retractor superiorly and sep-

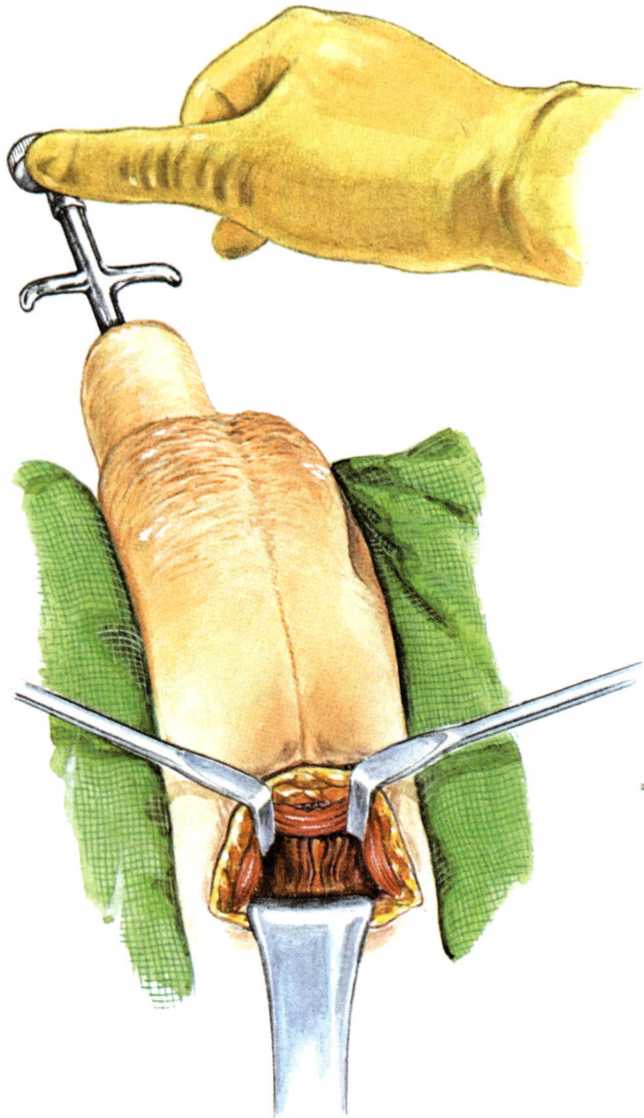

81-4

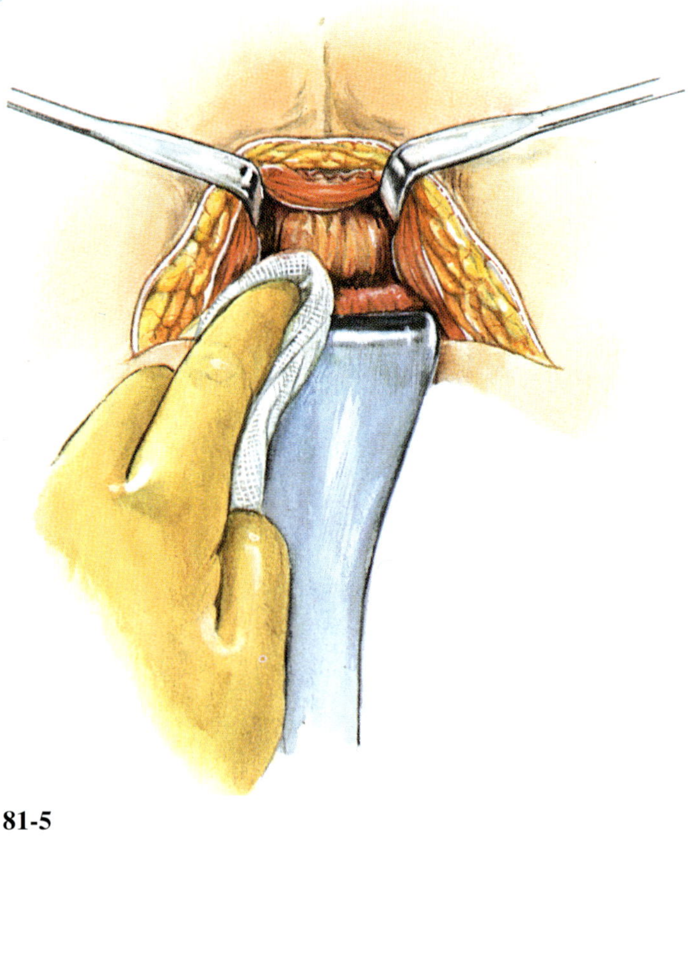

81-5

arating the rectum posteriorly. A sponge on a ring forceps is used in this maneuver. The dorsal aspect of the prostate can be further exposed, including the fascial layer overlying the seminal vesicles.

81-6. *The lateral aspect of the prostate is now dissected free* by moving the retractor handle sideways, so that the prostate is placed under tension away from the side of dissection. Blunt dissection is possible, using the dissecting sponge on a curved clamp. The same maneuver is now employed for dissecting the opposite lateral aspect of the prostate. Completion of both lateral prostatic capsular dissections exposes the vascular pedicles to the prostate. Each vascular pedicle is exposed and freed by blunt dissection on the lower aspect of the prostate. The vascular pedicles can be doubly clamped, divided, and ligated, or the ligation can be done later (81–8). Unlike the radical retropubic approach to total prostatectomy, total perineal prostatectomy avoids the lateral plexus of deep pelvic veins.

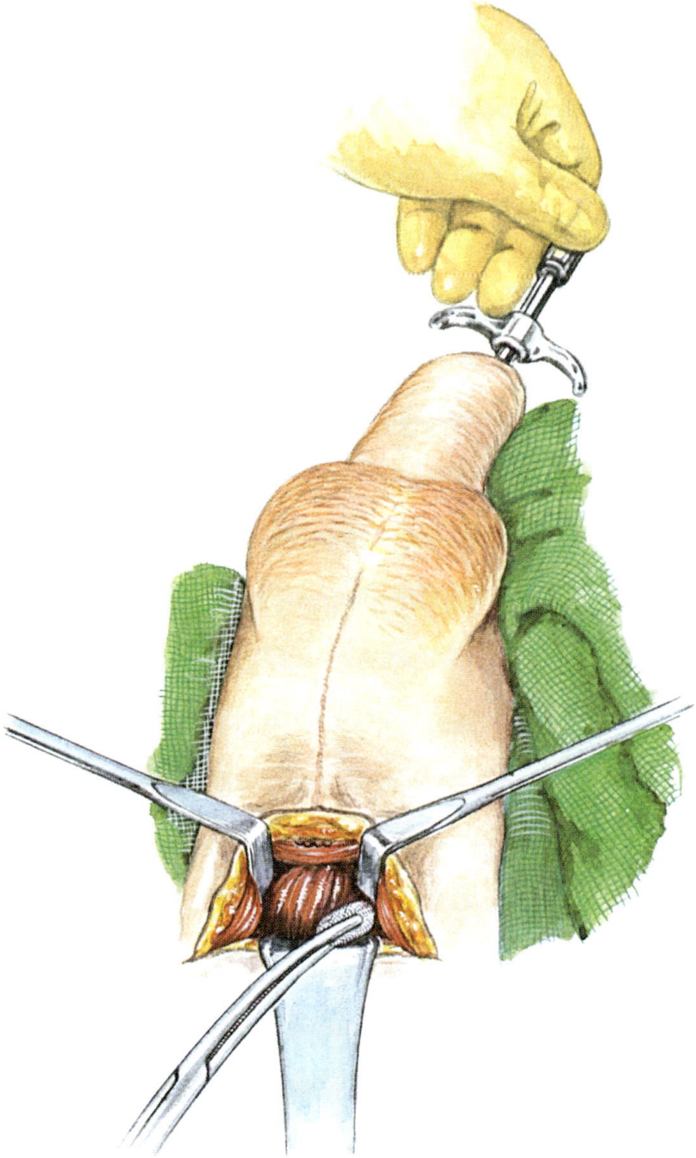

81-6

81-7. *The soft spot (verumontanum) can be located by palpation.* This landmark enables the surgeon to locate the border at the posterior apex of the prostate, where the membranous urethra begins. The border between the distal membranous urethra and the prostate is incised circumferentially for 180°, exposing the curved urethral retractor. The urethral retractor blades within the bladder are closed, and the instrument is withdrawn carefully. The remaining ventral urethra is transected in a horizontal plane.

81-8. *The straight urethral instrument is inserted perineally into the prostatic urethra and the bladder lumen.* The blades are opened and the entire prostate is lowered to expose the puboprostatic ligaments. A capsular vein has been ligated. The puboprostatic ligaments are incised away from the prostatic border. The vascular pedicles are now doubly clamped, divided, and ligated on the left. A suture (3–0 chromic catgut) can be used to secure hemostasis.

81-9. *The bladder neck area is now exposed* by placing traction on the prostatic retractor and moving the prostate and attached bladder neck into the wound area. The bladder neck at 12 o'clock is incised with the scalpel or the Bovie knife. An Allis clamp is used to mark the bladder neck on the patient's left at 5 o'clock. The Metzenbaum scissors can be inserted as an alternative. The bladder neck is transected laterally in two separate maneuvers, taking care to keep the blades of the scissors pointed vertically. The danger in cutting the bladder neck at 5 and 7 o'clock is angling the scissors towards the trigone and causing injury to the ureteral orifice. A catheter can sometimes be inserted as an alternative to replace the straight urethral retractor, and can be folded over the anterior prostatic border and through the bladder neck to provide traction as well. The deep

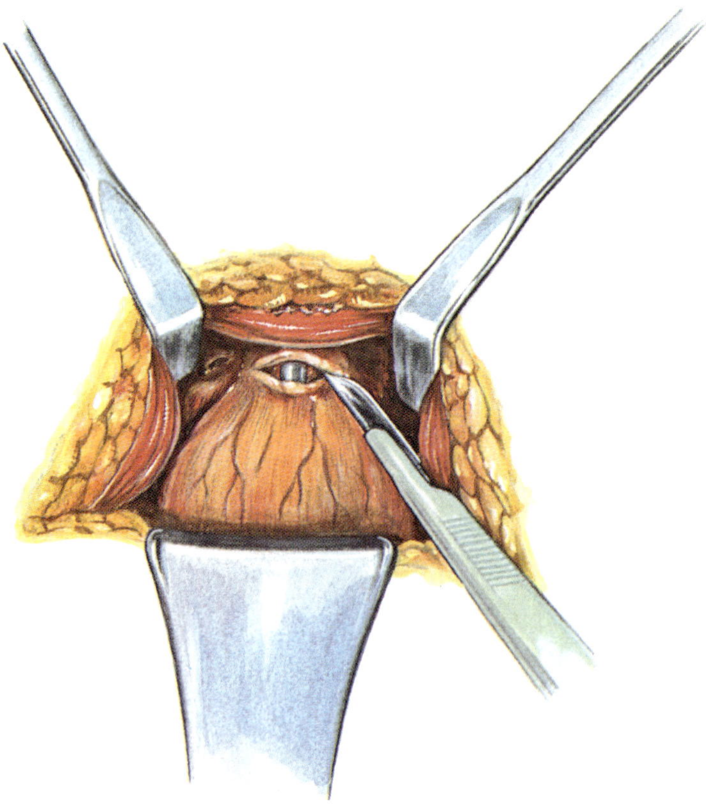

81-7

bladder neck area is incised distal to the trigone and ureteral orifice, leaving at least a 1.5 to 2 cm margin. A scalpel (15 blade) is used to incise the bladder neck at 6 o'clock.

81-10. *Gentle traction on the straight retractor will expose the anterior leaf of fascia covering the ventral surface of the seminal vesicles.* This space is incised and is used to further dissect the seminal vesicles and ejaculatory duct on each side. The entire seminal vesicle with the fascial covering is removed with the prostate. A right-angle clamp is used to free the right seminal vesicle. The ejaculatory duct is doubly ligated and divided on each side after exposure through the anterior leaf of the genital fascia. The ejaculatory duct and accompanying artery lie medial to each seminal vesicle. Sharp dissection now allows removal of the entire prostate, including the capsule and seminal vesicles.

81-11. After the specimen is removed, the bladder neck is identified. Allis clamps are used to grasp the bladder neck at four quadrants. Five mL of indigo carmine dye injected intravenously is helpful in the early identification of the ureteral orifices. *Interrupted chromic catgut sutures (2–0) are placed circumferentially to achieve hemostasis.* If the bladder neck is unusually wide, some type of closure must be effected to approximate the size of the membranous distal urethra. We believe that a vertical reapproximation or an inverted Y-shaped closure is effective. The branches of the inverted Y are at 5 and 7 o'clock, further protecting the orifices.

81-12. Before anastomosis of the bladder neck and urethra can be started, a 22 Fr indwelling catheter with a 30-mL bag is inserted through the urethral meatus. *The catheter*

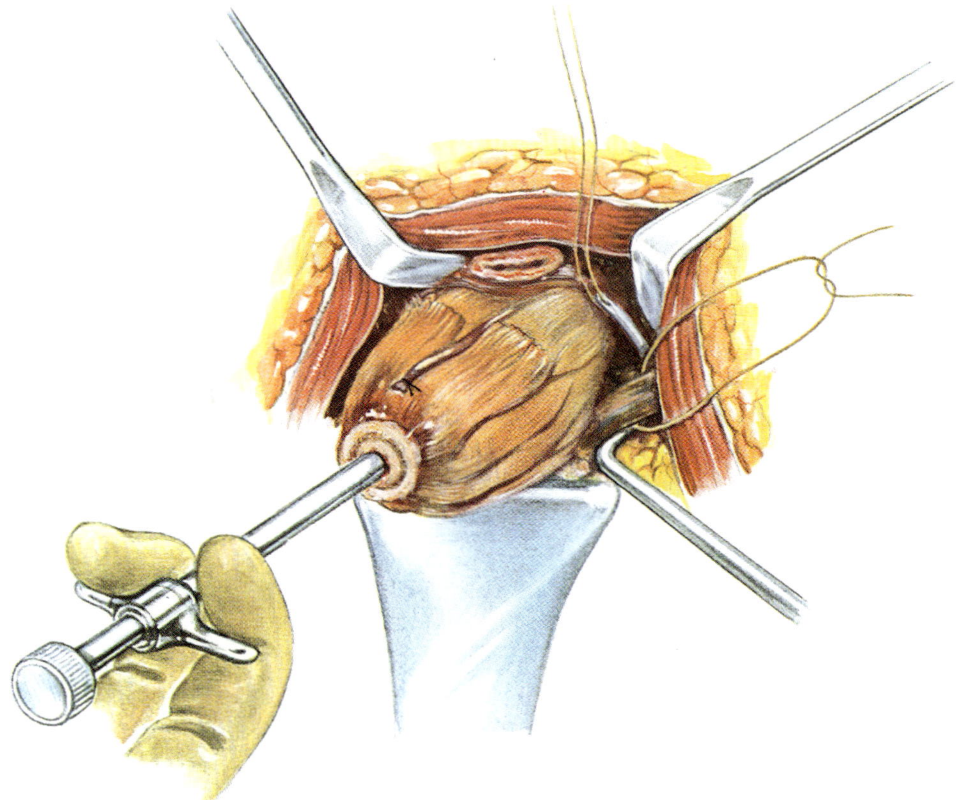

81-8

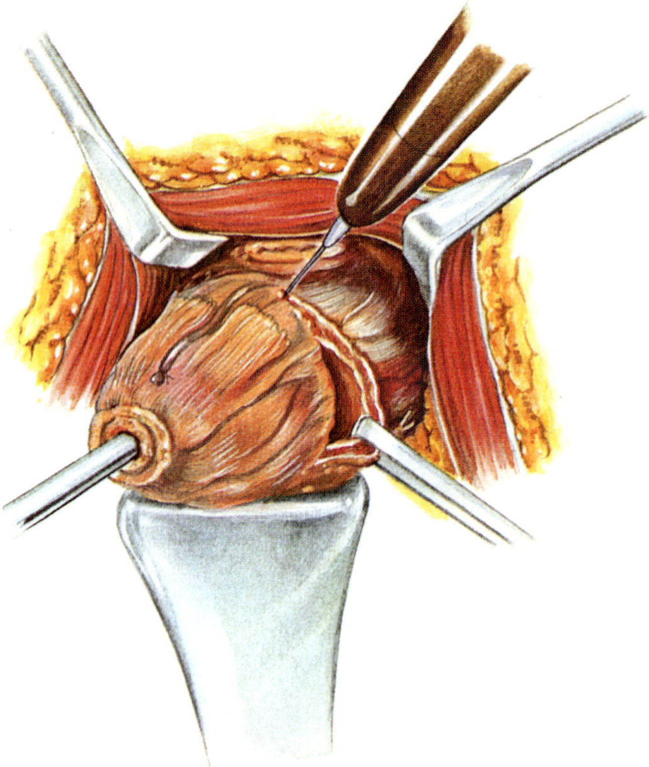

81-9

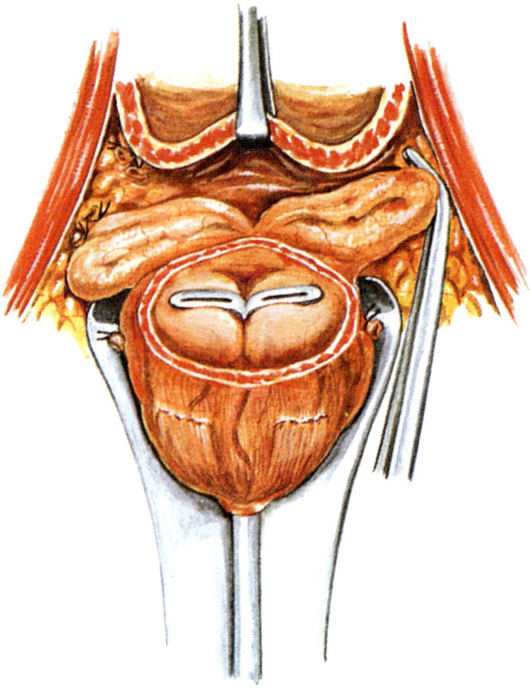

81-10

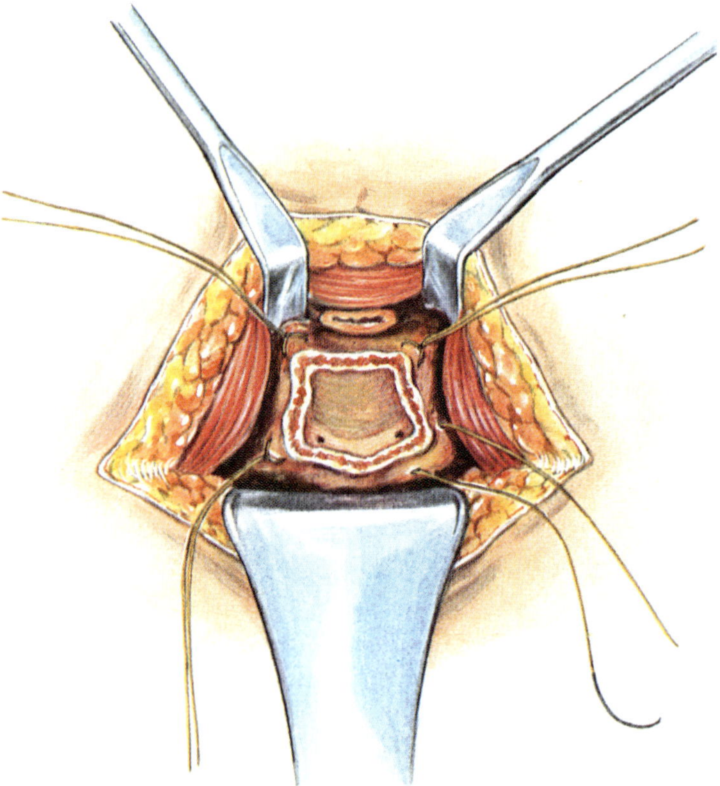

81-11

tip, reaching the cut membranous urethral end, *is pulled through for 7 or 9 cm and raised* (vertically) *superiorly.* A right-angle retractor (or deep lateral retractor) is placed against the catheter at the distal urethral interface and raised anteriorly, exposing the anterior end of the membranous urethra. This most difficult suture is placed horizontally through the urethra. The suture is also placed through the bladder neck at 12 o'clock. This suture is tied, bringing the urethra and bladder neck together.

81-13. The catheter tip is now inserted into the bladder and *the urethra is sutured to the bladder neck along the remaining quadrants.* Four to six sutures are placed to obtain a watertight closure. Excessive bladder neck has been reapproximated using a vertical closure.

The catheter bag is inflated and tested. Blood clots are removed from the bladder lumen by irrigation.

81-14. *Closure of the wound is now begun.* A drain, or a Jackson Pratt tube is brought from the anastomotic site to the skin edge. It is brought out to the skin through a separate stab incision. The levator ani muscles are reapproximated with 2–0 chromic catgut before subcutaneous tissue and skin closure.

81-15. *The anal sphincter has been protected.* The skin is reapproximated with 3–0 nylon sutures.

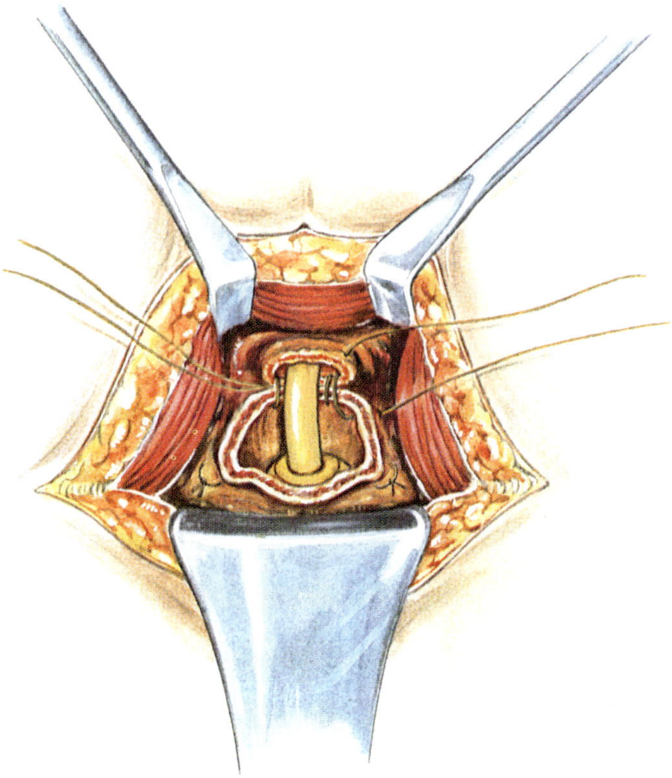

81-12

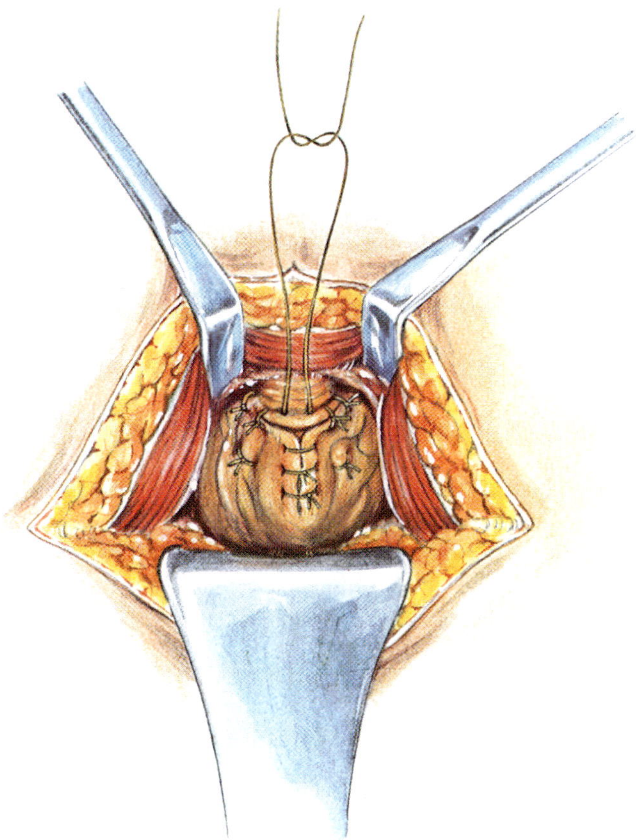

81-13

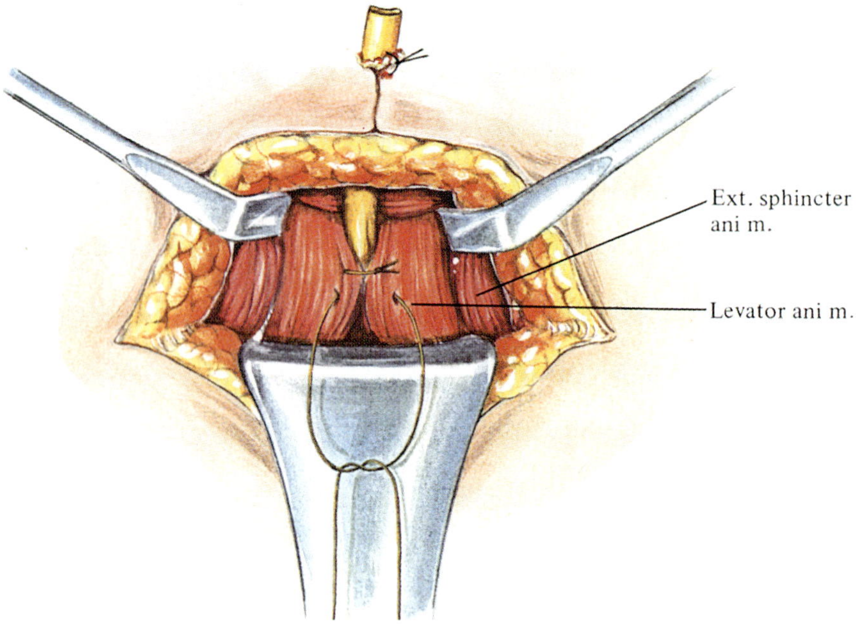

81-14

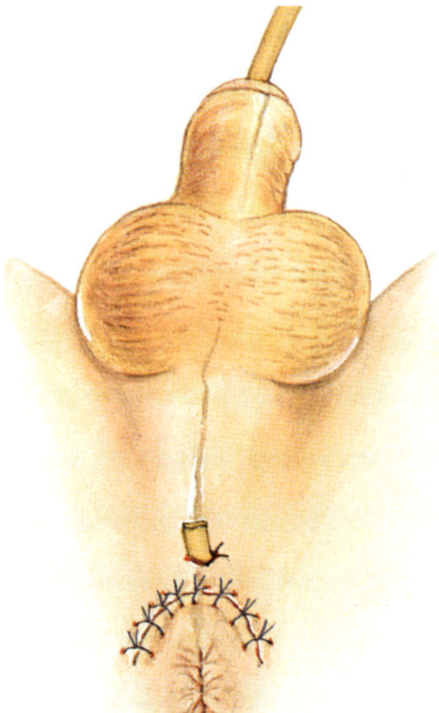

81-15

References

1. Cockett ATK, di Sant'Agnese PA, Gopinath P, Schoen SR, Abrahamsson P-A. Relationship of neuroendocrine cells of prostate and serotonin to BPH. Urology 42(5):512–519, 1993.
2. di Sant'Agnese PA, de Mesy Jensen KL, Churukian CJ, Agarwal MM. Human prostatic endocrine-paracrine (APUD) cells: distributional analysis with a comparison of serotonin and neuron-specific enolase immunoreactivity and silver stains. Arch Pathol Lab Med 109: 607–612, 1985.

Suggested Readings

Barry MJ, Fowler FJ Jr, O'Leary MP, Bruskewitz RC, Holtgrewe HL, Mebust WK, Cockett ATK, the Measurement Committee of the American Urological Association. The American Urological Association symptom index for benign prostatic hyperplasia. J Urol 148:1549, 1992.

Belt E. Radical perineal prostatectomy in early carcinoma of the prostate. J Urol 48:287, 1942.

Belt E, Ebert CE, Surber AC Jr. A new anatomic approach in perineal prostatectomy. J Urol 41: 482, 1939.

Cockett ATK, Barry MJ, Holtgrewe HL, Sihelnik S, Williams R, McConnell J. Indications for treatment of benign prostatic hyperplasia. The American Urological Association study. Cancer 70(suppl):280, 1992.

Flocks RH. The arterial distribution within the prostate gland: its role in transurethral prostatic resection. J Urol 37:524, 1937.

Millin T. Retropubic prostatectomy. A new extravesical technique—report on 20 cases. Lancet 2: 693, 1945.

Villers A, McNeal JE, Freiha FS, Boccon-Gibod L, Stamey TA. Invasion of Denonvilliers's fascia in radical prostatectomy specimens. J Urol 149:793–798, 1993.

Wacksman J, Gilbert A, Curtis AS. Results of the renewed extravesical reimplant for surgical correction of vesicoureteral reflux. J Urol 148:359–361, 1992.

Walsh PC. Radical prostatectomy for the treatment of localized prostatic carcinoma. Urol Clin North Am 7:583, 1980.

Walsh PC. Radial surgery for prostatic cancer. Cancer 45:1906, 1980.

Walsh PC, Donker PJ. Impotence following radical prostatectomy: insight into etiology and prevention. J Urol 128:492, 1982.

The Urethra

6

Surgical Anatomy

THE MALE URETHRA

The male urethra is a fibroelastic structure that extends from the internal urethral orifice at the vesical neck to the external urethral meatus at the tip of the glans penis. It is divided by the urogenital diaphragm into three parts: prostatic, membranous, and penile (Fig. 1). The prostatic urethra is the widest and is about 3 cm long in normal adults. The lumen of the urethra is distensible but normally is obliterated by elastic fibers causing apposition of its anterior and posterior walls. In prostatic lateral lobe hyperplasia, the urethral wall is changed into a wide anteroposterior fissure by encroachment of the enlarged lateral lobes upon the urethra.

The urethral crest extends along the posterior floor of the urethra from its origin on the vesical trigone to its bifurcated end. The prostatic sinus is a depressed fossa on each side of the crest and has many orifices from prostatic ducts (Fig. 2). The seminal colliculus (verumontanum) is the greatest prominence of the urethral crest, and the prostatic utricle opens in its central surface. The finer slitlike orifices of the ejaculatory ducts open beside the prostatic utricle.

The membranous urethra is the shortest, about 1.5 cm long, and passes through the urogenital diaphragm between its superior and inferior layers of fascia. This part of the urethra has no proper surrounding tissue but contains the circular fibers of the deep transverse perineal muscle, called the external urethral sphincter. This is a voluntary muscle controlled by the perineal branch of the internal pudendal nerve. Behind the membranous urethra, close to the inferior layer of the urogenital diaphragm, lie the bulbourethral glands of Cowper, which open into the penile urethra at its bulbous part on each side.

The penile urethra is the longest segment of urethra and is surrounded by the spongy body. It is about 15 cm long when the penis is flaccid and has a right-angled curve at the penoscrotal junction. The bulbous urethra is dilated and forms the perineal curve; openings of the bulbourethral glands of Cowper lie at its posterior wall. On the floor of the penile urethra are numerous small lacunas and mucous glands, the glands of Littre (Fig. 2). The external meatus is the narrowest part. The preterminal urethra next to the meatus has a dilated lumen known as the fossa navicularis.

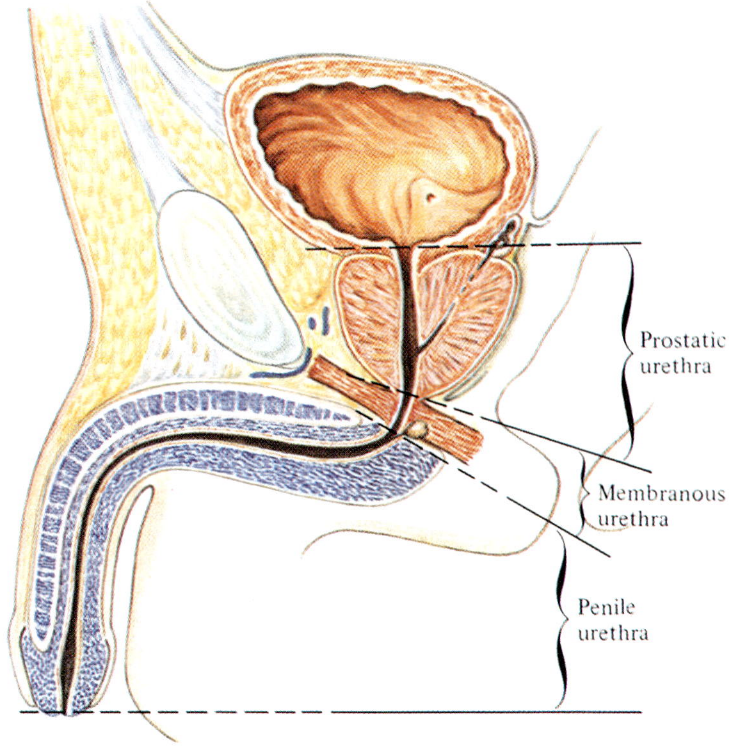

FIG. 1.
Anatomy of male urethra, midsagittal section.

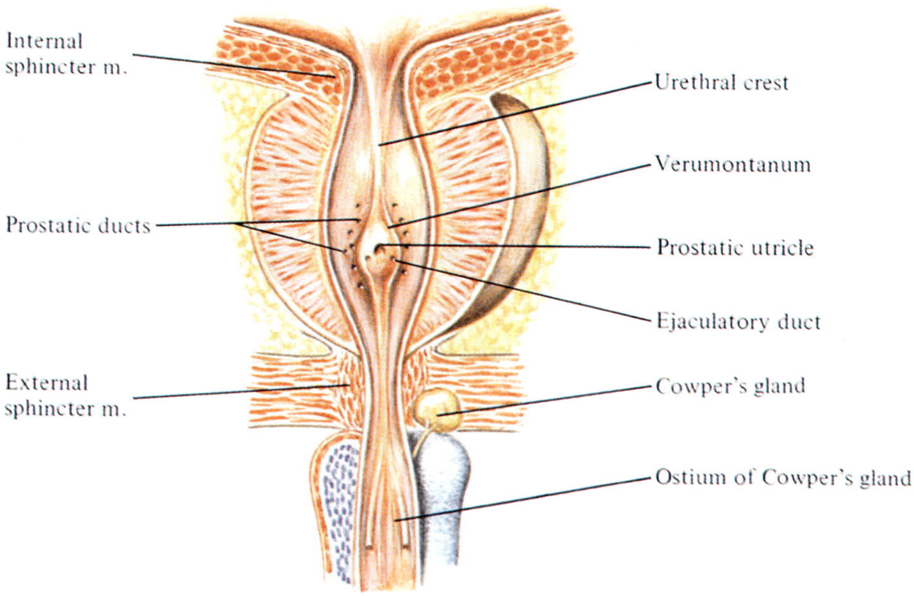

FIG. 2.
Prostatic and membranous urethra (anterior half of prostate has been unroofed).

The arterial supply to the urethra is derived from branches of the internal pudendal and inferior vesical arteries. Veins drain into the pudendal or perivesical plexuses. Lymphatic drainage is to the inguinal nodes and lymph glands along the iliac vessels.

THE FEMALE URETHRA

The female urethra is approximately 4 to 5 cm long and begins at the internal urethral orifice or vesical neck. It follows a slightly curved course downward and forward and terminates at the external urethral meatus on the roof of the vestibule.

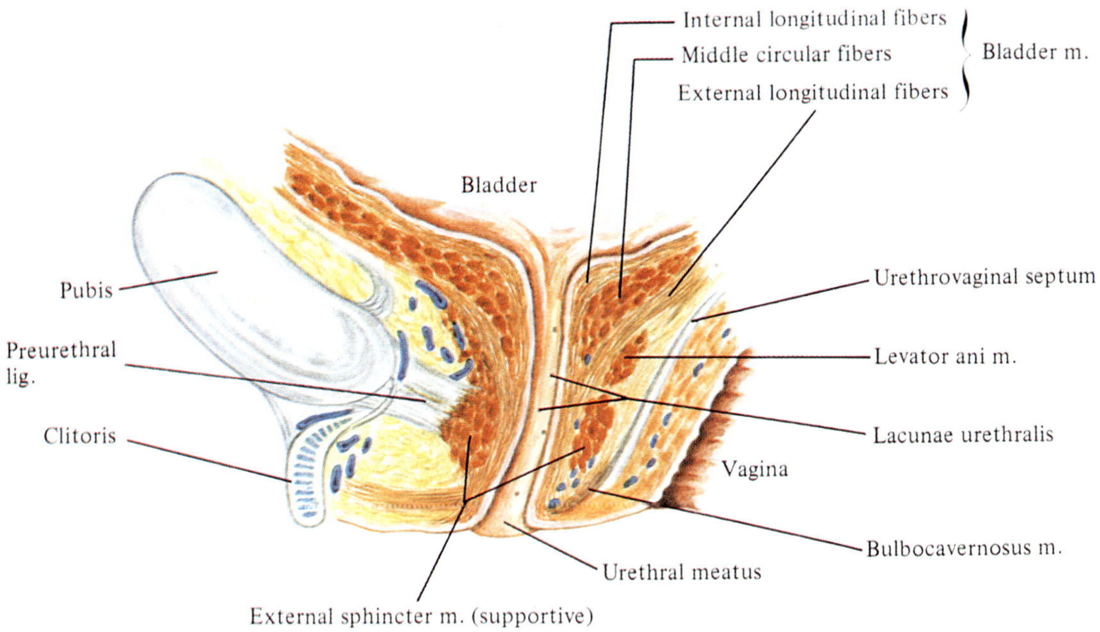

FIG. 3.
Female urethra, midsagittal section.

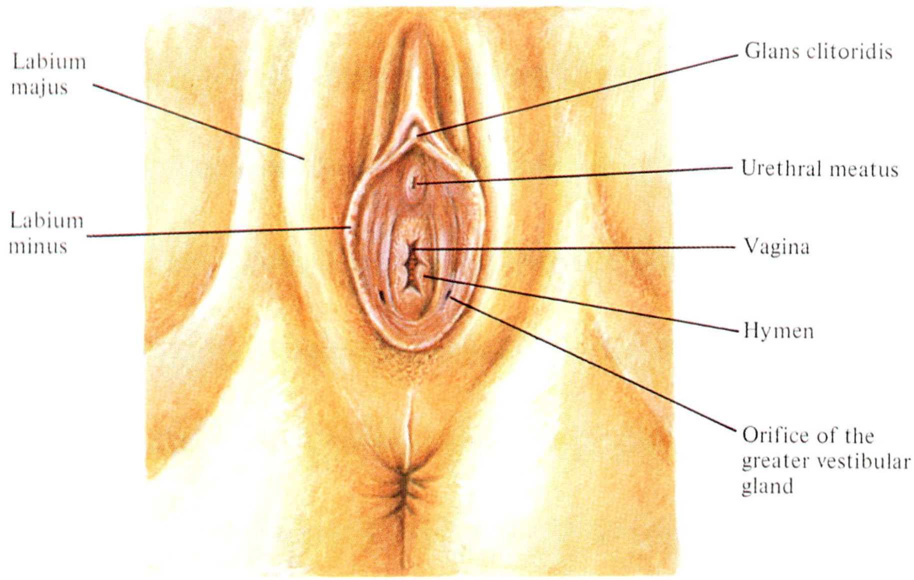

FIG. 4.
Female external genitalia.

The epithelium of the female urethra is squamous in its distal portion and transitional in its proximal segment. Numerous periurethral glands are embedded in the submucosal layer; the largest are the glands of Skene, which open just inside the meatus.

The longitudinal smooth-muscle layer of the bladder neck is prolonged to encase the urethra, but at the portion that pierces the urogenital diaphragm, it is surrounded by striated sphincter muscle, as in the male. The urethra also passes through the levator ani muscle before traversing the diaphragm and is supported by bulbocavernous muscle under the diaphragm.

Because the female urethra is short, care must be taken not to damage the urethral wall in operative procedures (Figs. 3 and 4). A distinct sphincter action is not always demonstrable in the female.

Operative Techniques

82. Surgical Repair of the Ruptured Urethra at the Distal Prostatic Junction

Complete rupture of the distal prostatic urethra is suspected if a male patient has suffered injury to the bony pelvis. The patient may present with fresh bleeding out of the urethral meatus.

The entire patient must be evaluated if multiple anatomic systems are injured. The cardiorespiratory system and the central nervous system take priority over the urologic system. Any penetrating wound of the abdomen also takes priority over the urologic system.

An intravenous infusion (double dose) urogram is obtained if one suspects renal injury. One should keep in mind that multiple-system injury is the rule in most patients involved in automobile accidents.

The physician in the emergency room is the first to see the patient. An attempt may be made to carefully insert a 16 French indwelling catheter into the bladder. If urethral disruption is complete, then the catheter will meet an obstruction. A retrograde urethrogram can assist in making the diagnosis.

Controversy exists regarding the best surgical treatment for reapproximating the severed urethral ends. Many clinicians feel that a suprapubic cystostomy is the treatment of choice at the outset. Drainage of urine from the perivesical lateral sites may be necessary. The belief is that extensive dissection must be avoided. This school believes that potency will be preserved, and a second-stage procedure 4–6 months later will allow easy reconstruction of the injured fibrosed urethra. We adhere to this concept.

The other, larger group of clinicians believes that early reapproximation of the urethra is indicated. This surgical technique is illustrated. The patient is in a supine position. His thighs are separated and elevated over sandbags so that the perineal area is accessible.

82-1. *The bladder is entered by cystotomy.* Double interlocking sounds are carefully placed. The area of prostatic disruption is seen from this midsagittal view. The special metal sound entering the pendulous urethra also has a perforation on its tip.

82-2. The metal sound from distal urethra, which has met the proximal sound, is guided into the bladder lumen. A straight soft rubber 18 Fr catheter is tied to the metal tip, and the rubber catheter is withdrawn.

82-3. *The rubber catheter is attached outside the urethral meatus to an indwelling silicone rubber catheter* (22 or 20 Fr, depending on the size of the patient).

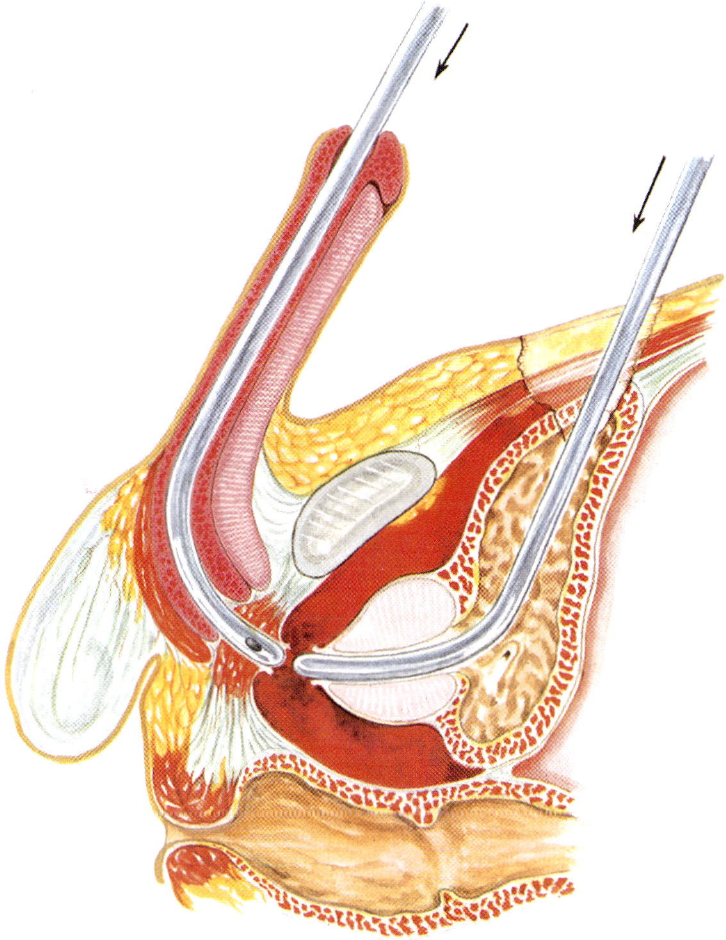

82-1

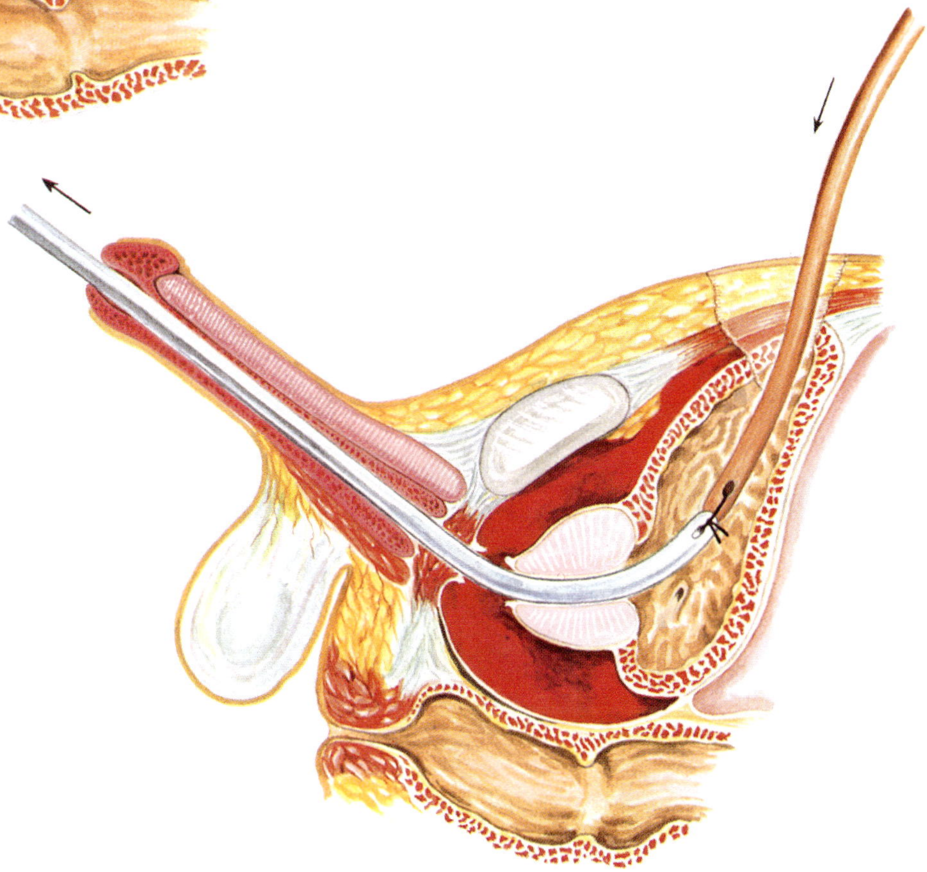

82-2

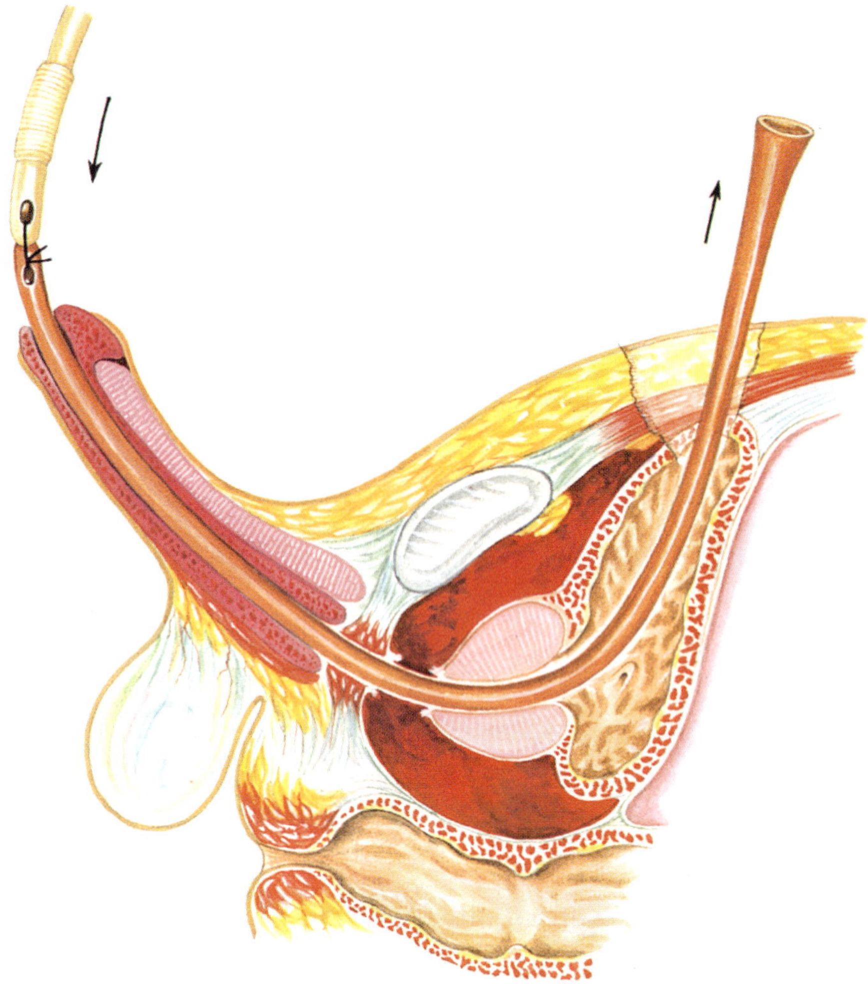

82-3

82-4. *The indwelling catheter is inserted and secured* (30 mL in the balloon). A suprapubic tube (Malecot tip, 24 Fr) is inserted. The bladder is closed in two layers. We now use a Jackson-Pratt closed drainage tube to discourage infection. The compressible bulb on the distal end provides a negative pressure, thus allowing the tissue fluid to collect in the lumen of the bulb or the closed drainage bag.

Traction-like (Vest type) perineal sutures (0–0 nylon) may be used; they extend from the prostatic capsule anterolaterally through the perineum. Each suture is secured over a button for 2 to 3 weeks. The alternative is to place a 2.2-pound (1-kg) weight on a pulley. The catheter emerging from the penile urethra is attached to the raised weight on an overhead pulley at a 45° angle from the horizontal. Care must be taken to ensure that the line of traction is secure at all times. Such traction is usually applied for a minimum of 3 weeks.

Prevention of urinary tract infection is important. Urine is cultured at least once each week from the suprapubic tube. Ceftriaxone is a broad spectrum cephalosporin that can be given intravenously or intramuscularly. Depending on the size of the patient, the initial dose can be 1 g in an average adult or 1.5 to 2 g in a large adult. At 12 hours following intramuscular administration, the blood levels are in the 50% range from the initial dose of 1 g. The antibiotic is continued or changed to an oral broad spectrum antibiotic.

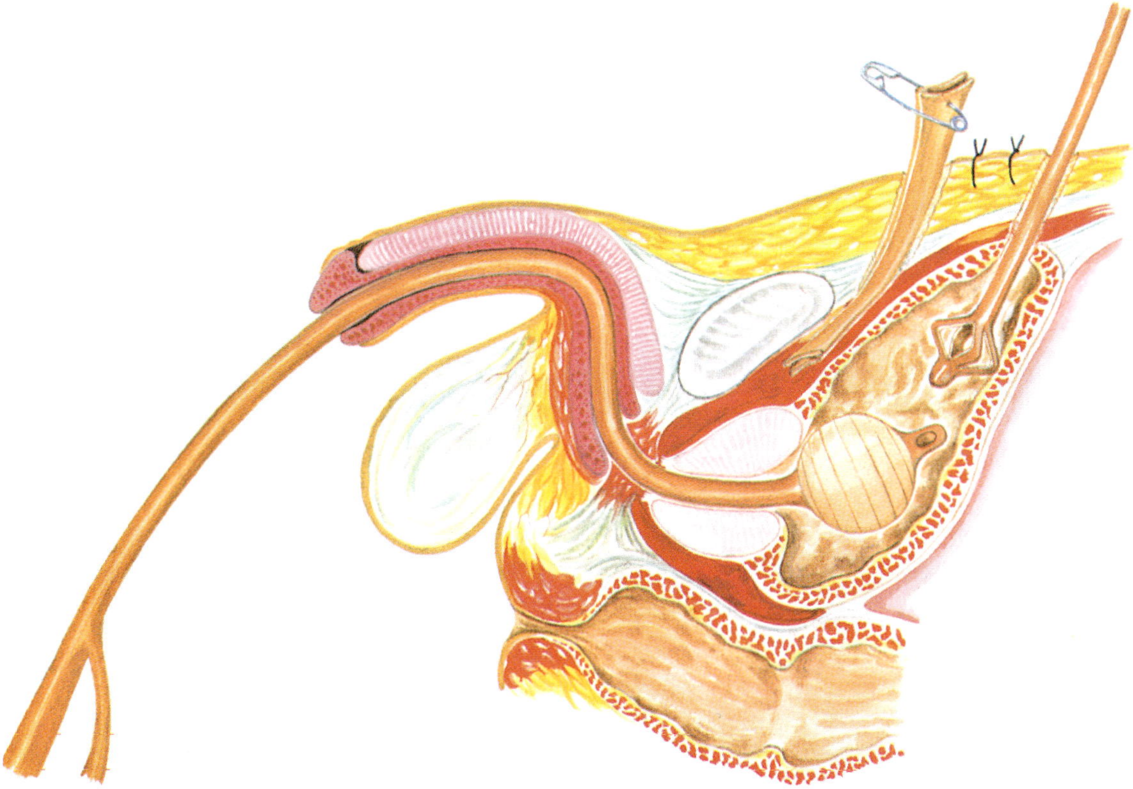

82-4

83. Perineal Urethrotomy: Removal of a Large (1.5 cm) Calculus

83-1. The calculus can be palpated. *The skin, musculature, and underlying perineal urethra is incised.* Stay sutures are placed to identify and expose urethral lumen if the margins are not distinct.

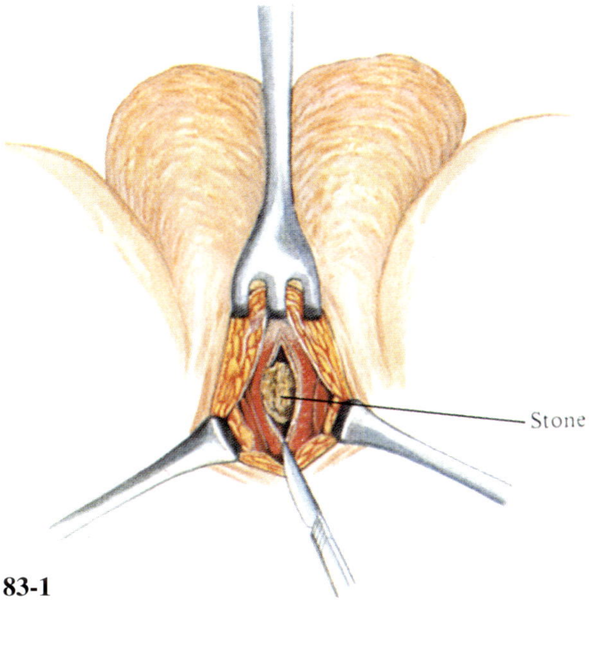

83-1

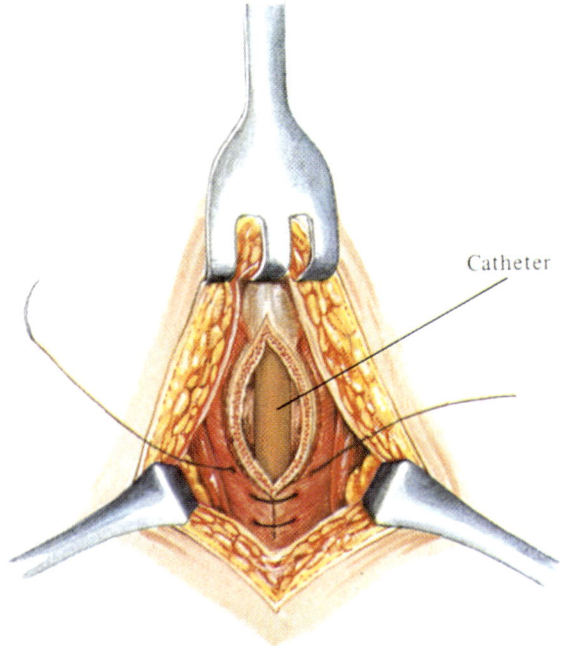

83-2

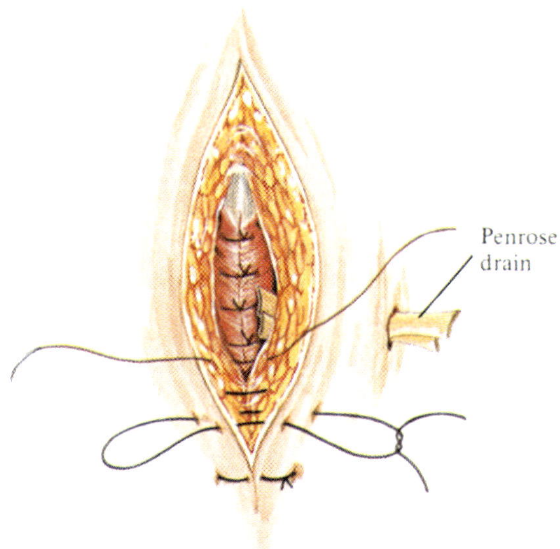

83-3

83-2. *An indwelling catheter,* 18 or 20 Fr (5-mL bag) *is inserted.* The urethra is reapproximated using 3–0 chromic catgut.

83-3. *Closure of the urethra is complete.* A flat tubular drain is brought out laterally through a separate skin incision. The subcutaneous tissue and skin are reapproximated (3–0 chromic catgut).

84. Transurethral Removal of Stone or Foreign Body

84-1. Under anesthesia *a straight clamp is inserted into the pendulous urethra, and the calculus is removed.* The thumb and forefinger assist in preventing migration of the foreign body.

84-2. A moderate-sized calculus (1.5 to 2 cm) can obstruct the prostatic urethra. *A Van Buren sound* (24 Fr) is used to dislodge the calculus into the bladder. The resectoscope (26 sheath) can also be used to dislodge the calculus into the bladder.

84-3. *The loop of the resectoscope can be used to trap the calculus,* and the entire instrument (including the sheath and resectoscope) can be removed through the urethra.

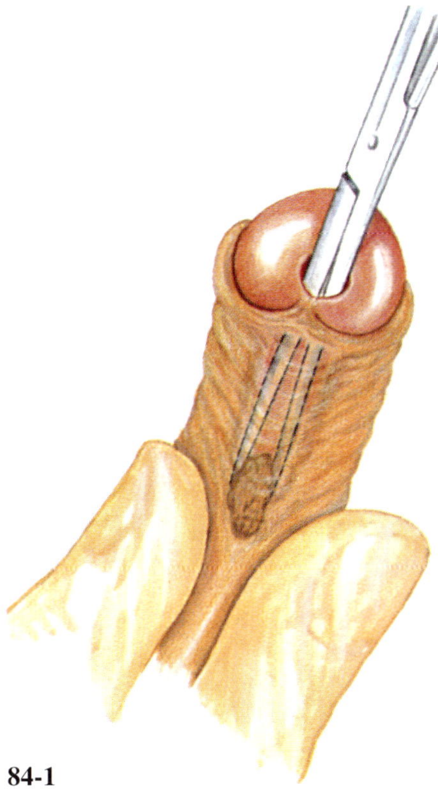

84-1

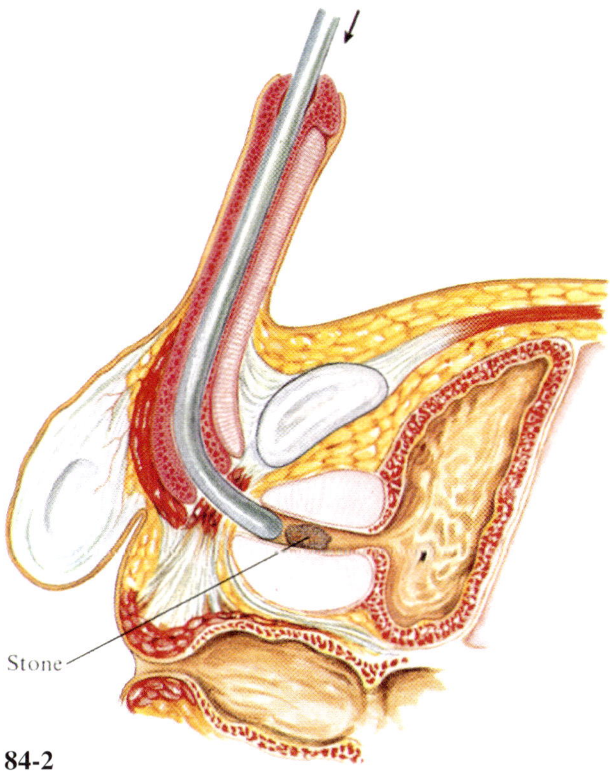

84-2

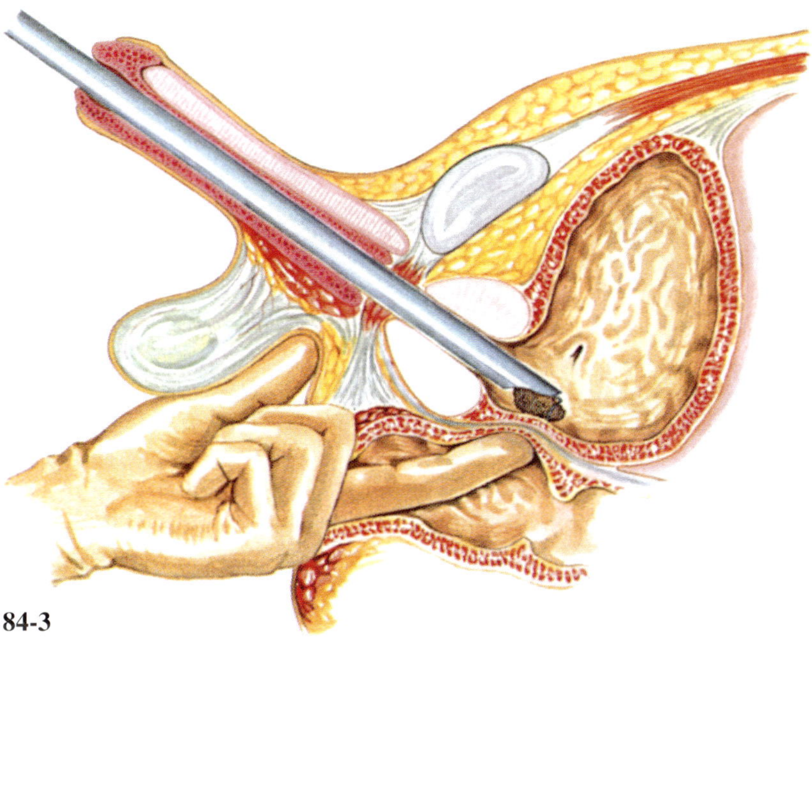

84-3

The gloved index finger on the left is used to trap the calculus. If the calculus is too large, then the lithotrite should be inserted, and the calculus pushed into the bladder should be crushed into smaller fragments. Care must be taken to ensure that all fragments are removed by means of copious irrigations.

Urethroplasty

85. First-Stage Urethroplasty—Turner-Warwick Procedure

A previous retrograde urethrogram has demarcated the severity and the extent of stricture formation. In our experience, many patients have been dilated for many years, usually at intervals of a few months. They now request reconstructive urethral surgery.

Spinal or general anesthesia can be used. The patient is placed in the lithotomy position. Stirrups afford better exposure than the thigh-leg braces used in transurethral surgery.

85-1. We inject a dilute solution of methylene blue dye (15 mL) through the urethral meatus to stain the strictured areas. *An incision is made (dotted line)* for a bulbous urethral stricture.

85-2. The bulbocavernous muscle is incised longitudinally. The urethra is similarly incised, and the cut edges are retracted. A special-retaining retractor assists in the procedure.

85-3. *Scrotal skin is used to form the broad-based floor of the opened urethra.* The scrotal skin is tested to be sure it will reach the open urethra without tension. Stay sutures assist in the proper orientation.

85-4. *The scrotal skin is shaped into a funnel,* and the nylon (3–0) stay sutures are brought out through the new opening in the midscrotum (*at right*). Care is taken to place the most difficult sutures at the innermost and inferior margins. An untied suture has been placed in this difficult area. Several more sutures should be placed on each side of the apex to provide a good healing margin.

85-5. *A special nasal speculum adapted for urethroplasties* is helpful in placing the deep sutures near the membranous urethra. We agree with Turner-Warwick that the membranous urethra can be incised at 6 o'clock and the scrotal inlay can be taken to prostatic urethra when necessary. Special Reverdin needles adapted by Turner-Warwick are useful for the purpose of securing the deep sutures.

85-6. *In the completed first-stage urethroplasty,* with long tails on the nylon 3–0 sutures, the vertical perineal incision is closed transversely. A flat tubular drain can be placed at each angle if deemed necessary. Both ends of the new urethrostomies should accommodate 30 to 32 Fr urethral sounds.

An indwelling urethral catheter is brought out through the new opening and left in place for 4 to 5 days. Before the patient is discharged from the hospital he is carefully instructed in the art of inserting urethral suppositories through each of the urethrostomies. In our opinion, fibrinous adhesions can form at the distal urethrostomy if the patient is inattentive. He is instructed to insert a urethral suppository in each direction on a daily basis.

The patient is followed regularly in the office. We will dilate both urethrostomy sites at 7- to 10-day intervals during the first month (24 to 28 Fr).

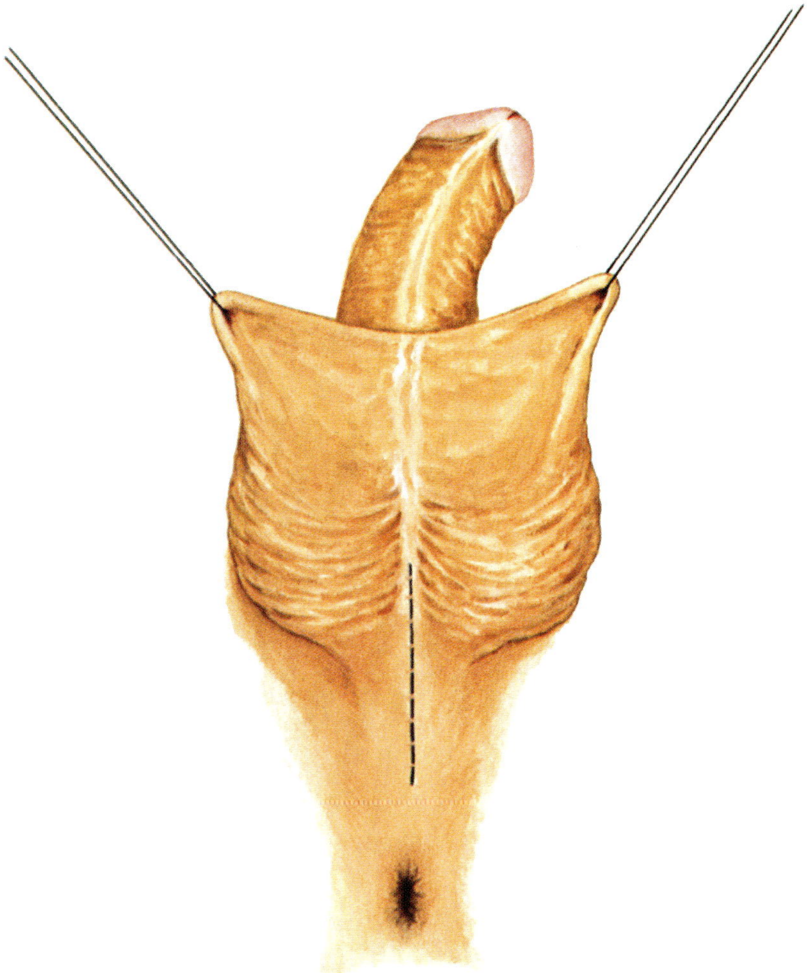

85-1

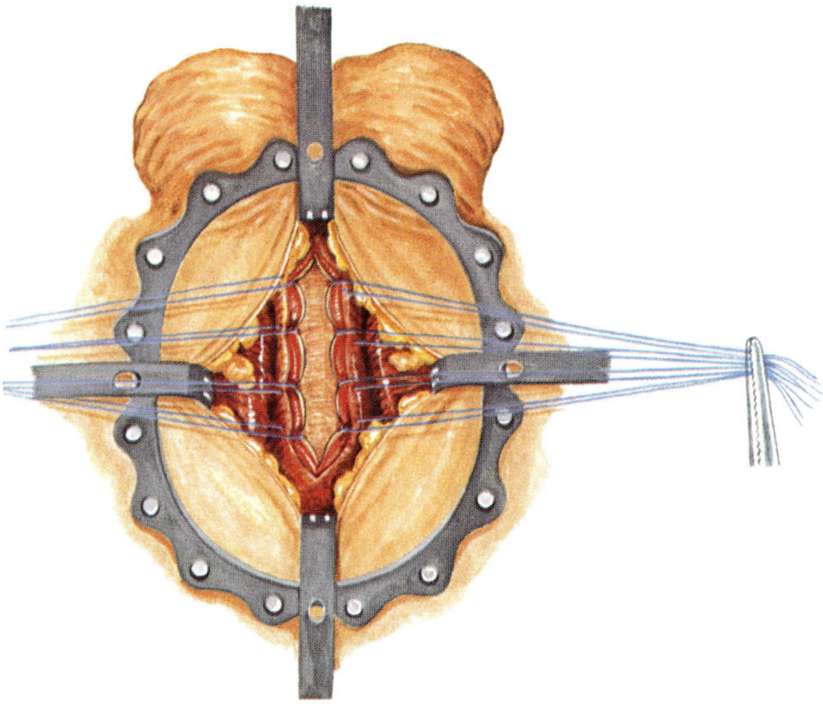

85-2

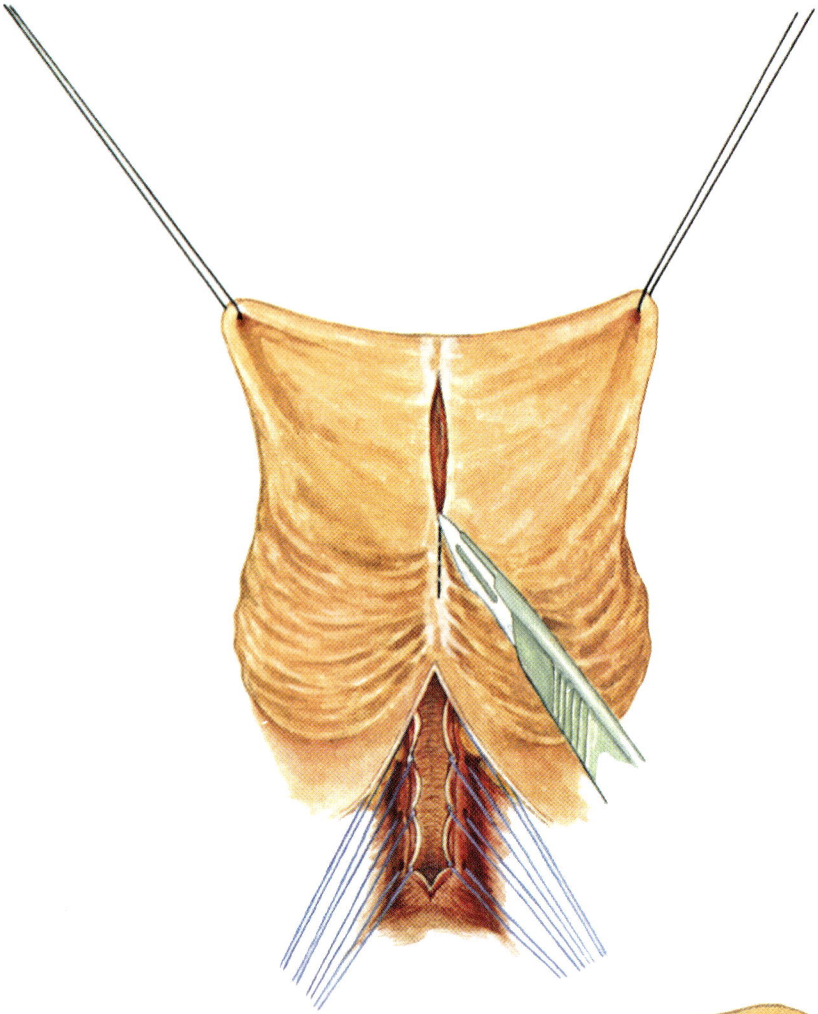

85-3

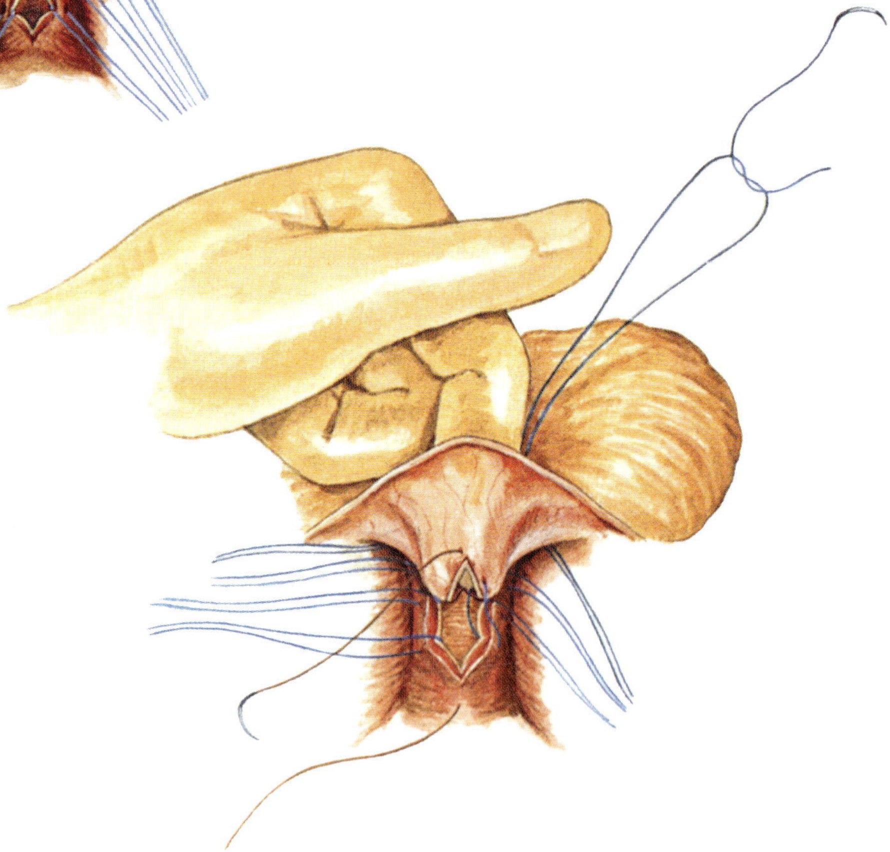

85-4

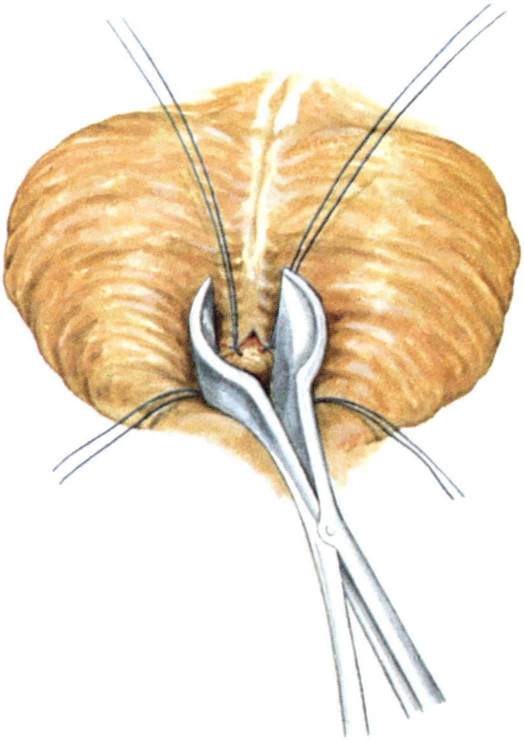

85-5

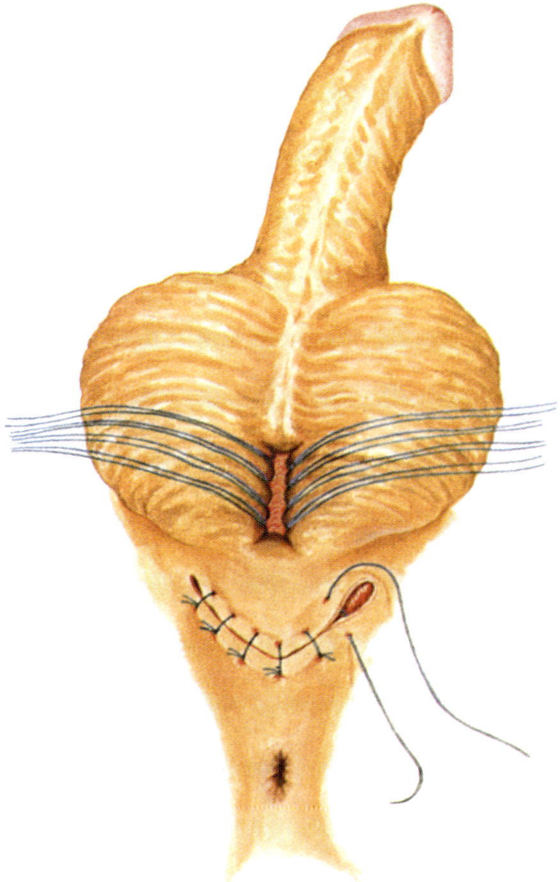

85-6

At 1 month in the postoperative period the patient is hospitalized (1 day short-term admission) and anesthetized. The position for cystoscopy is used. Residual hairs in the scrotal inlay are removed by epilation. Gentle traction is maintained on each hair while the fine needle is inserted beside it to the follicle. We use the 12-volt DC apparatus currently used by plastic surgeons for removal of eyelashes. Only a few seconds are necessary before each hair is released from its follicle.

The nylon sutures are removed with a small knife blade at the deep scrotal-urethral interface. Cystoscopy is performed to be sure benign prostatic hypertrophy (BPH) or bladder neck obstruction is not also present. If the prostate is significantly enlarged, then transurethral resection of the prostate is performed during a subsequent admission. Both urethrostomies are carefully calibrated and dilated (24 to 28 Fr distally, 28–34 Fr proximally).

If transurethral resection of the prostate is indicated, then this procedure is scheduled in the interim, and the second stage urethroplasty is not performed until 4 to 5 months have elapsed.

86. Second-Stage Urethroplasty—Turner-Warwick Procedure

The patient is placed in the lithotomy position. We prefer the stirrups for elevation of the lower extremities. General or spinal anesthesia may be used.

86-1. *A special sound perforated on its tip* (26 Fr) *is inserted.* A small suprapubic skin incision is made and carried in the midline through the fascia of the rectus abdominis muscle. Tenting upward on the sound allows easy identification of the bladder wall.

86-2. The perforated tip of the sound allows *an indwelling urethral catheter* (20 Fr, 5-mL inflatable bag) *to be secured.* Heavy silk (1–0) is used to approximate both tips. The catheter is drawn into the bladder and out the proximal urethra.

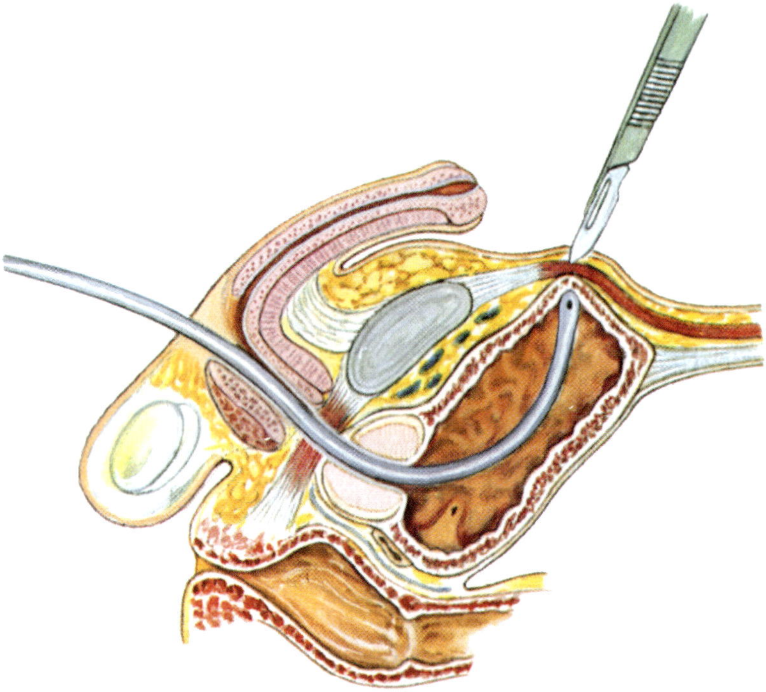

86-1

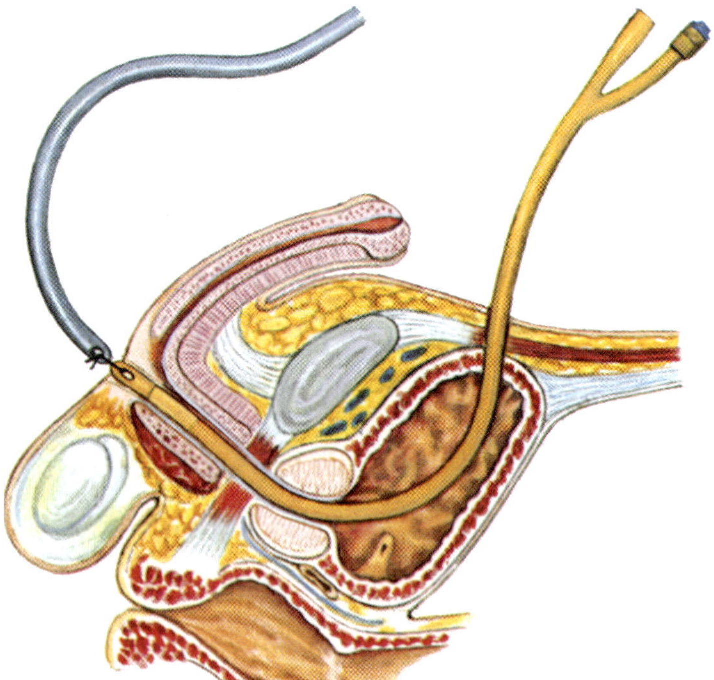

86-2

86-3. The tie is released and the catheter is carefully retracted into bladder lumen. *The bag is inflated* and the catheter is irrigated to be sure that its tip is in the bladder lumen. The suprapubic cystostomy should take only a few minutes.

86-4. We believe that *the border of the new urethra should be marked (broken line).* Stay sutures often assist in proper orientation.

86-5. The *new tube of skin has been freed.* The outer skin margin must be undermined so that a second layer of closure can be reapproximated without tension.

86-6. *A continuous stitch is used to tubulize the new urethra* (3–0 chromic catgut). The suture line does not include the skin edge but is subcuticular in its location. After completion of the new urethra, subcutaneous tissue is brought over the urethra to provide a partial middle-layer closure.

86-7. *The skin is reapproximated with interrupted 4–0 nylon sutures* as a second covering layer. The suprapubic tube is secured to the skin.

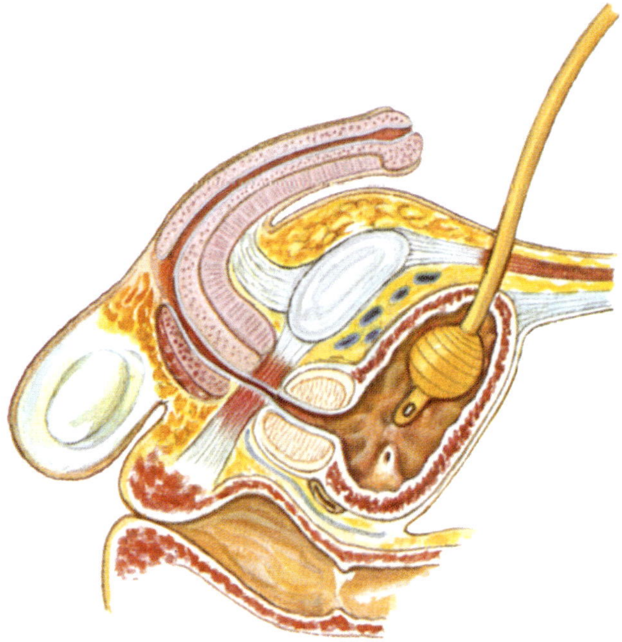

86-3

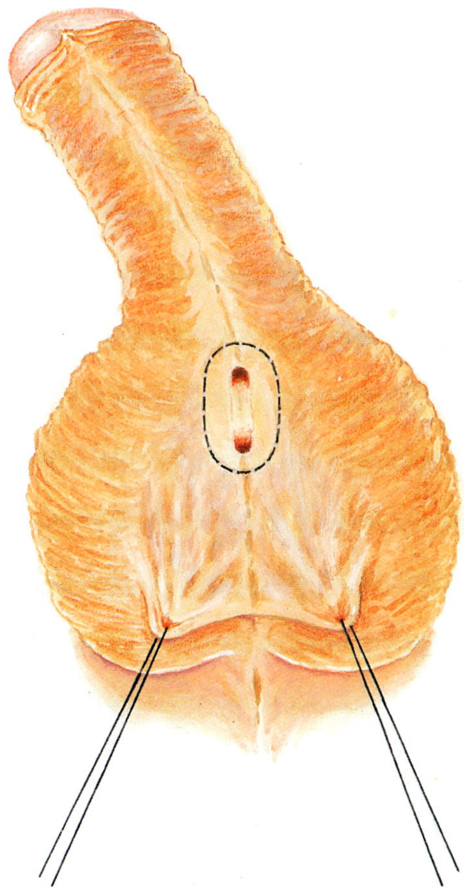

86-4

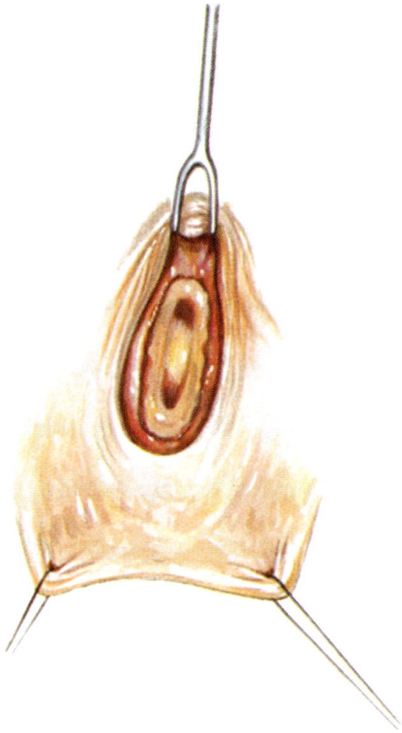

86-5

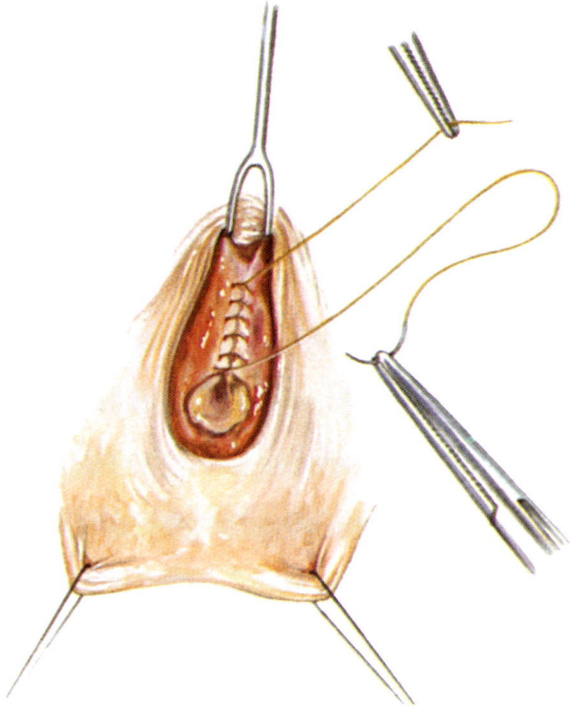

86-6

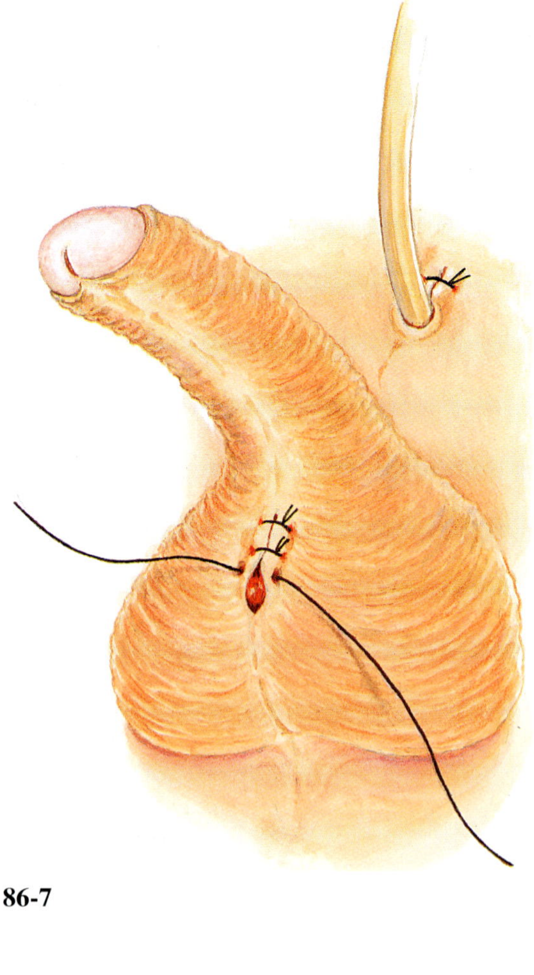

86-7

87. One-Stage Urethroplasty (Blandy Procedure)

There are obvious advantages to the use of a one-stage surgical procedure. In this operation Professor Blandy describes the use of a scrotal flap which is incorporated so that a urethroplasty can be formed.

87-1. The incision is a standard upside-down U-shaped scrotal flap. The incision should end just in front of the ischial tuberosities on each side. To obtain access to the bulbous urethra, one has to start the flap sufficiently far back as shown. In this way there should be no difficulty when one sutures the flap in the appropriate position. As we have emphasized, in most operations the key to success is having good access to the anatomic area and the stricture.

87-2. After the flap has been raised, the ischial bulbospongiosus muscle is brought into position as shown. The illustration depicts the reflection of the bulbospongiosus muscle as it is reflected from the bulbous urethra. The retractors expose the area.

87-3. The urethra is opened with a bougie in place. The bougie in this instance is just distal to the stricture.

87-4. The corpus spongiosum is oversewn to control bleeding and the stricture is now incised proximally. The bulbospongiosus muscle is dissected from the bulb and is reflected on either side as shown. The urethra is extended to the bougie and one can now insert a 4–0 catgut suture on either side to close the spongy tissue. This prevents loss of blood as shown in the illustration. The surgeon then carries the incision forward until healthy tissue is encountered. He/she also carries the dissection backwards and up toward the verumontanum until the stricture is completely divided. As the surgeon makes

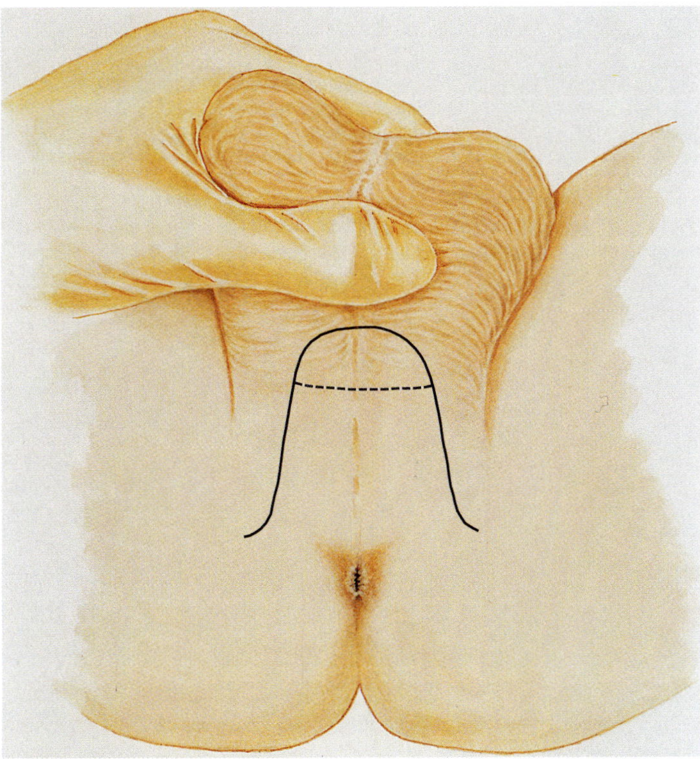

87-1

the incision in the midline, he/she must control the bleeding. We recommend the use of running hemostatic stitches down each side of the split corpus spongiosum. It is important to be sure that one has dissected beyond the stenosed strictured area. The best way to be sure that one has gone beyond the stricture is to insert the forefinger past the stenosed area. One now gains easy access into the prostatic urethra. If you cannot insert your finger, then more dissection needs to be carried out.

87-5. Next, insert the nasal speculum, which is upside down. The insertion is carried out until one sees the verumontanum. The cut edge of the healthy urethra should be just distal to the adjacent lower edge of the prostate.

87-6. The patch is now formed. The patch originates from the tip of the scrotal flap and it is provided with its own dartos pedicle if one undermines the flap appropriately. The flap should not be too wide. Remember that scrotal skin can be stretched and one can wrap it around a 26 Fr bougie. Be sure that you have not made the scrotal strip too large or wide.

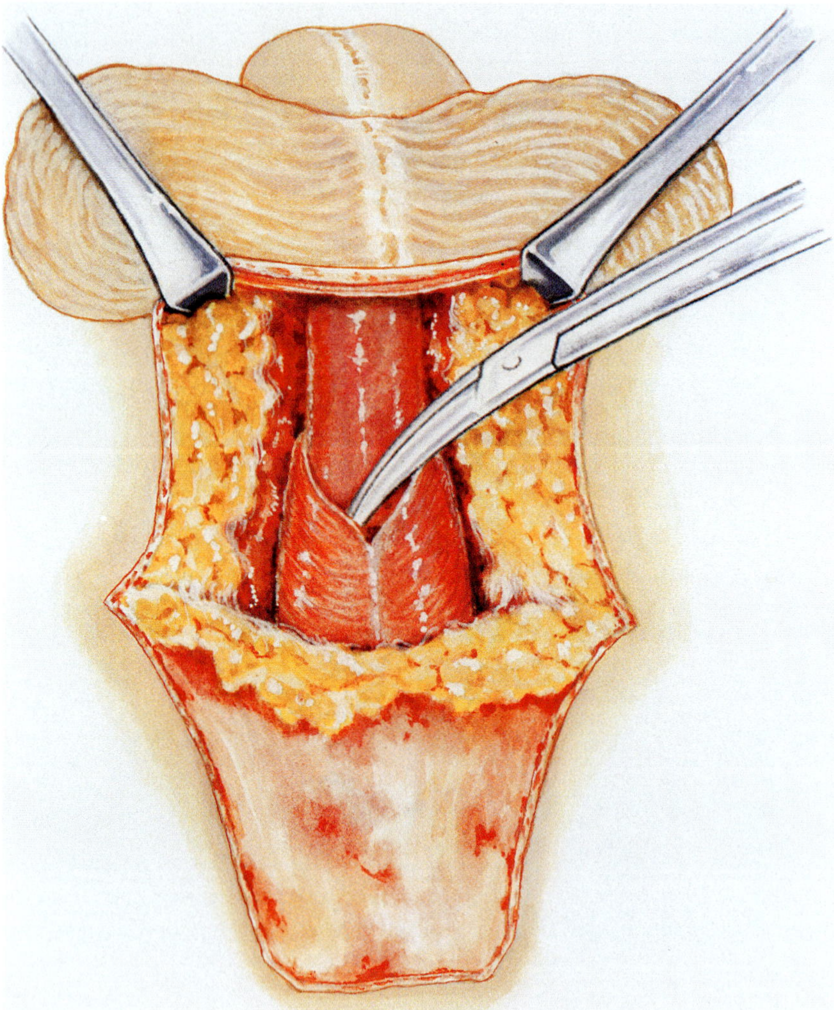

87-2

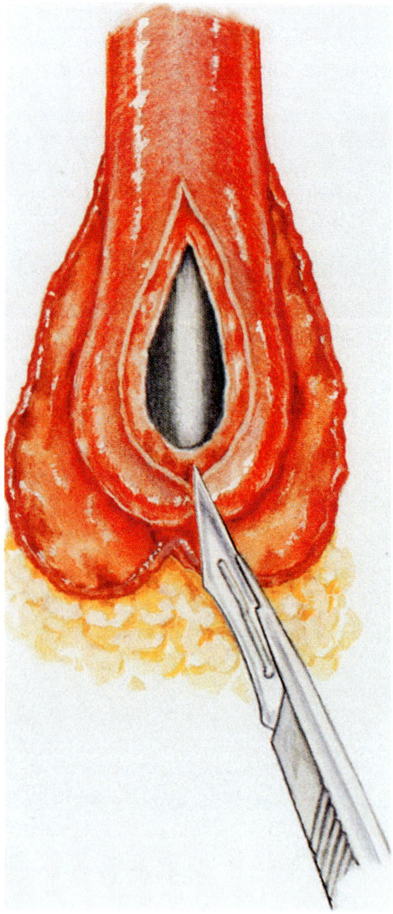

87-3

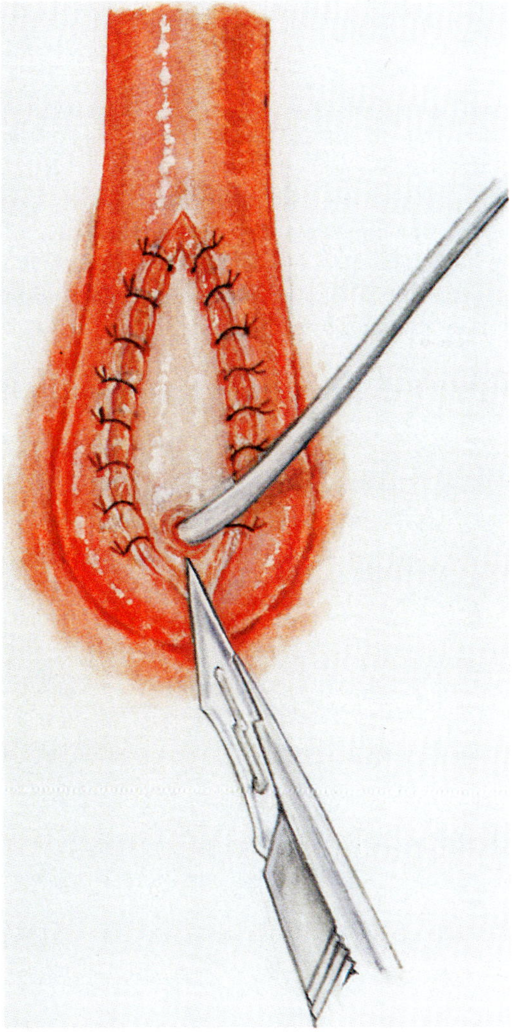

87-4

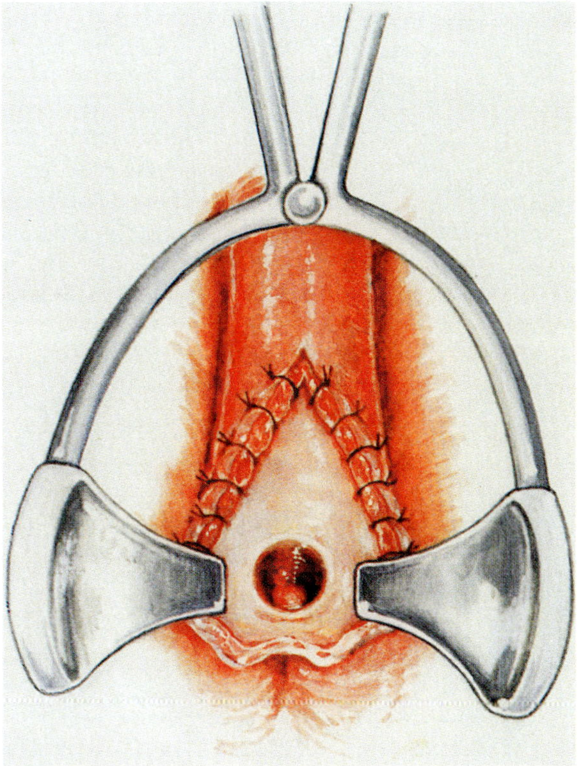

87-5

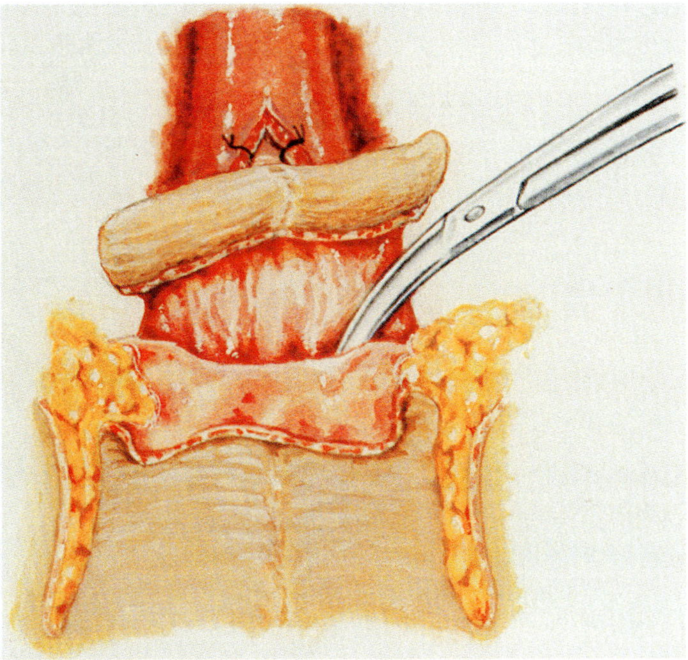

87-6

The patch is appropriately trimmed and, using 3–0 chromic catgut on a reverse cutting needle, one places three interrupted sutures between the tip of the patch and the upper end of the incision.

87-7. This portion will become the urethra. The sutures are tied so that the end of the flap can be inverted into the defect in the urethra.

87-8. The remaining sutures are now placed one after the other, between the edge of the flap and the cut edge of the urethra. In our experience, it is better to use interrupted sutures. After one places 2 to 3 sutures on each side, one can remove the speculum and the remaining stitches for the flap can be inserted under direct vision.

87-9. It is important to use a 14 Fr or 16 Fr Silastic catheter in the newly constructed urethra.

The bulbospongiosus muscle is loosely approximated over the dartos pedicle. The skin is brought together with very fine everting nylon-type sutures. If drainage is slightly excessive, then one can use a small Jackson-Pratt drainage tube which is part of a closed system. Bleeding needs to be controlled. A very firm compression dressing is appropriate under a T bandage. One can use foam to assist in putting pressure on the operated site to prevent a hematoma.

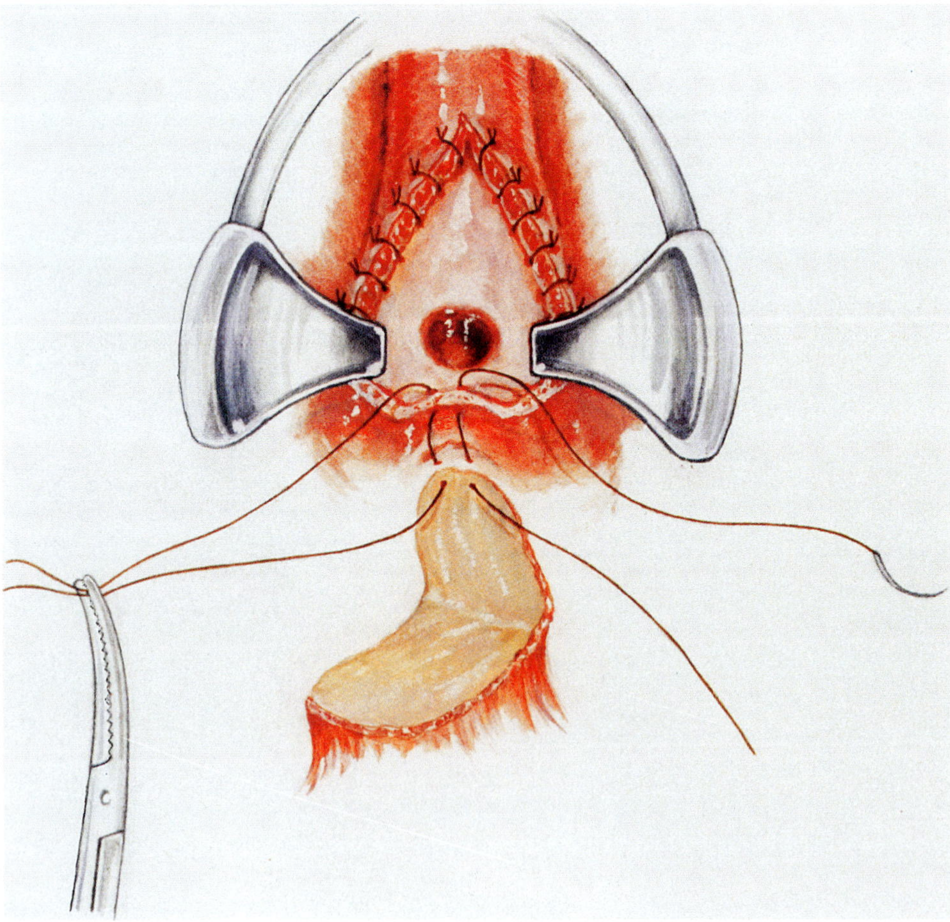

87-7

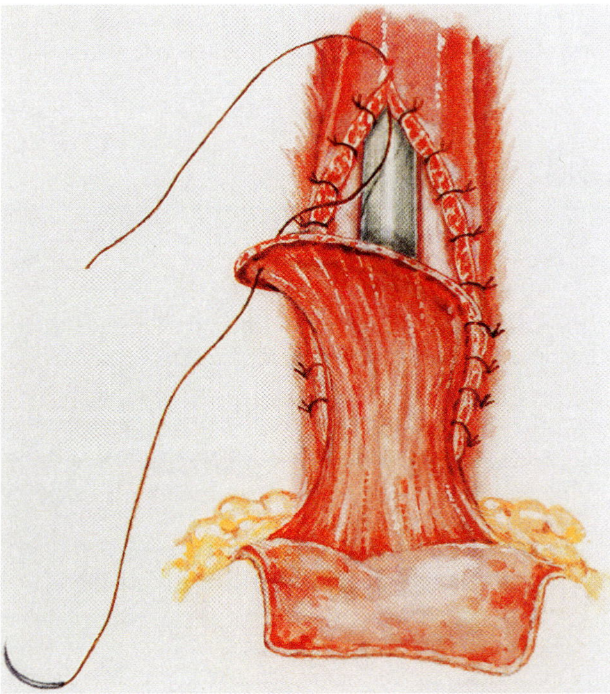

87-8

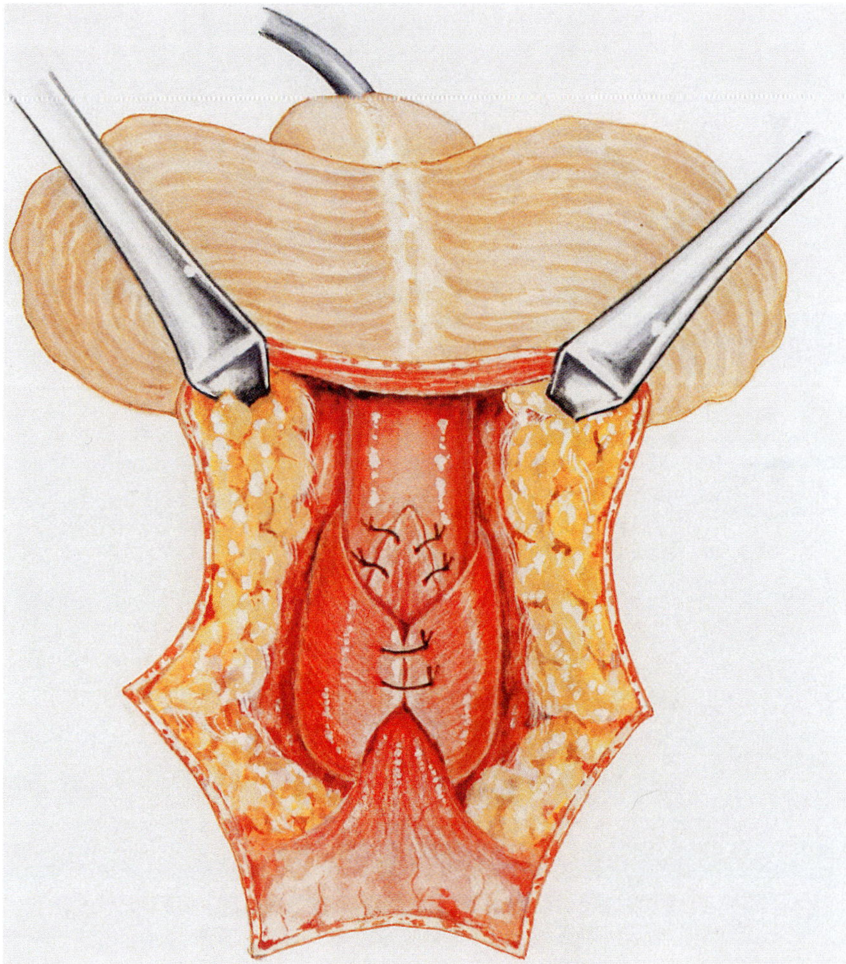

87-9

It is important to keep the patient on appropriate antibiotics for at least 5–6 days. In our view, ampicillin and gentamycin may be appropriate, although one of the new cephalosporins may also be an appropriate choice.

Perineal Urethroplasty

88. First-Stage Urethroplasty

Subtle differences exist between the Leadbetter technique described in 1960 and the Gil-Vernet technique reported in 1966. The technique presented here resembles the procedure described by Gil-Vernet.

Spinal or general anesthesia may be used. The patient is in a slightly exaggerated lithotomy position. A urethrogram has been obtained, and the strictured area is in the deep bulbous urethra and extends distally.

88-1. When a long stricture is present, *an inverted U incision is made (dotted lines).* The vertical arm of the incision across the scrotum is employed in this procedure.

88-2. The perineal flap is freed. *The bulbocavernosus muscle is divided in the midline, and the urethra is incised beyond the strictures.* Stay sutures assist in providing exposure. Hemostasis must be maintained. Figure-of-eight sutures in the muscle may be needed to secure hemostasis.

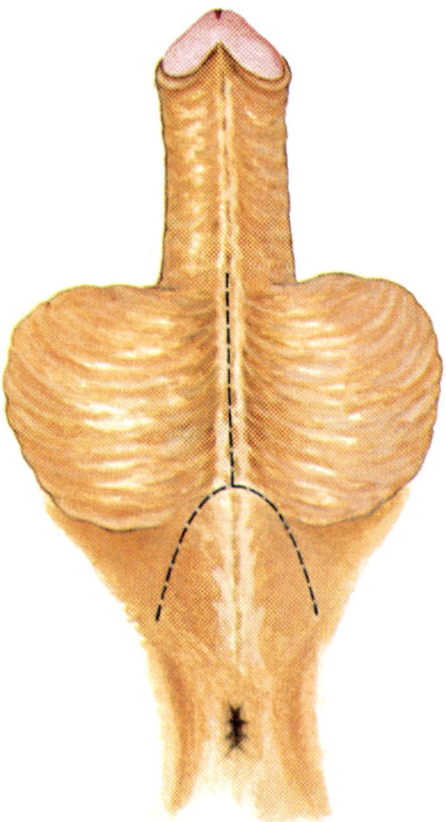

88-1

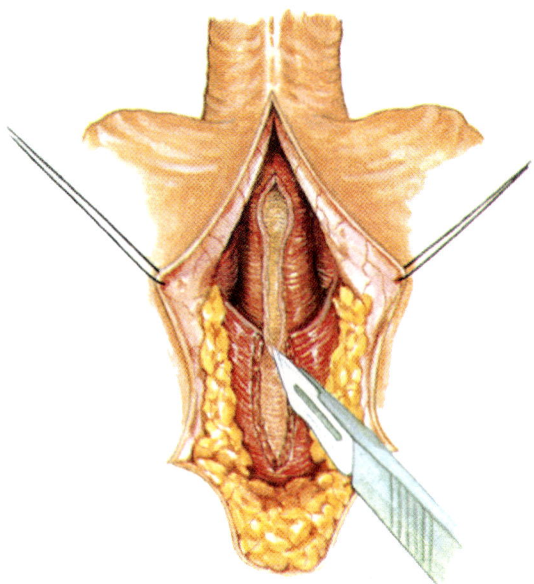

88-2

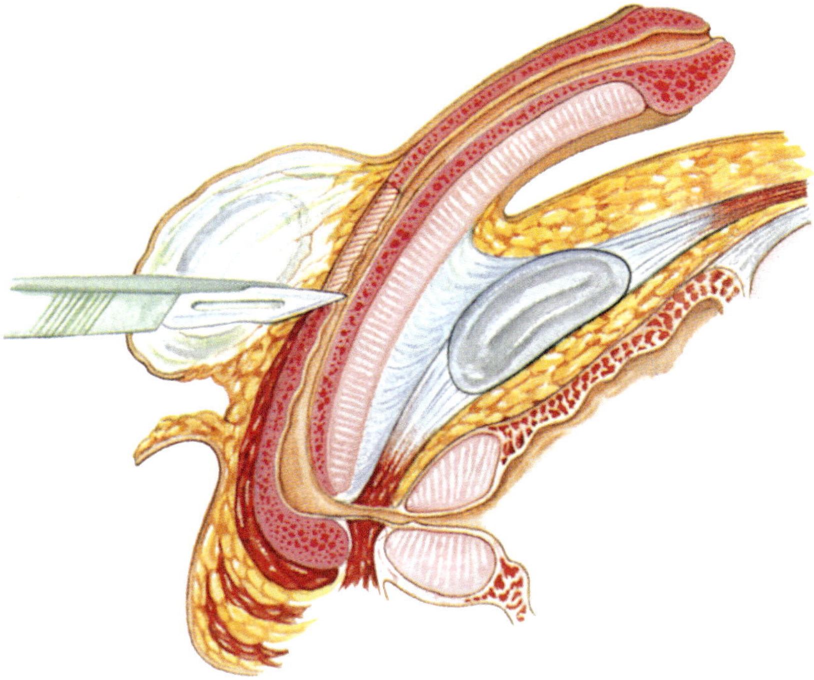

88-3

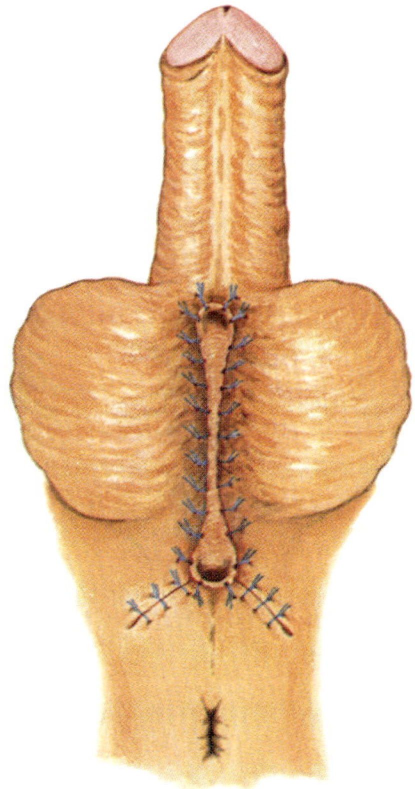

88-4

88-3. The schematic demonstrates *the long stricture (undulations) in the involved urethra.* The perineal flap is seen.

88-4. *The posterior flap is laid into the floor of the proximal urethra.* The edges at the interface are sutured with 3–0 nylon. The entire urethra is sutured to skin margins as demonstrated. A catheter into the proximal urethra is inserted and maintained for 4 to 5 days. Stitches are removed in approximately 2 weeks.

89. Second-Stage Urethroplasty

Before the second-stage urethroplasty is performed, the patient is cystoscoped to rule out significant prostatic hypertrophy. Transurethral resection of the prostate, if deemed necessary, is completed before the second-stage urethroplasty. A suprapubic catheter may be inserted (see 86-1 through 86-3). The patient is positioned as usual.

89-1. *The new urethral tube to be formed is carefully marked (dotted line).*

89-2. *The tube of new skin is sutured, in part, over a stenting urethral catheter* (22 Fr). It is important to undermine both skin edges so closure can be accomplished without tension (3–0 chromic catgut).

89-3. *A second layer of subcutaneous tissue is fashioned to cover the new urethra.*

89-4. *The skin is reapproximated with interrupted 3–0 nylon sutures.* We prefer removal of the urethral catheter since a suprapubic catheter is inserted at the beginning of this procedure.

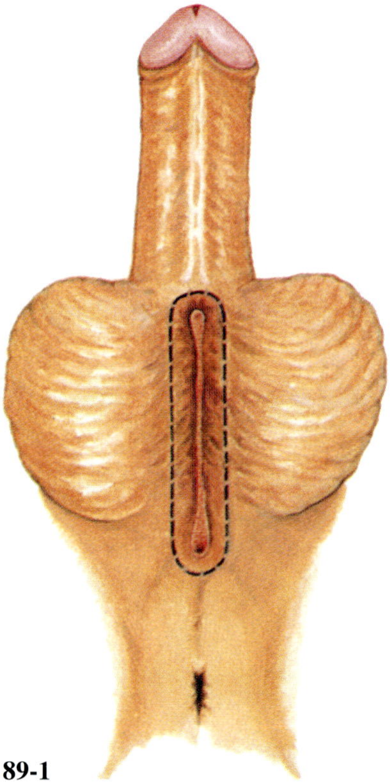

89-1

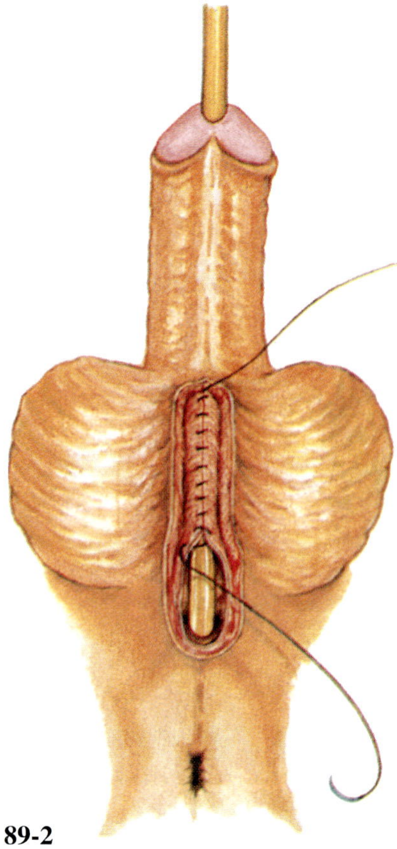

89-2

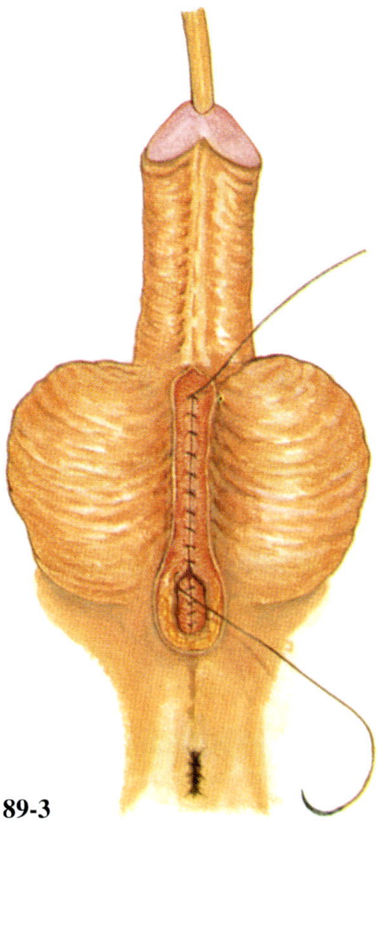

89-3

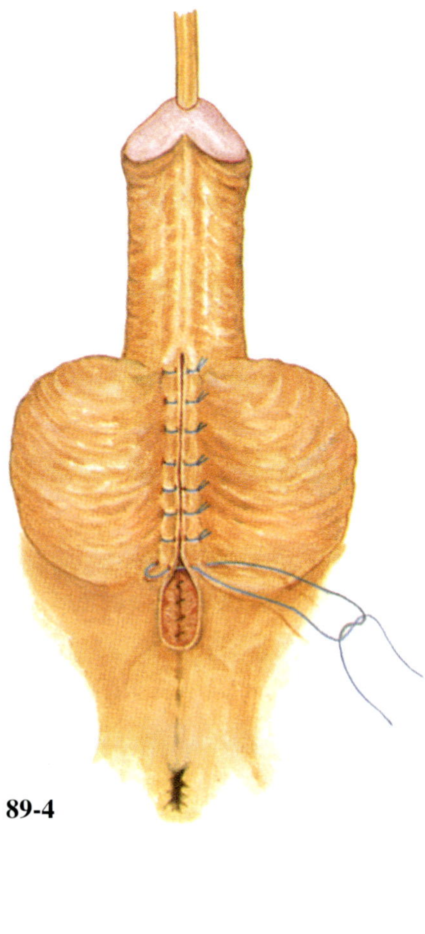

89-4

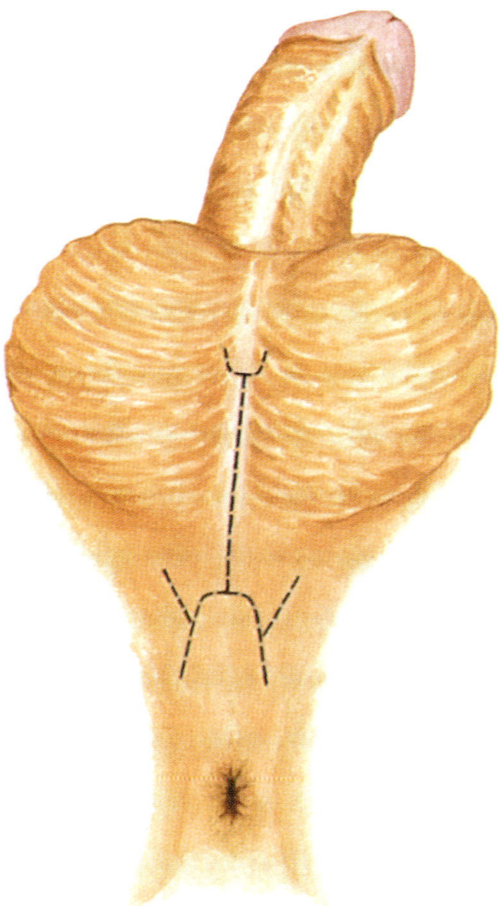

90-1

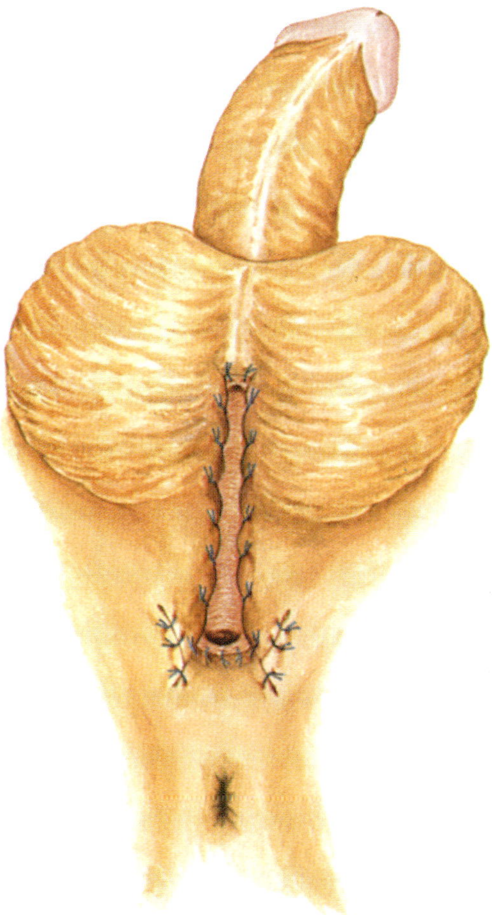

90-2

90. Modified First-Stage Perineal Urethroplasty

Pierce has described his experience with difficult perineal urethral strictures. His procedure is similar to the techniques described by Leadbetter and Gil-Vernet.

90-1. We have modified the posterior perineal flap technique of Pierce so that mobilization is provided at the proximal and distal urethrostomy sites, where stenosis usually may occur. *The lines of incision* are marked.

90-2. *The 3–0 nylon sutures are placed in interrupted fashion.* Our modification at the proximal stoma allows greater relaxation than that obtained with Pierce's method.

Multiple-Stage Repair of Hypospadias With Chordee Removal

Hypospadias is a congenital deformity. Incomplete development of the urethra is the basic defect. This anomaly occurs in about 2 of 500 births. The etiology is unknown.

The prepuce is usually deficient ventrally. A redundant dorsal hood is present. A broad band of fibrous tissue extends from the abnormal meatus to the glans and shortens the ventral aspect, causing the familiar curvature—chordee.

The usual classification of hypospadias is based on the anatomic location of the urethral meatus:

1. Ventral location of urethra in the glans penis or juxtaglandular urethral location
2. Distal penile or coronal
3. Proximal penile
4. Penoscrotal junction
5. Scrotal
6. Perineal

The operation to correct the hypospadias should be performed after 2 years of age. If the penis is exceedingly small, then the operation is delayed another 6 months.

91. First-Stage Hypospadias Repair

91-1. In a midscrotal type of hypospadias *the line of incision is circular (dotted line).*

91-2. Several stay sutures are placed through the glans penis. A silk stay suture may be preferred. *The fibrous tissue comprising the chordee is excised.* Note the lateral boundaries of chordee. The proximal border is the urethral stoma.

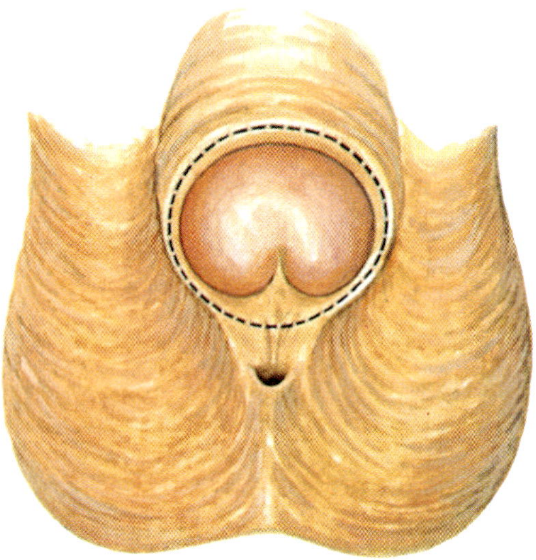

91-1

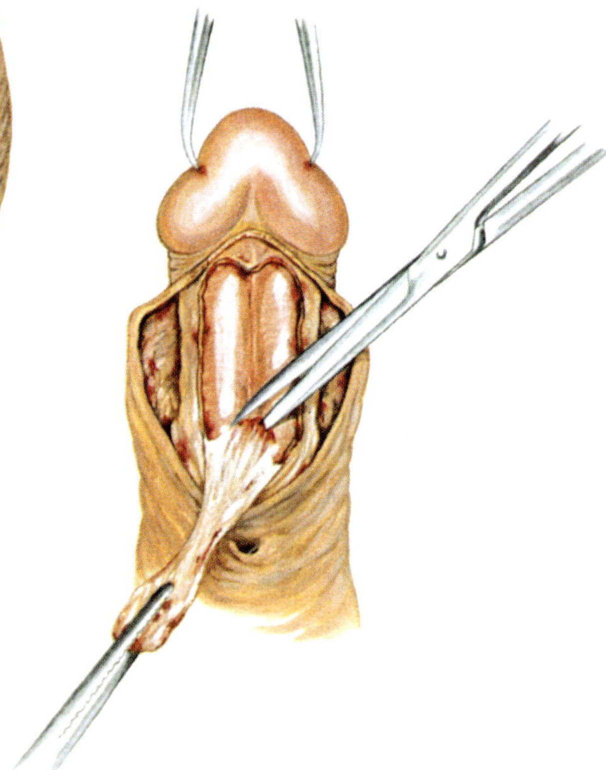

91-2

91-3. The chordee has been removed to the urethral opening. *The skin flap and hood are elevated with skin hooks.* A window made in the dorsal skin will slip over the glans penis.

91-4. The dorsal hood with the window has been slipped over the glans penis. *Allis clamps provide orientation.* The new skin margin and the skin edge around the corona are reapproximated with 4–0 chromic catgut. The rectangular flap of skin will be used to create a distal urethra.

91-5. *The new tube of distal urethra is fashioned* and the glans penis is also tunneled to allow placement of the distal tubular urethral flap at the tip.

91-6. *A stent* (10 Fr silicone or rubber tube) *is left in place.* The new floor of the ventral penis is formed by suturing the edges. A scrotal catheter is inserted into the bladder and left indwelling for 5 to 6 days.

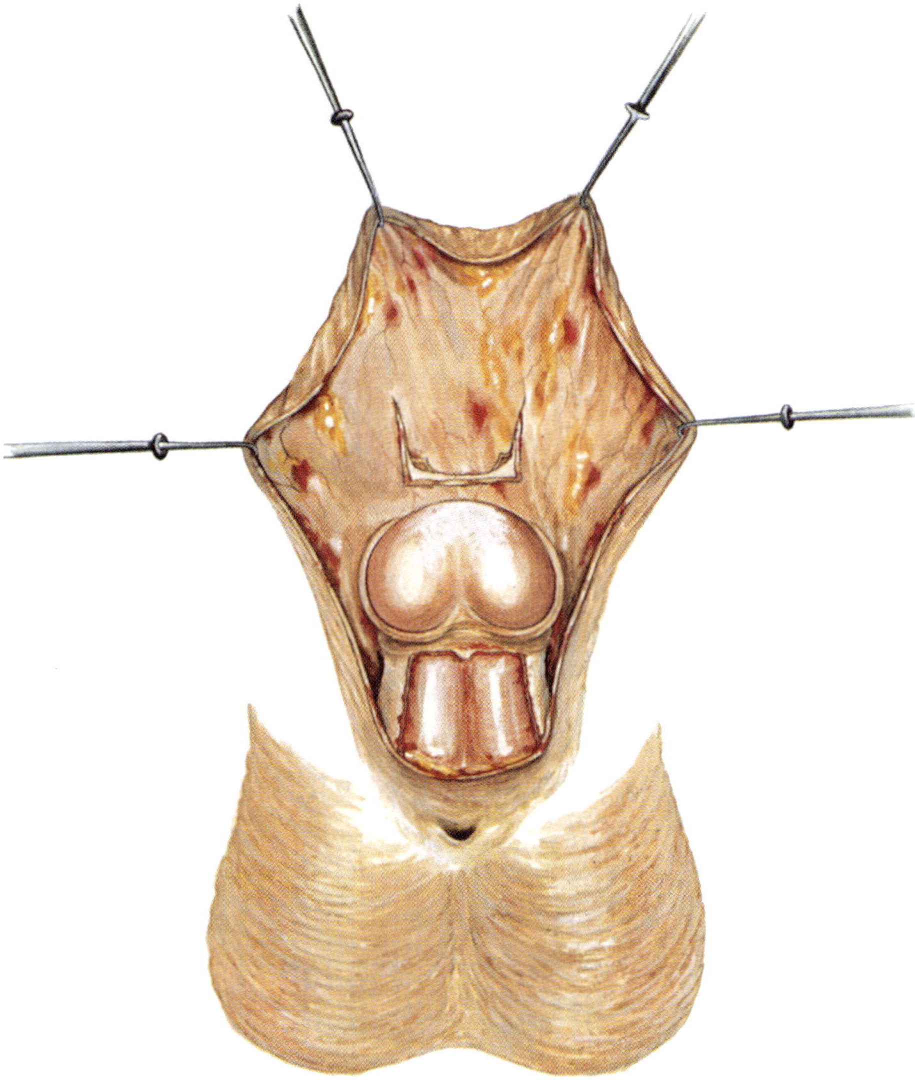

91-3

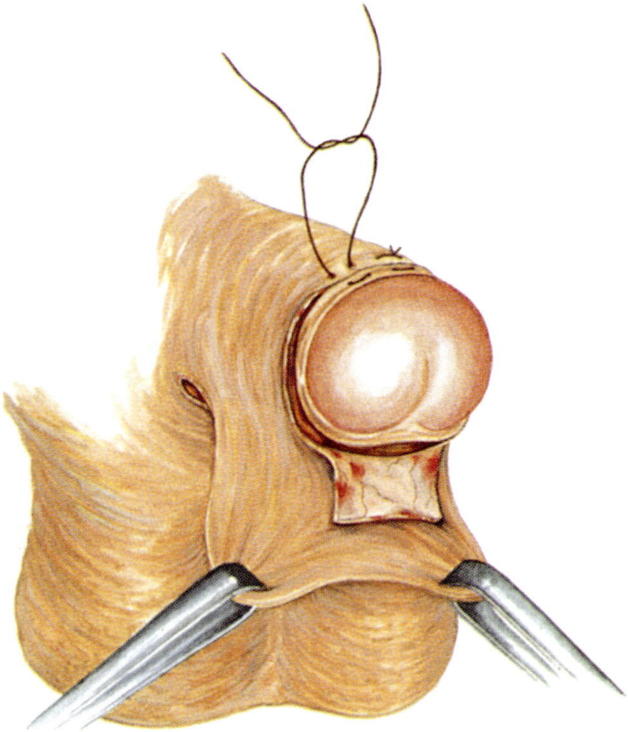

91-4

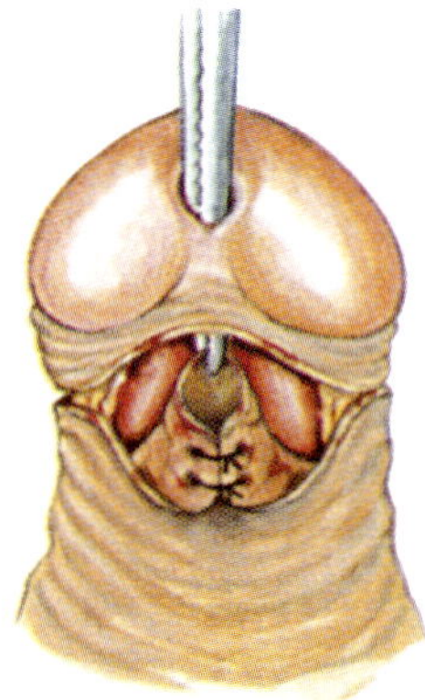

91-5

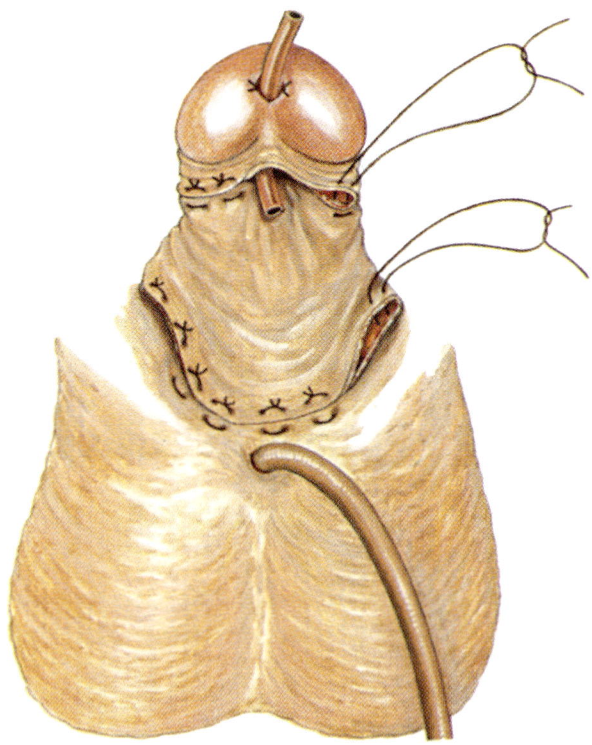

91-6

92. Second-Stage Hypospadias Repair (Abundant Skin Available)

An interval of at least 4 months is allowed before a second-stage hypospadias repair is undertaken.

92-1. Adequate penile skin is available. *The skin to be used in fashioning a new urethral tube is incised.* A stay suture through the glans penis is helpful in the operation. Note the horizontal extension of the skin incision at the corona.

92-2. *A urethral catheter serves as a stent* (8 Fr in a child). The inner tubular skin flap is reapproximated around the stent. A running inverting suture is used to place skin edge in apposition on the interior (3–0 chromic catgut).

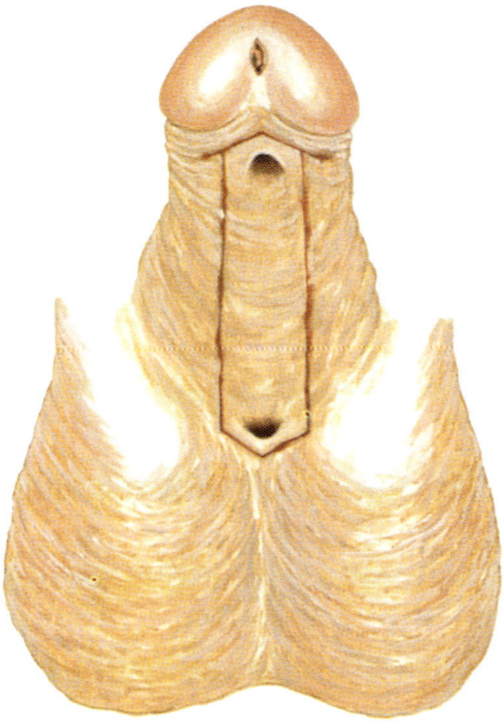

92-1

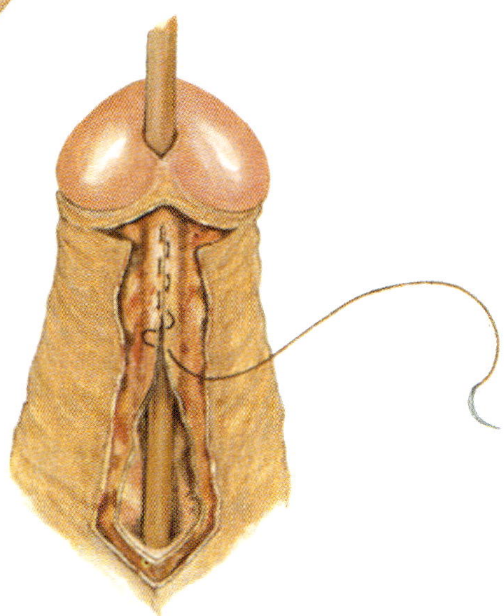

92-2

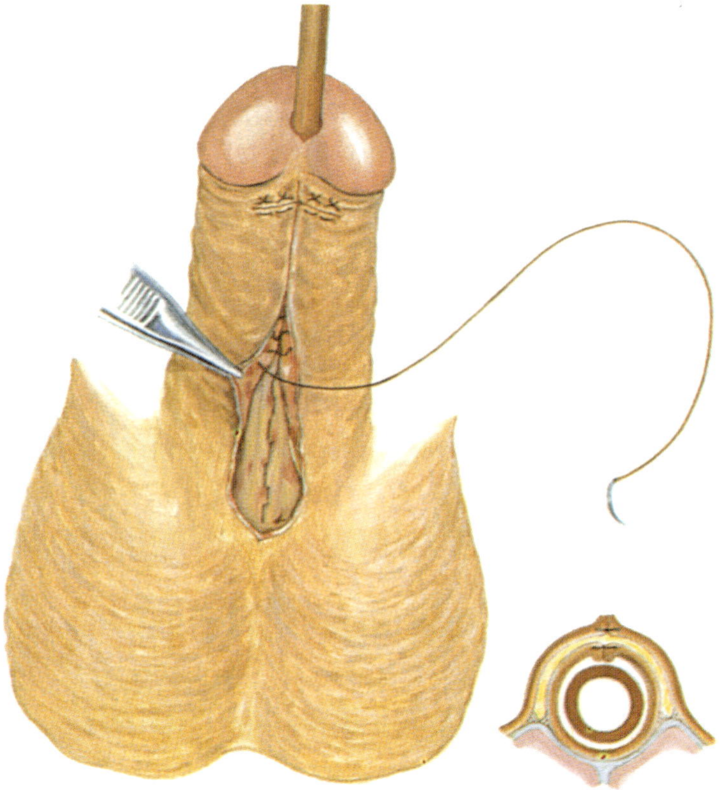

92-3

92-3. The second layer of skin closure is accomplished with a running subcuticular suture (3–0 chromic catgut). The transverse distal penile skin closure has been made to relieve the urethra of undue tension. The cross-sectional insert reveals the double-layer closure. The catheter within the urethra is shown in dark brown (*see insert*). An indwelling catheter (10 or 12 Fr) is left in the bladder for at least 7 days.

93. Second-Stage Hypospadias Repair (Marginal Skin Available, D. Browne Technique)

A perineal urethrostomy or suprapubic cystostomy is completed prior to the repair (14 Fr catheter).

93-1. *The skin is incised for tubulization.* A one-layer closure is effected by using a single-layer closure (3–0 chromic catgut).

93-2. The stent is helpful in bringing together both skin edges. *The subcuticular closure is started at the glans.*

93-3. To complete the second-stage hypospadias repair, *the final remaining suture proximally is brought through the skin and tied.* The stent is removed. *A cross section shows the paucity of skin and the single-layer closure around the catheter (see insert).*

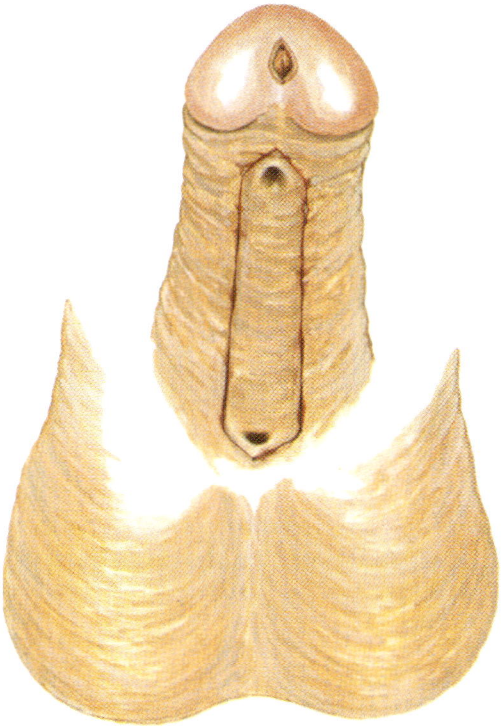

93-1

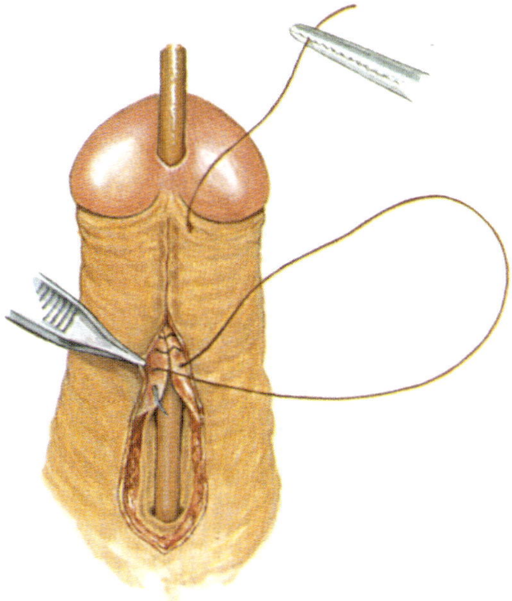

93-2

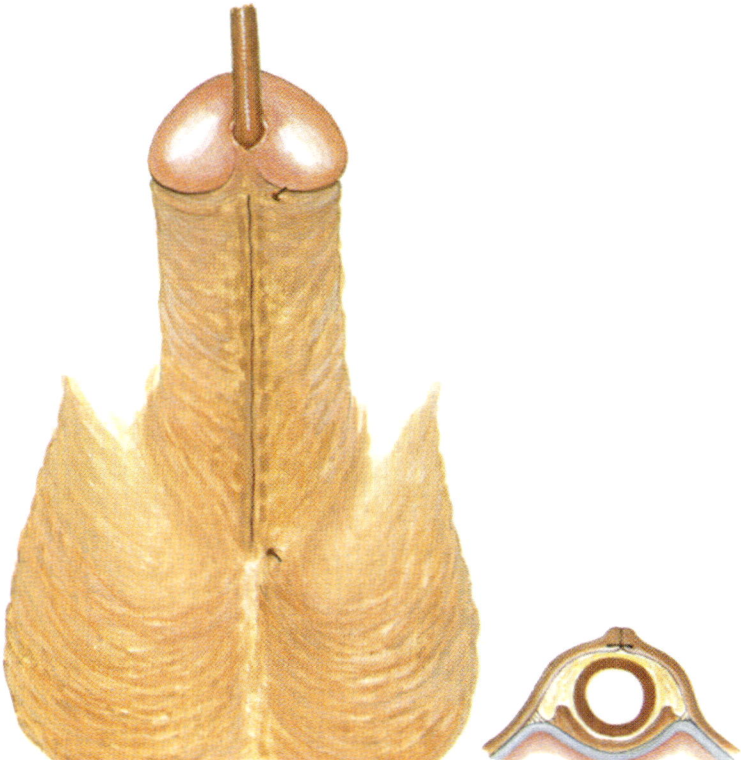

93-3

94. One-Stage Repair of Hypospadias

The Devine-Horton modification of the Mustarde operation is used for a distal penile location of the urethra.

94-1. *A stay suture is placed through the glans penis and a tourniquet is around the base of the penis.* A small needle (24 gauge) is inserted into the right cavernous body and saline is injected to produce an erection. The extent of chordee formation can be appreciated after this maneuver. The dotted lines form the boundaries of several skin flaps. A circumferential incision is also made around the coronal skin margin.

94-2. The skin edges on the ventral surface of the penile shaft are raised and elevated with skin hooks. *The fibrotic tissue representing chordee is removed by sharp dissection down to the glistening fascial sheath.* The glans penis sits as a cap on the distal penile shaft.

94-3. *Three triangular flaps of glans penis and underlying tissue are created* by sharp dissection. (The flaps are held by skin hooks.) Care is necessary to keep the flaps thin and yet viable. Hemostasis must be meticulously controlled at all times. The lateral borders where chordee has been removed are visible.

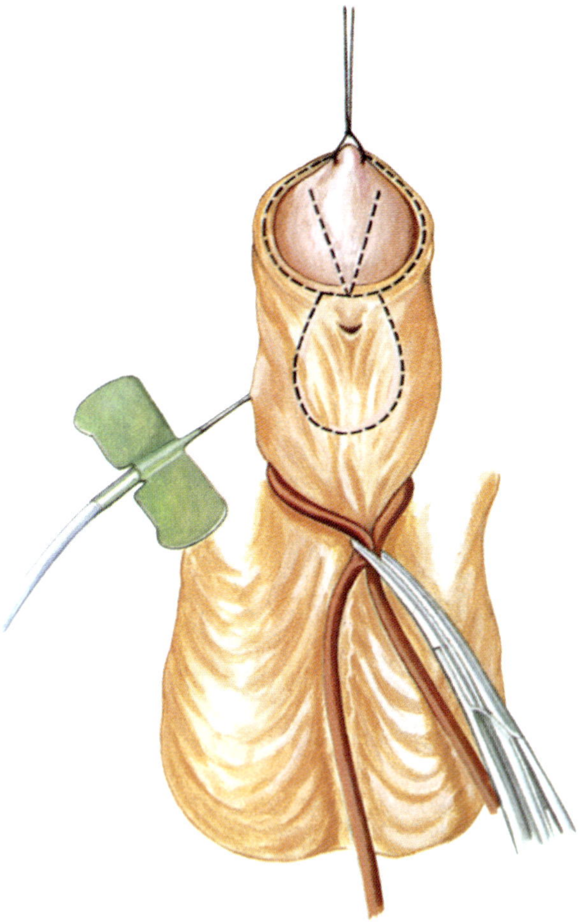

94-1

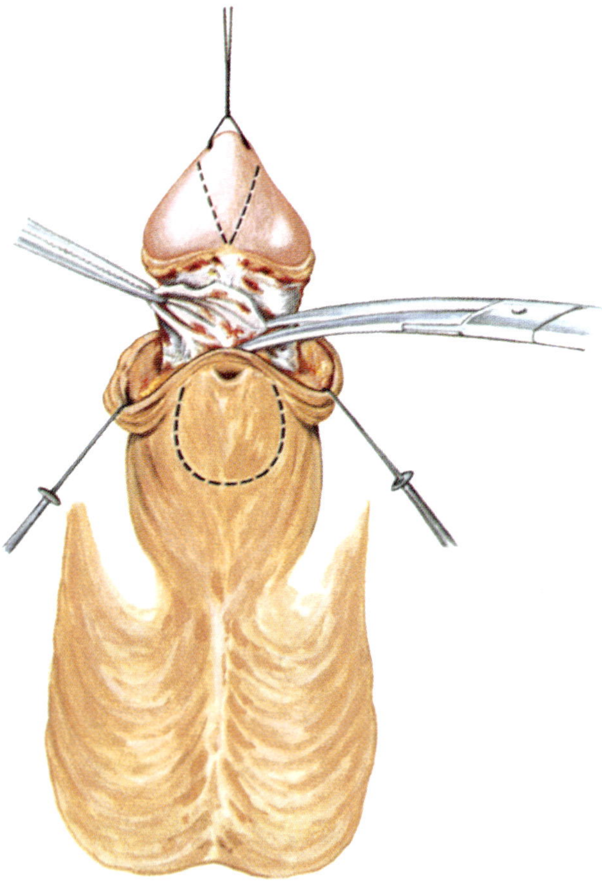

94-2

94-4. *A flap of skin attached to the urethral meatus is fashioned* by sharp dissection so that it may be flipped up. Care is necessary to avoid making "buttonholes" in the flap. A sound or stent can be inserted to check the urethral walls when necessary. Skin hooks aid in freeing this flap. The triangular flaps formed from the glans penis are also visible.

94-5. *The flap extending distally from the urethra is tubulized,* using 3–0 chromic catgut, starting proximally and extending within 1 cm from the end. The middle triangular flap is then tucked proximally and sewn to the remaining centimeter of tubular flap to ease the tension and widen the stoma.

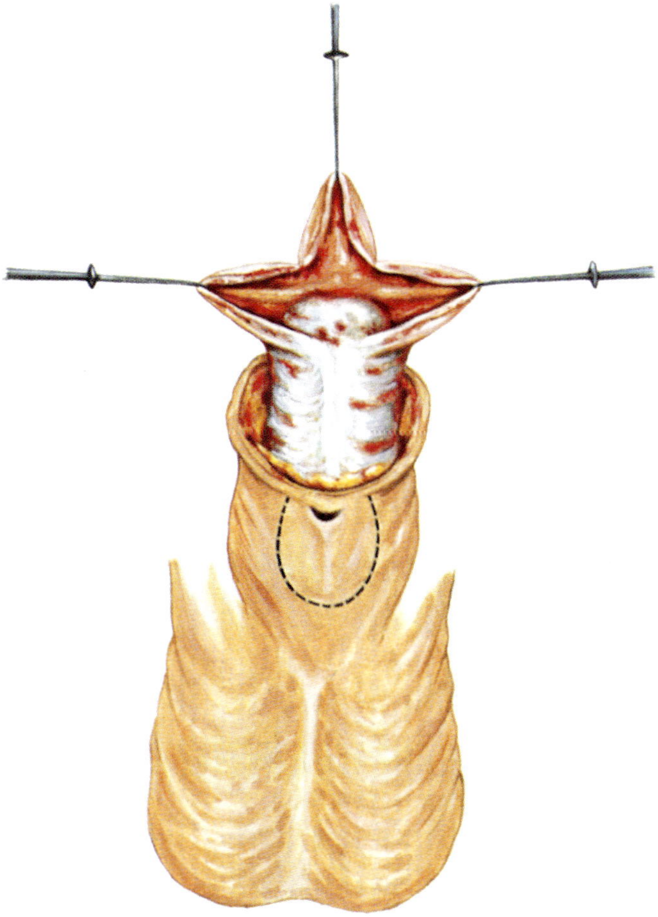

94-3

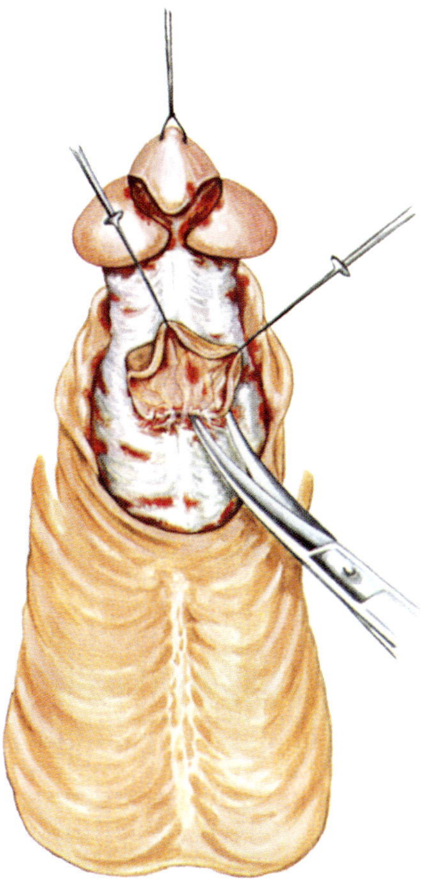

94-4

94-6. *The remaining two triangular flaps are secured around an indwelling straight Robinson catheter* (10 Fr) and sutured to the adjacent margins. The dorsal penile skin is then incised longitudinally for about 4–6 cm and each skin edge is brought laterally to the ventral aspect of the penile shaft. Hemostasis must be judiciously maintained at all times.

94-7. *The skin on the shaft of the penis is closed.* The coronal skin edge attached to glans penis is reapproximated to the skin flaps with 3–0 chromic catgut, and the stay suture in the glans penis is used to secure the straight Robinson catheter. The catheter is left in place for 5 days. A special slightly compressive dressing surrounded by elastic bandage (Elastoplast) is created around the penile shaft, pointing vertically from the horizontal suprapubic skin margin. This helps control some of the ooze.

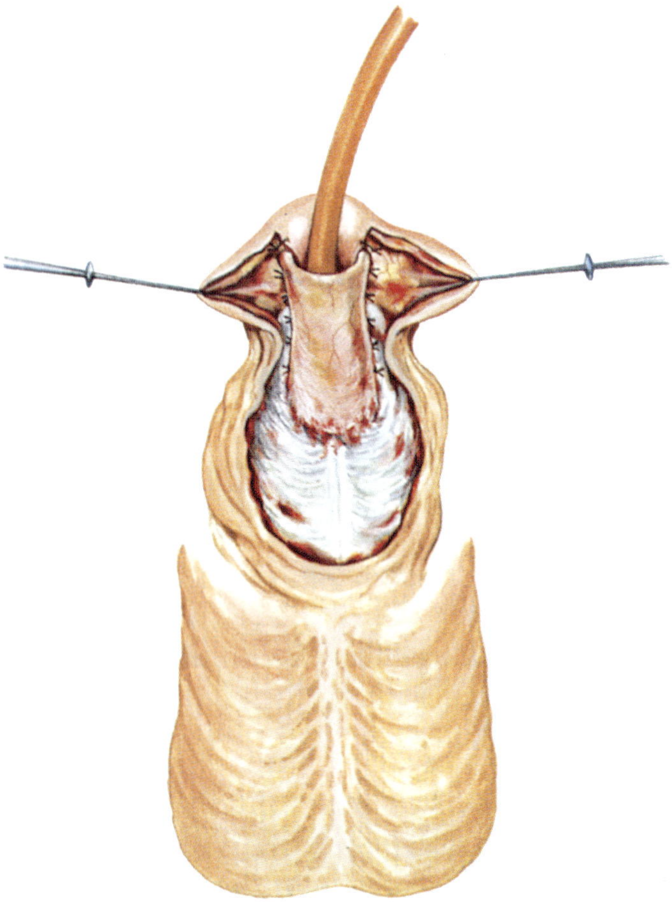

94-5

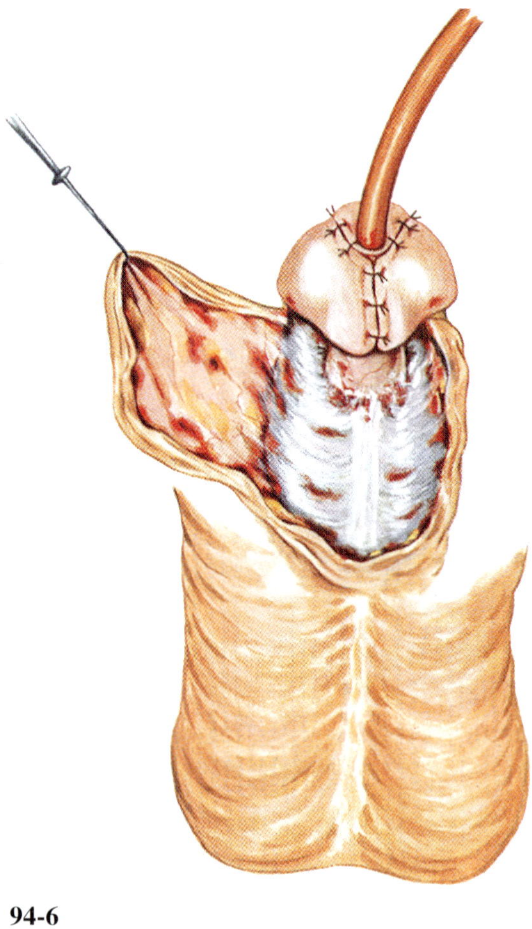

94-6

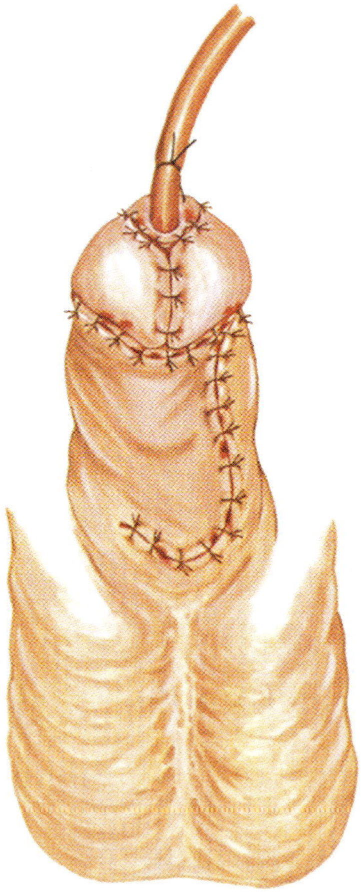

94-7

95. One-Stage Repair of Perineal Hypospadias

In this technique a full-thickness tubular graft is formed from preputial skin to bridge the gap. A suprapubic cystostomy tube is inserted at the outset to divert urine away from the area of reconstruction.

95-1. *The lines of incision into skin edges.* Although not shown, we place a silk suture through the glans penis to aid in the orientation.

95-2. The oval skin flap around the proximal urethra is seen. The skin margins are separated and skin hooks are placed at the distal corners. *The preputial skin, which has been measured around a 12–16 Fr catheter* (depending on age of the patient), *is incised transversely.* Note that the fibrous tissue representing chordee has been excised from a wide rectangular area. Hemostasis has also been meticulously controlled. *The preputial skin is fashioned into a tube around the appropriate catheter, with the raw surface on the outside (see insert).*

95-3. *The proximal flap is formed into a tube by suturing the edges* (3–0 chromic catgut). The triangular flaps in the glans penis have been fashioned. Skin hooks assist in the dissection.

95-4. *The tubular skin graft is fitted into place and shortened if necessary.* The proximal anastomosis of tubular graft to urethra is made on a bias to widen the anastomotic site. The triangular flap of glans penis is placed proximally into part of the distal tubular graft, again to widen this distal anastomotic margin.

95-5. *The remaining triangular flaps of glans penis are brought around the stent and secured by sutures* (3–0 chromic catgut). The skin edges are reapproximated. The stent is removed after the compression dressing covered by elastic bandage has been secured around the penile shaft.

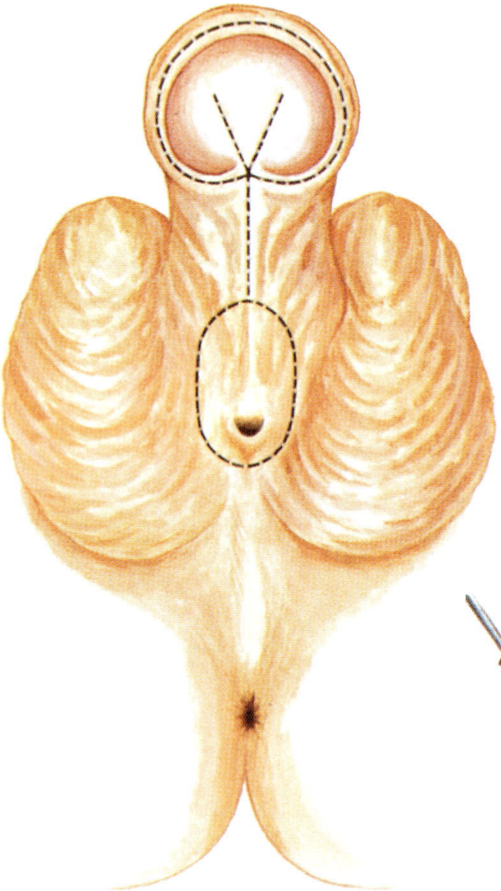

95-1

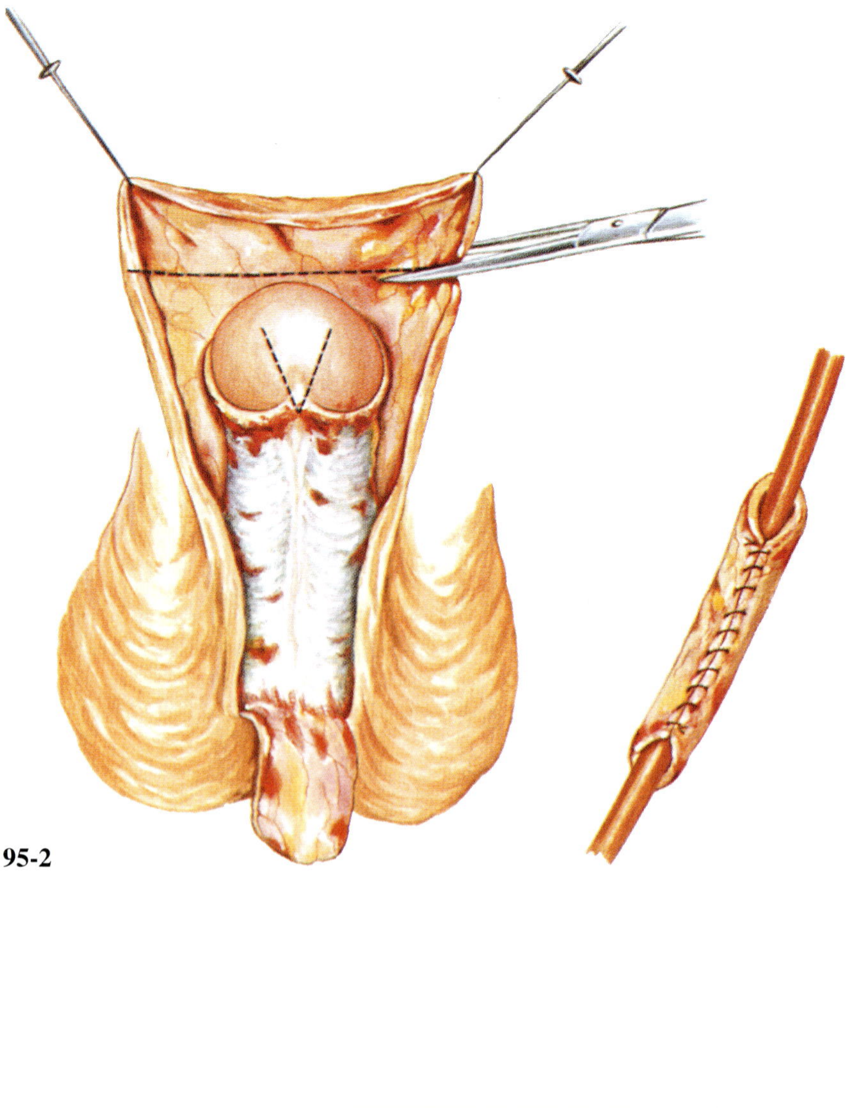

95-2

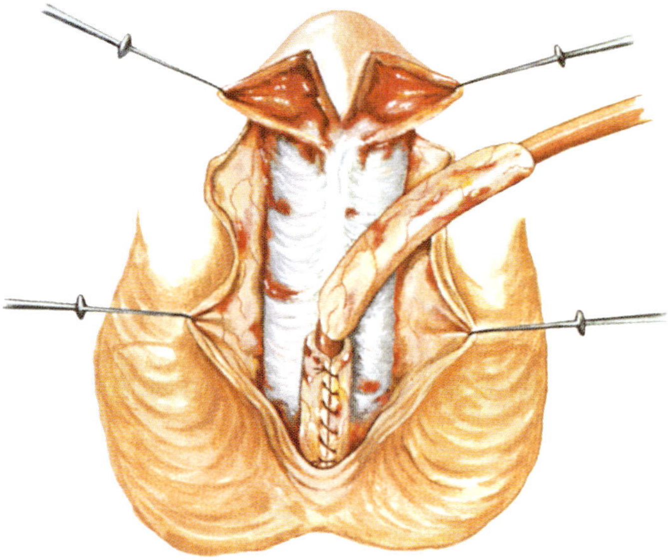

95-3

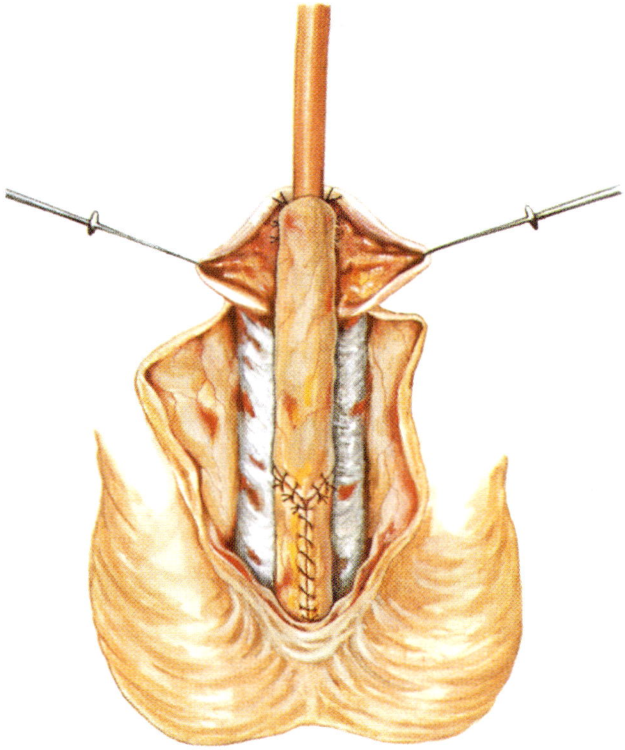

95-4

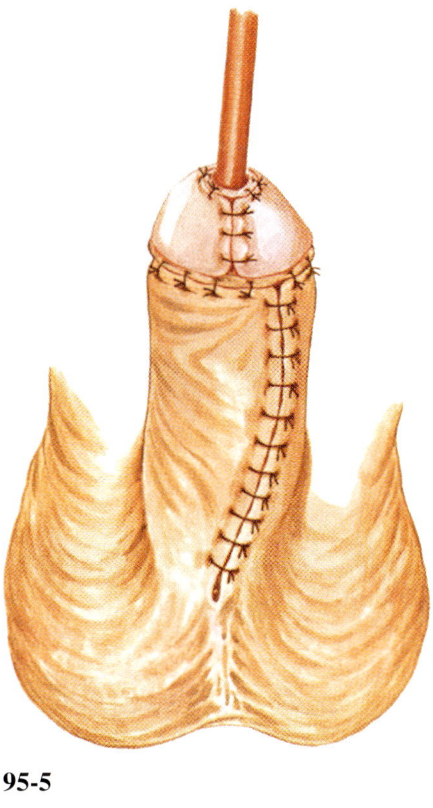

95-5

Surgical Procedures of the Female Urethra

96. Surgical Treatment of Urethral Disease in the Female

The patient is placed in a lithotomy position. Light anesthesia or local anesthesia is employed.

96-1. A urethral caruncle extrudes from and involves the distal urethra. *A urethral catheter (18 Fr Foley) is inserted* and the bag is inflated. A guillotine tie is placed proximal to the lesion, around the normal urethra. The lesion is grasped with forceps and the ligature (2–0 silk) is tightened.

96-2. *Removal of the catheter 2 days later* will usually include the urethral lesion.

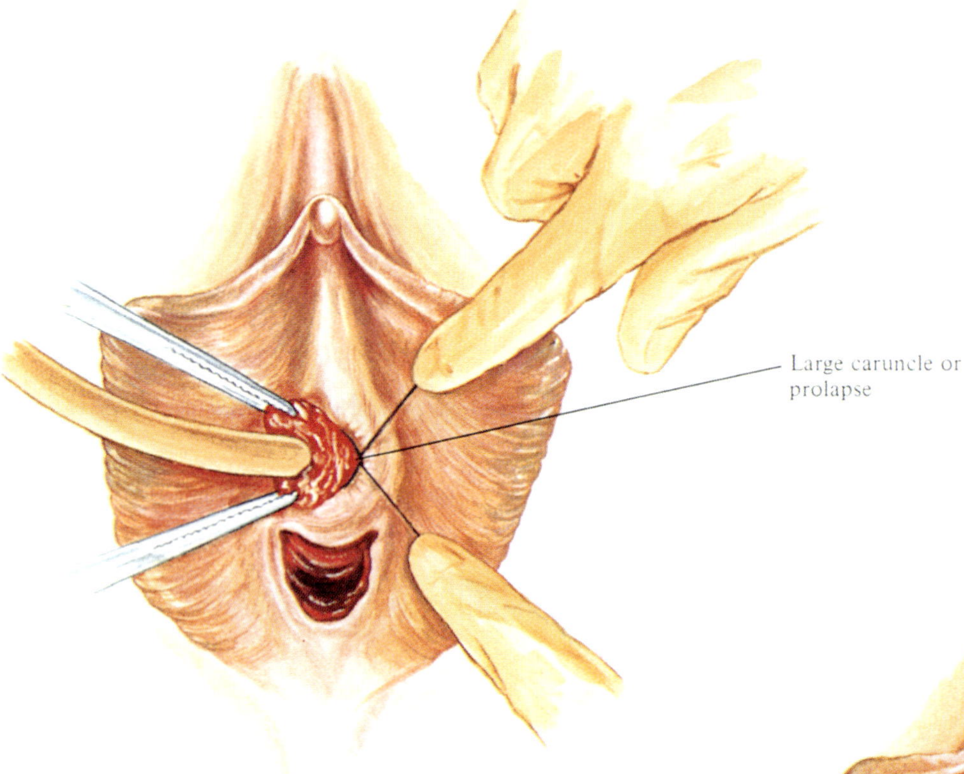

96-1

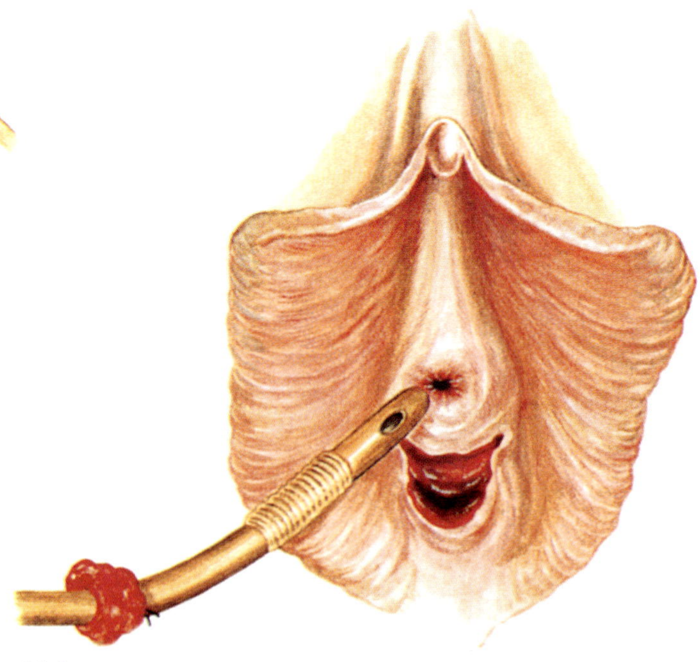

96-2

97. Removal of Distal or Midurethral Lesions

A urethral diverticulum can be diagnosed at the time of pelvic examination. Careful elevation of the roof of the vagina overlying the urethra, moving from a proximal to a distal direction, may produce a slight gush of purulent fluid. Fullness may also be palpated at times, but this is more difficult to corroborate. A urethrogram with a double balloon attachment can also assist in the diagnosis.

97-1. *The labial and vaginal edges are secured in each quadrant. The incision (dotted line) creates an anterior vaginal flap.* A weighted vaginal speculum is inserted to increase exposure.

97-2. *The lesion is removed* in this instance by means of a cutting current on a probe.

97-3. *Reapproximation of the urethra and anterior vaginal wall* is completed in separate distinct layers; 3–0 chromic catgut is used. An indwelling catheter may be left for 4–6 days.

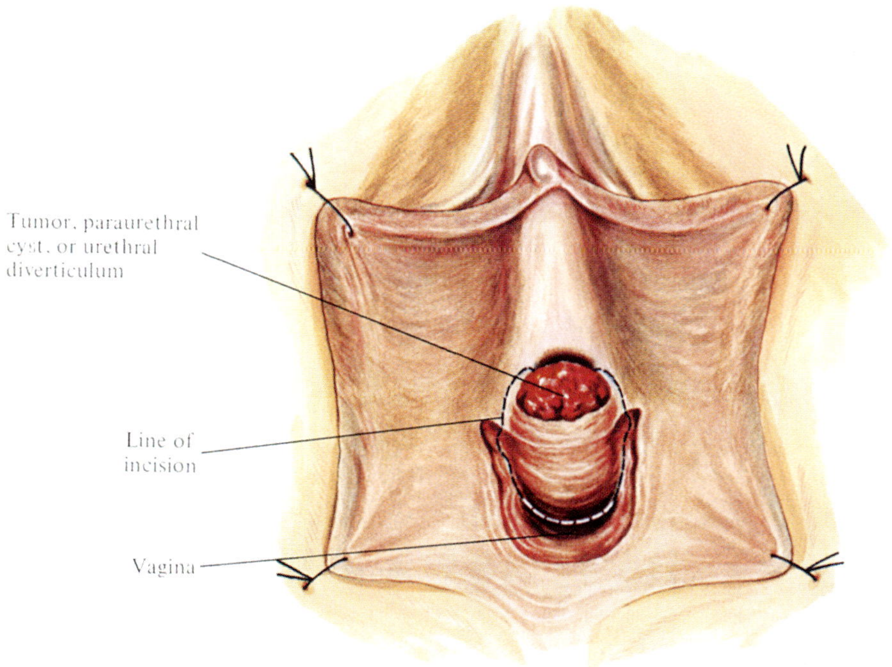

97-1

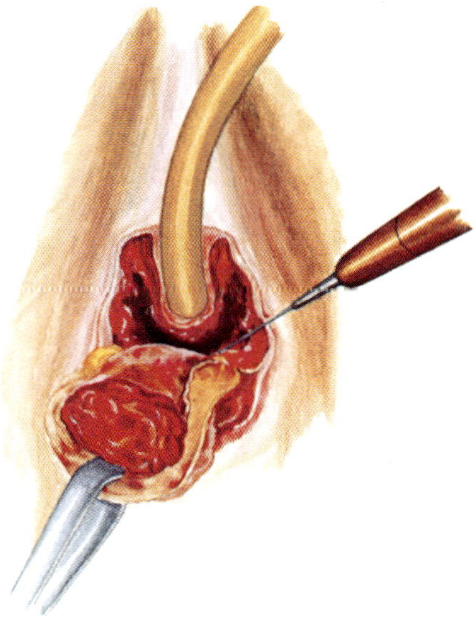

97-2

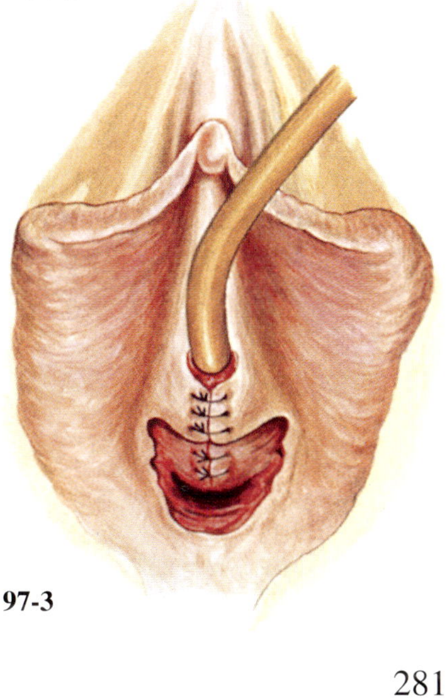

97-3

Suggested Readings

Browne D. An operation for hypospadias. Proc Roy Soc Med 42:466, 1949.

Devine CJ Jr, Horton CE. A one stage hypospadias repair. J Urol 85:166, 1961.

Gil-Vernet JM. Un traitement des stenoses traumatiques et inflammatoires de l'uretére postérieur. Nouvelle méthode d'urétroplastie. J Urol Nephrol 72:97, 1966.

Leadbetter GW Jr. A simplified urethroplasty for strictures of the bulbous urethra. J Urol 83:54, 1960.

Pierce JM Jr. Urethroplasty for anterior urethral stricture. J Urol 109:422, 1973.

Turner-Warwick R. The repair of urethral strictures in the region of the membranous urethra. J Urol 100:303, 1968.

The Penis

7

Surgical Anatomy

STRUCTURE

The penis is a pendulous, erectile organ with a posterior fixed base or root and is supported by the suspensory ligament, an extension of the linea alba. The main erectile body of the penis is composed of three cylinder-like masses of cavernous tissue—the left and right cavernous bodies and the spongy body of the urethra (Fig. 1).

The cavernous bodies originate at the midportion of the ischiopubic rami and firmly attach to the periosteum of the descending pubic rami and the inferior surface of the urogenital diaphragm. The bodies are united, side by side, in the body of the penis and have blunt ends at the base of the glans penis. At its root they are separated by the penile crura (Fig. 2). The perineal portion of the cavernous bodies is covered by ischiocavernous muscle and the bulb of the urethra is covered by bulbocavernous muscle (Fig. 3).

The spongy body is slender and erectile and lies along the ventral groove of the paired cavernous bodies. Posteriorly, at the root, the spongy body expands to form the bulbous urethra, which is invested by bulbocavernous muscle. Anteriorly, at the end of the penis, the spongy body enlarges to form the glans penis and covers the ends of the cavernous bodies.

The spongy body serves as an envelope around the urethra from the urogenital diaphragm to the external urethral meatus, which opens at the glans. The glans penis is coated by a semimucous membrane rich in sebaceous glands and terminal nerve fibers.

Each erectile body is surrounded by a dense elastic connective tissue sheath called the tunica albuginea (white integument); trabeculas of this sheath surround the vascular spaces of the spongy structure.

All the penile bodies are invested together by a thin layer of Buck's fascia, which encases them from the base of the glans to the root of the penis. It fuses the suspensory ligament and inferior surface of the urogenital diaphragm. Colles's fascia invests the penis between the skin and Buck's fascia and is continuous with the same layer of fascia over the perineum (Figs. 3 and 4).

The skin of the penis is thin and loosely attached to the underlying structures and is devoid of adipose tissue and hair except at its base. It is continued forward as the prepuce (foreskin), which forms a cuff covering the glans. The internal surface of the pre-

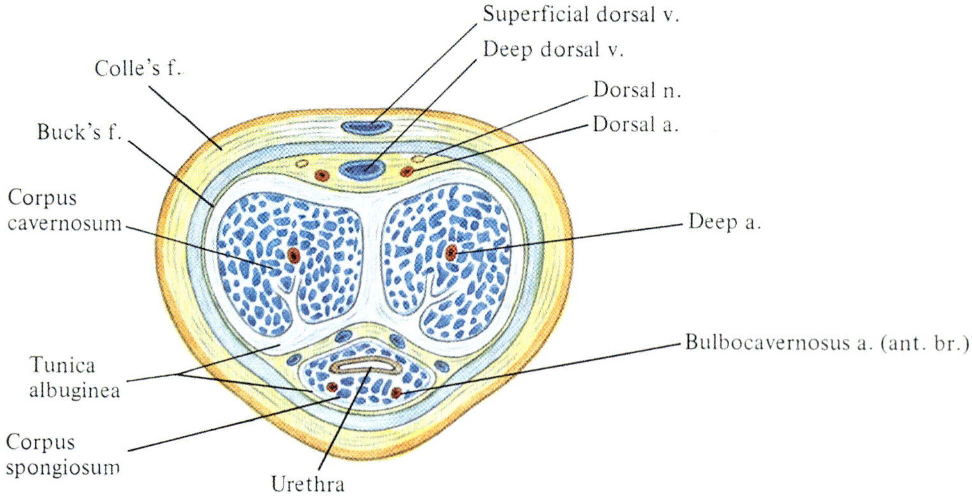

FIG. 1.
Cross section of penis.

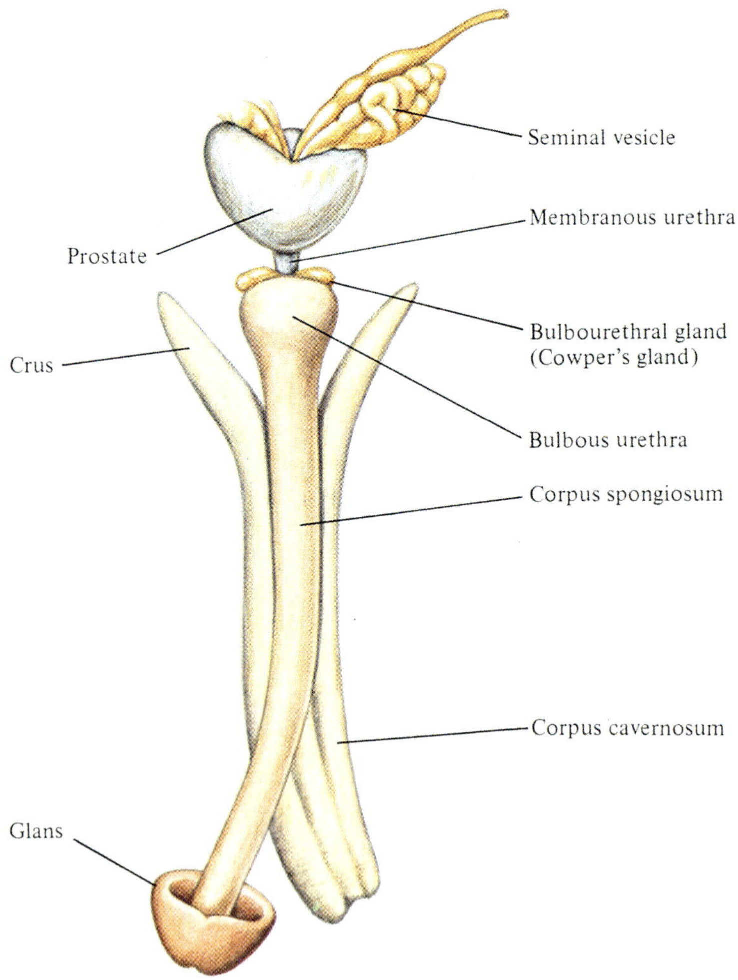

FIG. 2.
Erectile bodies of penis.

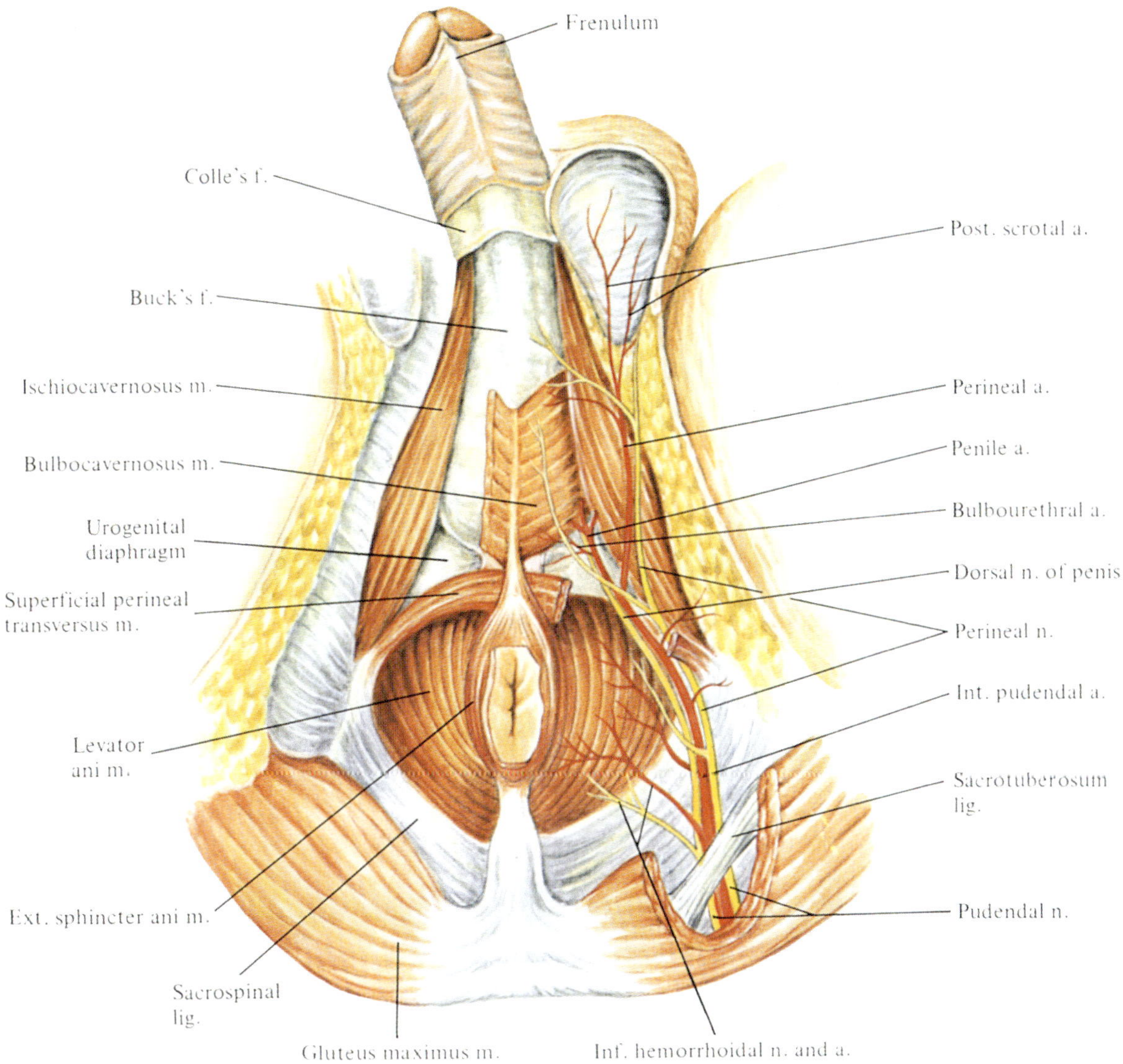

FIG. 3.
Superficial structures of male perineum.

puce is a semimucous membrane similar to that covering the glans and contains sebaceous glands which secrete smegma. On the ventral aspect of the glans, the frenulum, a well-defined median fold of skin, is attached from the lower angle of the urethral meatus to the prepuce. The frenulum contains a small artery, which may bleed profusely if transected during circumcision.

VASCULAR SUPPLY

The arterial supply of the penis is derived from the internal pudendal artery. This artery divides into three paired branches at the base of the urogenital triangle: the dorsal, cavernous (deep), and bulbourethral arteries. The dorsal arteries of the penis course along the dorsal surface of the penile bodies between Buck's fascia and the tunica albuginea, one on each side of the deep dorsal vein. The dorsal nerve lies lateral to the artery. These arteries supply the body of the penis and terminate in the glans. The cavernous arteries

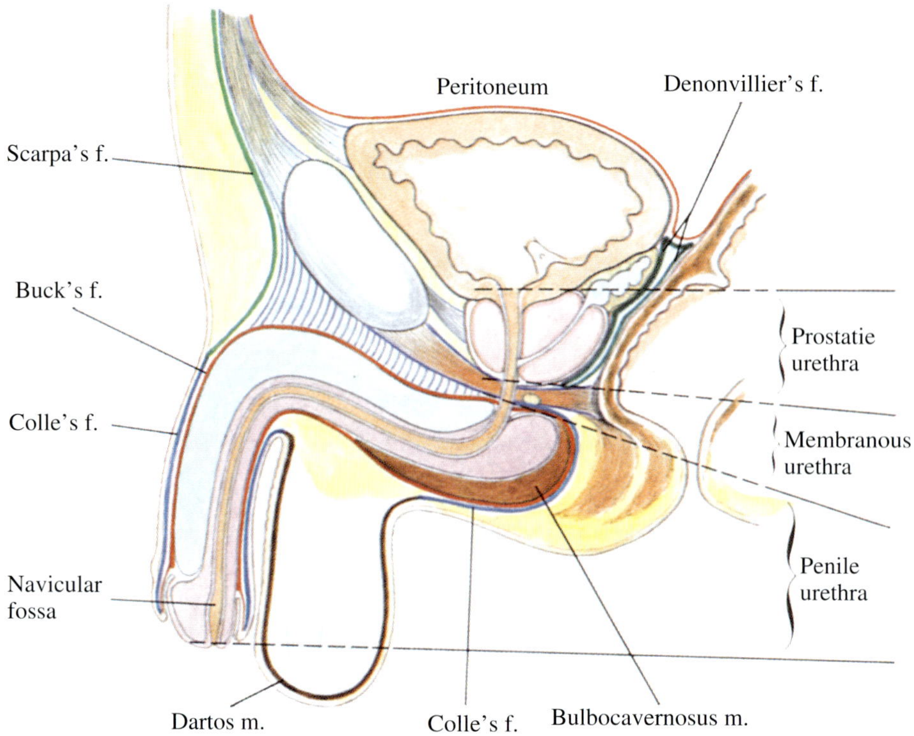

FIG. 4.
Fascial coverings of male genital system and urethra, midsagittal section.

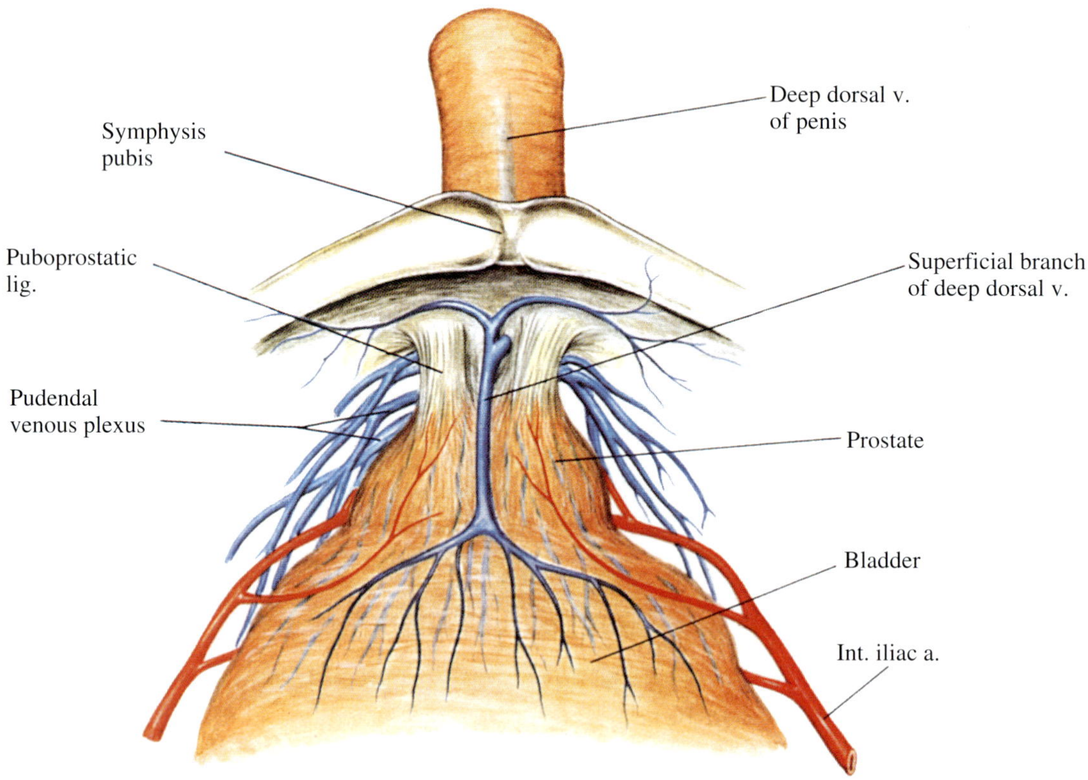

FIG. 5.
Venous supply to prostate.

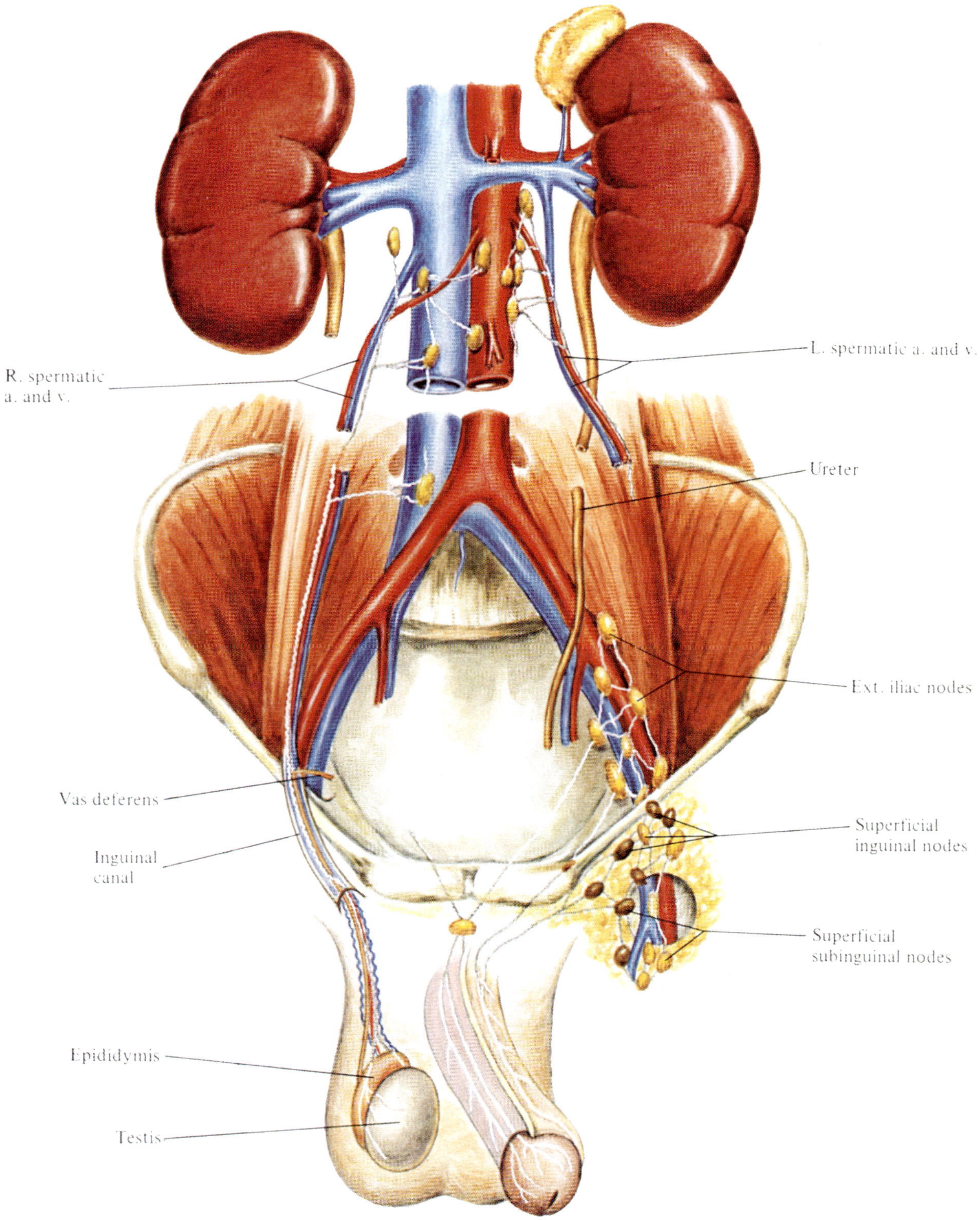

FIG. 6.
Lymphatic drainage of penis and testis.

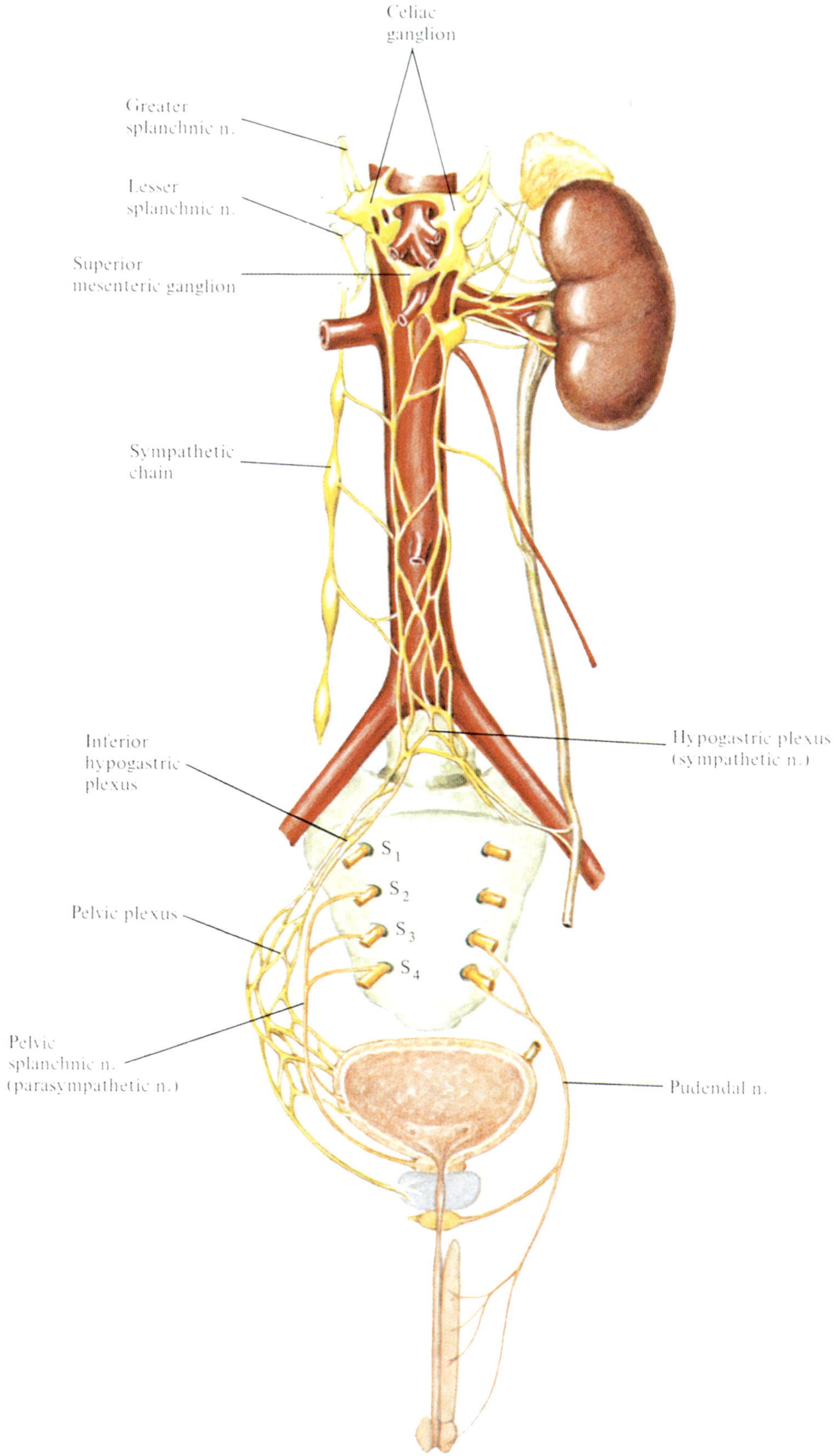

FIG. 7.
Autonomic and somatic nerve supply to male urogenital system.

pierce the medial aspect of each crus, distribute branches, and run forward in each cavernous body.

The bulbourethral arteries course along the urethra to the glans and there anastomose with the terminal branches of the dorsal arteries.

The veins of the penis comprise a superficial and a deep group. The superficial veins drain the prepuce and skin of the penis, form a network in the subcutaneous tissue, and empty into the superficial dorsal vein. The latter vein is easily seen through the skin. It runs proximally and terminates by dividing into right and left branches, which drain into the external pudendal veins in the thigh.

The deep dorsal vein begins at the base of the glans, courses proximally in the median line between Buck's fascia and the tunica albuginea, and drains the glans and all cavernous bodies. It terminates by joining the venous plexus around the prostate (Fig. 5).

The lymphatics of the penis are divided into two main groups—superficial and deep. The superficial lymphatics from the skin of the penis join to larger lymphatic trunks that follow the dorsal vein of the penis and drain mainly into the external iliac nodes.

The deep lymphatics from the glans and the penile body drain into the deep inguinal nodes, medial femoral nodes (including the sentinel node), and also external iliac nodes.

There are also anastomoses between the lymphatics of the bulbar and membranous urethra that drain into the internal iliac nodes via the trunks accompanying the internal pudendal vessels.

Lymphatic drainage of the penis is of great importance in the management of a penile malignancy (Fig. 6).

NERVE SUPPLY

Sympathetic nerve fibers of the pelvic plexus are also distributed to the seminal vesicles, prostate, and urethra. The somatic innervation of the pudendal nerve distributes motor fibers to the external sphincter and perineal muscles and sensory fibers to the perineal tissues, urethra, and penis (Figs. 3 and 7).

Operative Techniques

98. Circumcision

In the adult male, this procedure can be performed under local anesthesia or it may also be performed under general anesthesia as part of a short-term admission.

98-1. The patient's penis and scrotal area are cleansed. *The redundant prepuce is incised* over the corona in a circumferential fashion.

98-2. *A dorsal incision can now be made to the site of the coronal incision.*

98-3. *Redundant foreskin is excised on the ventral aspect.* Care is taken to preserve some of the frenulum to allow a better cosmetic result.

98-4. Careful hemostasis must be maintained. We like the disposable, battery-operated coagulation device, which can be held in the hand and is widely available. *The skin edges are reapproximated with interrupted 3–0 chromic catgut sutures.*

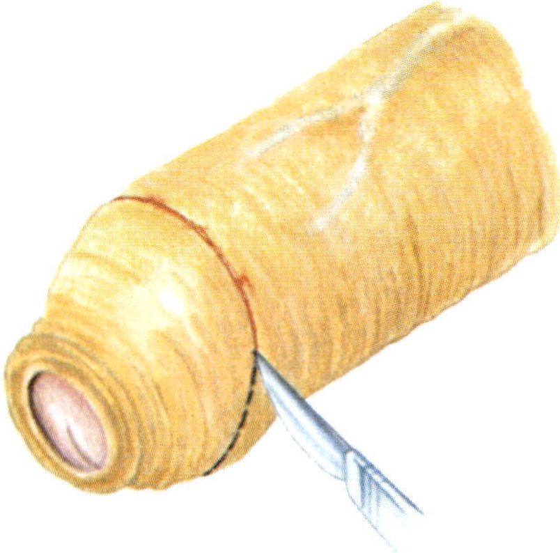

98-1

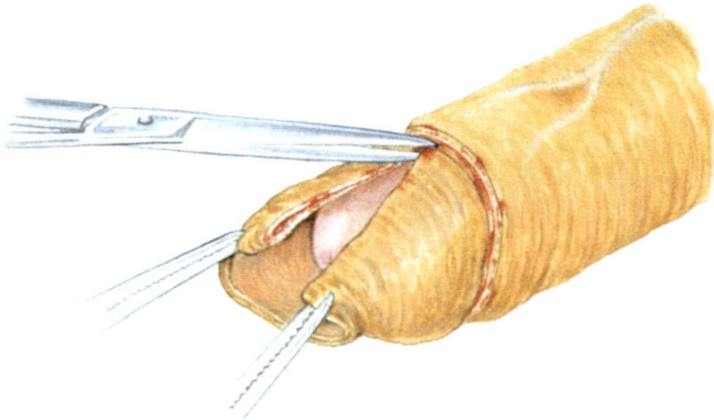

98-2

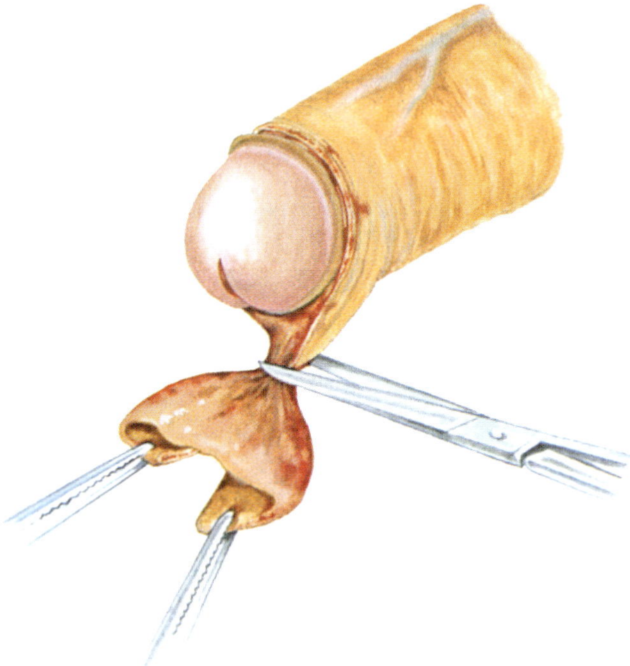

98-3

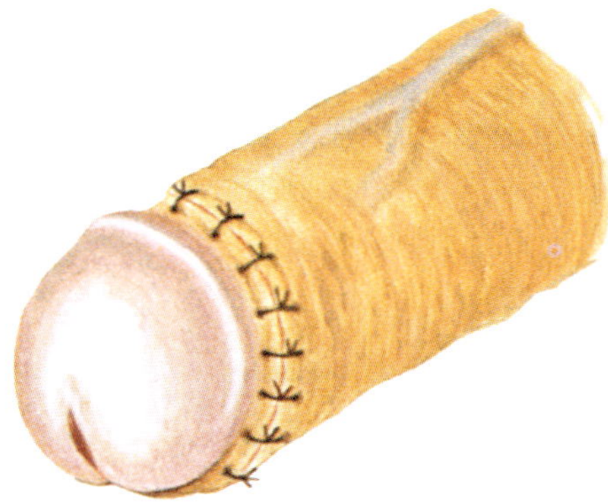

98-4

99. Circumcision in Infancy

Infant circumcision may be carried out within a day or two after birth if cultural custom so requires. The Yellen clamp helps to accomplish the procedure with ease and rapidity.

99-1. *A dorsal slit is made to the border just distal to the coronal margin.* Retracting the prepuce on both sides by clamps is helpful.

99-2. The bell-shaped Yellen clamp comes in several sizes. *The proper-sized hollow Yellen clamp is placed over the glans penis.* Stay sutures assist in the procedure.

99-3. *The external attachment to the Yellen clamp is secured* with the hollow ringlike base placed over the lower margin of the bell-shaped internal attachment. *A circumferential incision is made.* We usually wait 10 minutes before releasing the clamp.

99-4. *Redundant prepuce is excised,* leaving an excellent sealed margin.

99-5. *The bell-shaped attachment is removed.* Hemostasis is not needed and no sutures are required.

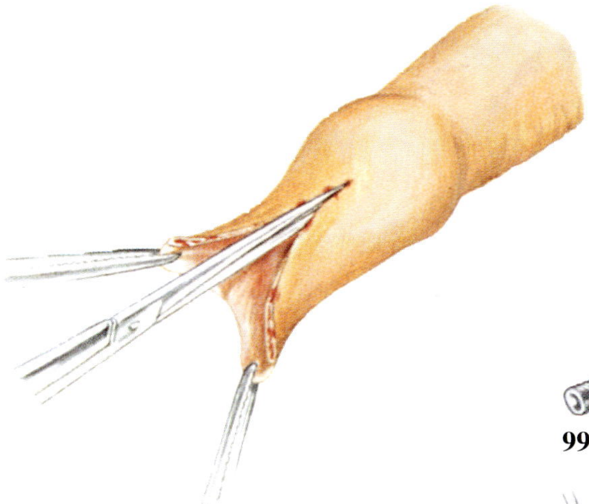

99-1

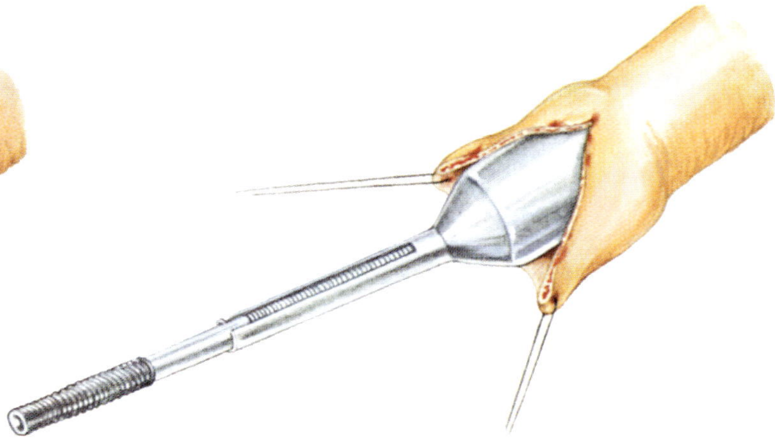

99-2

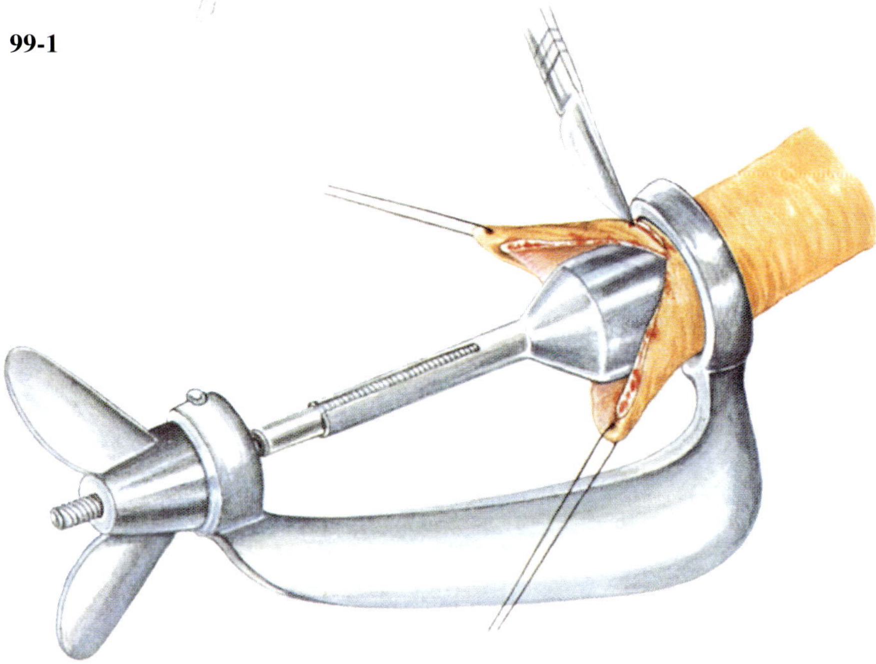

99-3

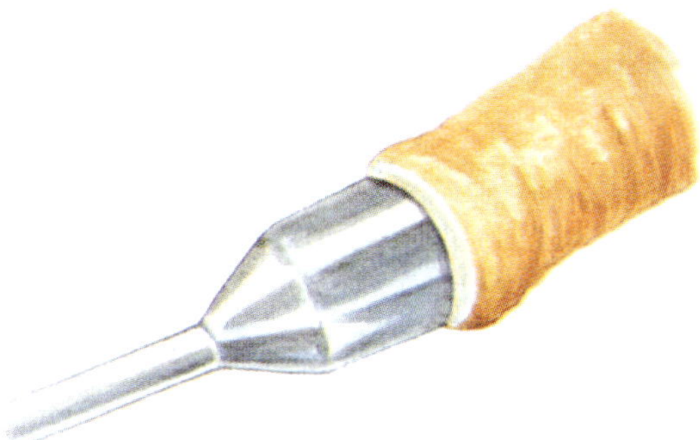

99-4

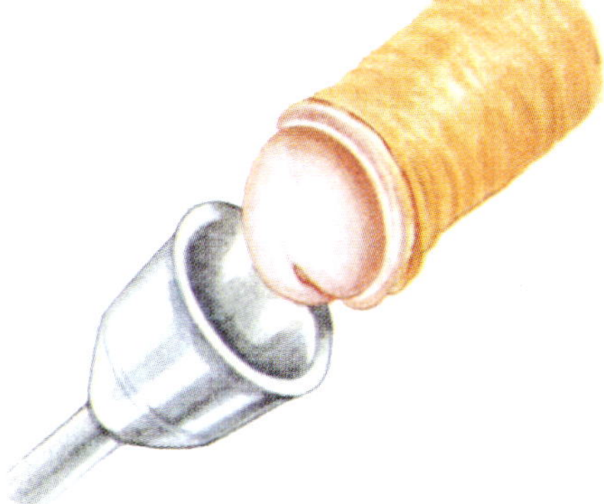

99-5

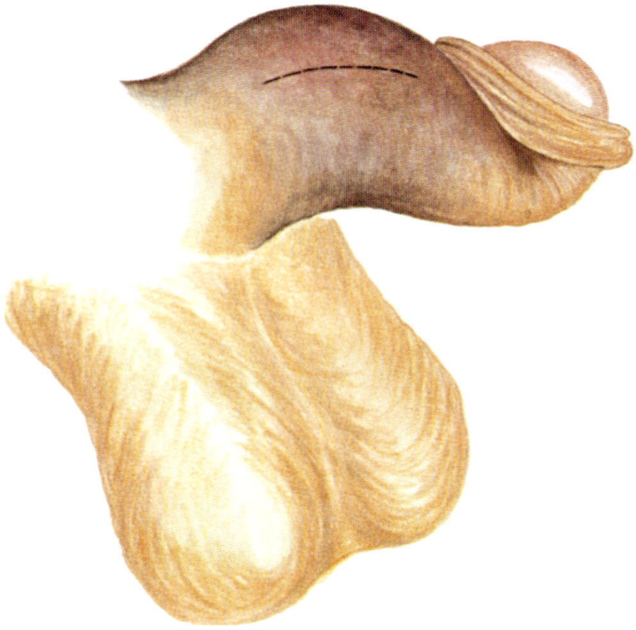

100-1

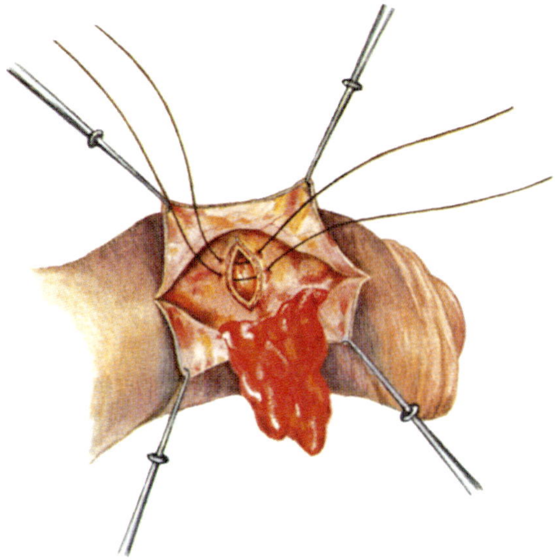

100-2

100. Trauma to the Penile Shaft

The penile shaft may be injured from an external source during erection. Koshiba treated 5 cases and collected 56 other cases in Japan. The injury occurred most often in the second decade and was noted following sexual intercourse or masturbation. The urethra was not injured. The patient usually complains of severe pain.

100-1. *A large hematoma forms at the ruptured area.* Forty-two of 56 cases underwent repair of the fascia and evacuation of the hematoma. Impotence was not a problem. Hemorrhage may be superficial beneath Colles' fascia but external to Buck's fascia. In the case illustrated, trauma has been severe and hemorrhage extends beneath Buck's fascia (see Fig. 1).

100-2. The skin and Colles' fascia are incised. Buck's fascia is opened transversely and *the hematoma is evacuated.* Hemorrhage is controlled. Chromic catgut sutures (3–0) are used to reapproximate the fascial edges. Skin hooks assist in exposure of the injured area.

101. Covering an Extensive Skin Defect on the Penile Shaft

This injury is seen frequently on the farm. The clothing covering penile skin may be entrapped in a conveyor type belt or wheel. Whenever possible, the denuded penis, and the testis when appropriate, should be covered with skin within 8 to 10 hours.

Split-thickness skin grafts are an acceptable method for covering the defect caused by avulsion of the penile skin. The injured area must be cleansed and débrided thoroughly. Dirt and hair are removed. Hematomas are incised and removed. We have found the inner thigh skin area to be a useful donor site (the skin graft is 0.02 inches thick).

An alternative can also be employed, as follows.

101-1. *The penile shaft is débrided* and hemostasis is achieved. The scrotal skin appears healthy. The incision (dotted line) will serve to create the new collar of tissue around the corona of the penis. The subcutaneous scrotal skin can be tunneled to allow the penis to be buried.

101-2. *The corona of the penis is approximated to scrotal skin,* and the defect in the anterior superior scrotal area is reapproximated. At least several months are allowed for healing to take place.

101-3. *The new scrotal skin to be used in covering the penile shaft is outlined.* Stay sutures can be placed at the inferior corners to improve the surgeon's orientation.

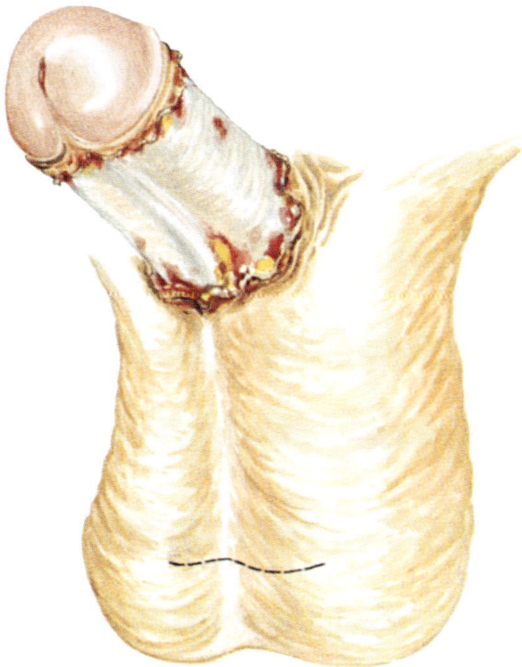

101-1

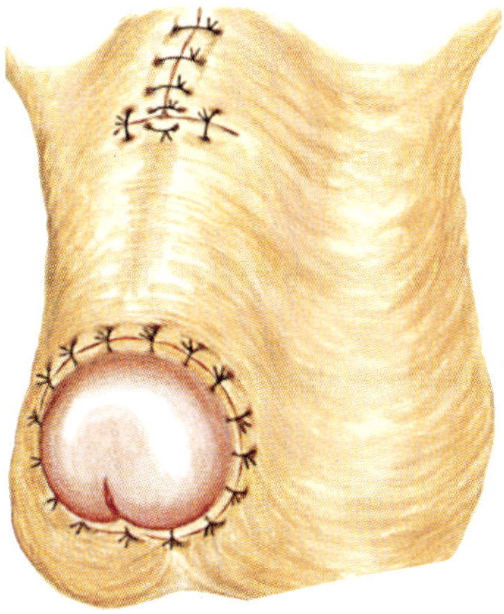

101-2

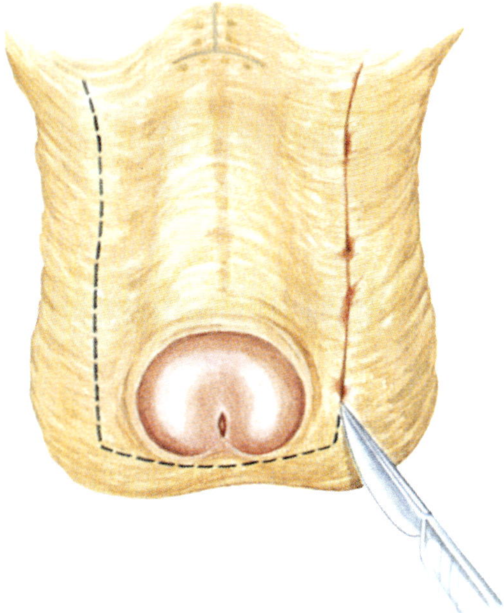

101-3

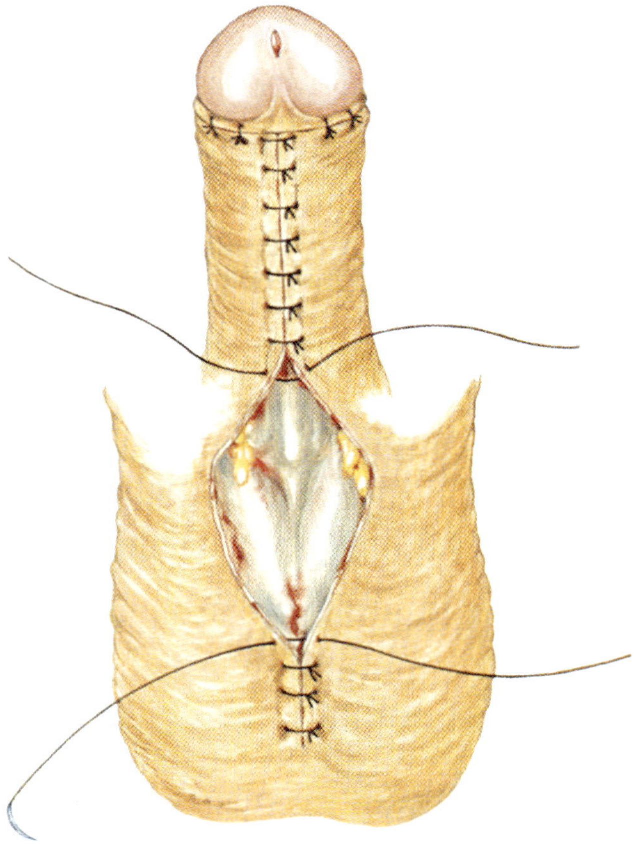

101-4

101-4. *The penis and attached scrotal skin are released.* The skin margins and the inferior scrotal skin are reapproximated. As an alternative, the scrotal skin margins at the penoscrotal junction can be closed transversely if that approach is deemed appropriate.

Correction of Priapism and Organic Impotency

Priapism is a condition characterized by abnormally prolonged and distressing erection of the penis. It is usually painful to have intercourse with priapism. The commonest cause in the black male is a sickle-cell disorder. Priapism rarely resolves spontaneously. Medical or surgical measures are needed to treat this condition.

Priapism is relatively infrequent. Those seeking more detail on the pathophysiology of this condition are referred to the studies by Farrer and Goodwin and by Winter.

102. Anastomosis of the Cavernous Body to the Spongy Body

102-1. A new, highly successful procedure consists of creating two oval windows—one in the cavernous body and a second lying in apposition, in the spongy body. *Both erectile bodies are prepared and dissected.* They are still covered by fascia.

102-2. *It is important that a running suture (3–0 chromic catgut) be placed between the fascia of both bodies.*

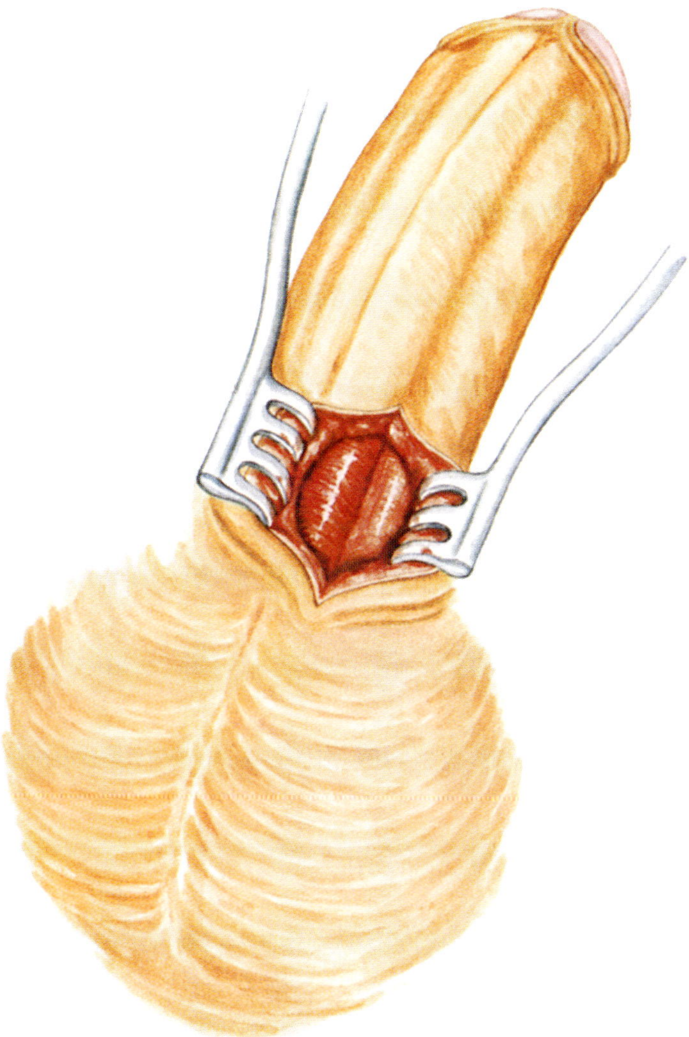

102-1

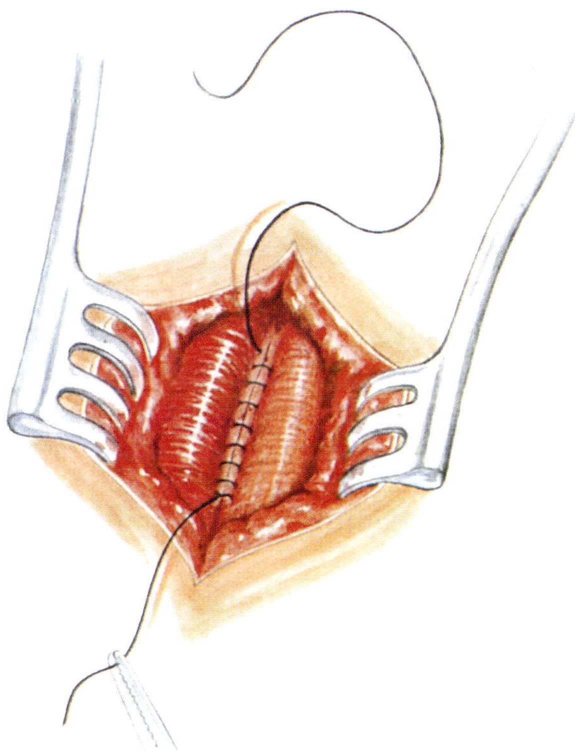

102-2

102-3. *Oval windows are fashioned* by removing the fascial walls in both bodies and both bodies are vigorously irrigated to remove the clot.

102-4. *Side-to-side anastomosis is completed* with a running 3–0 chromic catgut suture. The skin and subcutaneous tissue are reapproximated in the usual fashion.

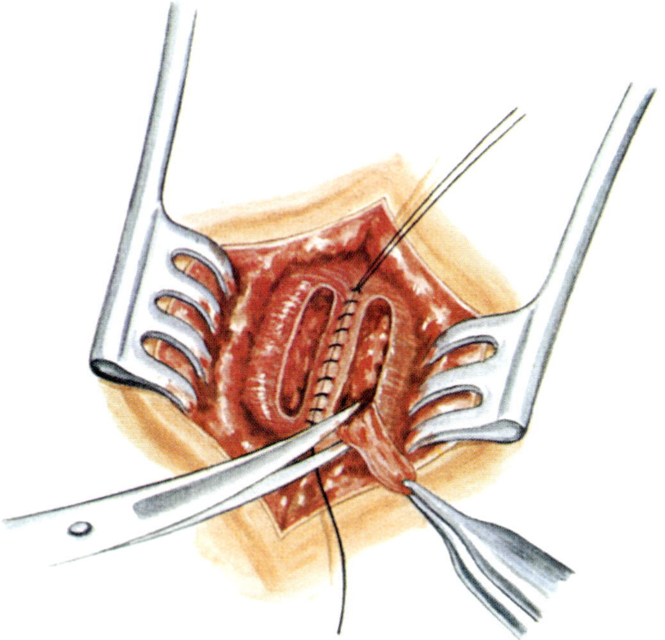

102-3

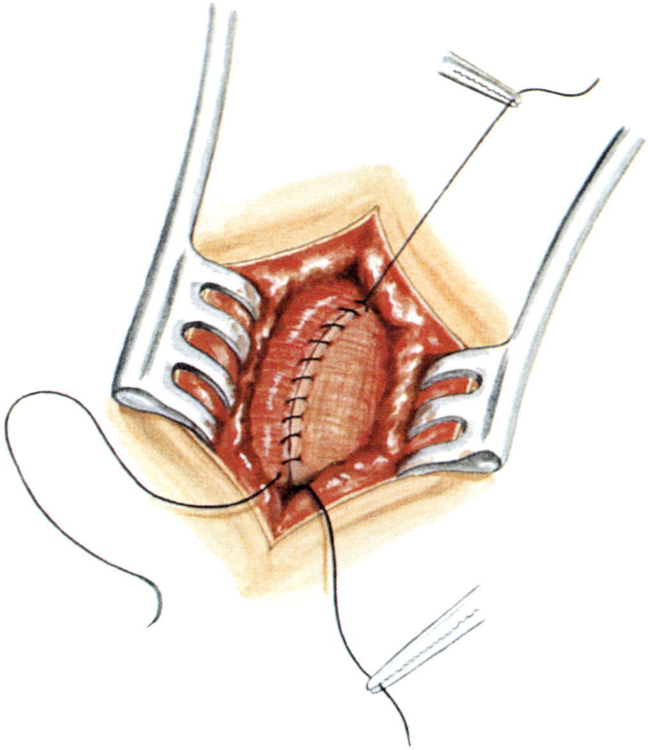

102-4

103. Anastomosis of the Right Saphenous Vein to the Cavernous Body

103-1. Two incisions are necessary in this procedure. *The saphenous vein is isolated and the distal margin is ligated.* Approximately 6–8 cm of vein is freed. A tunnel is made beneath the skin to allow the vein to reach the base of the penis. The lateral aspect of the cavernous body is dissected, exposing the fascial covering. An end-to-side anastomosis of vein to the cavernous body is made. Closure of both wounds is by layers in the usual fashion. A bilateral saphenous-vein-to-cavernous-body procedure is sometimes indicated.

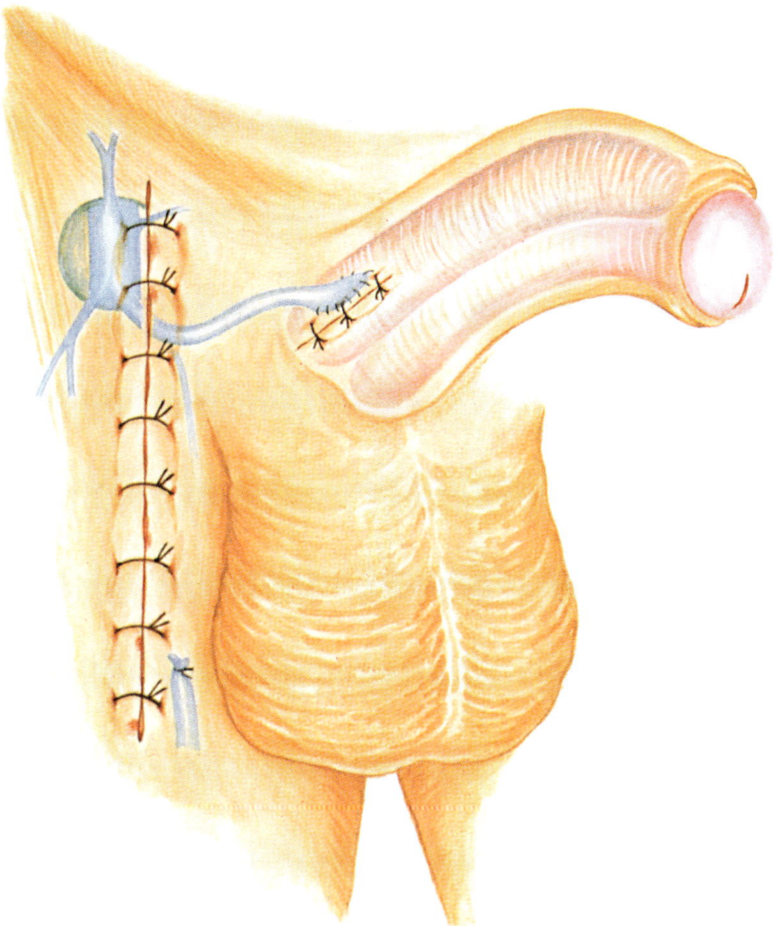

103-1

104. The Winter Technique

Priapism is an infrequent but important complication that many physicians encounter. Urologists see this problem in increasing numbers, and we should be aware of the early intervention and management of priapism.

One of the early problems encountered by urologists is the excessive delay between the onset of priapism and surgical intervention. This usually occurs when the primary care physician is unaware of the need for early intervention and waits too long before obtaining urologic consultation. The etiologies of priapism are 1) sickle-cell disease in Blacks, 2) trauma, 3) neoplasia, 4) leukemia, or 5) papaverine/phentolamine injections particularly to obtain erections. Usually the papaverine is injected in a higher, inappropriate dose.

The pathophysiology of priapism may be due to hypoxia with accompanying edema and penile swelling. Most often it becomes irreversible when thrombosis and fibrosis are long standing. A sustained thrombosis can lead to fibrosis. The common clinical presentation is a prolonged penile erection which is sustained. The neurovasomotor apparatus that produces spasm in the outlet or at the penile vessels is due to stagnation of blood in the corpora cavernosa. The corpora lose oxygen and develop an increase in carbon dioxide content. These chemical changes promote edema and, eventually, thrombosis can occur if treatment is delayed.

104-1 and 104-2. The most effective treatment is the creation of the corpora cavernosa/spongiosa shunt as shown by the use of the needles. This is a special needle that actually cuts through the corpora cavernosa as shown in the sagittal view. Years ago a biopsy needle was used, but more recently a special needle has been developed which provides much better communication between the appropriate glans penis and the corpora cavernosa. After the shunts are produced in the hospital examining area, more definitive exchange and evacuation of clots can be performed.

The operating room may be the appropriate place for treatment. The penis is first cleansed with povidone iodine and pentane analgesia can be administered to the patient through a Duke type inhaler. One percent lidocaine is injected into the glands penis and the distal ends of both corpora cavernosa.

The corpora are then aspirated and irrigated with saline until all the stagnant blood has been removed. A Travenol biopsy needle is introduced twice through the end of the glans penis and two cores of tissue are removed from the septum separating the glands from the two corpora cavernosa. Thus, by creating the two fistulas, one allows blood to escape from the cavernosa system into the spongioidal compartments.

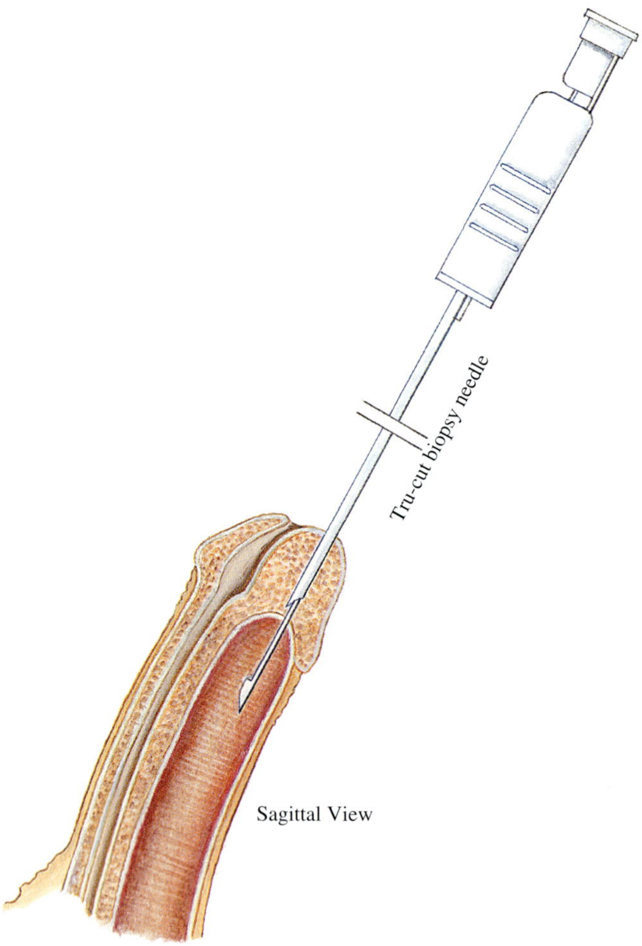

104-1

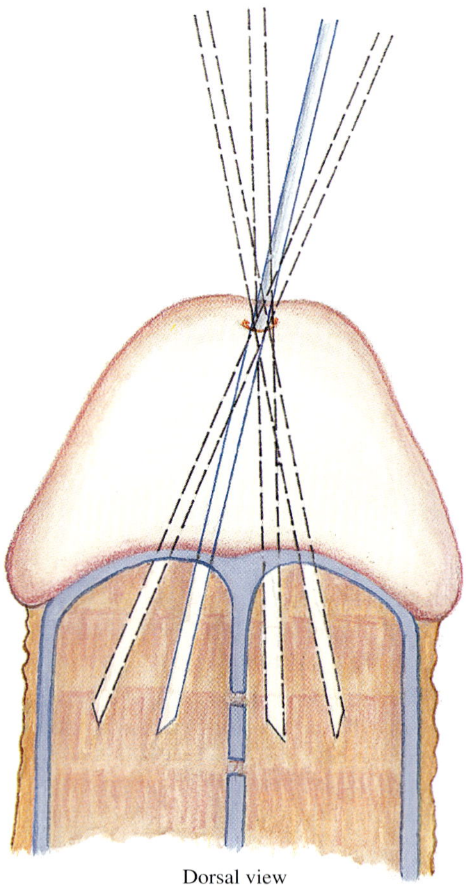

104-2

Correction of Organic Impotency

105. Small-Carrion Procedure

A silicone rubber prosthesis is inserted into the cavernous body (Small-Carrion procedure) bilaterally.

Candidates for this procedure have organic impotency. Patients who have undergone radical perineal prostatectomy or total cystectomy and prostatectomy are candidates. Selected patients with diabetes mellitus and impotency are also good candidates. We have seen a few neurologic disorders causing impotency, and the procedure using the prosthesis is indicated for these few patients, as well as for those in whom trauma or priapism resulted in impotency.

The patient is placed into the slightly exaggerated lithotomy position and prepared and draped to allow adequate exposure of the perineum. We keep all lengths of the paired prosthetic rods with the tapered curved ends (see Fig. 105–5). After an appropriate pair of rods has been selected, we soak the silicone rubber prosthesis in an erythromycin solution (1 g in 500 mL saline).

105-1. *A vertical skin incision is made from a point inferior to the scrotal perineal junction* and extends for 6–8 cm. A sound (24 French) is passed into the urethra and bladder to help identify the bulbous urethra.

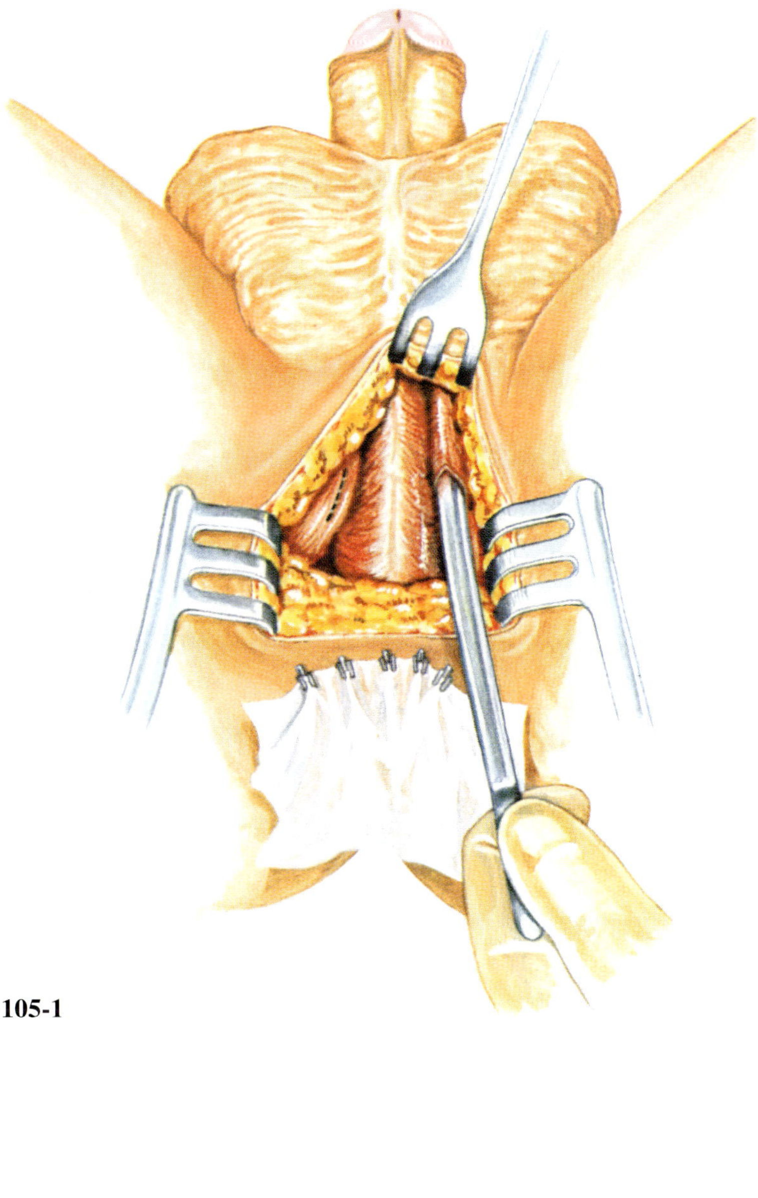

105-1

The bulbocavernous muscle overlying the urethra is carefully exposed. The connective tissue overlying each ischiocavernous muscle is freed and wiped laterally, exposing the fascial covering.

A longitudinal incision is made through the fascial layer of ischiocavernous muscle, exposing the interior of the cavernous bodies. Stay sutures are placed to keep the fascial margins separated. This incision is approximately 4–6 cm superior to the ischial tuberosity on the right. Hegar dilators are then inserted (gradually increasing sizes from 8 to 16 Fr are used) to dilate the cavernous bodies from the incision to their distal ends at the coronal penile margin.

105-2. The dilator is also reversed in its direction so that the inferior proximal cavernous body is also dilated. The procedure is repeated on the opposite side.

105-3. The surgeon can usually determine the appropriate prosthetic length and diameter of the shaft after dilatations have been completed. The *appropriate silicone rubber rod is selected and inserted.* The distal tip should rest against the glans penis, slightly raising the glans. The tapered narrower end is inserted pointing toward the ischial tuberosity.

105-4. *The fascial layers are reapproximated with 3–0 chromic catgut.* We usually leave a urethral indwelling catheter (16 Fr) in the bladder for 24 hours.

105-5. *The paired silicone rubber rods are checked for proper alignment and position.* Note the slight groove under the glans penis. Note also that the tapered curved posterior ends point toward the ischial tuberosity.

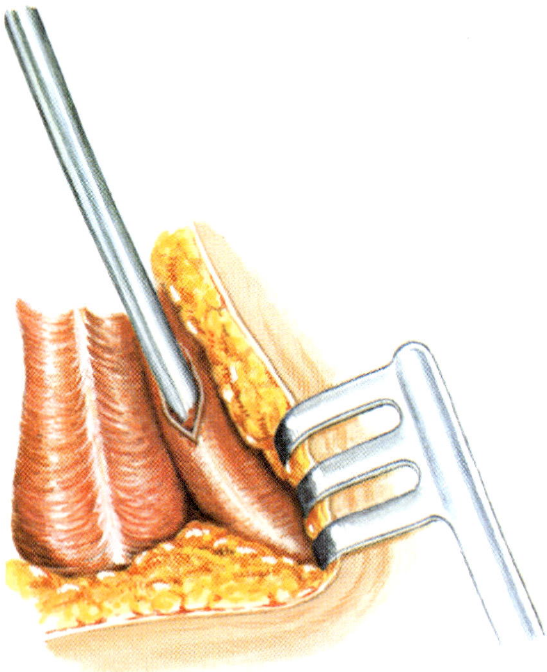

105-2

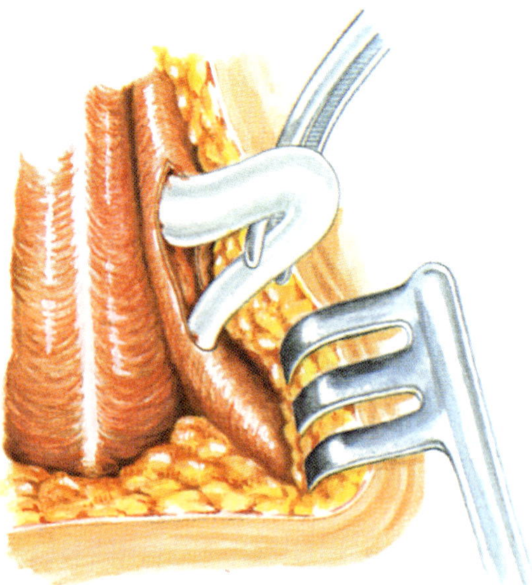

105-3

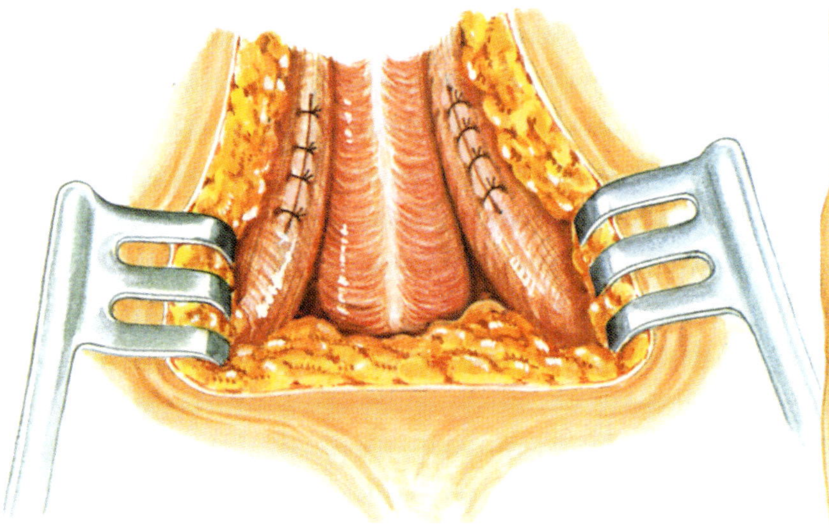

105-4

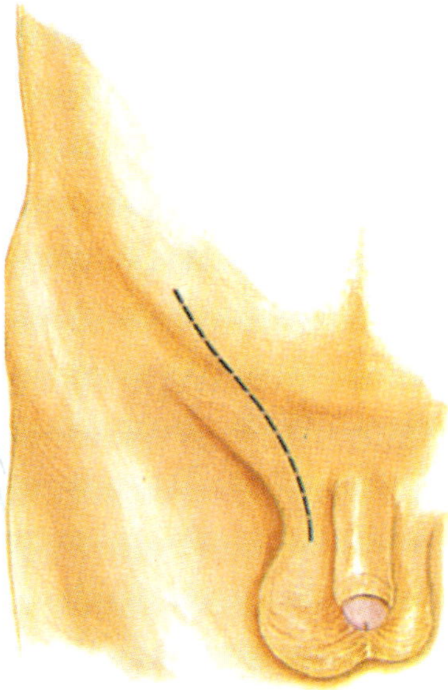

105-5

106. Dorsal Incision Technique

Implantation of paired penile prosthesis in corpora cavernosum

106-1. A vertical, dorsal incision is made in the proximal penis as shown. Care is taken to avoid the dorsal subcutaneous vein or its tributary.

106-2. An incision is made into the wall of the right corporal cavernosal tissue. Stay sutures are used (4–0 silk or 4–0 Prolene) after exposing the right dorsal wall of the corpora cavernosum.

106-3. A small Hegar dilator is introduced into the lumen of the corpora cavernosum, and the luminal tissue is progressively dilated in the right corpora cavernosum as shown so that the prosthesis can be accommodated.

106-4. Dilatation is also carried out proximally and progressively so that the appropriate proximal end of the prosthesis can be accommodated. Although not shown, a similar incision is made into the left anterior wall of the corpora cavernosum and stay sutures are also placed. Progressive dilatation is also carried out on the left.

106-5. The right flexible penile prosthesis has been inserted distally to the corona and the proximal temporary U-shaped bend in the penile prosthesis is formed so that the proximal tip can be inserted and accommodated. A similar procedure is performed on the left side. Hegar dilators are again used. The flexible penile rod is inserted in the left lumen distally first and then proximally.

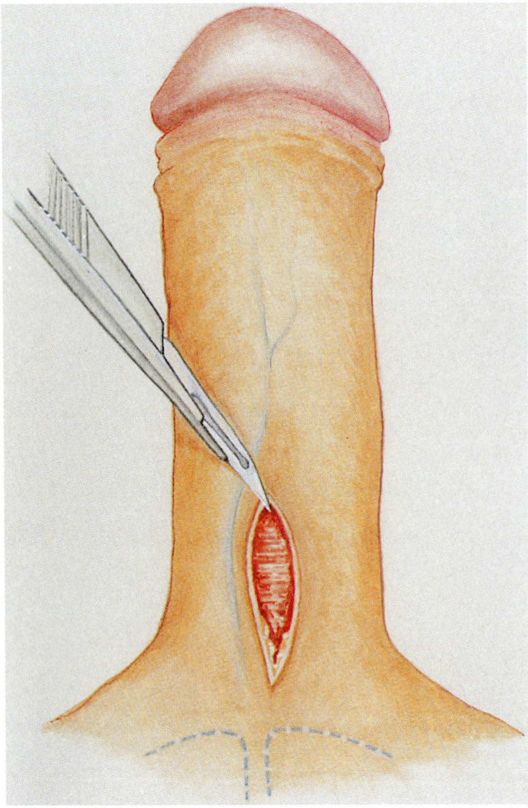

106-1

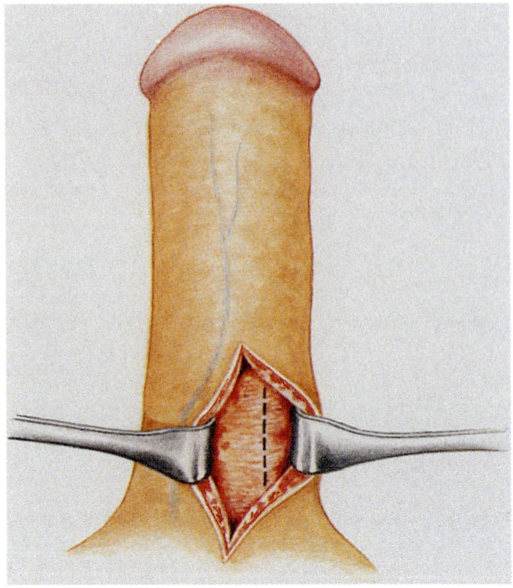

106-2

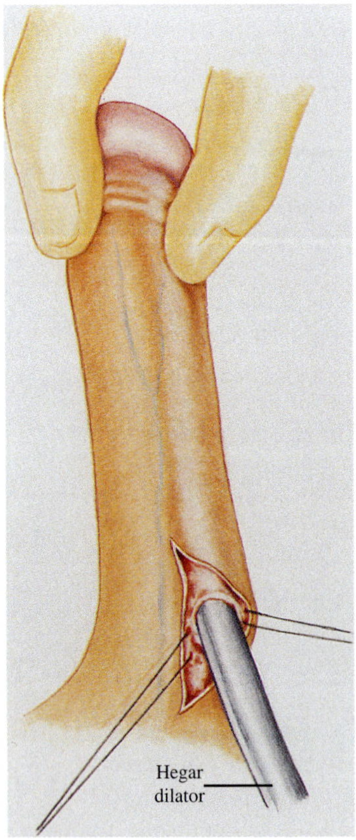

106-3

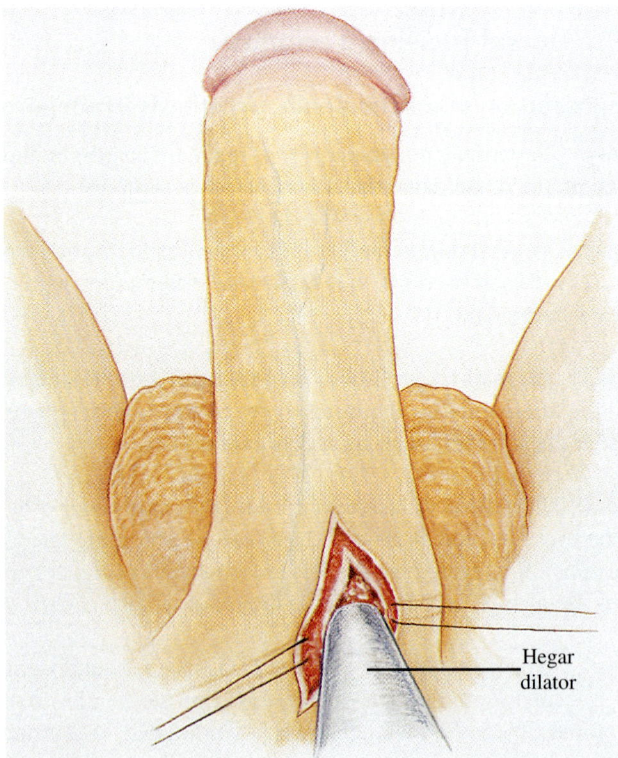

106-4

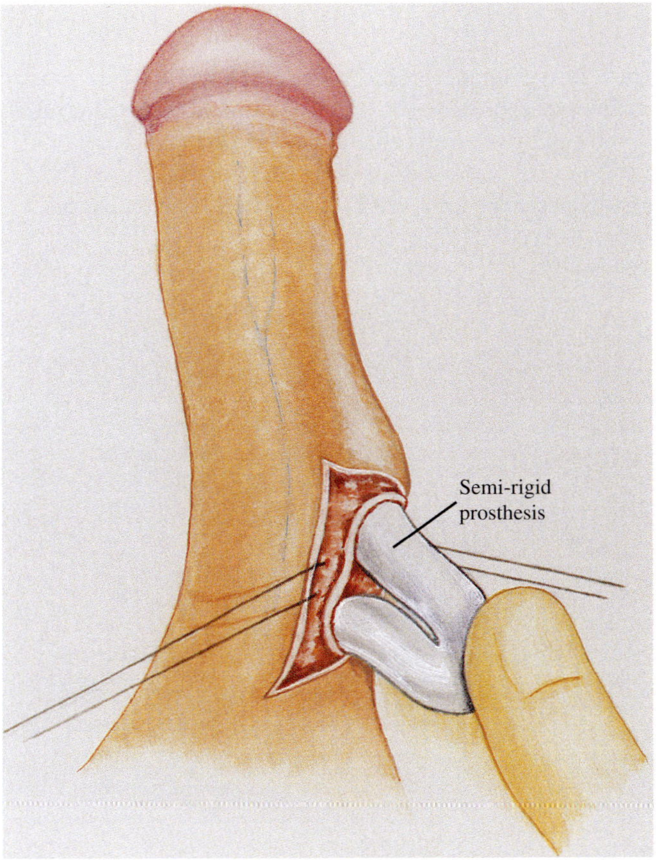

106-5

Both corporal incisions are closed separately with 4–0 Prolene or chromic catgut sutures. The penile skin can be closed with interrupted 4–0 catgut sutures. A urethral Foley type indwelling catheter is inserted so that urine is easily passed. The patient is sent home the next day with the indwelling catheter. If he is a diabetic person, then management of the diabetes mellitus is necessary. The catheter can be removed several days later in the office. Antibiotics, wide spectrum type, are useful and indicated.

The paired inflatable, penile prosthesis may last a few years. It can also erode with time. The implant needs to be removed if pain occurs. If one-half of the prosthesis leaks through the expansible membrane, the erect penis may be deformed and insertion may be difficult. A reimplantation may be necessary.

107. Jonas Procedure for Penile Implants

A modification of the dorsal incision technique has been described by Jonas, in Germany.

107-1. A coronal semicircular incision is made just proximal to the glans penis on the anterior surface. The fascial covering of cavernosal tissue is incised, first on one side, then the other. Stay sutures are used to expose the luminal compartment on each side. The Hegar dilators are used on each side to dilate the lumen progressively so that the flexible penile prosthesis can be accommodated.

107-2. The distal end of the prosthesis is about to be carefully inserted into the lumen with a twisting motion.

107-3. The index finger is helpful in applying a twisting motion as the prosthesis slips into the lumen proximally.

The corporal cavernosal wall is reapproximated with interrupted Prolene sutures. The coronal-subcutaneous tissue is reapproximated with 4–0 chromic catgut interrupted sutures. Again, a Foley type indwelling urethral catheter (16 Fr) may be necessary. Antibiotics are given perioperatively, and oral wide spectrum antibiotics are used for 4 to 6 days after discharge. The catheter can be removed in 1 or 2 days as an outpatient.

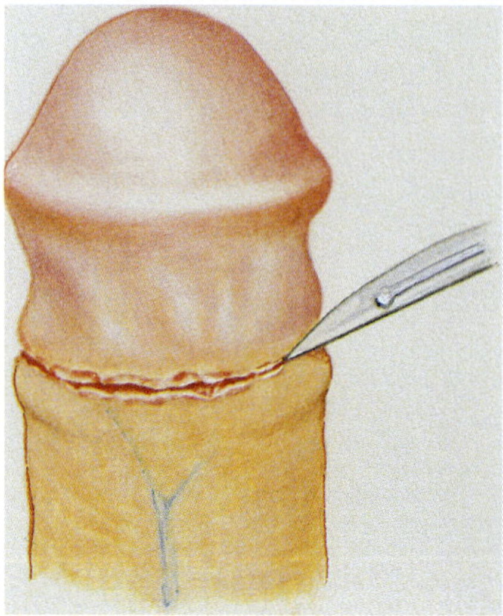

107-1

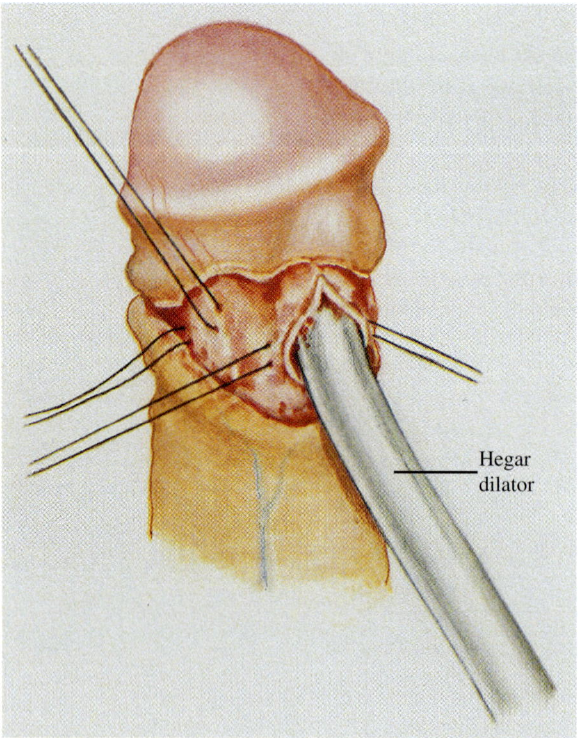

107-2

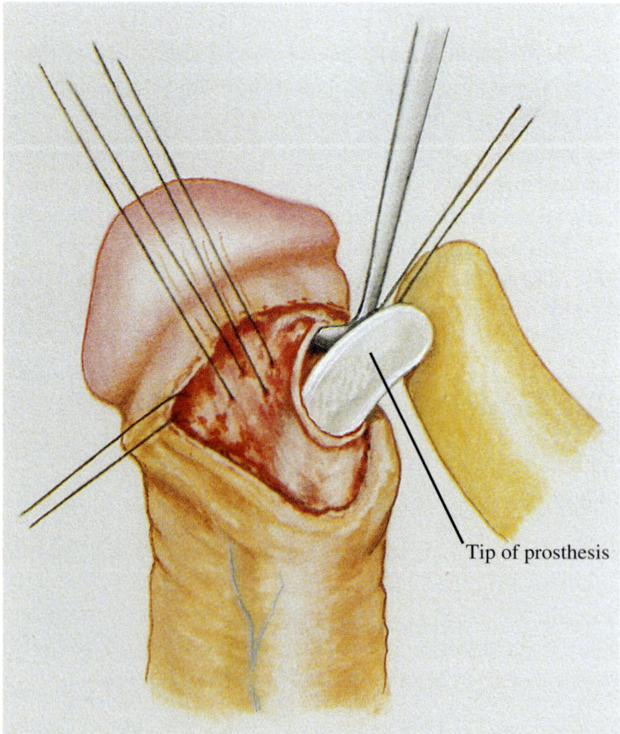

107-3

Suggested Readings

Creecy AA, Beazlie FS Jr. Fracture of the penis: traumatic rupture of corpora cavernosa. J Urol 78:620, 1957.

Farrer JR, Goodwin WE. Treatment of priapism: comparison of method in fifteen cases. J Urol 86:768, 1961.

Lugg JA, Gonzalez-Cadavid NF, Rajfer J. The role of nitric oxide in erectile function [Review]. J Andrology 16:2,1995.

Meares EM Jr. Traumatic rupture of the corpus cavernosum. J Urol 105:407, 1971.

Small MP, Carrion HM, Gordon JA. Small-Carrion penile prosthesis. Urology 5:479, 1975.

Winter CC. Cure of idiopathic priapism. New procedure for creating fistula between glans penis and corpora cavernosa. Urology 8:389, 1976.

Winter CC. Priapism. In: Glenn JF, ed. Urologic Surgery. Hagerstown: Harper & Row, 1975.

The Scrotum and Its Contents

Surgical Anatomy

STRUCTURE OF THE SCROTUM

The scrotum is a contractile cutaneous pouch containing the testes and the inferior part of the spermatic cords. It has a bilateral origin: the left and right scrotum are fused together in the midline forming the median raphe. This septum divides the scrotal cavity into two compartments. The scrotal wall consists of skin, muscle, and connective tissue. The skin of the scrotum is thin and elastic and usually lies in folds. It is deeply pigmented and contains many sebaceous glands and hair follicles.

Immediately beneath the skin is the dartos tunic, a thin layer of involuntary muscle and connective tissue that contracts with cold and relaxes with heat. It is supplied with sympathetic nerve fibers. Anteriorly it is continuous with the superficial fascia of the abdominal wall; laterally it is attached to ischiopubic rami; and posteriorly it is prolonged into the superficial perineal Colles's fascia.

A layer of loose connective tissue lies between the dartos layer and the deeper layers. The tissue is sufficiently loose to permit the scrotal contents to move about freely in the scrotal cavity. This layer presents a good plane of cleavage when the scrotum is being approached surgically. It is in this loose layer that extravasations and hematomas from the perineal region accumulate; the extravasation may spread superiorly under Scarpa's fascia and the superficial fascia of abdominal wall.

Besides the above three layers, there are another three complete layers that invest the testis and cord. All of them are derived from the anterior abdominal wall.

The most superficial is the external spermatic fascia, an extension of the external oblique fascia.

The middle layer is the cremaster muscle layer, which is derived from internal oblique muscle. By contraction of this layer, the testis is drawn toward the external inguinal ring. The cremasteric reflex is produced by strong contractions of these muscle fibers if the skin or medial thigh is scratched.

The deepest is the internal spermatic fascia, an extension of the transversalis fascia. It is composed of loose connective tissue and closely invests elements of the spermatic cord and testis.

The tunica vaginalis of the testis is a serous membrane that covers most of testis and

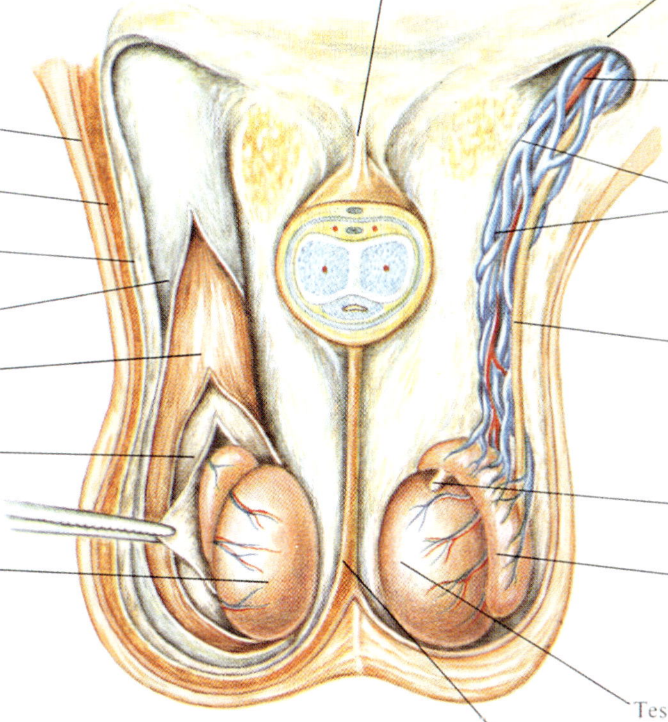

FIG. 1.
The scrotum and its contents (frontal view).

epididymis. Developmentally it is derived from the vaginal process of the peritoneum. The remainder of the funicular portion of the process, the vaginal ligament, lies among elements of spermatic cord from the internal inguinal ring to the tunica vaginalis. Like all other serous membranes, it forms a cavity that contains a film of fluid and it divides the tunica vaginalis into parietal and visceral layers. The parietal layer is closely adherent to the internal spermatic fascia. It reflects forward at the posterior wall of the scrotum and becomes continuous with the visceral layer, which is closely adherent to tunica albuginea, the fibrous covering of the testis and epididymis (Figs. 1 and 2).

STRUCTURE OF THE TESTIS, EPIDIDYMIS, AND SPERMATIC CORD

The testis is a paired oval glandular organ that lies in either side of scrotal cavity. It is loosely suspended by the spermatic cord and its investing tunic layers. It is also attached to the base of the scrotum by the gubernaculum.

The testis is coated by a pearly white fibrous layer, the tunica albuginea. It becomes thicker at the posterior border, forming the mediastinal testis, from which numerous incomplete fibrous septa pass inward to subdivide the testis into many lobules. Each lobule of the testis is filled with convoluted seminiferous tubules; the proximal end unites with the ends of other lobules to form a network called the rete testis at the mediastinal testis. From this network about 20 efferent ductules arise and enter the head of the epididymis from the upper pole of the testis (Fig. 3).

The function of the testis is to produce sperm from the seminiferous tubules and to secrete androgen from the interstitial or Leydig cells.

The epididymis is a long narrow body surmounting the posterior border of the testis. It is divided into three parts: head, body, and tail. The head of the epididymis is enlarged and attached on the upper pole of the testis. The body is separated from the testis and the tail is attached to the testis again at its lower end.

The head is composed of efferent ductules that emerge from the testis. The ductules converge into a convoluted single duct system in the epididymal body that connects with the vas deferens at the tail. The function of the epididymis is to collect sperm from the testis and allow them to mature.

The spermatic cord is a long, rounded bundle that originates at the internal inguinal ring and terminates at the upper pole of the testis. It consists of the vas deferens, blood vessels, lymphatics, and nerve fibers to the cord and testis. All these structures are loosely united by connective tissue elements and ensheathed by the same fascial coverings of the testis.

VASCULAR SUPPLY

The blood supply of the scrotal wall is mainly derived from the external and internal pudendal arteries. The veins follow the arteries. The lymphatics of the scrotal wall form an exceedingly rich network and drain into the inguinal and femoral nodes.

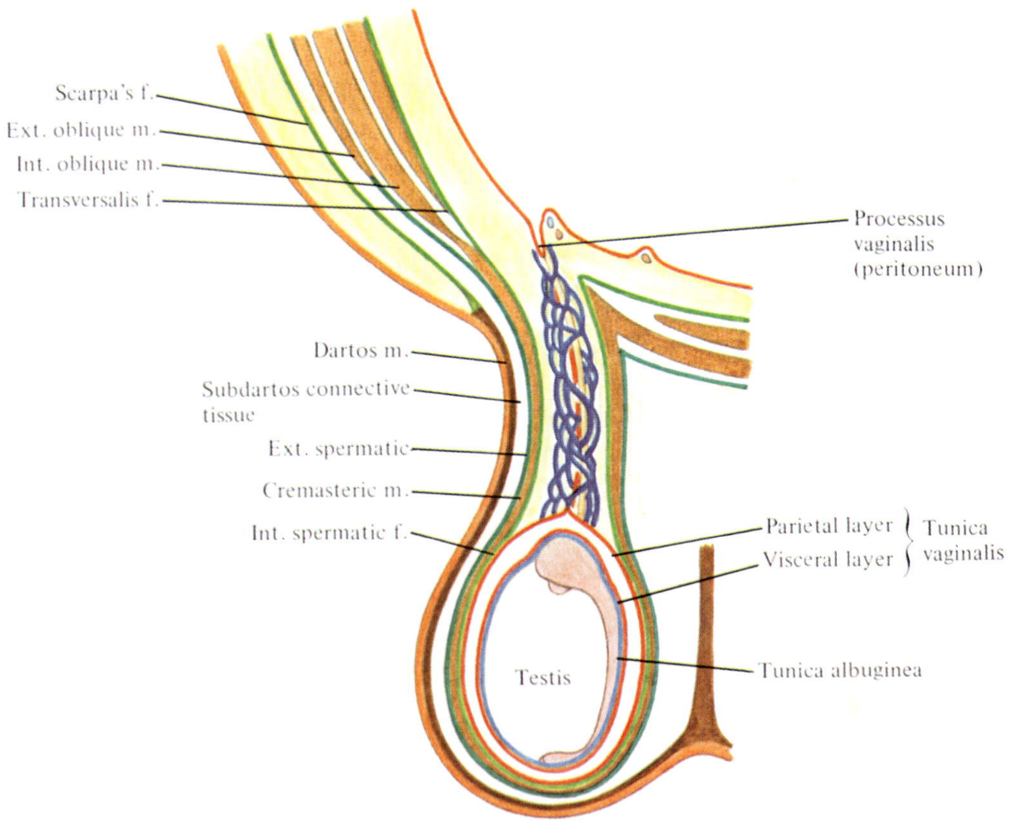

FIG. 2.
The scrotum and inguinal region (schematic of frontal view, right half).

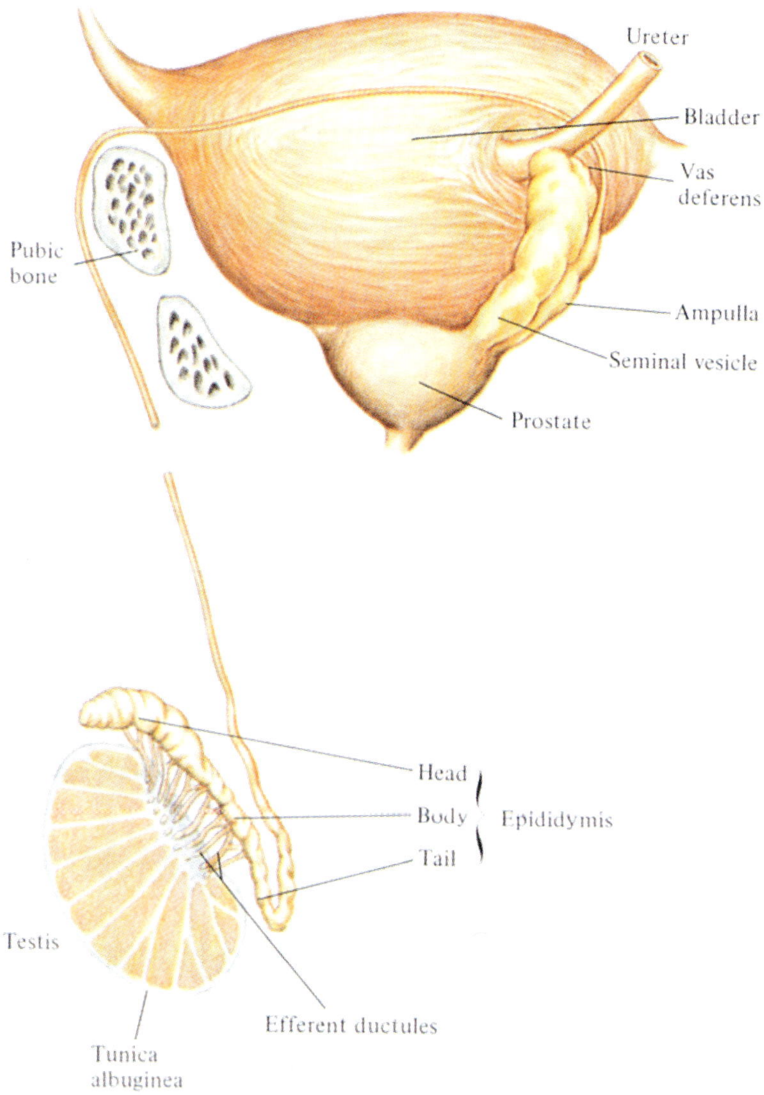

FIG. 3.
Male reproductive system (lateral view).

There are two arteries in the spermatic cord: the internal spermatic artery and the artery of the vas deferens. The latter artery is derived from the superior or inferior vesical artery, runs along the vas, and supplies it before branching to the epididymis and testis.

The internal spermatic artery, the main supplying artery of the testis, arises from the abdominal aorta just below the renal arteries, distributes a branch to the ureter, and joins the spermatic cord at the internal inguinal ring. It enters the testis at the mediastinum testis, distributing a branch to the head of the epididymis.

These two arteries are anastomosed together at their distal ends; hence, damage to any one will not compromise the testis at the distal end. One must be careful in working at the head of the epididymis because the testicular artery can be damaged, resulting in loss of function. In addition to these, a cremasteric artery, which is derived from the inferior epigastric artery, supplies coverings of the cord.

The veins of the testis and epididymis form the pampiniform plexus in the spermatic cord. This plexus is grossly divided into anterior and posterior groups; the former surrounds the spermatic artery and the latter surrounds the vas deferens.

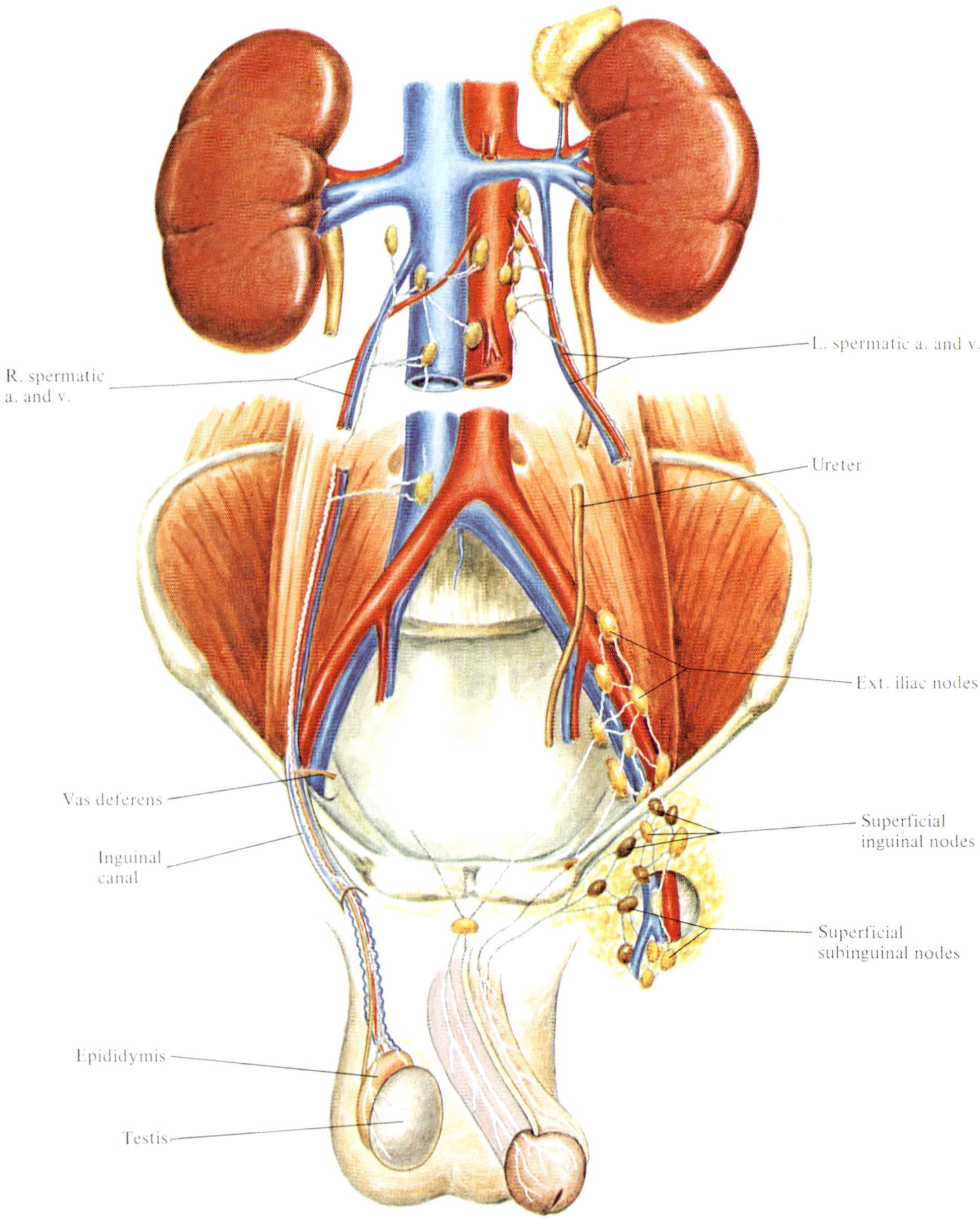

FIG. 4.
Lymphatic drainage of penis and testis.

As the veins ascend, they decrease in number but increase in size and finally converge into the spermatic vein at the internal inguinal ring.

The right vein drains directly into the inferior vena cava at an oblique angle near the renal pedicle.

The left vein is valvular and drains into the left renal vein almost at a right angle. This fact may explain the increased incidence of varicoceles on the left side, as compared with the right.

The lymphatics of the scrotal contents follow the spermatic vessels throughout their course and drain into the lumbar nodes near the aorta and inferior vena cava. There is no direct connection with the inguinal nodes, an important factor in the treatment of malignant tumors of the testis (Fig. 4).

NERVE SUPPLY

Sympathetic fibers to the testis and epididymis are derived from the renal and aortic plexus, accompanied by the spermatic artery and vas deferens. The pudendal nerve

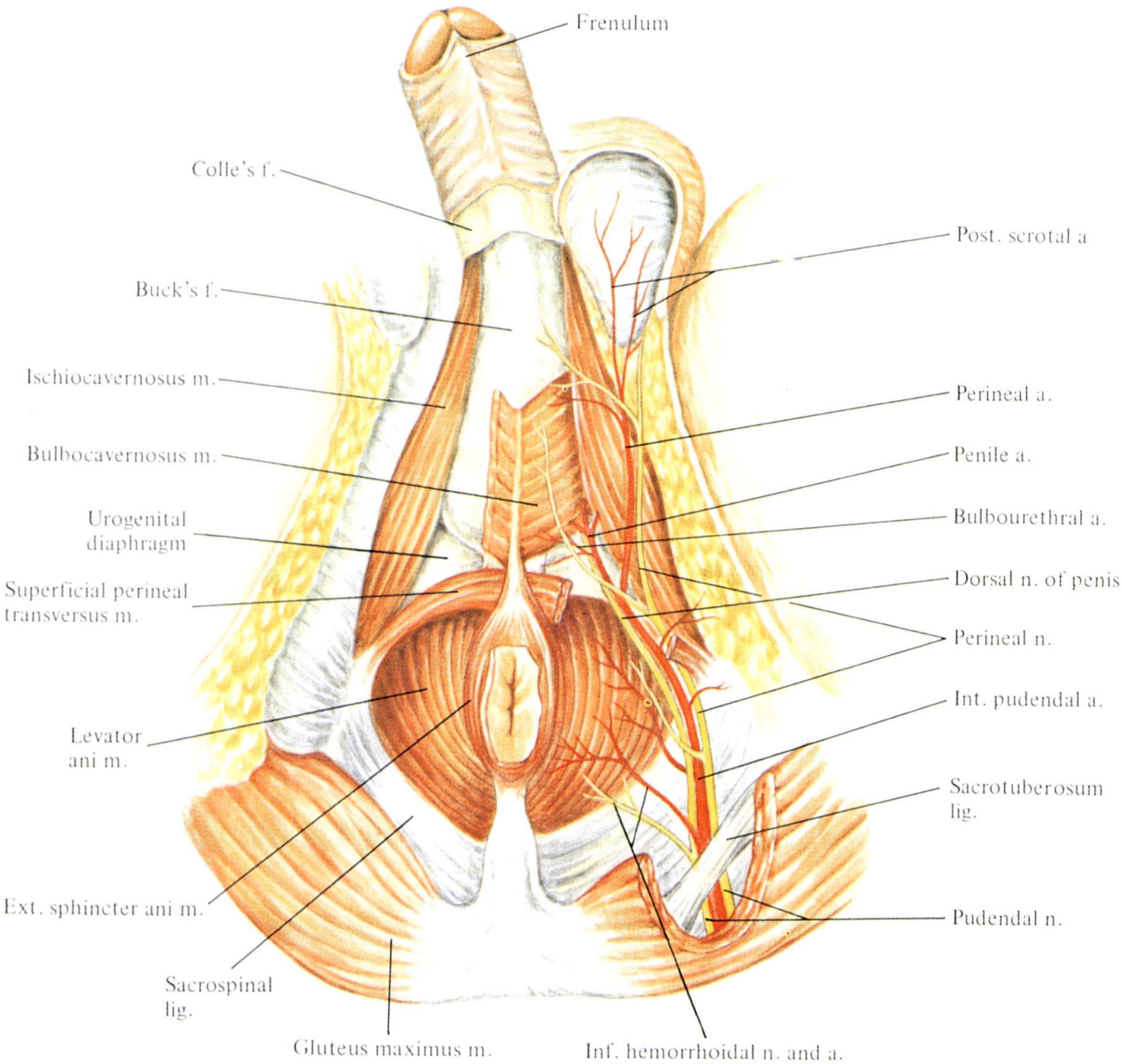

FIG. 5.
Superficial structures of the male perineum.

sends some branches of motor and sensory fibers to the skin and muscles of the scrotum (Fig. 5).

Surgical Anatomy of the Seminal Vesicle and Vas Deferens

The seminal vesicles are paired lobulated sacs lying at the base of the bladder, superior to the prostate and anterior to the rectal wall and fascia. Each vesicle is a tubular structure with a blind end that constitutes a diverticulum of the lower end of the vas deferens. The seminal vesicle has a histologic structure similar to that of an ampullated end of the vas deferens, a secreting type of epithelium. In the adult, it is about 4–5 cm long, but the length of the tube will reach 10–15 cm when uncoiled (Fig. 6). The open end of the sem-

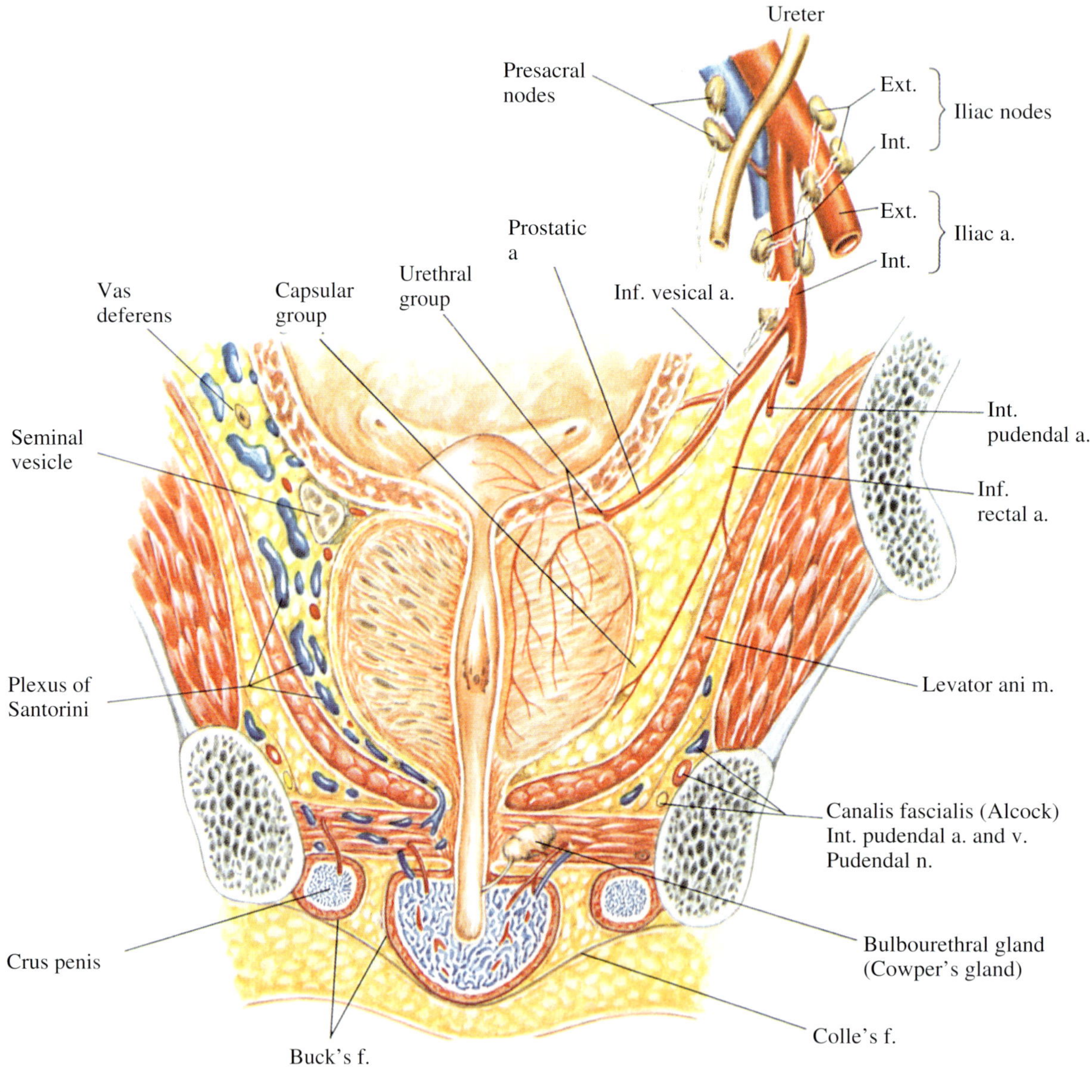

FIG. 6.
Coronal section of prostate and bladder floor; adjacent muscle groups are shown.

inal vesicle joins the vas deferens at the base of the prostate to form the ejaculatory duct. The latter pierces the prostate between the posterior and median lobes and enters the prostatic urethra through the seminal colliculus (verumontanum).

The vas deferens passes along the base of the bladder, along the medial aspect of the seminal vesicles, and across the terminal part of the ureter; it is covered by peritoneum, hooks around the origin of the inferior epigastric artery, joins with other constituents of the spermatic cord in the inguinal canal, and connects the lower end of the epididymis at the dependent scrotal end (Fig. 3).

The blood supply to each seminal vesicle is derived from the inferior vesical and the middle hemorrhoidal arteries. Veins drain into the vesicoprostatic plexuses. The artery is closely attached to the vas wall. The artery runs from the base of the bladder to the epididymis and anastomoses with the testicular artery.

Operative Techniques

108. Left Hydrocelectomy in the Infant

A hydrocele is a collection of fluid within the tunica vaginalis and usually surrounds a testis. It can extend superiorly up the cord.

108-1. A scrotal incision is made and carried through the dartos, external, and internal spermatic fascia. *The hydrocele sac including testicles is delivered outside the skin margin.* We usually explore the anteromedial cord proximal to the hydrocele to rule out the presence of an indirect hernia. If a hernial sac is also present, then the incision is extended up into the inguinal area, and a herniorrhaphy is completed.

The line of incision through the hydrocele sac is indicated by the dotted line.

108-2. *Excessive sac is excised.* The edges and remaining sac are reversed so that the newly cut edges of sac are reapproximated around the lower cord and epididymis with 3–0 or 4–0 chromic catgut.

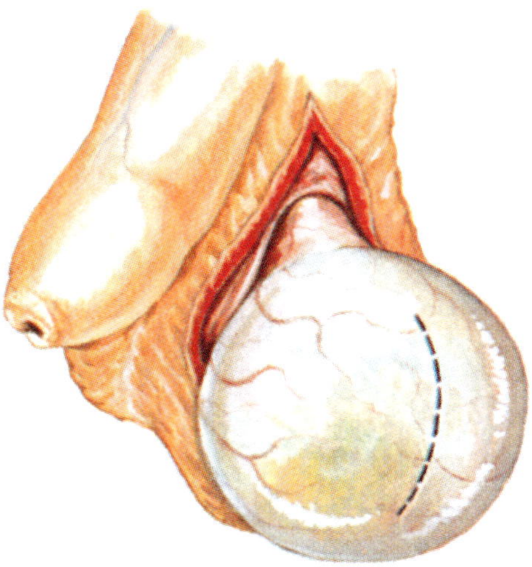

108-1

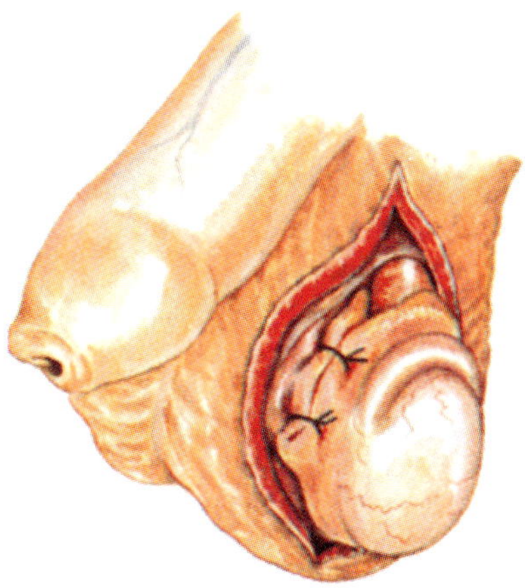

108-2

109. Hydrocelectomy in the Adult

109-1. *The hydrocele is delivered outside the scrotal incision.* The sac is opened and the borders are retracted with clamps. Excessive sac is excised (dotted line).

109-2. *The edges of the tunica vaginalis are reversed around the cord* so that the inner surfaces are now exteriorized. The edges are sutured with 3–0 chromic catgut.

109-3. When the tunica vaginalis is thickened and indurated, it may not easily be closed around the lower cord. In this instance, continuous right and left sutures (3–0 chromic catgut) are placed around the edges of the sac to ensure hemostasis.

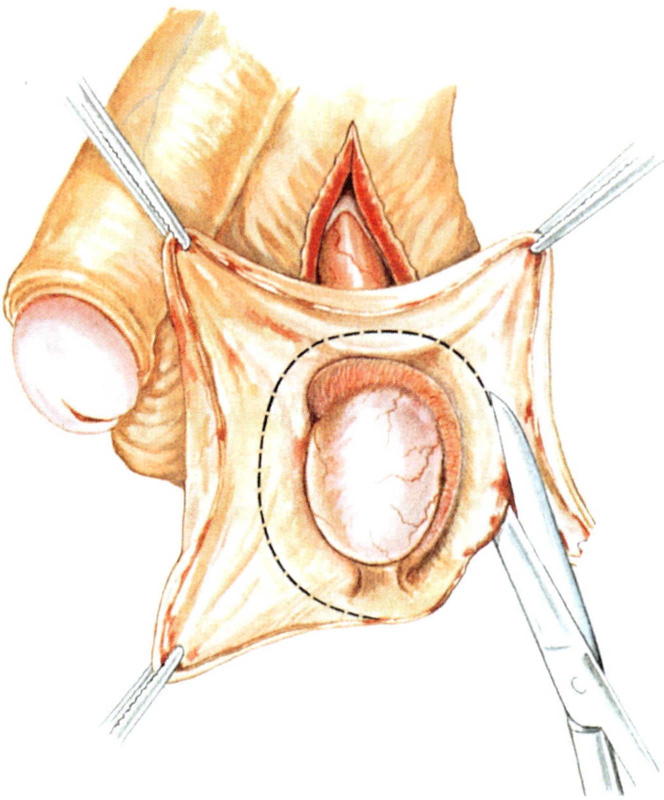

109-1

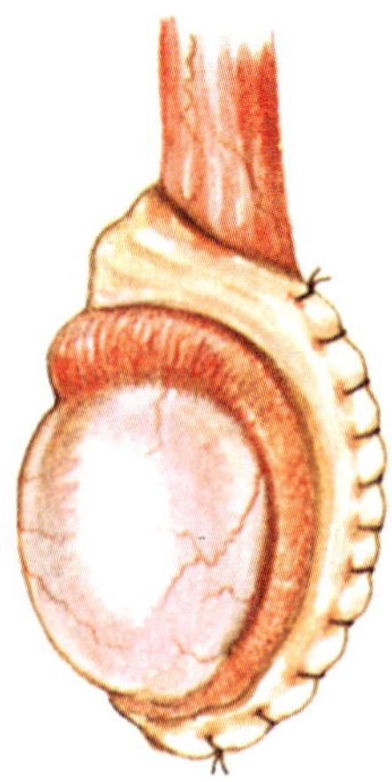

109-2

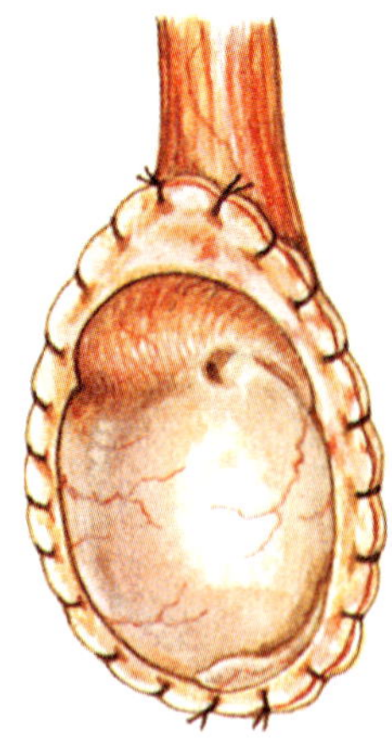

109-3

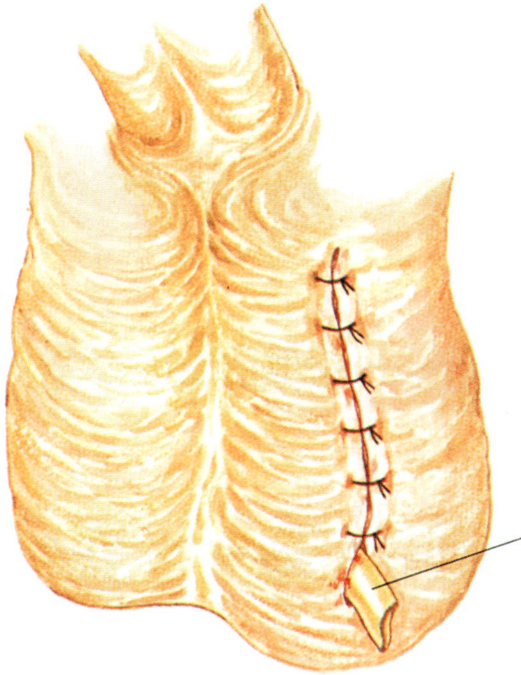

109-4

109-4. *Closure is by layers.* The internal and external spermatic fascia can be closed as a single layer (3–0 chromic catgut). The dartos and skin are reapproximated with interrupted 3–0 chromic catgut. A drain from the wound may be placed in the inferior margin of the skin in selected instances. It is secured separately with a safety pin and is removed in 24 hours if drainage is minimal. A compression dressing is a better alternative than a drain.

110. Spermatocelectomy in the Adult

A spermatocele is a retention cyst of small tubules within the head of the epididymis. The differential diagnosis of a small (2–3 cm) mass in the scrotum is often difficult. A hydrocele, if large, covers the entire gonad. It will transilluminate artificial light. A spermatocele is located near the head of the epididymis (superior location) and will not transilluminate light.

110-1. The testis, cord, and epididymis are exposed. *The spermatocele is grasped with forceps and carefully excised.* Note its location in relation to the head of the epididymis.

110-2. *The spermatocele sac is circumscribed at its base* and its attachments to the head of the epididymis are exposed. A ligature is placed around the tubular attachments to the head of the epididymis.

110-3. *The spermatocele is excised.* Closure is in the usual fashion (see 110-4). A flat tubular drain is not necessary.

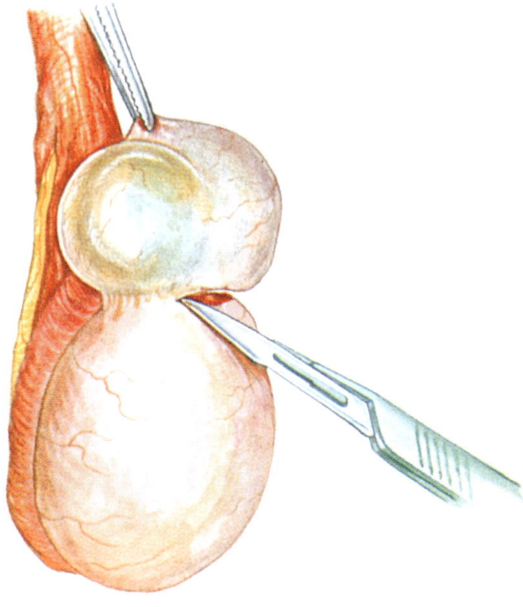

110-1

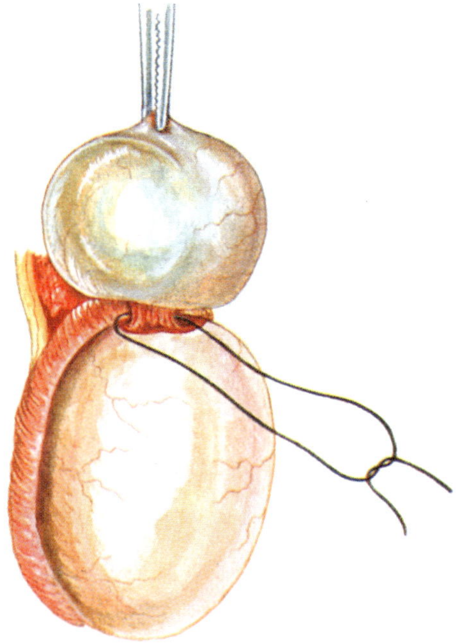

110-2

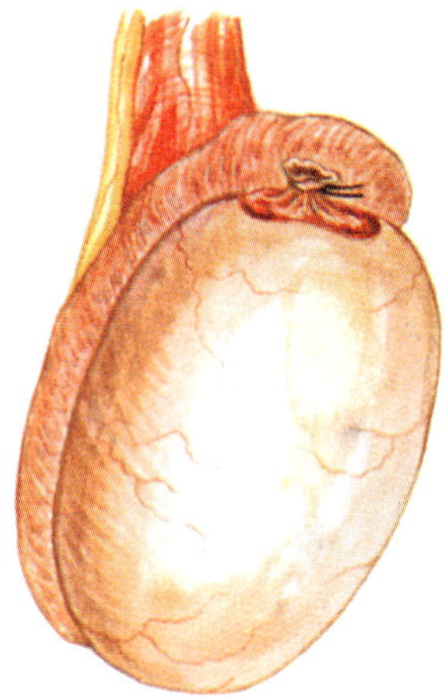

110-3

111. Left Varicocelectomy

A left varicocele is a condition characterized by dilation and tortuosity of the deep veins of the pampiniform plexus. A symptomatic varicocele may be treated surgically if the male patient is proved to be infertile. In our experience, three semen analyses will show a low motility score and 20 to 25% immature and tapered sperm forms on morphologic examination.

111-1. We use a high left-sided slightly oblique line of incision.

111-2. *The approach to the left spermatic vein is extraperitoneal.* The muscles are separated between muscle fibers. In an obese patient only the external oblique muscle is incised along the horizontal plane. Added exposure can also be gained by incising the lateral left border of rectus sheath.

111-3. *The deeper muscles are separated by blunt dissection.* The edge of the rectus abdominis muscle can be seen on the medial aspect. The illustration includes the internal oblique and transversus abdominis muscles. By using narrow Deaver retractors medially, one can easily reach the floor of the cavity. *The psoas major muscle is exposed* by wiping the peritoneal lining and its contents medially. Usually a sponge on a ring forceps is useful in gaining appropriate exposure.

111-4. By exposing the psoas major muscle medially, one comes upon the transversalis fascia, which serves as an envelope around the spermatic vein. Careful dissection through this envelope will reveal at least one and, in most instances, two or more spermatic veins. Our rule is that if we find an exceedingly large pencil-sized spermatic vein, then we may find only one or two other veins coursing superiorly away from the varicocele. At times we have found three and even four veins in this region. After the *veins* are exposed they *are doubly ligated and transected in between.* The ureter is not exposed by carefully following this approach. In this illustration we have shown the ureter for orientation. If one wishes to locate the ureter, then one simply needs to take the narrow Deaver retractor and move more medially and posteriorly where the ureter can be easily seen running superiorly and inferiorly. The ureter is often slightly adherent to the posterior parietal peritoneum.

This incision can be used to approach the left mid-ureter for removal of a calculus.

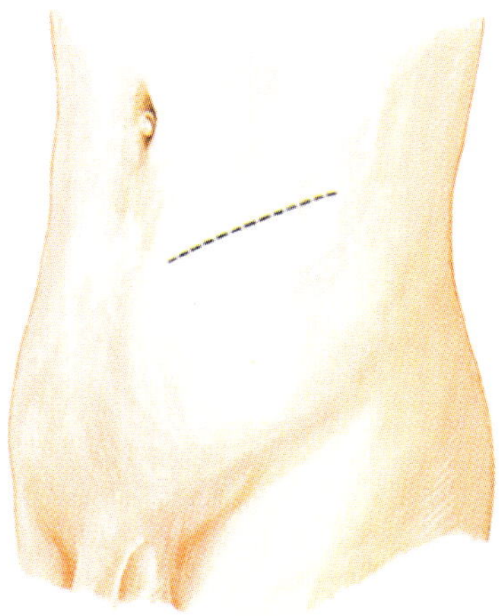

111-1

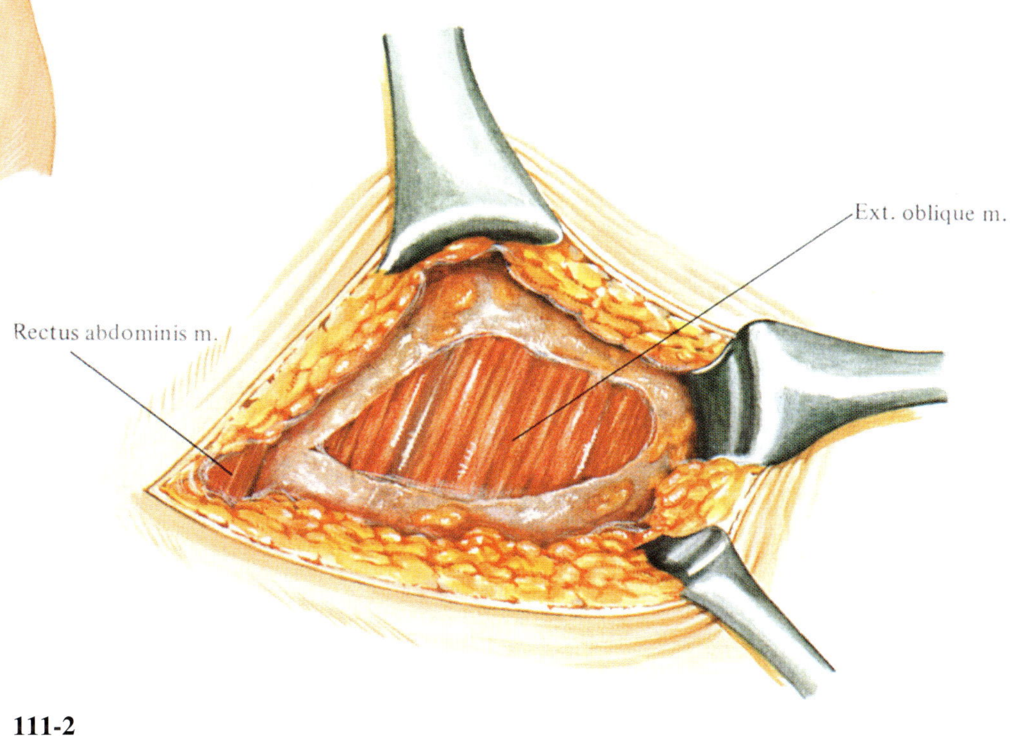

111-2

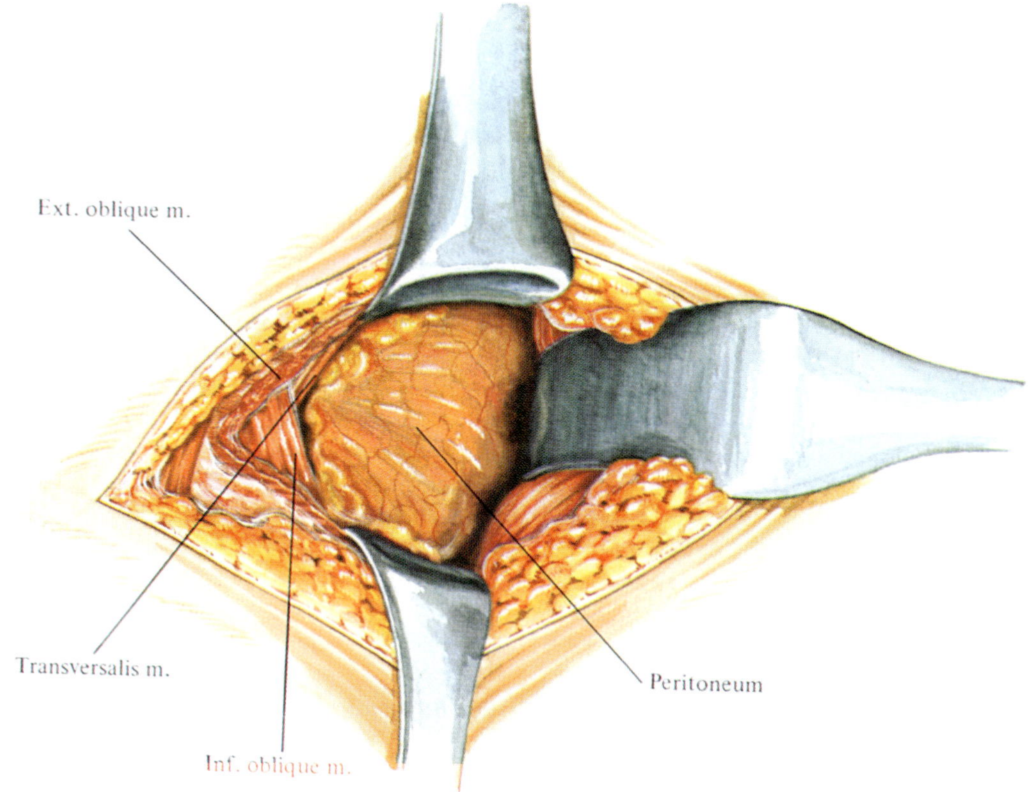
Ext. oblique m.
Transversalis m.
Peritoneum
Inf. oblique m.

111-3

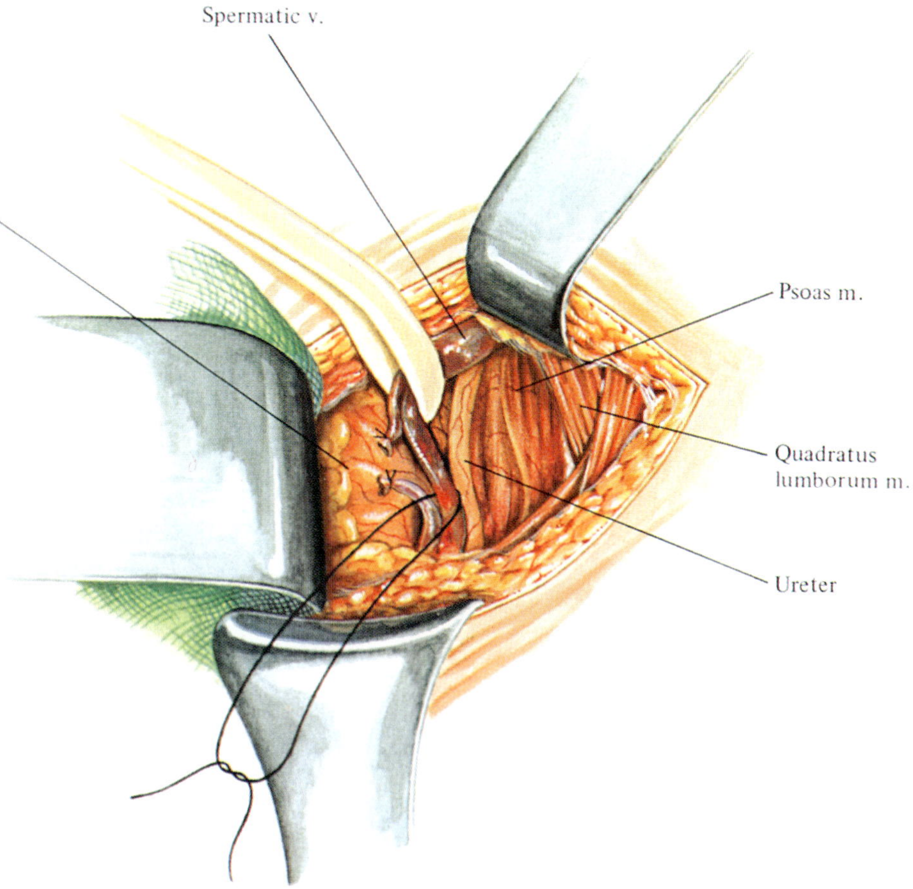
Spermatic v.
Peritoneum
Psoas m.
Quadratus
lumborum m.
Ureter

111-4

112. Orchiopexy for Undescended Testis (Ombredanne Procedure[1])

We believe that the procedure for cryptorchidism should be performed prior to age 5 years. If delayed into puberty, we believe the patient's fertility potential will be reduced.

112-1. *An inguinal incision is made on the right.* The testis is found in the inguinal canal. A stay suture is placed through the gubernaculum. The testis, including the cord, is brought down to the outer border of lowermost scrotum.

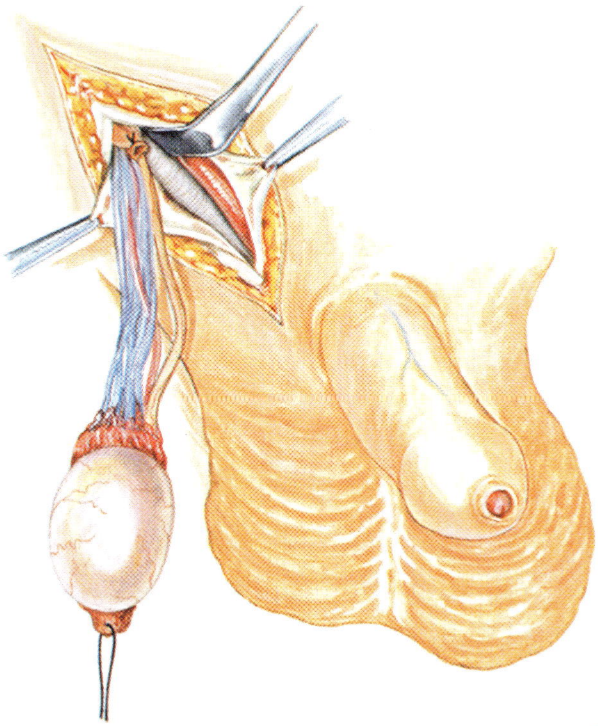

112-1

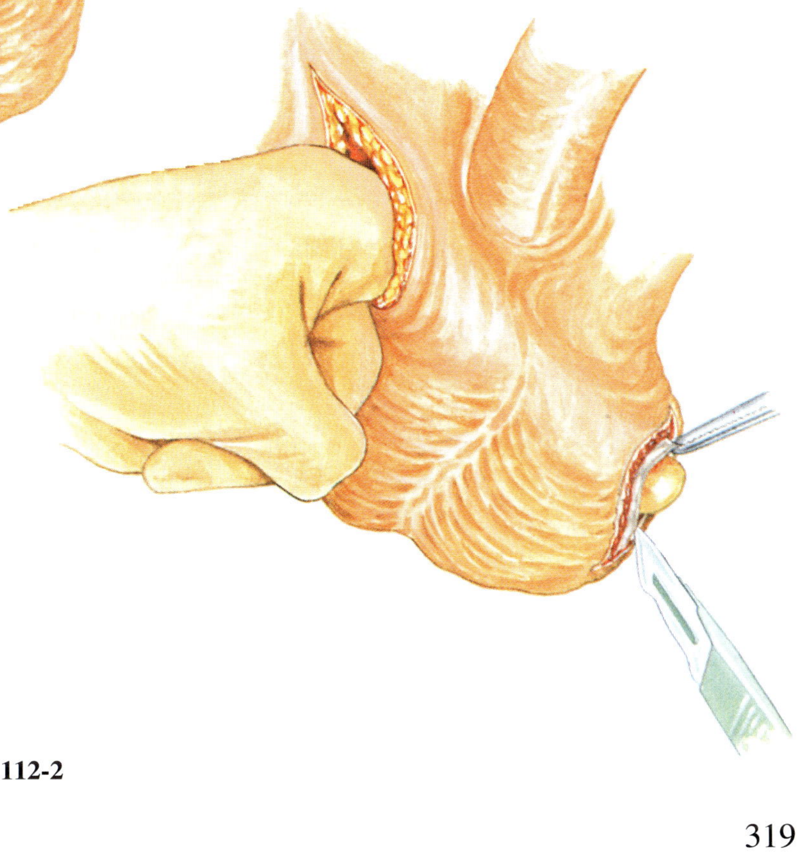

112-2

112-2. *A tunnel is made by the index finger.* The scrotal septum is tented to the opposite scrotal margin. The skin, fascia, and intrascrotal septum are incised.

112-3. A curved clamp is tented against the tip of the index finger and brought upward to the lower inguinal skin incision. The gubernaculum is grasped and *the right testicle is brought out through the left scrotal skin margin without tension.* The intrascrotal septum is closed with 3–0 chromic catgut to prevent the testis from retracting to the right lower inguinal area.

112-4. *The final resting place of the right testicle* is demonstrated schematically. The septum is indicated in brown and the skin incisions can be seen.

112-5. After a few months, the gross appearance on examination of the scrotum is remarkable. *Each testis is located in a lateral aspect of the scrotum.* The schematic shows the true fascial relationships.

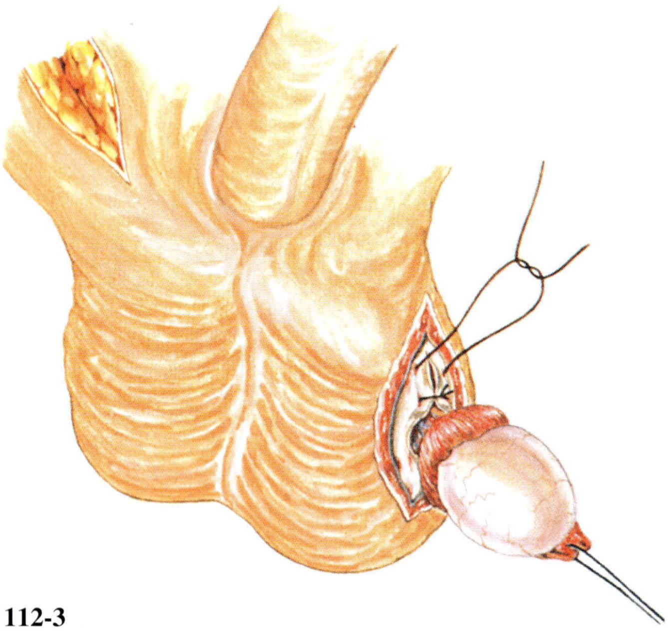

112-3

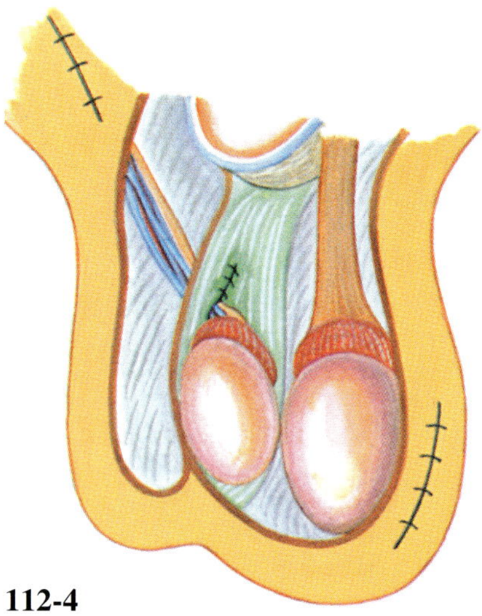

112-4

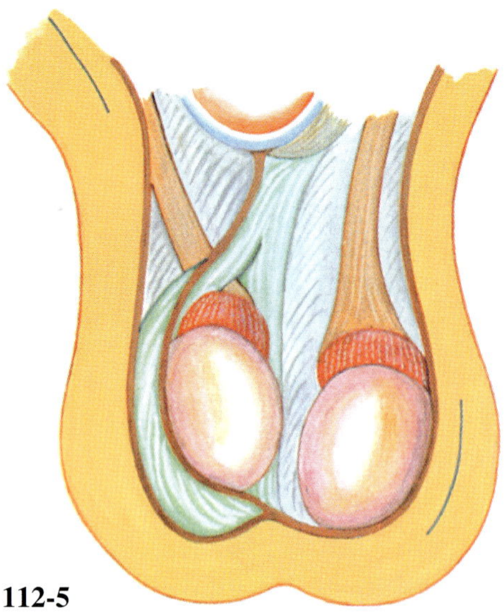

112-5

113. Subdartos Technique for Orchiopexy of Undescended Testicles

Pediatric Urology

The first part of the operation consists of exploring the inguinal area, isolating the right testicle and its cord. Every effort is made to preserve the blood supply. Equally important is freeing and straightening the cord so that increased length of the cord has been assured.

113-1. The subdartos technique is shown. This layer can be dissected free as shown. It is important to also make a distal transverse incision in the inferior right scrotum so the subdartos compartment can be more easily freed.

113-2. The testicle has been placed into the new scrotal compartment and fixed to the subdartos-scrotal tissue. The inferior incision is closed. The superior scrotal incision is closed with 5–0 Prolene sutures. Care is taken to fix the cord without interfering with the blood supply and the vas deferens.

113-3. This reveals the sagittal diagram with emphasis on the dartos and the compartment where the testicle now resides.

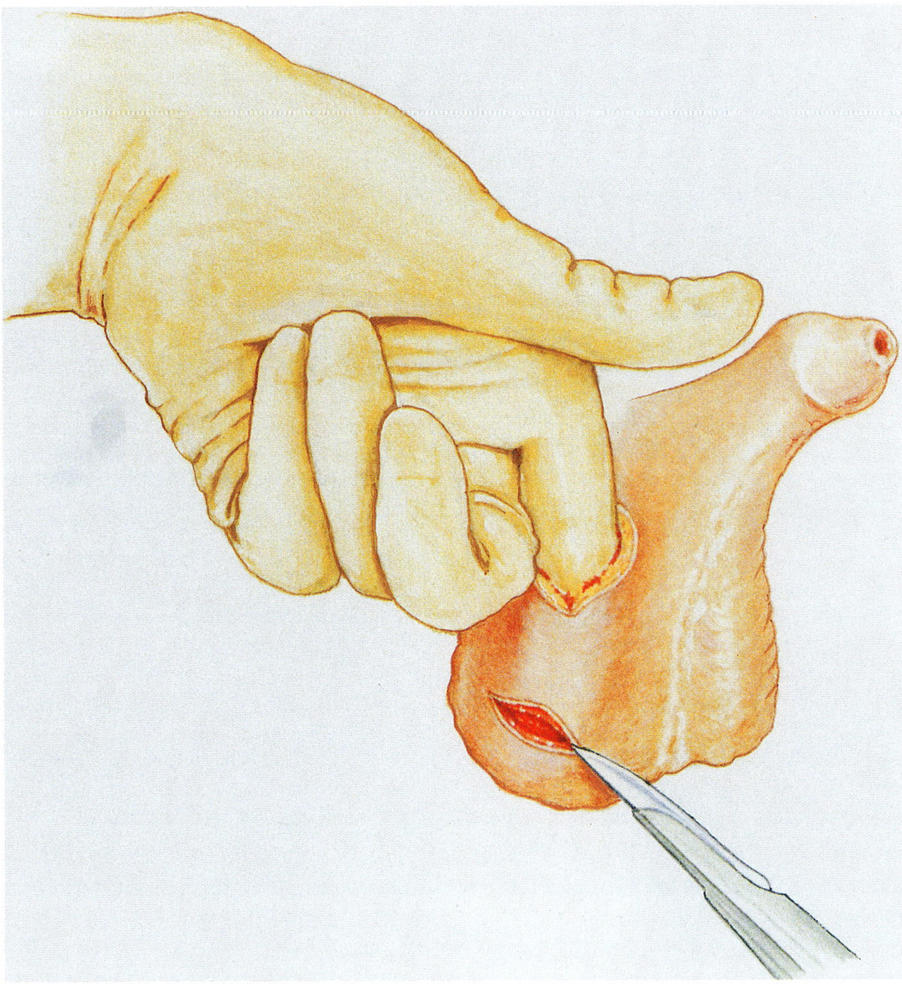

113-1

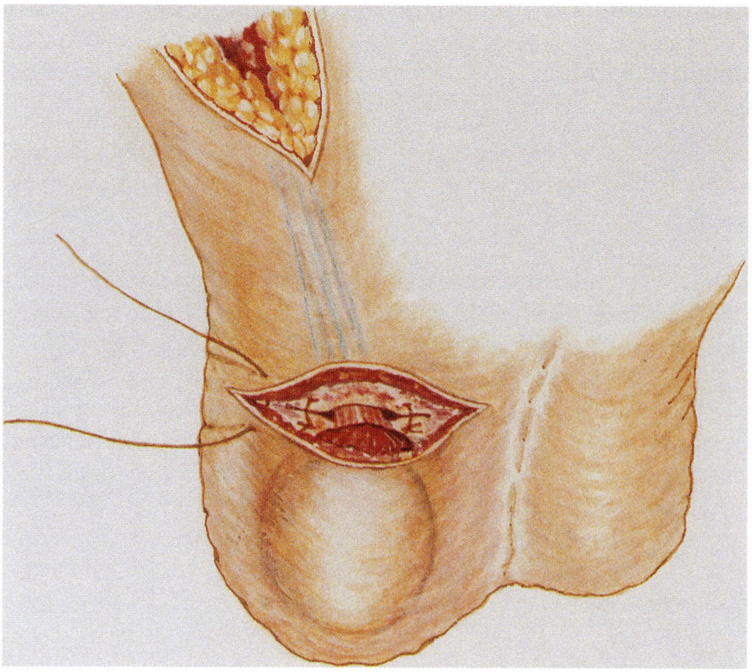

113-2

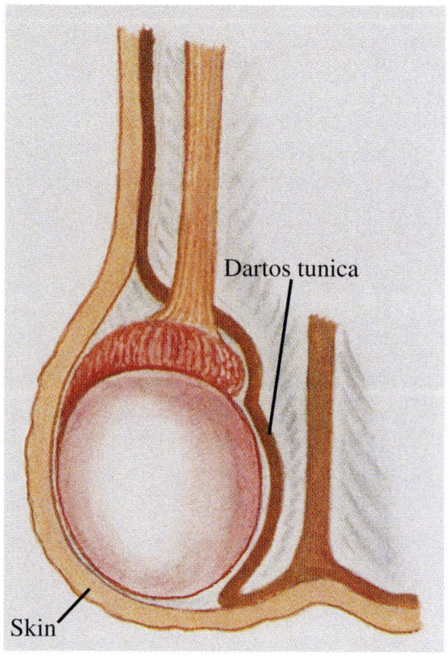

113-3

114. Subcapsular Castration

An alternative to a complete orchiectomy on each side is the technique for subcapsular castration. These procedures would be used as palliative treatment for stage D adenocarcinoma of the prostate. Estrogen therapy is also continued in this selected group of patients.

114-1. The appropriate testis is grasped firmly and immobilized. *A vertical incision is carried down to the tunica albuginea.*

114-2. *The testis is delivered outside the scrotal incision.* The tunica albuginea is incised, and both margins are grasped. The seminiferous tubules are removed meticulously.

114-3. *The tubules located at the head of the epididymis are grasped with clamps.* A ligature is placed at the neck and secured.

114-4. *The margins of the tunica albuginea are reapproximated.* The scrotum and underlying fascia are closed by layers (Fig. 109-4). A drain is not needed since a compression dressing can be used if needed.

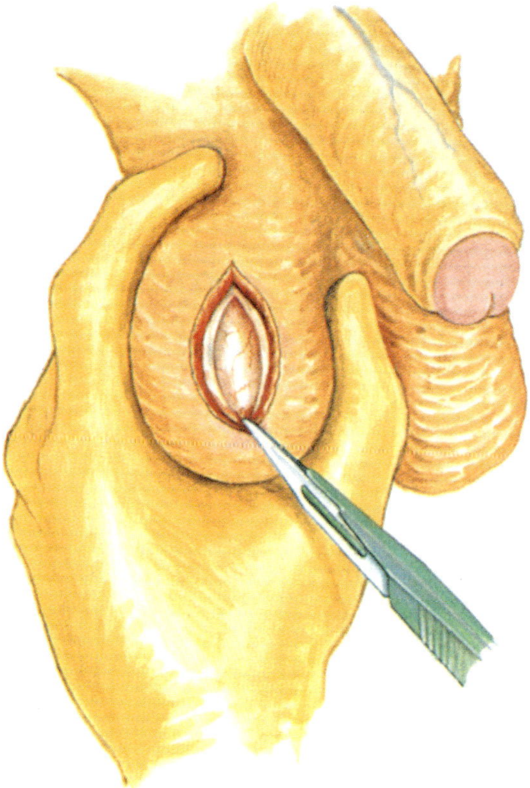

114-1

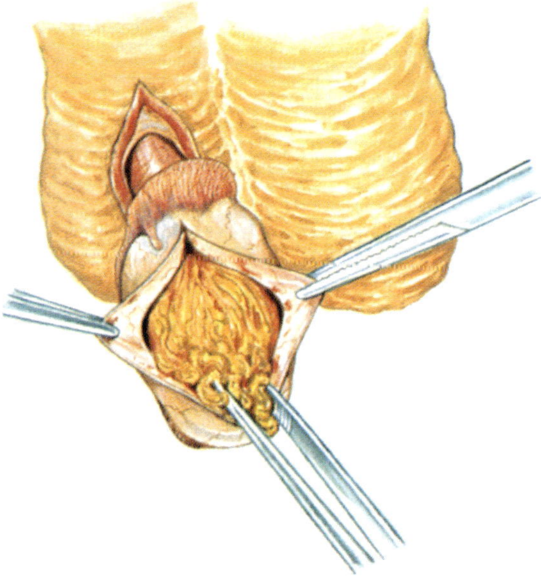

114-2

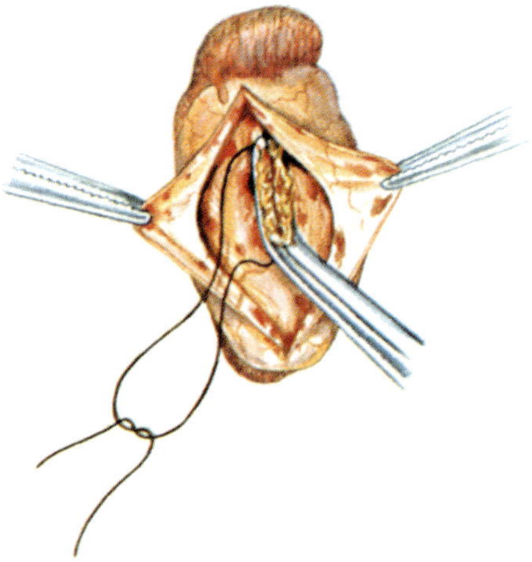

114-3

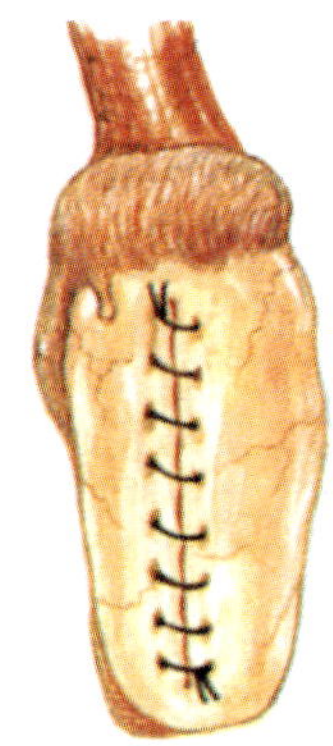

114-4

115. Right Radical Orchiectomy

Enlargement and induration of a testis may be secondary to neoplasia. A variety of germinal cell tumors can occur in the male between 18 and 35 years of age. There is no history of trauma in the case of neoplasia, although an acute injury may bring the involved testis to the physician's attention.

In nonseminomatous germinal tumors, biochemical markers in the blood may serve as useful prognostic indicators; these are considered in the discussion of bilateral retroperitoneal lymph node dissection (see section 116).

115-1. *The inguinal incision extends from internal ring down to the superior portion of the right scrotum* (dotted line).

115-2. The external oblique aponeurosis is incised and retracted. The entire spermatic cord is dissected free, starting near the external inguinal ring. A flat tubular drain is used to isolate the cord, exposing the internal oblique muscle. The proximal cord is clamped with a rubber-shod clamp before delivering the testis into the wound. The scrotal incision can be extended inferiorly if the testicular mass is moderately enlarged.

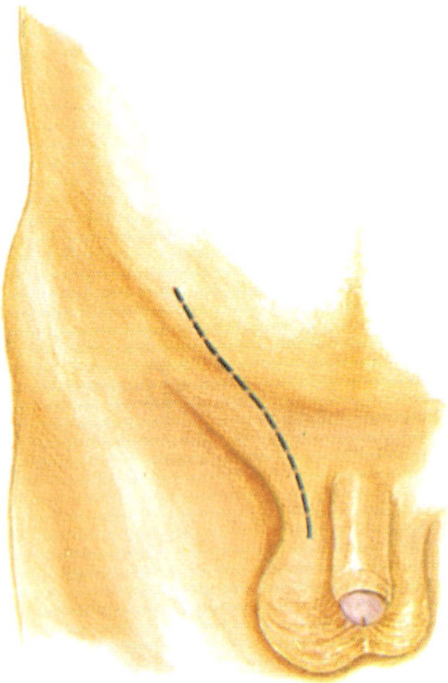

115-1

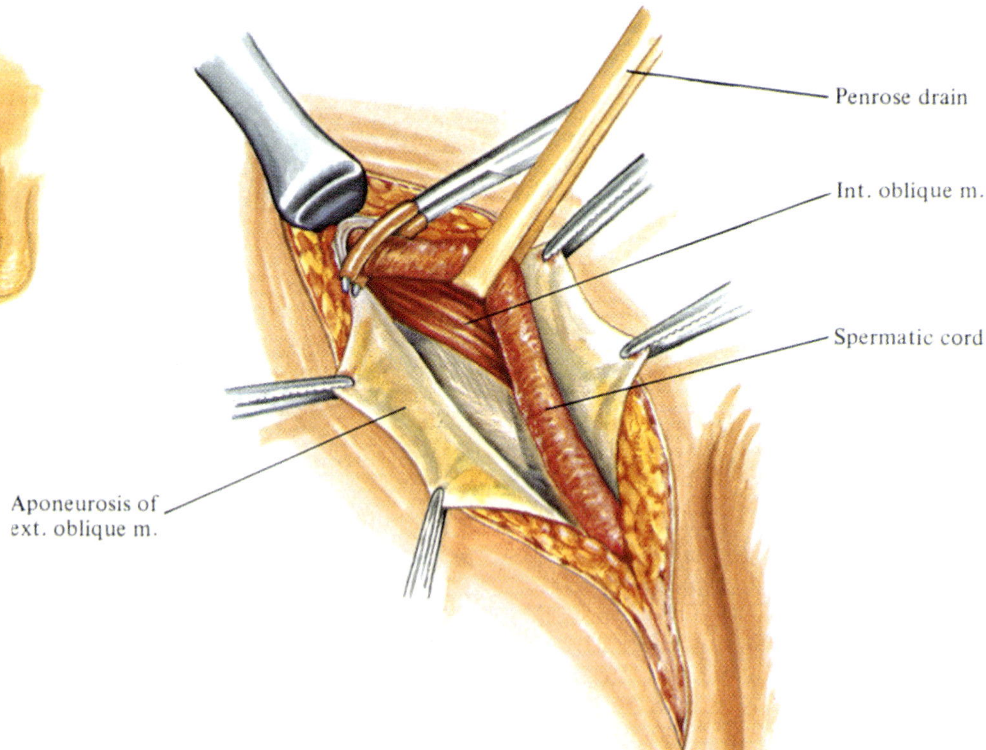

115-2

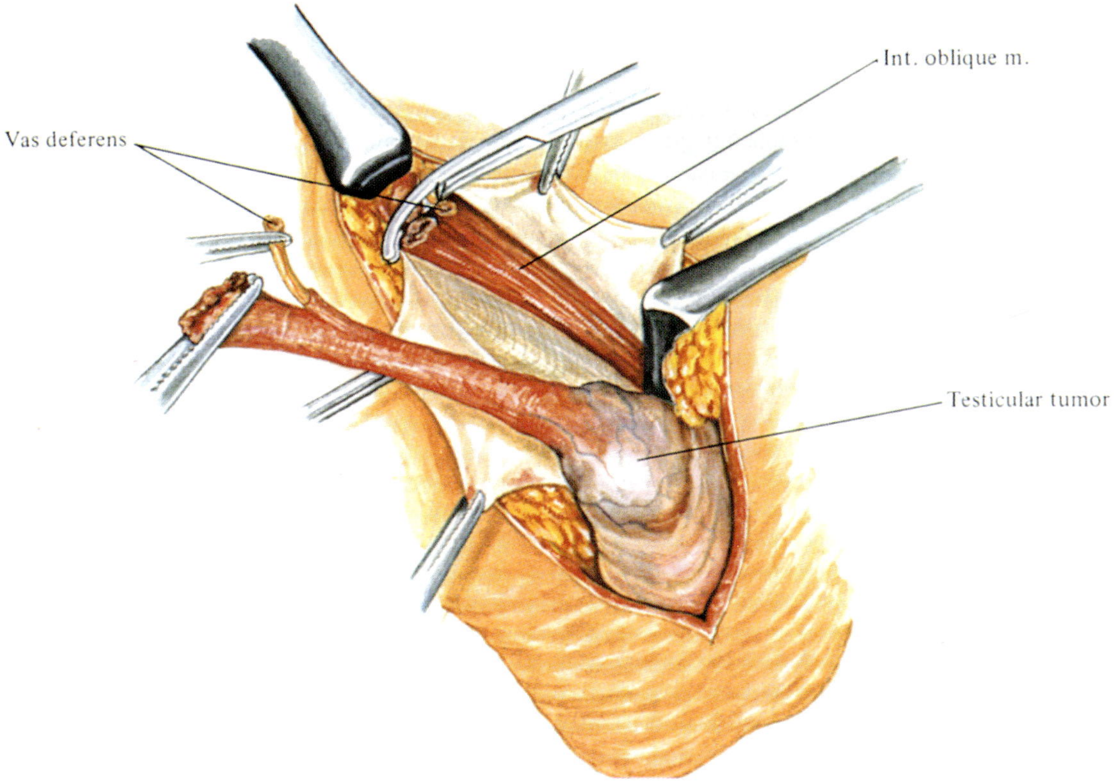

115-3

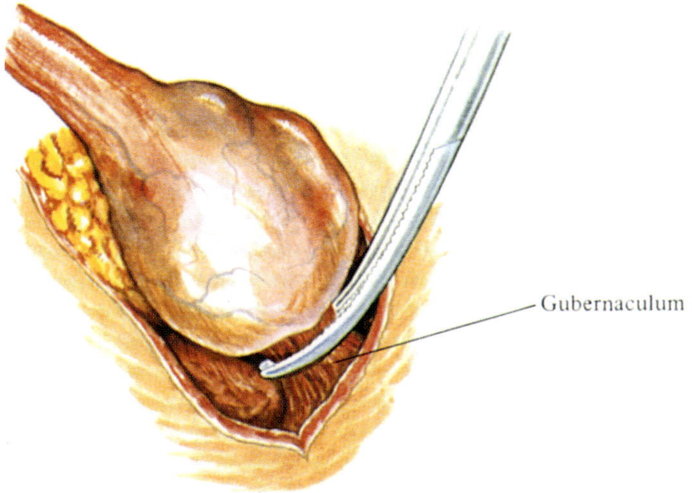

115-4

115-3. *The spermatic cord is doubly clamped.* Care is taken to separate the vas deferens from the vascular and lymphatic structures. Separate clamps are used during transection of the cord. Separate ligatures (2–0 silk) are placed around the proximal cord and vas deferens.

115-4. *The gubernaculum is freed and clamped.* The testis and attached spermatic cord are removed.

116. Bilateral Retroperitoneal Lymph Node Dissection

Before lymph node dissection is undertaken, it is worth determining if the tumor has extended beyond the inguinal canal. Certain diagnostic studies are indicated.

Pedal lymphangiography has been recommended in a few instances. It is often useful in demarcating areas of lymph node metastasis (80%). We agree with Skinner,[2] however, who has stated that the contrast medium employed interferes with the ease of surgical dissection. We no longer obtain lymphangiography routinely.

A chest study with tomography is useful to rule out the presence of tumor metastasis.

An intravenous urogram is obtained if a recent study has not already been performed. We now believe that the computed tomographic scan (with contrast media in the kidney), focusing on the retroperitoneal node sites between aortic bifurcation and renal pedicles, is the most definitive study for evaluating the presence of positive lymph nodes. We have been impressed by its usefulness, particularly around the great vessels at the renal pedicle.

In nonseminomatous germinal tumors the biochemical markers in the bloodstream are also useful. Elevated titers of human chorionic gonadotropin (beta subunit) and/or alpha fetoprotein are indicative of lymph node metastasis.

116-1. *A midline incision is employed, extending from the xiphoid to the symphysis pubis.* The abdomen is explored. If nodes are enlarged above the renal pedicle, then the case is inoperable and only a biopsy is taken. Tumor sites are marked with silver clips.

116-2. *The retroperitoneal space is fully explored* by mobilizing the entire left colon and retracting it to the right. The transverse colon is protected and placed on the superior abdominal wall over a moist drape. The small intestines are placed in a plastic bag and the noose is tightened at the root of the mesentery. The small bowel is placed on the right lateral abdominal wall.

The duodenum is mobilized medially and superiorly to expose the right renal pedicle.

116-3. *Dissection of the ipsilateral renal pedicle (left) is begun.* All lymphatics and areolar tissue are removed circumferentially around the renal vein and artery, extending superiorly to the superior mesenteric artery. The spermatic artery near its origin and the vein are dissected on the left, doubly ligated, and transected in between. The dissection is carried anteriorly over the aorta and to the inferior vena cava. The dissection is now extended circumferentially, around the right renal vein and renal artery. Fatty tissue from the lateral portion of the vena cava is dissected free en bloc. Lumbar veins behind the vena cava and below the renal pedicle may be doubly ligated with small-size hemoclips. An umbilical tape, carefully placed superior to the right renal vein and behind the vena cava, assists in the dissection posterior to the vena cava. A second umbilical tape is now placed around the aorta above the crossing of the left renal vein. This maneuver assists in the dissection between the two great vessels and behind the aorta. All the lymphatic and areolar tissues are removed from around and between both great vessels. The lateral borders for the dissection are the longitudinal course of each ureter. The dissection is carried down past the bifurcation of the aorta. We usually ligate and transect the inferior mesenteric artery to assist in the complete dissection.

Dissection is usually continued distally to the bifurcation of the common iliac artery on the contralateral side. On the side of the tumor, the spermatic artery and vein, along with the cord (the vas deferens coursing from the prostate), are dissected and removed en toto to the internal inguinal abdominal ring.

After completion of the dissection, the aorta can be lifted from its posterior bed except for the posterior attachments of the lumbar arteries, major tributaries, superior

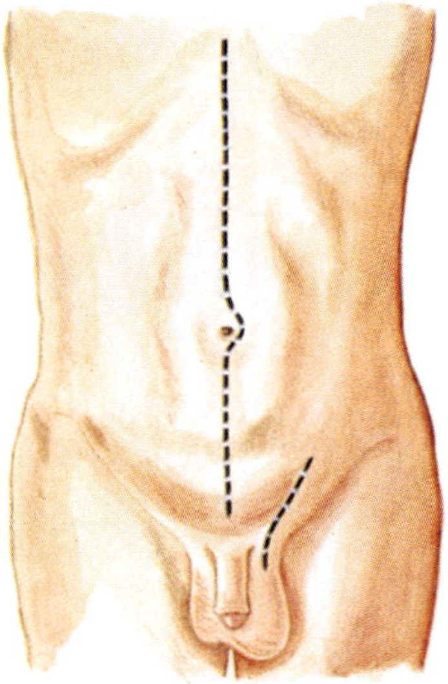

116-1

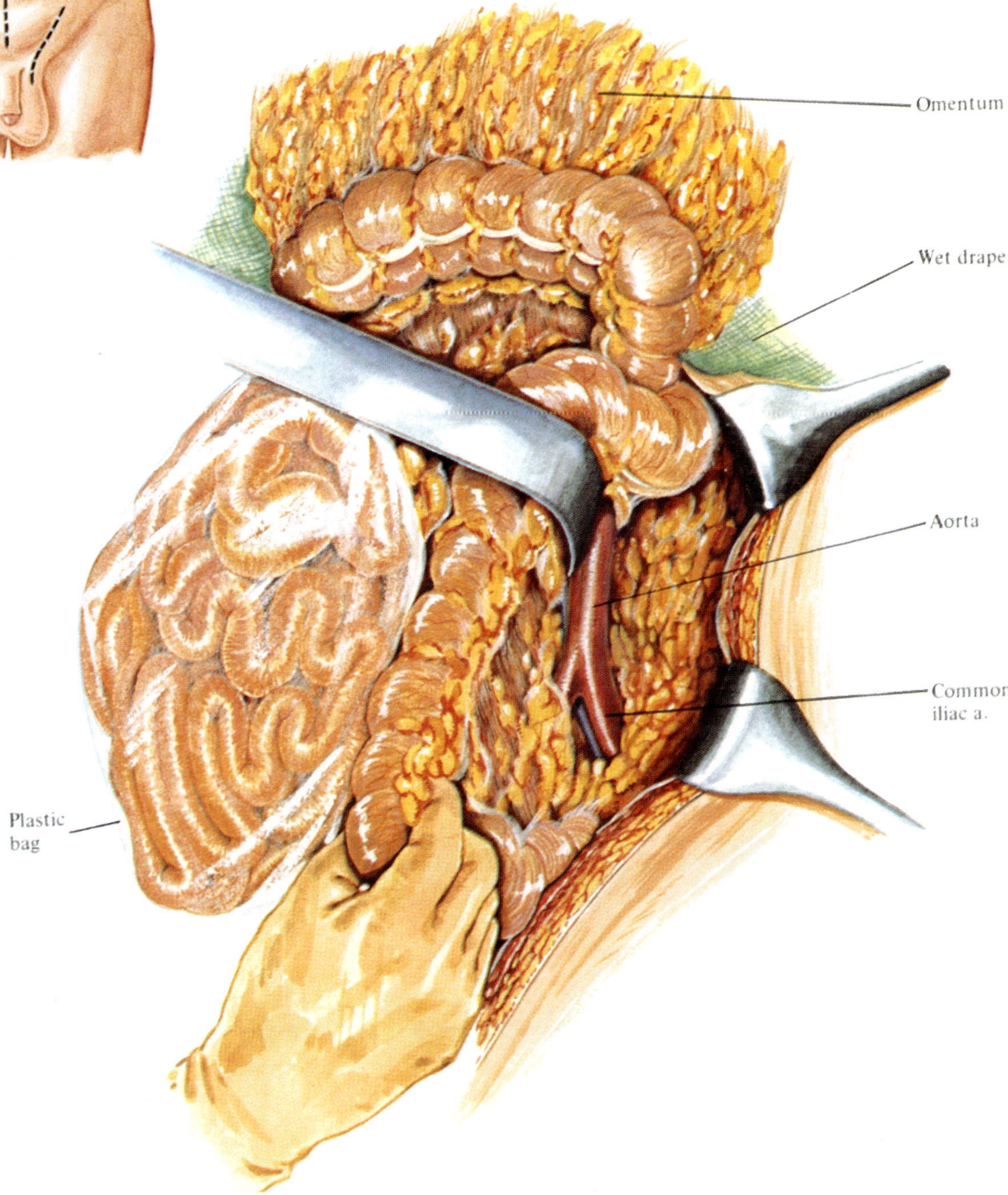

116-2

mesenteric artery, and both renal arteries. The inferior vena cava can be similarly elevated. No areolar or lymphatic tissue is seen when the great vessels are moved in various directions.

After the dissection is completed, the mobilized duodenum and left descending colon are replaced in their original location and sutured to the parietal peritoneum. A routine appendectomy is not usually performed.

Closure is by layers. We use 0–0 nylon interrupted sutures on the fascia instead of wire. A flat tubular drain is not necessary.

116-4. *The lymph node dissection for a right-sided nonseminomatous germinal tumor is completed.* The vena cava is retracted laterally. Both renal pedicles can be seen. The right spermatic vein is ligated proximally. The ureters can be seen on each side. The inferior mesenteric artery has been preserved in this instance.

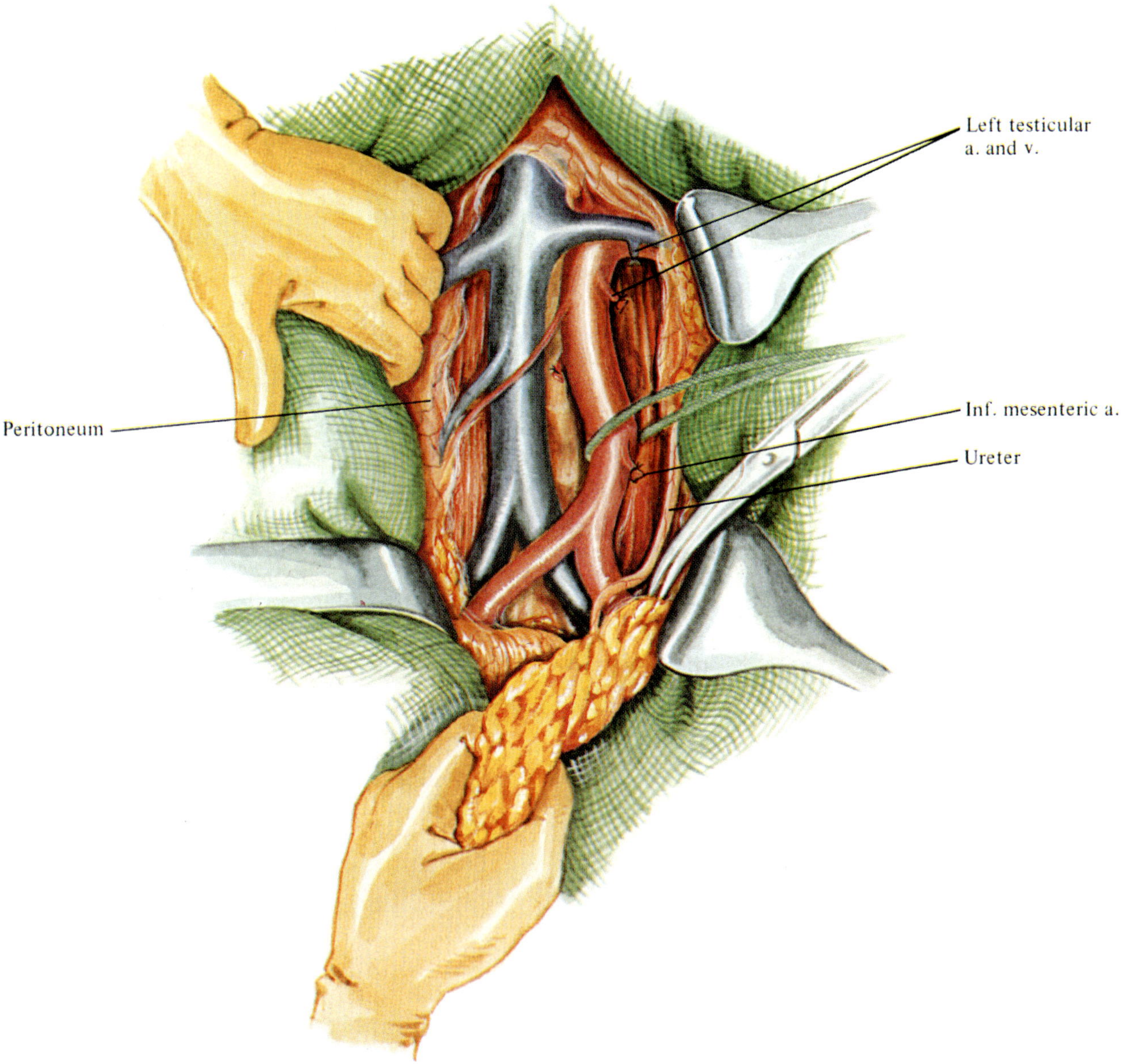

116-3

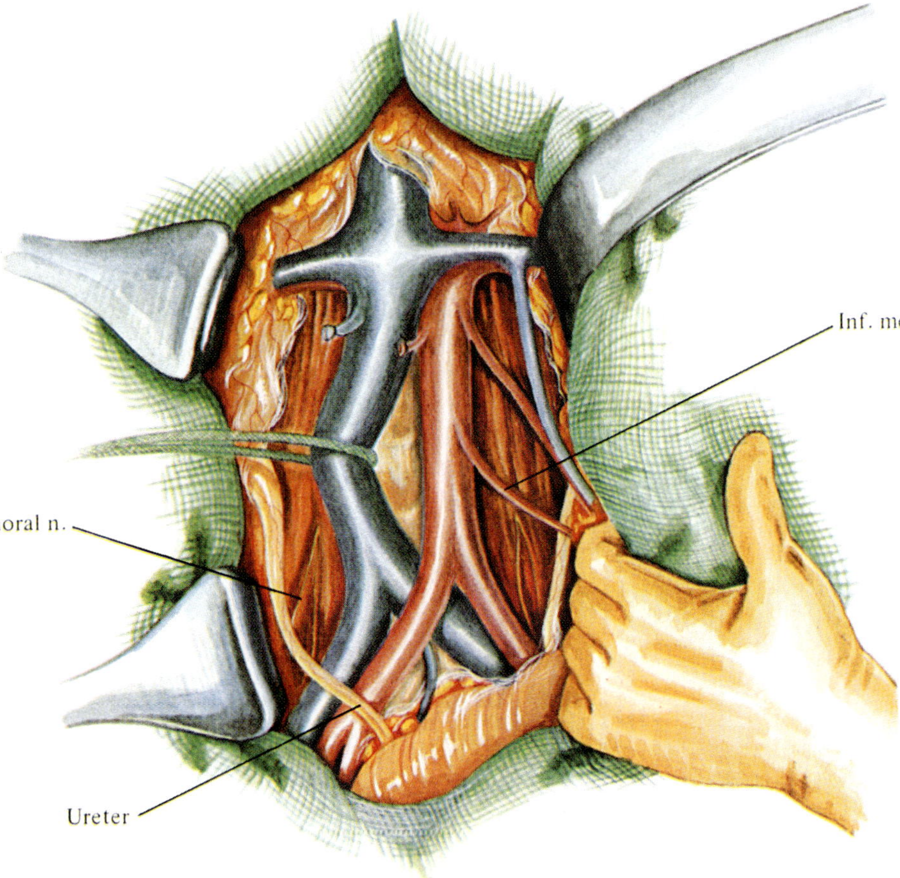

116-4

117. Nerve Sparing Technique

In a report by Donohue et al.,[3] the feasibility of nerve sparing (sympathetic nerve sparing) postganglionic fibers in the lumbar region has been reported. Keeping intact the postsympathetic nerves or postejaculatory branches are important.

Most of the patients (73 of the 75 men) had testicular neoplasms, i.e., teratocarcinoma, clinical stage I disease. A smaller group (14 men) had pathological stage II cancer. Of importance is the fact that none of the men were treated with adjuvant chemotherapy after the nerve sparing retroperitoneal lymphadenectomy. Only 4 of the 14 with stage II disease had a relapse and they are now free of cancer following chemotherapy and/or surgical rescue.

Preservation of Emission

From recent reports[4] it would appear that lumbar sympathetic, postganglionic fibers—lumbar fibers 1 to 4—are important for emission and subsequent antegrade ejaculation. The other important aspect relating to the template for dissection needs emphasis. Paraaortic tissues below the inferior mesenteric artery must be carefully dissected and removed. The postganglionic fibers below the inferior mesenteric artery must be preserved. These sympathetic postganglionic fibers ultimately course inferiorly and contribute to the hypogastric plexus. This hypogastric plexus terminates in the seminal vesicle and the ampulla of the vas.

117-1. This illustration includes the anatomic structures that surround the retroperitoneal lymph nodes. The inferior mesenteric artery at its origin is seen. The chain of lymph nodes are also seen. For purposes of discussion, the lumbar sympathetic chain is shown laterally on the abdominal aorta. The location of the chain is posterior to the aorta and is between the great vessels.

117-2. (Illustration from Donahue et al. J Urol 144:287, 1990.) When the tumor is on the right side, the right template is the area of dissection. In our experience it is always a good idea to place a small Penrose drain around and above the aorta and vena cava to control inadvertent bleeding from an obscure lumbar branch. A similar Penrose drain is placed around the vena cava and aorta below the area of dissection.

The template for dissection on the left side is also shown. The retroperitoneal dissection includes the retroperitoneal-para-aortic and para-venacaval nodes. The postganglionic-sympathetic nerves must be preserved.

Dr. John Donohue from Indiana has the largest experience with surgery for testicular neoplasms that also have lymph node involvement in the retroperitoneal area.

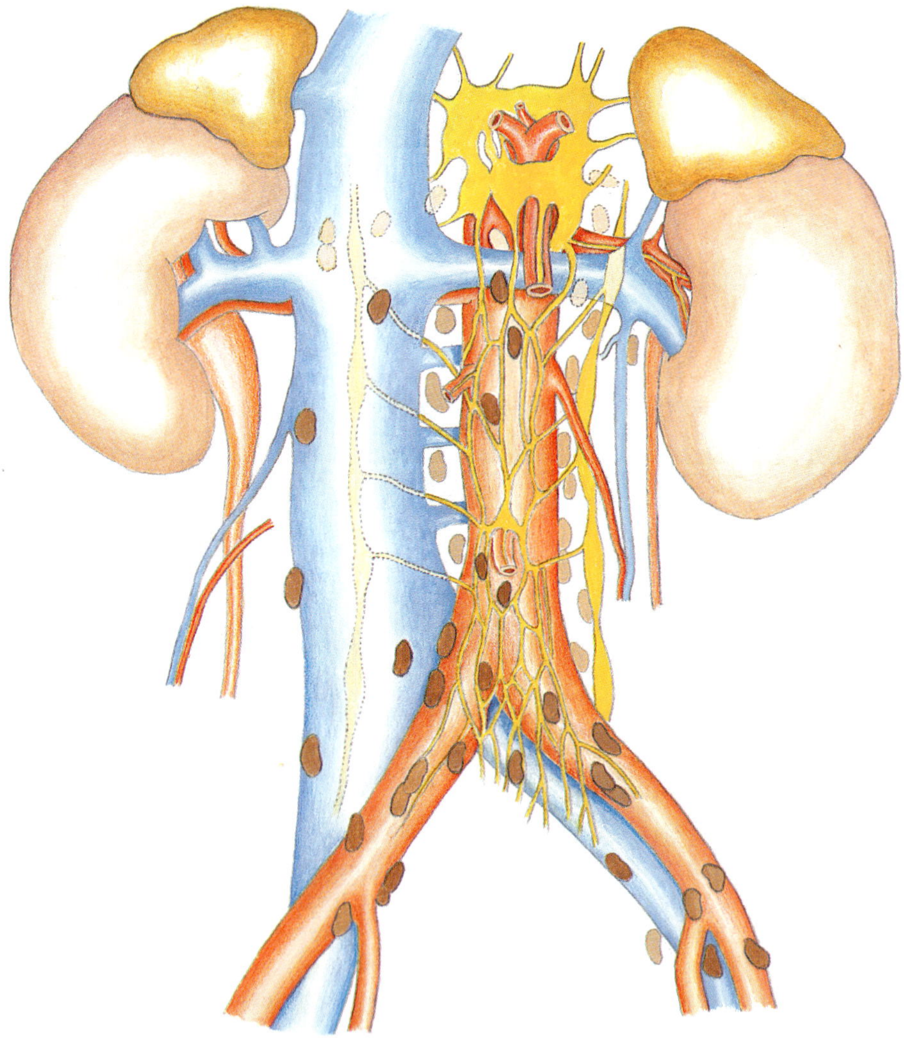

117-1

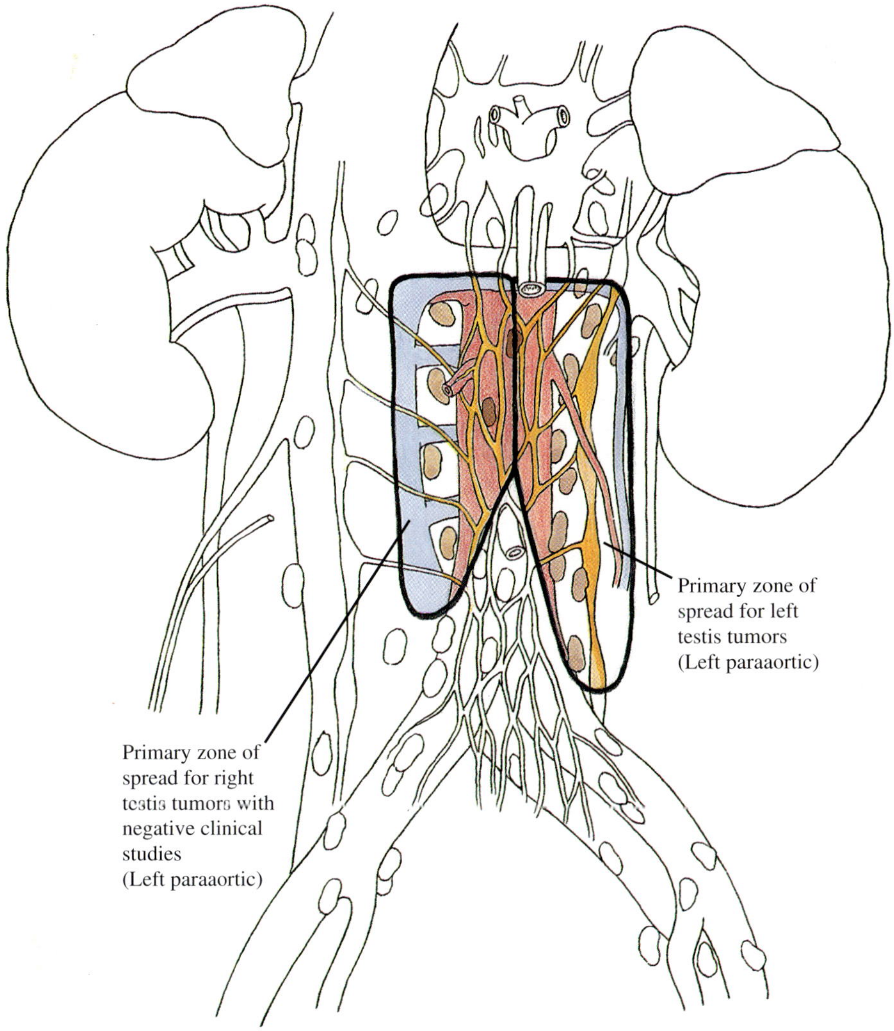

117-2

Chemotherapy is usually needed to shrink or render lymph nodes noncancerous. A nerve sparing technique in the retroperitoneum is important to preserve emission and ejaculation. Donohue's large experience of nerve sparing lymphadenectomy with preservation of ejaculation is worthy of restatement.

In the illustration for 117–1, the major lymph nodes are shown particularly medial and adjacent to the inferior vena cava, the lower abdominal aorta and the retroperitoneal sites in between these great vessels and lateral to the vessels. The pathways are shown focusing on the lumbar sympathetic nerves.

Lymph node dissection in the retroperitoneum requires surgeons to have knowledge of the map outlining the lumbar vessels generally in younger men with testicular neoplasms. During dissection, the template of dissection is determined by the clinical stage and intraoperative findings.

The illustration 117-2 can be divided into two regions retroperitoneally. For right testicular neoplasm (nonseminomatous type), the primary zone of lymph node spread is in the right para-aortic region.

In left testicular neoplasms (nonseminomatous neoplasms), the area of dissection is the left para-aortic zone. The template includes the area to the left of the retroperitoneum as shown. The left para-aortic nodes must be removed. The sympathetic nerve—postganglionic fibers in the lumbar region—must be preserved.

Epididymal and Spermatic Cord Surgery

118. Epididymectomy

Inflammation of the epididymis secondary to bacterial infection may leave a slightly enlarged and tender epididymal body. If the patient is past the third decade of life and is symptomatic, an epididymectomy may be indicated.

118-1. *The testis surrounded by its fascial investments is delivered outside the scrotum.* The tunica vaginalis of the testis is opened. The edges are retracted. Care must be taken in dissecting the head and body of the epididymis from the testis. As the dissection proceeds, the testicular branch and epididymal branch of the internal spermatic artery can be isolated. The testicular branch must be preserved.

The vas deferens can be divided superiorly and ligated on both sides.

118-2. *The tunica vaginalis of the testis can then be loosely reapproximated* with interrupted 3–0 chromic catgut sutures.

118-3. *Scrotal skin closure is completed.* A flat tubular drain is optional, depending on the amount of inflammation and drainage encountered. The drain is removed in 24 hours.

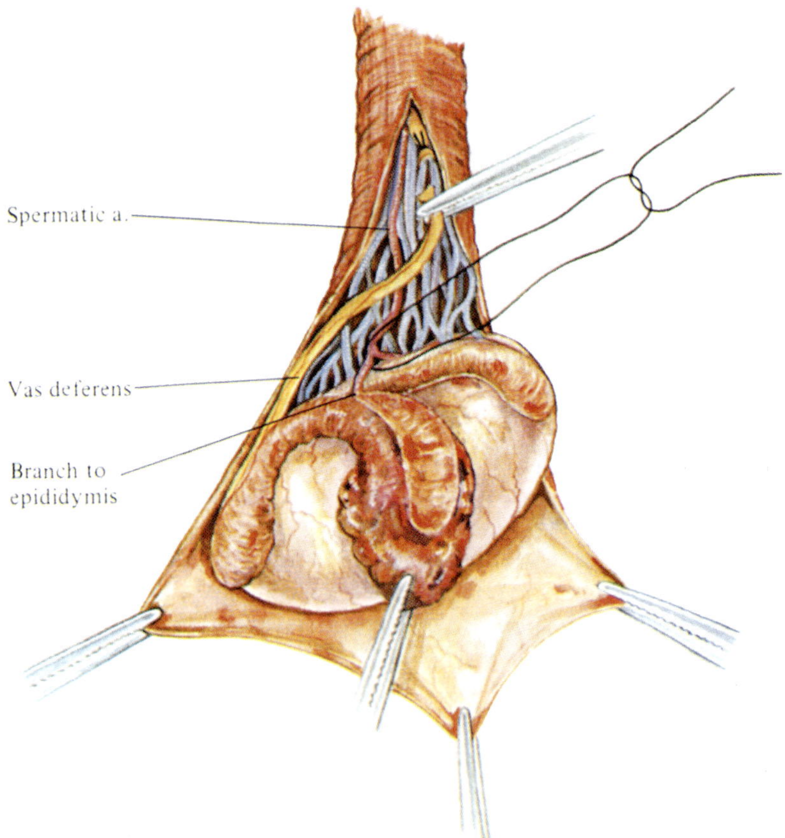

118-1

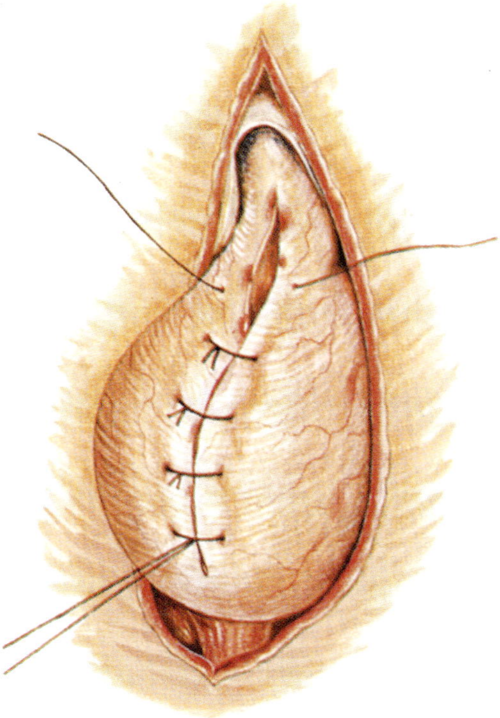

118-2

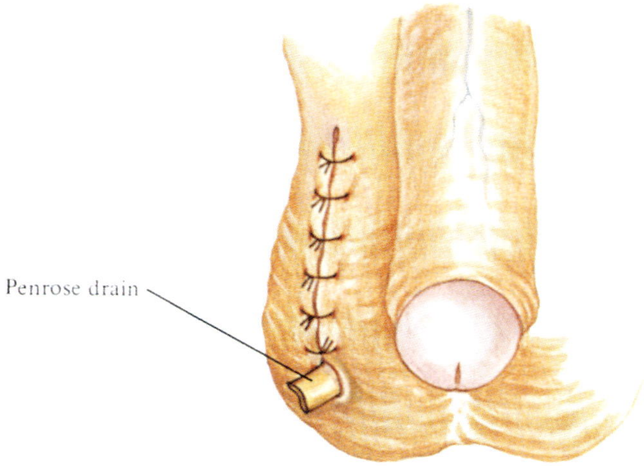

118-3

119. Epididymovasostomy

The indication for this procedure is the finding of a selective block or fibrosis in the distal tail of the epididymis. Tests indicate that the patient is azoospermic and a distal vasogram demonstrates the site of blockage.

119-1. The body of the epididymis near the tail is freed. The vas deferens near the tail is also freed. It is important that the tubular ramifications in the body of the epididymis be incised so that an artificial reservoir is created. *Elliptical incisions are made in each structure.* A plastic (Silastic) stent attached to a 24-gauge needle assists in the alignment of both structures. Microvascular instruments and a dissecting microscope are helpful.

119-2. *Side-to-side anastomosis is completed* with 7–0 nylon sutures. The needle is removed and the superior end of the stent is left in the lumen of the vas deferens about 3 cm from the new opening. The inferior end of the stent, attached to a button, is secured outside the skin incision. This allows easy removal of the stent after 12 to 14 days.

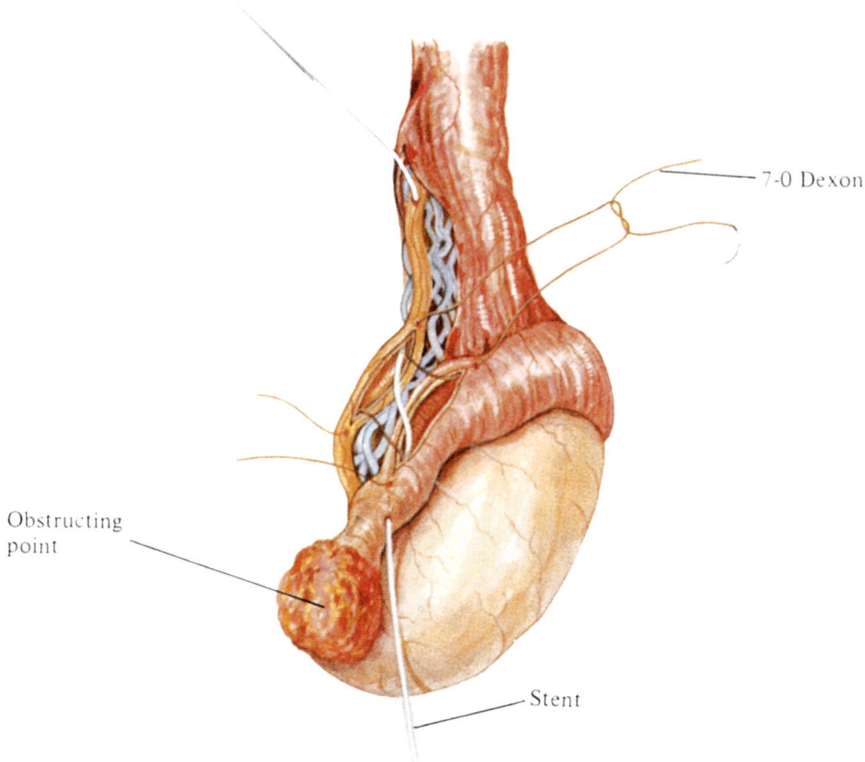

119-1

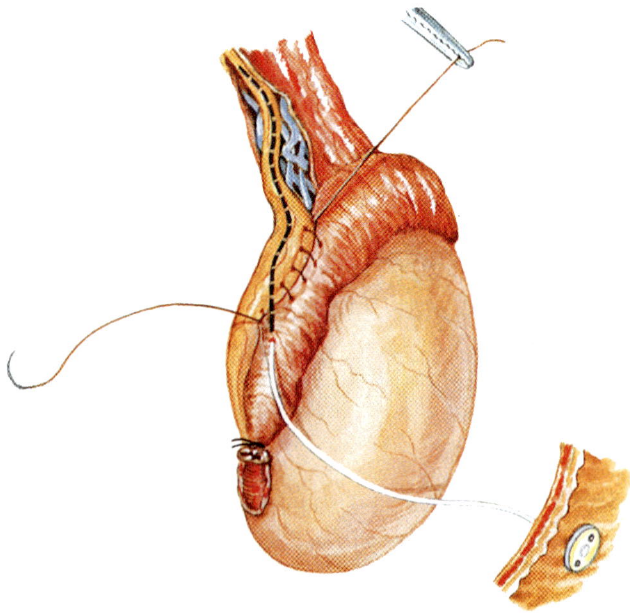

119-2

120. Torsion of the Spermatic Cord

Torsion of the spermatic cord (torsion of the "testis") occurs because of faulty embryogenesis that allows free rotation of the testis. It can be a bilateral problem. In the normal male a fascial attachment exists between the testis-epididymis and the inner wall of the scrotum.

The diagnosis of torsion is based on exclusion and a high index of suspicion. Epididymitis in the acute phase will manifest itself as part of an acute or subacute prostatitis. Pyuria will be seen in the urine specimen. Scrotal pain is severe. There may be elevation of the testis on the affected side because of torsion. Radioisotopic imaging studies of the scrotum are useful in making the diagnosis. One would expect to find a good vascular response with technetium pertechnate (^{99m}Tc) or similar isotopes in the normal testicle. A compromised vascular pedicle would show vascular insufficiency by isotope uptake studies.

120-1. A scrotal incision is made and carried through the fascial investments. *The tunica vaginalis of the testis is opened.* The cyanotic, twisted testis may be found. We believe that early exploration within 6–10 hours after onset of symptoms will result in a higher salvage rate of such affected testes.

120-2. *The spermatic cord is untwisted.* If the tunic is adherent to the scrotum, it is freed, and three sutures are placed to anchor the testicle. The sutures must include dartos if the tunic is mobile.

The contralateral testis should be similarly corrected.

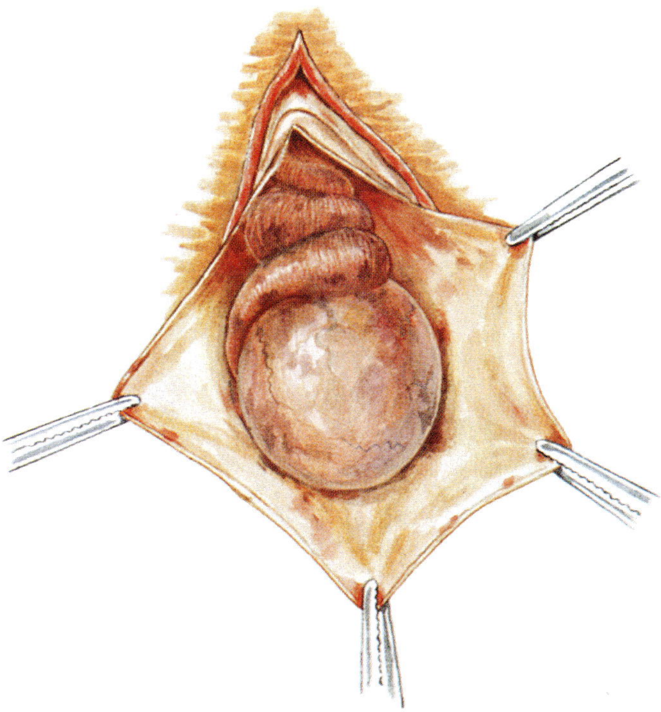

120-1

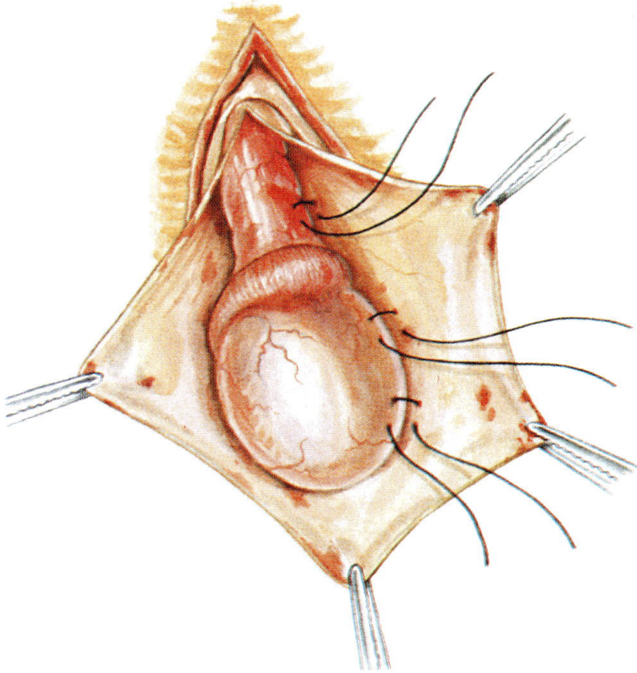

120-2

121. Bilateral Vasovasostomy

The usual candidate for bilateral vasovasostomy has undergone bilateral partial vasectomy 1 to 8 years previously. He is now married for the second time, often to a younger woman, and the couple desire to start a second family.

The problem of sperm autoantibodies arising in the male is still unsettled. We have been impressed at the poor semen quality in patients who have undergone vasectomy more than 5 years prior to vasovasostomy. In most instances, the numbers of sperm following surgery are adequate (more than 20 million per milliliter).

Although the procedure is illustrated on the left side, a bilateral approach through separate incisions is employed.

121-1. *A skin incision is made over the vas deferens.* An Allis clamp is used to grasp the vas deferens.

121-2. The fibrosed, diseased vas deferens enmeshed in a granuloma is excised. Stay sutures assist in exposing both ends of the remaining vas deferens. Sperm coursing from the epididymis can usually be expressed from the lumen.

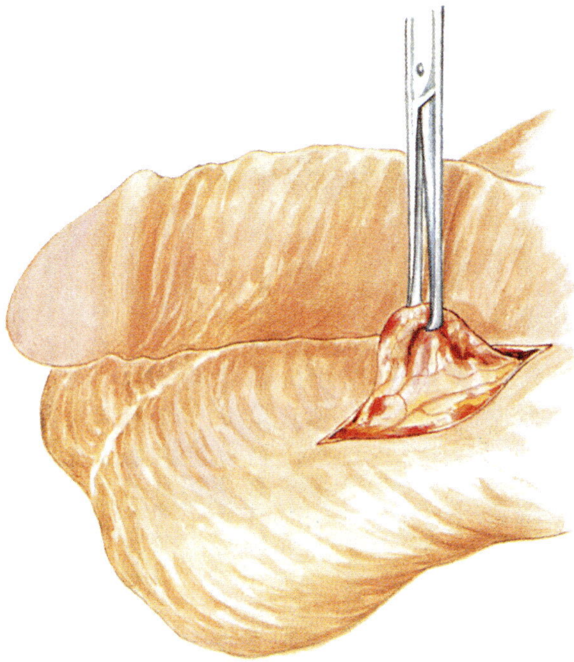

121-1

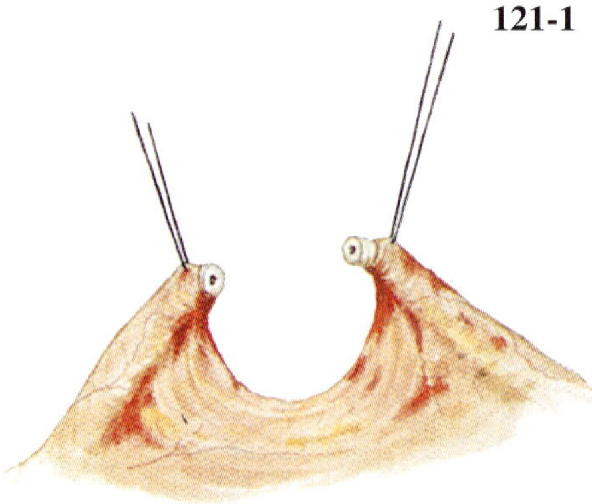

121-2

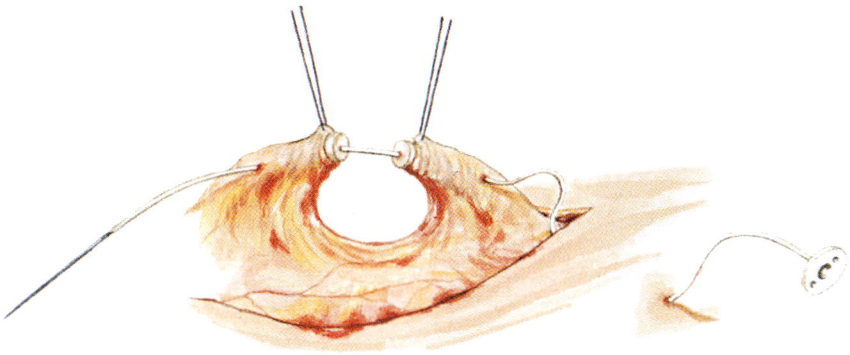

121-3

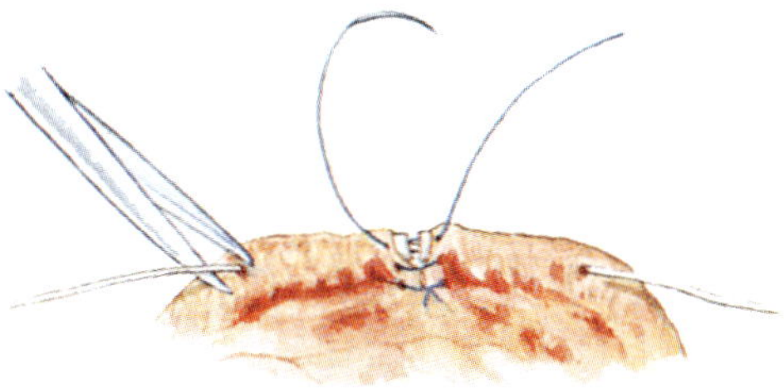

121-4

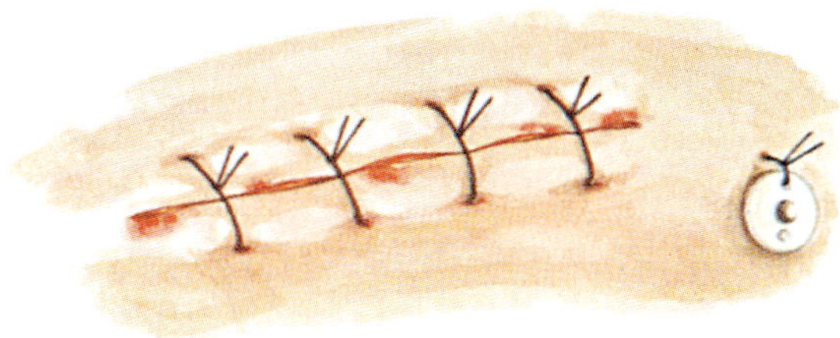

121-5

121-3. We have devised a silicone rubber (Silastic) stent with a 22-, 24-, or 26-gauge needle glued to each end of small stents in three sizes. Both blunt needles can be used to enter the lumen in opposite directions from each interrupted end of the vas deferens. The plastic (Silastic) button is attached to the stent on the superior side outside the skin by using a special sterilized tube of silicone glue.

121-4. *The end of each vas deferens is reapproximated* with 8–0 nylon sutures (four to six). Care is taken to place the sutures, including the mucosa, at right angles. The stent on the inferior side is cut just prior to skin closure; the end of the stent is allowed to lie in lumen. Loupes are helpful during the anastomosis. A second layer excluding the opithelium is helpful.

121-5. *The fascial layers and skin are closed separately.* The plastic button is secured to the skin. We keep the stents in place for 2 to 4 days.

122. Microscopic Vasovasostomy to Reestablish Transport of Viable Sperm

The typical male patient has usually fathered a family (1–2 children) with his first wife. Following a divorce, the male usually meets and finally marries a younger second wife. She is insistent that she wants to bear children for her new husband.

Usually, a regional anesthetic can ensure a pain-free scrotal area. The operative technique is as follows: the scrotum on one side is opened at the site previously marked. This site includes both ends of the ligated vas deferens.

The ligated vas deferens on each side, superior and inferior ends are carefully freed, taking care not to destroy the blood supply of the artery to the vas deferens.

122-1. After freeing the vas deferens on both sides, a holding clamp is placed. Note that the inferior end has a larger lumen due to increased luminal pressure as the testicle and epididymis attempt to transport sperm.

122-2 and 122-3. The smaller lumen is dilated to the size of the larger lumen. We use interrupted 7–0 or 8–0 Prolene sutures. Loupes can be used to magnify the lumen at this stage and 5 to 6 sutures of interrupted Vicryl (or Prolene) can be used to anastomose the mucosal lining of the lumen.

122-4 through 122-8. The first mucosal suture is placed and tied (knot on submucosal layer). Several mucosal sutures are placed (122–5). In 122–6 another submucosal suture completes the initial layer of closure. In 122–7 and 122–8, the second layer of sutures is placed as shown.

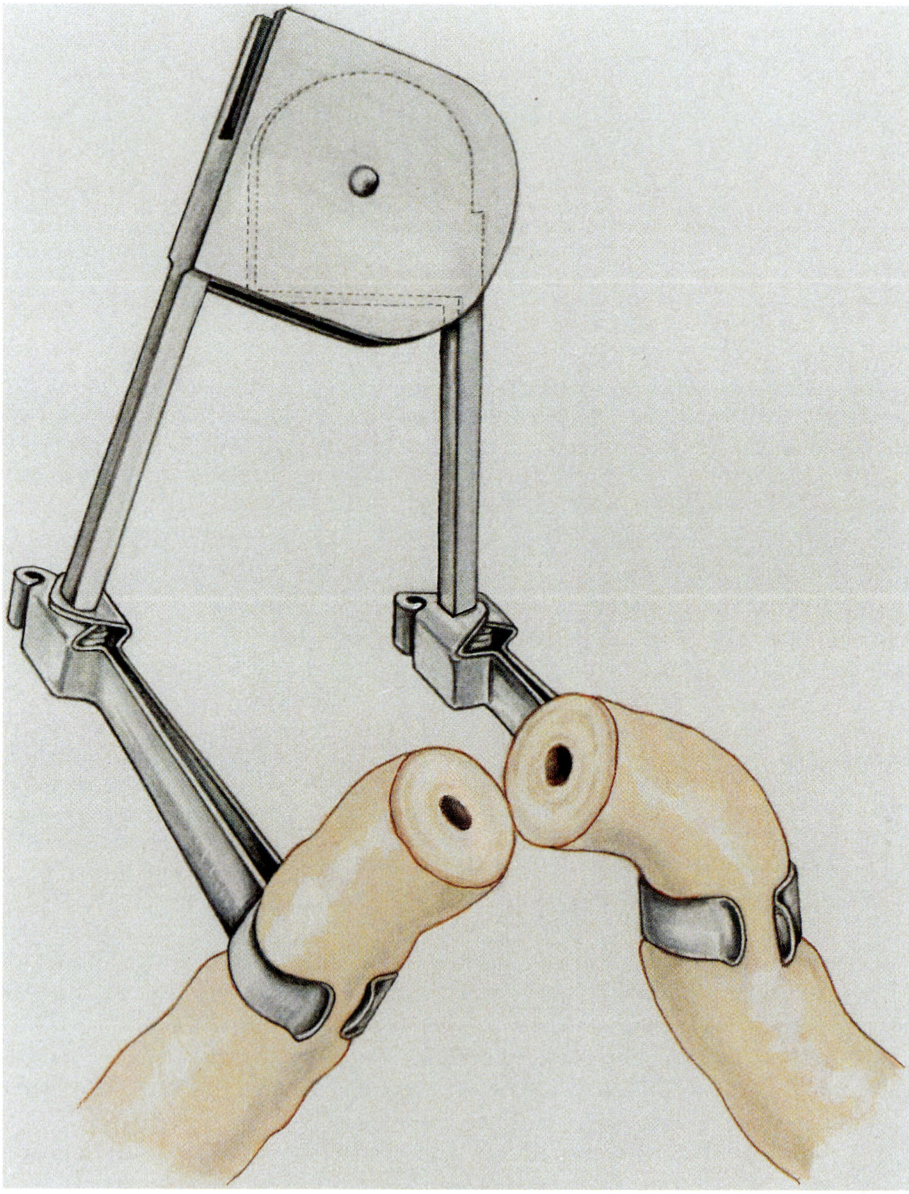

122-1

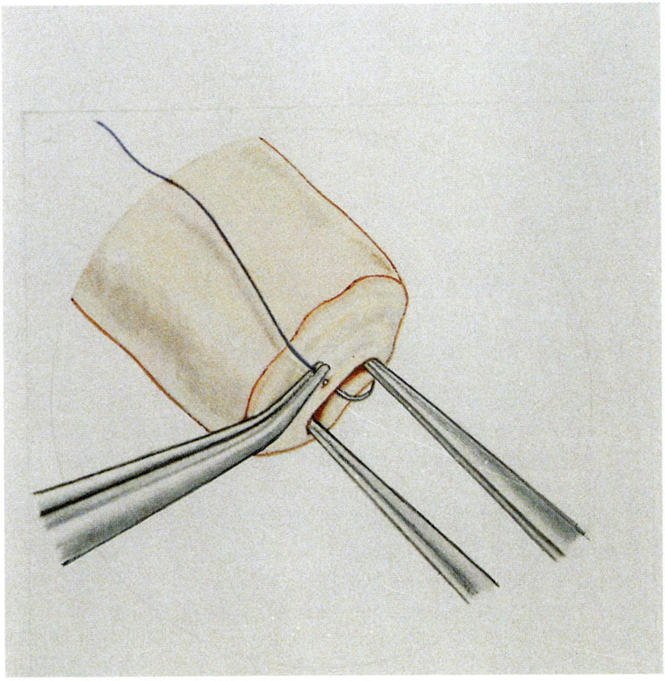
122-2

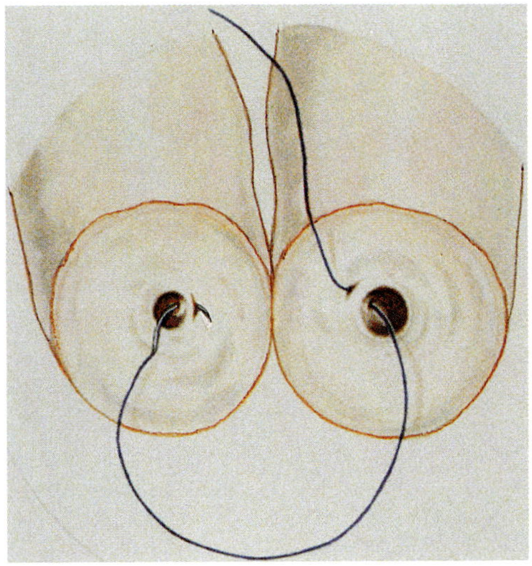
122-3

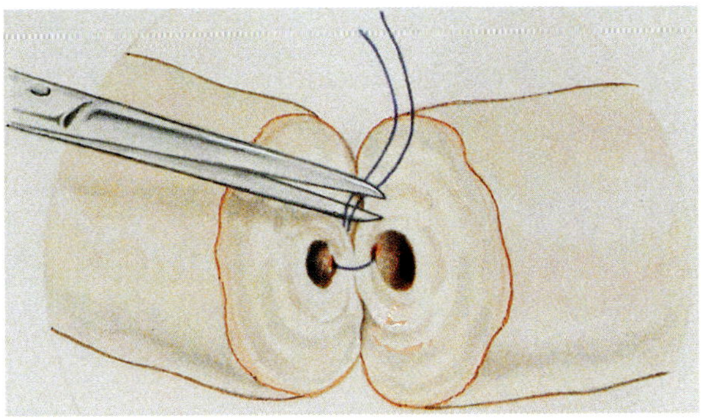
122-4

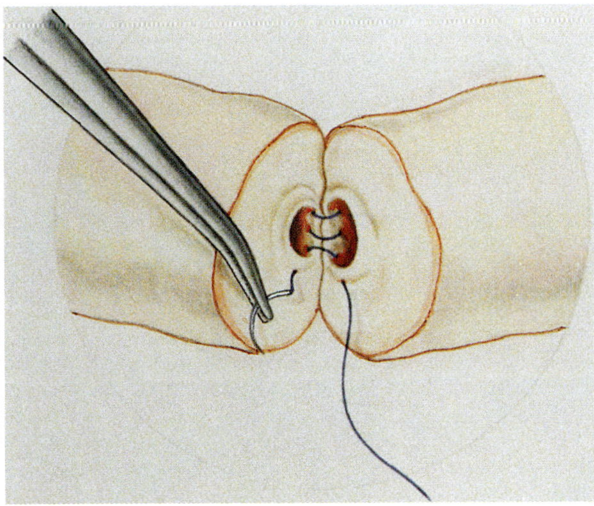
122-5

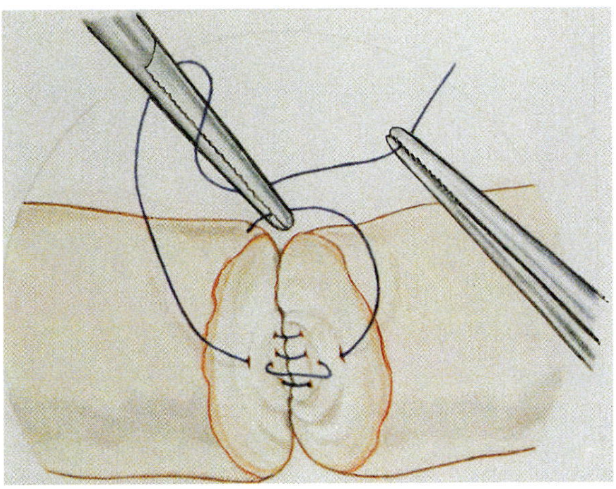
122-6

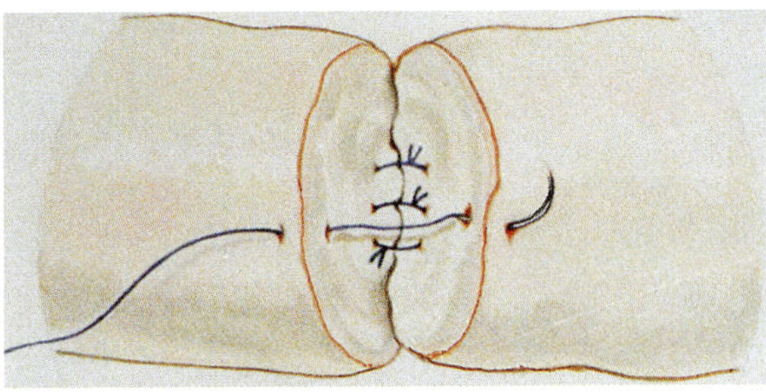
122-7

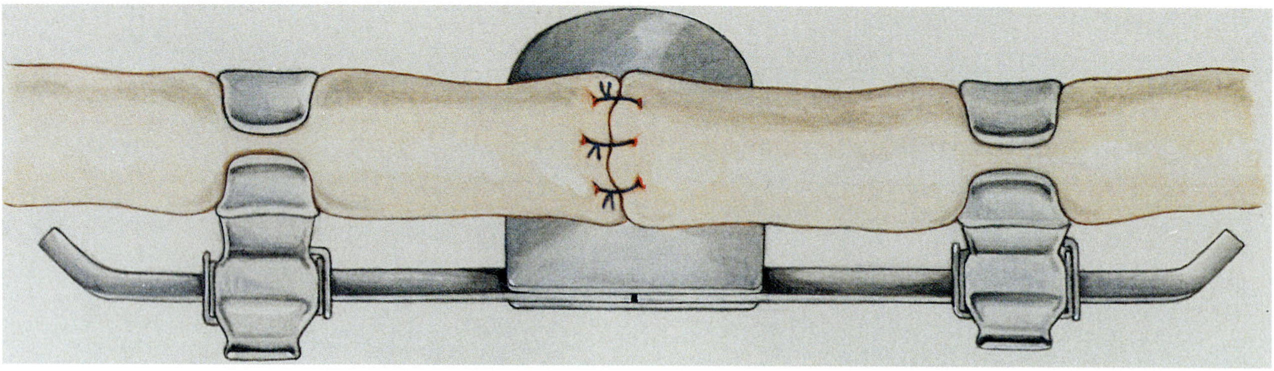

122-8

References

1. Ombredanne L. Indication et technique de l'orchidopexie transscrotale. Presse Med 18:745, 1910.
2. Skinner DG. Considerations for management of large retroperitoneal tumors use of the modified thoracoabdominal approach. J Urol 117:605, 1977.
3. Donohue JP, Foster RS, Rowland RG, Bihrle R, Jones J, Geier G. Nerve-sparing retroperitoneal lymphadenectomy with preservation of ejaculation. J Urol 144:287–292, 1990.
4. Baniel J, Foster RS, Donohue JP. Surgical anatomy of the lumbar vessels: implications for retroperitoneal surgery. J Urol 153:1422–1425, 1995.

Endoscopic Surgery

9

The urologist must be keenly aware of the anatomy within and surrounding both kidneys. We have drawn two illustrations (L2 level and L3 level) that clearly demonstrate the important structures on transverse section. The major vessels can be seen on cross section. The right kidney, adjacent to the liver and gallbladder, can be seen in the first view (Fig. 1). The L3 transverse view now depicts, in the crosssection, part of the ascending colon and the descending colon (Fig. 2).

Figure 3 is a cross section that depicts the anatomic axis. The coronal plane—30°—is demonstrated. In Figures 4A and 4B, Brödel's line on the right and Hodson's line on the left are shown.

Percutaneous Stone Manipulation

Endourology—percutaneous, renal pelviocalyceal removal, or fragmentation of stones—is a proven technique to extricate stone fragments from the appropriate kidney. In the United States, Dr. Ralph Clayman, now a professor of urology at Washington University Medical School in St. Louis, and Professor W. Castaneda-Zuninga, Professor of Radiology at University of Minnesota School of Medicine, published a manual that is a landmark in endourology.[1]

All of the techniques a urologist-endourologist needs to understand are clearly demonstrated in the manual. Today, many urologists will work as part of a team with an experienced radiologist, who is more adept at placing the needle in the appropriate posterior calyx or the appropriate entry point to the renal pelvis.

In the United States, some urologic centers have developed in-house expertise to deal with stones. In other countries outside the United States, e.g., Japan, experience has been obtained by dedicated urologists who have gained the expertise to introduce the appropriate instruments, starting first with a long percutaneous needle with an obturator. Our color atlas provides several examples.

In the "classic" left kidney, the calyces can be numbered from 1 to 8 (Fig. 5). Calyces 1 and 8 are compounded polar calyces. The anterior calyces are 2, 4, and 6. The

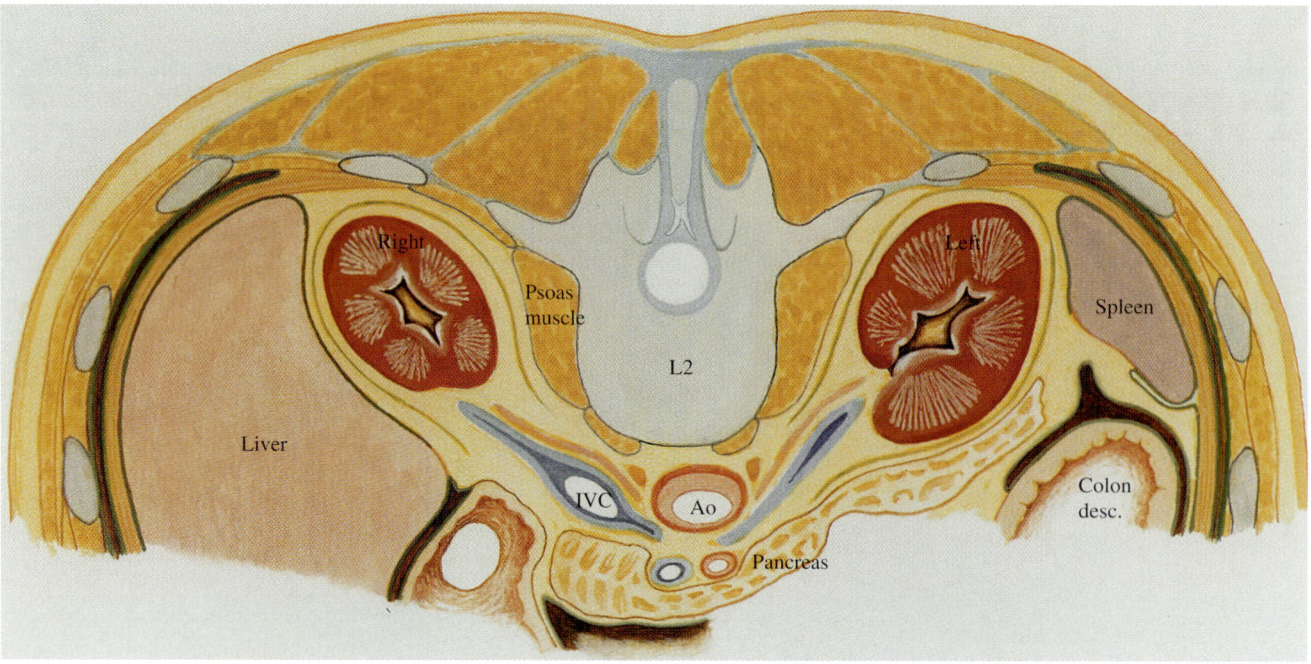

FIG. 1.
Cross section of the anatomy of the human body at lumbar 2. The kidneys are clearly shown. The arterial and venous blood vessels to the kidney are also shown. Also, the aorta and vena cava are seen. Spleen and liver are shown in part. A portion of the large bowel is seen on each side.

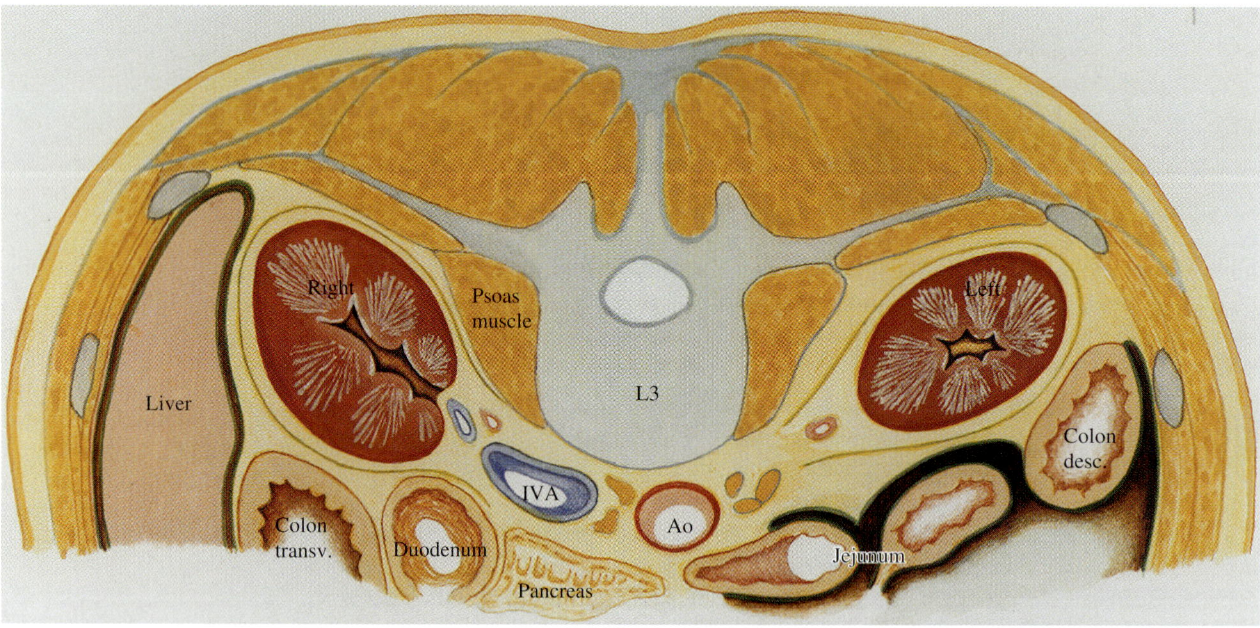

FIG. 2.
The cross section is at L3. Again, the kidneys are shown. The intestines, including the large bowel, are seen in the cross section.

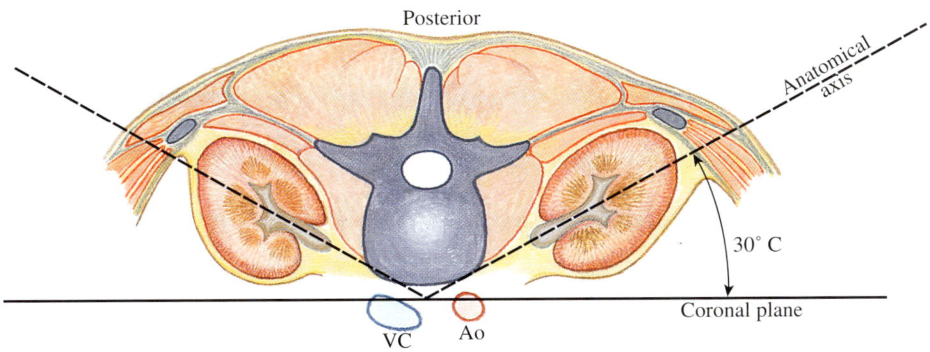

FIG. 3.
Cross section through the kidneys. The anatomical axis through the kidney levels is demonstrated. A 30° angle from the coronal plane is seen on the left kidney. Experienced urologists appreciate this anatomic pathway and have good experience with this approach.

posterior calyces are 3, 5, and 7. When a renal pyelogram is shown on an x-ray view box, the kidney is rotated so that the anterior calyces appear more lateral.

It is important to illustrate the arterial blood supply to the kidney from an anterior and posterior view. Brödel's white-line or avascular plane can be demonstrated (Fig. 6).

The single renal artery courses into the renal hilum. The renal vein is anterior; the renal pelvis lies posteriorly. Generally, the renal artery branches into five segmental arteries. Each of these five branched arteries supply a major renal segment. There is no cross communication of arteries between segments.

The first branch of the renal artery is the posterior segment and, generally, it arises medial to the renal hilum. As shown, the posterior branch passes laterally and posteriorly before crossing the posterior upper part of the renal pelvis and the posterior aspect of the upper pole—the infundibulum (Fig. 5).

The other four branches cross anteriorly and continue across the anterior aspect of the renal pelvis. These four branches supply the apical, upper anterior, middle anterior, and lower renal segments. As illustrated, the apical and lower polar segments supply blood to the apical or end segments that cover the anterior and posterior margins (Fig. 5).

The endourologist must develop an appreciation for the avascular junction between the anterior and posterior branches of the renal artery (Fig. 6). This avascular plane—Brödel's line of incision— is important in the removal of a staghorn calculus. The plane is usually 1 to 1.5 cm posterior to the lateral margin.

POSITIONING THE PATIENT FOR PERCUTANEOUS NEPHROSTOMY

Renal calculi are most commonly located in the pelvis or in the posterior, middle, or lower calyces. Note the 30° elevation or tilt of the patient (Fig. 6). The posterior lower pole calyx lies at an 80° angle to the fluoroscopy table. When properly positioned, the nephrostomy needle can be aligned directly over the calyx as shown. This perpendicular approach allows entry into the posterior calyx and spares the renal papilla.

Diagrammatically the needle enters calyces 5 and 7 and passes below the 12th rib. The pleural cavity is not entered. The advantages when a posterior calyx is selected are as follows:

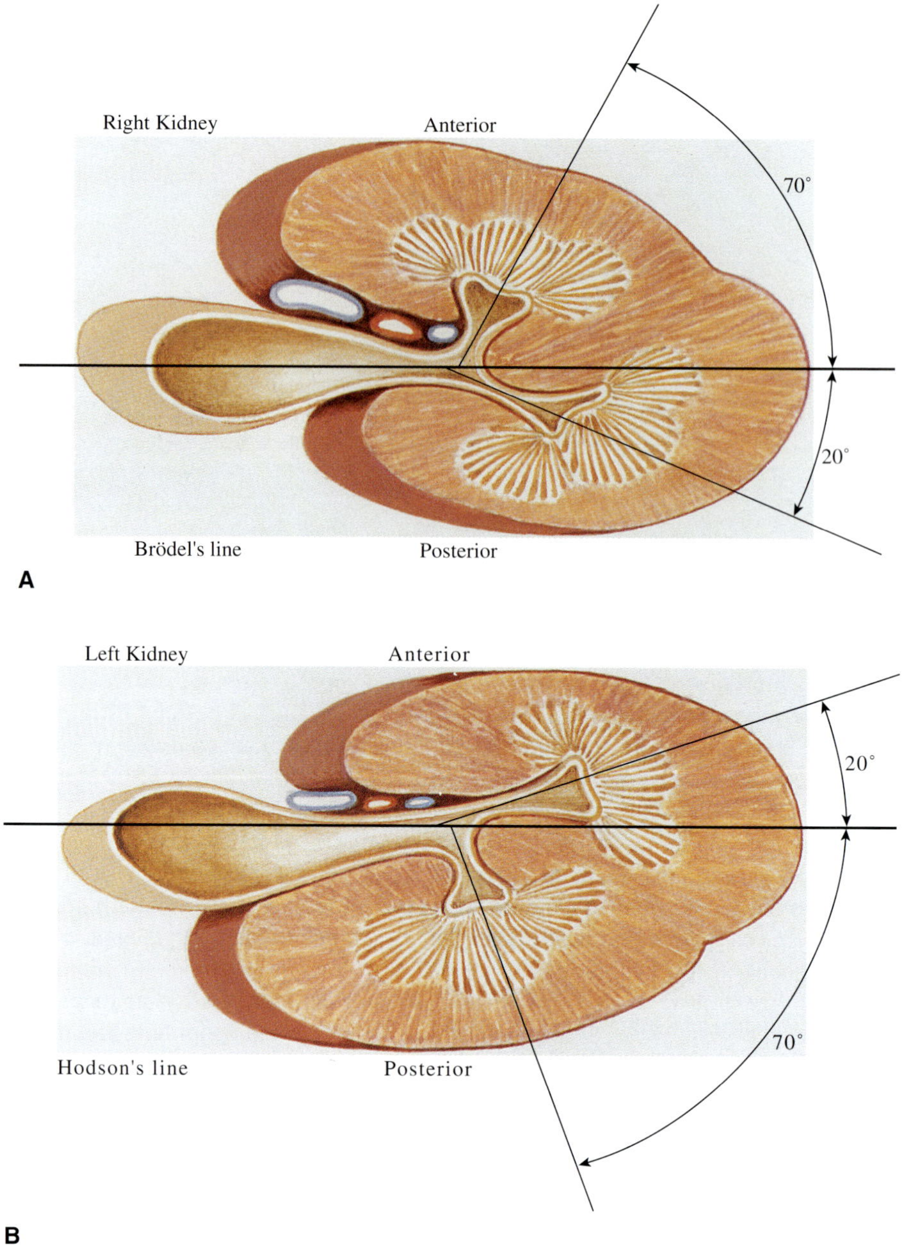

FIG. 4.
A. This demonstrates differences in the angle of the major calyces in the right kidney and the left kidney. Brödel described the posterior calyces in the right kidney pointing to a line a little posterior to the convex border of the kidney. The more anterior calyces are pointed straight forward into the convex part of the kidney. The anterior calyces project 70° from the frontal (coronal) plane of the kidney. The posterior calyces are longer and project 20° behind the frontal plane. **B.** Hodson suggested that the typical left kidney was an exact mirror image with a prominent posterior hilar lip and the posterior calyces faced the mid posterior portion of the kidney. The anterior calyces were longer and projected just anterior to the convex lateral renal margin.

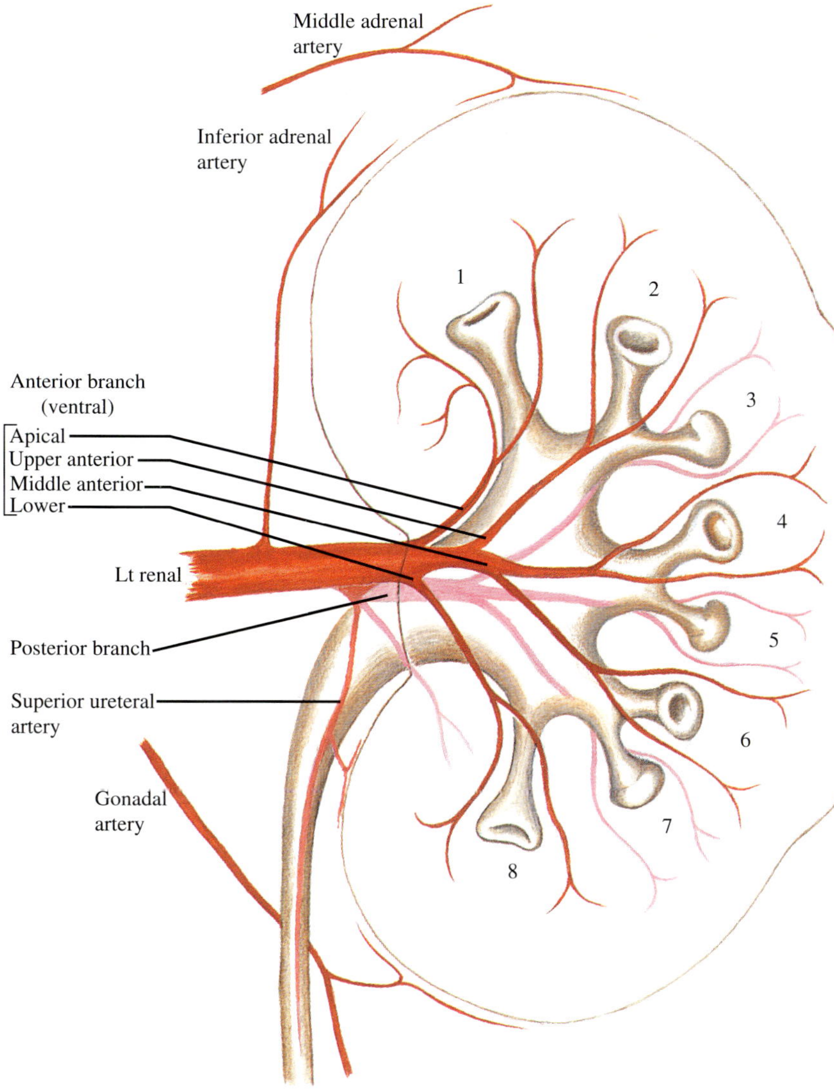

FIG. 5.
Arterial supply in the left kidney (classic).

1. Better access to the renal pelvis and ureter;
2. An avascular plane is encountered;
3. The anterior, divisional branches of the renal artery are avoided; and
4. The pathway is inferior to the posterior segmental renal artery.

Once the percutaneous nephrostomy has been established, the procedure can begin.

123. Percutaneous Nephrolithotripsy

In most urological centers, expertise is available for fragmentation of impacted stones in a posterior calyx.

It is important to obtain special ultrasonic localizing devices. The ultrasound device allows a long percutaneous needle and its obturator to be passed into the appropriate posterior calyx. Rotation of the patient along the longitudinal axis has been mentioned previously.

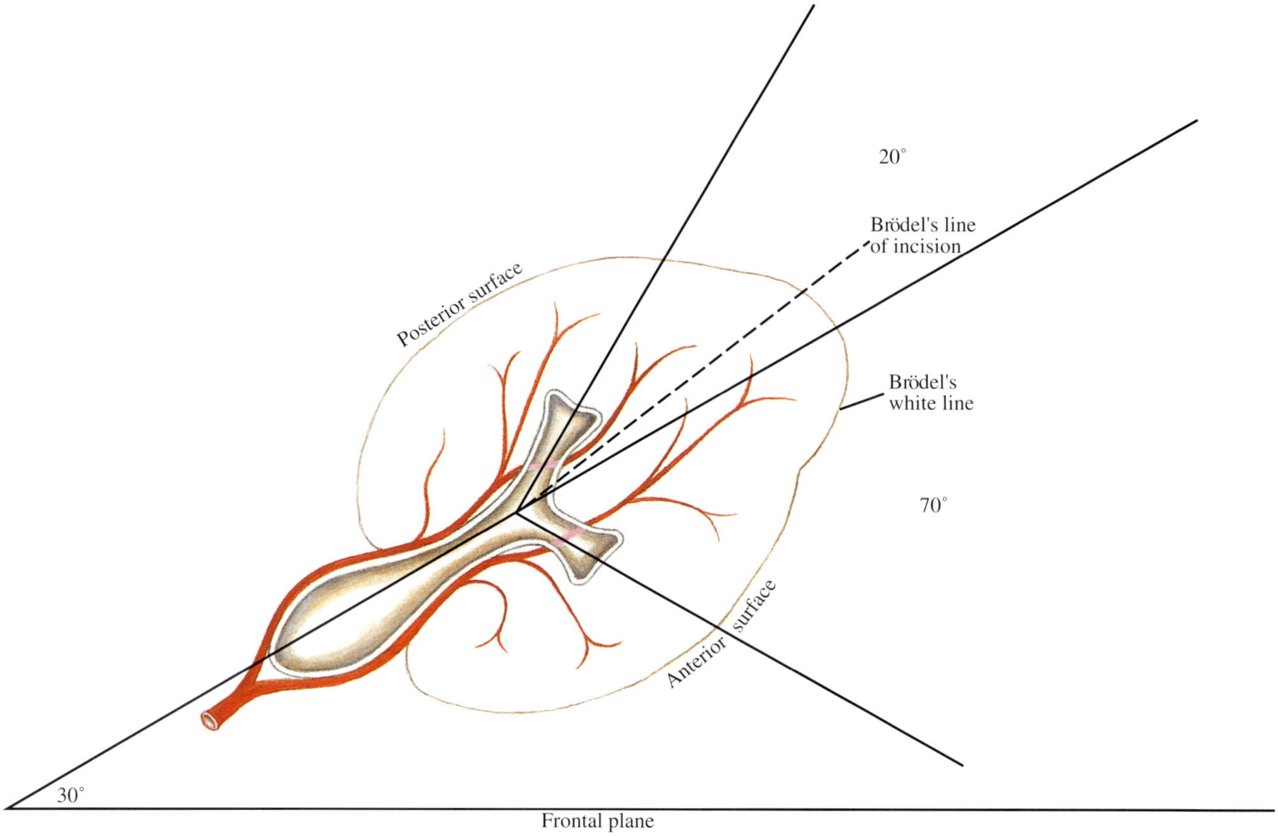

FIG. 6.
Crosssection of the left kidney to show the Brödel's lines (classic).

123-1. The needle is passed as shown into the calyx. After the obturator within the needle is removed, a wire with a flexible tip is passed through the lumen of the needle and the needle is removed. The flexible tip of the wire should be in the midureter.

123-2. At this point, special dilators with a tapered or narrow tip are passed over the wire to dilate the percutaneous and musculofascial structures, the renal calyx, and its junction with the pelvis. During this stage the ultrasonic device is used to monitor the progressive dilation of the calyx, infundibulum, and pelvis as the structures surrounding the stone are dilated. Amplatz dilators allow dilation through the area where the stone is lodged (see 123-2). A second flexible tip wire is inserted for safety before the first wire is removed.

The ultrasonic device is repositioned and larger Amplatz dilators are inserted if the dilation is following the path to the renal pelvis and major calyx. Successive larger Amplatz dilators are carefully used to dilate the calyx and infundibulum so that the nephroscope can be accommodated. A second wire with a less flexible tip may be passed so that the nephroscope will easily enter the calyx and infundibulum to make contact with the stone.

123-3. When the stone is clearly seen, an ultrasonic tip that can fragment stones is passed through the appropriate portal and the stone is broken. Irrigation through the nephroscope is important in helping remove debris from the fragmented stone.

123-4. A balloon technique with expansion prevents stone fragments from migrating down the ureter. At the onset the balloon ureteral catheter (7 French) is inserted up the appropriate ureter. The balloon is inflated prior to stone manipulation and fragmentation.

123-5. The nephroscopic approach in a superior calyx.

123-6. A close-up view of the ultrasound disintegrator device.

123-7. This illustration demonstrates a variety of small grasping forceps to retrieve broken stone fragments.

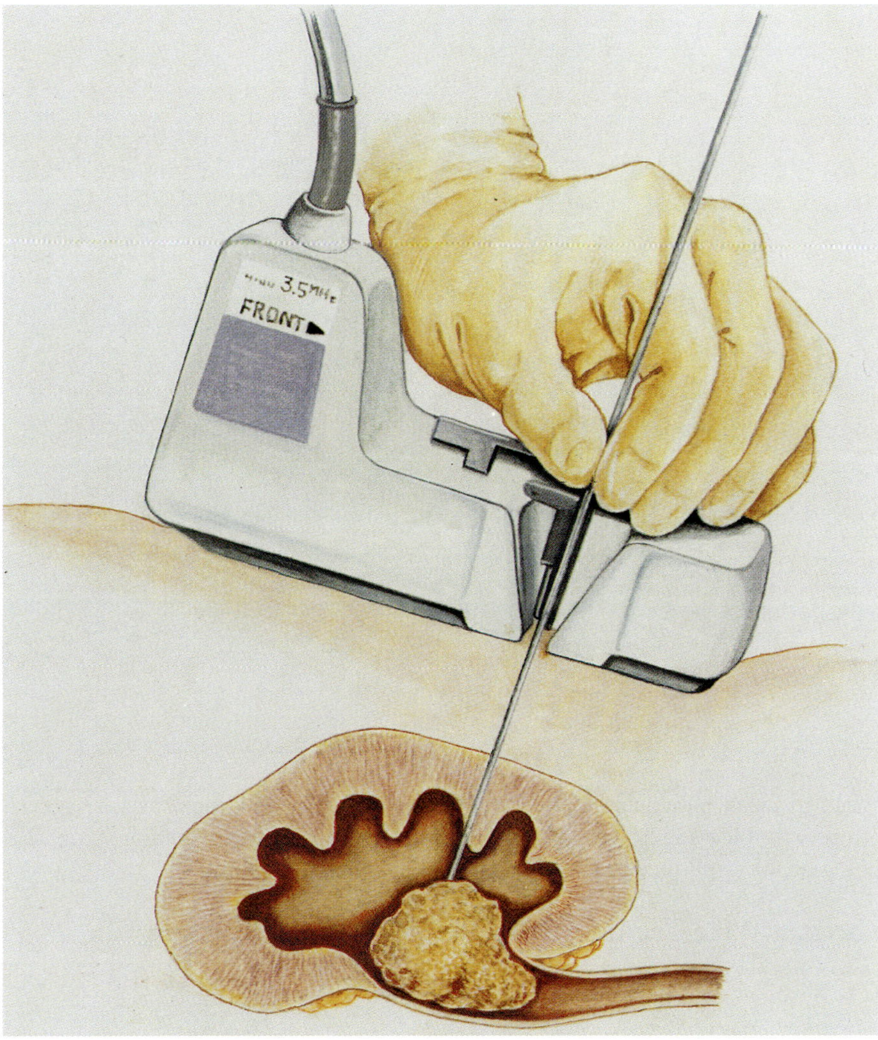

123-1

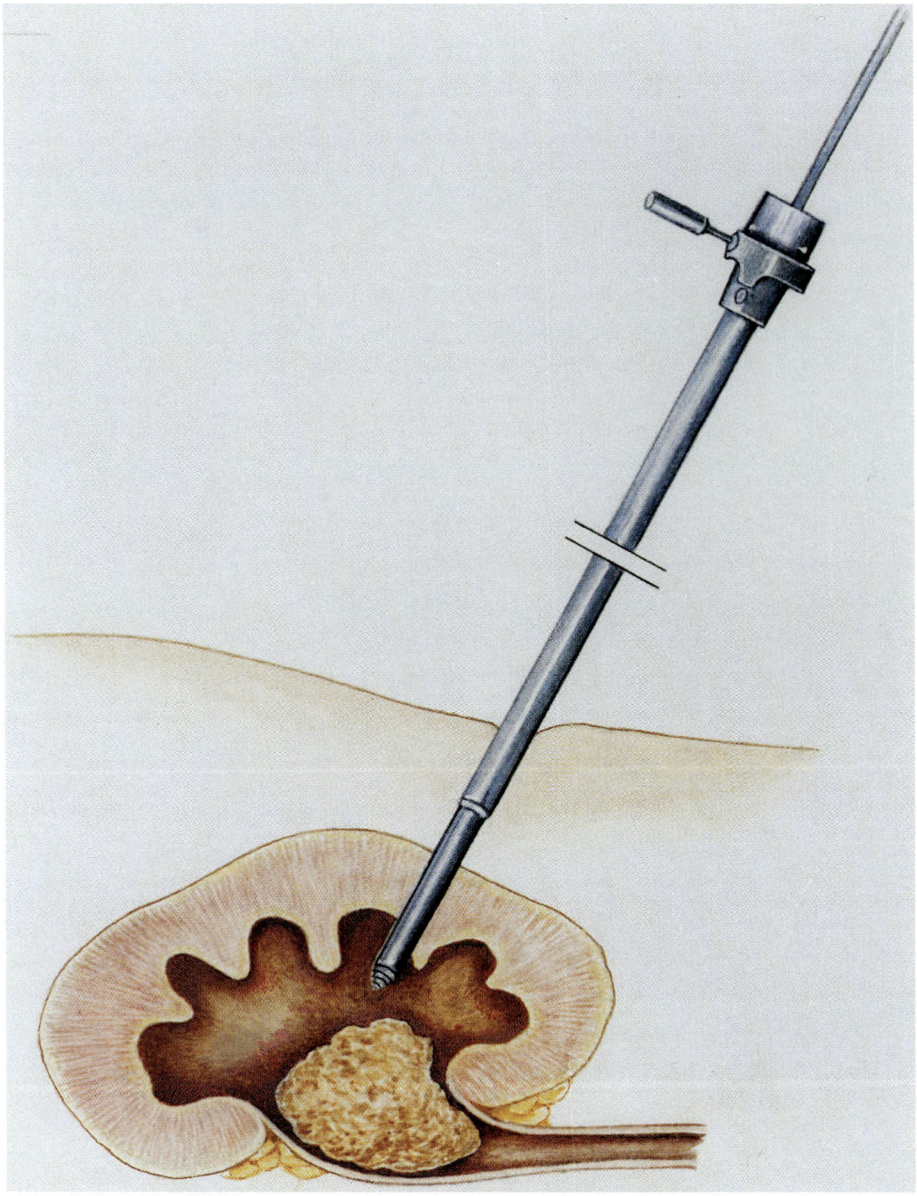

123-2

When the stone fragments have been removed, we leave a nephrostomy tube in place to prevent bleeding and to allow drainage. The size is approximately 10 or 12 Fr depending on the nephroscope used.

124. Rocket Wire Technique for Retrograde Nephrostomy and Percutaneous Stone Removal

In 1985 Hunter et al.[2] described a new technique for a urinary retrograde approach to the appropriate calyx and the exterior. Nephrostomy and percutaneous removal of cal-

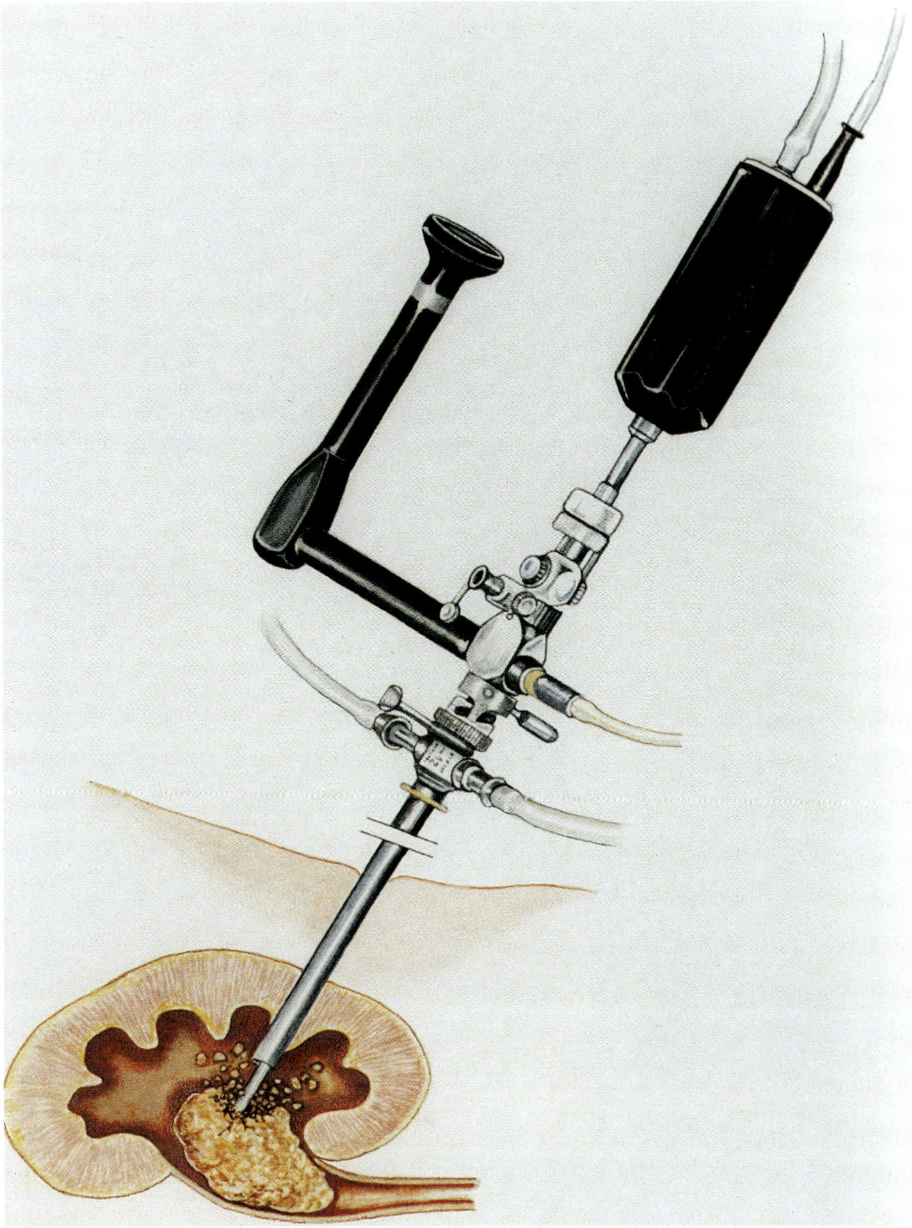

123-3

culi can be simplified by this technique. Thirty patients underwent the procedure by the group from Gainesville, Fla.

In most of the 22 patients, intravenous sedation and local anesthesia were employed. Eight required general anesthesia. Twenty men and 10 women were included. All patients had radiodense calculi, and all but one had a nondilated pelviocalyceal system.

The procedure is *contraindicated* if a urinary tract infection is present. Bleeding abnormalities are a contraindication. Prophylactic antibiotics and IV fluids are administered during the procedure.

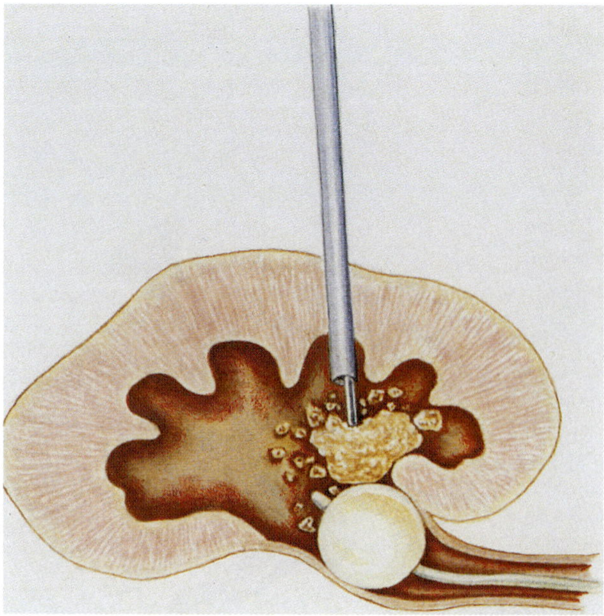

123-4

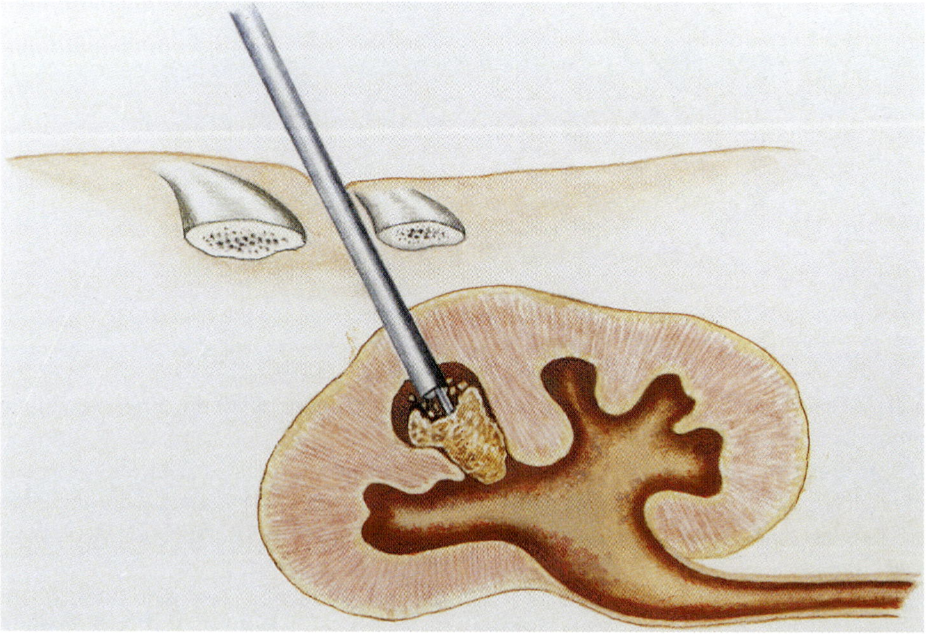

123-5

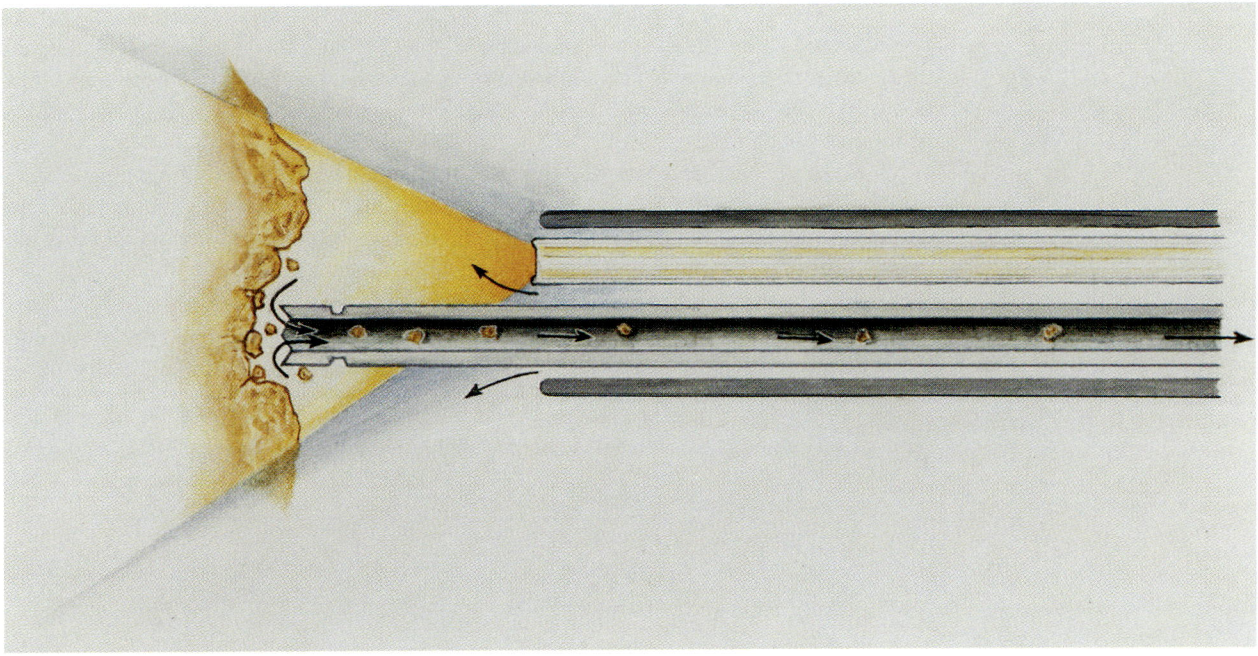

123-6

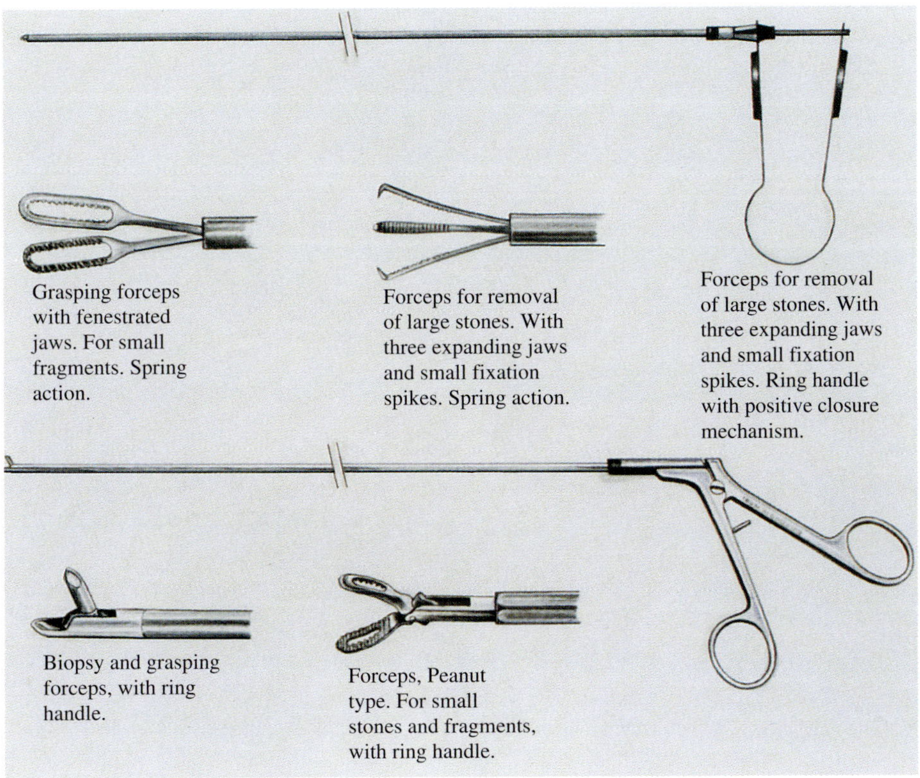
Grasping forceps with fenestrated jaws. For small fragments. Spring action.
Forceps for removal of large stones. With three expanding jaws and small fixation spikes. Spring action.
Forceps for removal of large stones. With three expanding jaws and small fixation spikes. Ring handle with positive closure mechanism.
Biopsy and grasping forceps, with ring handle.
Forceps, Peanut type. For small stones and fragments, with ring handle.

123-7

Preoperatively, the urologist reviews the most recent x-rays and/or an intravenous pyelographic study (IVP) study to determine the anatomy of the collecting system and the location of the calculi. The nephrostomy site is based on review of x-rays and location of the calculi. In general, the calyx that provides optimal access to the calculus to be removed is chosen.

Retrograde Nephrostomy: Cystoscopy, fluoroscopy, and fluoroscopic guidance are mandatory. Sixteen patients underwent cystoscopy and fluoroscopic guidance in the radiology department. A conventional x-ray tube-under-table fluoroscopy apparatus was employed.

In the obese patient, it is important to examine the patient fluoroscopically. Visualizing the calculus in an obese patient is mandatory. If fluoroscopic visualization is unclear, then a conventional x-ray film or retrograde study is mandatory. Anterior-posterior or oblique films are also necessary in these obese patients.

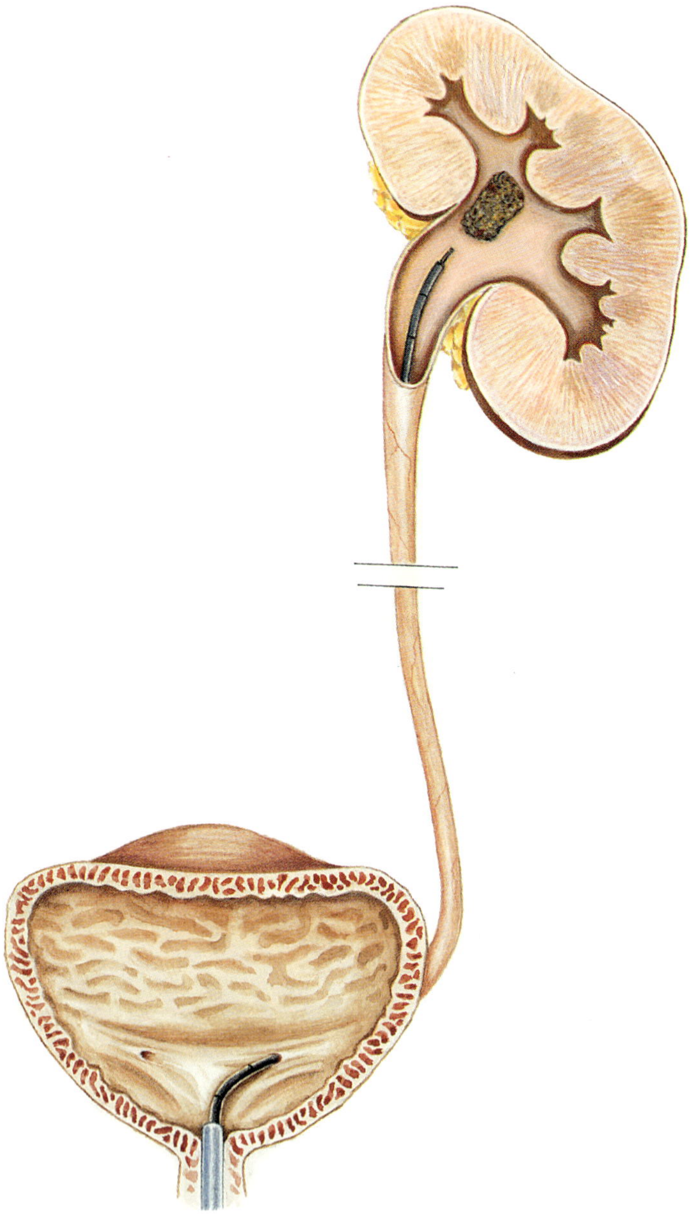

124-1

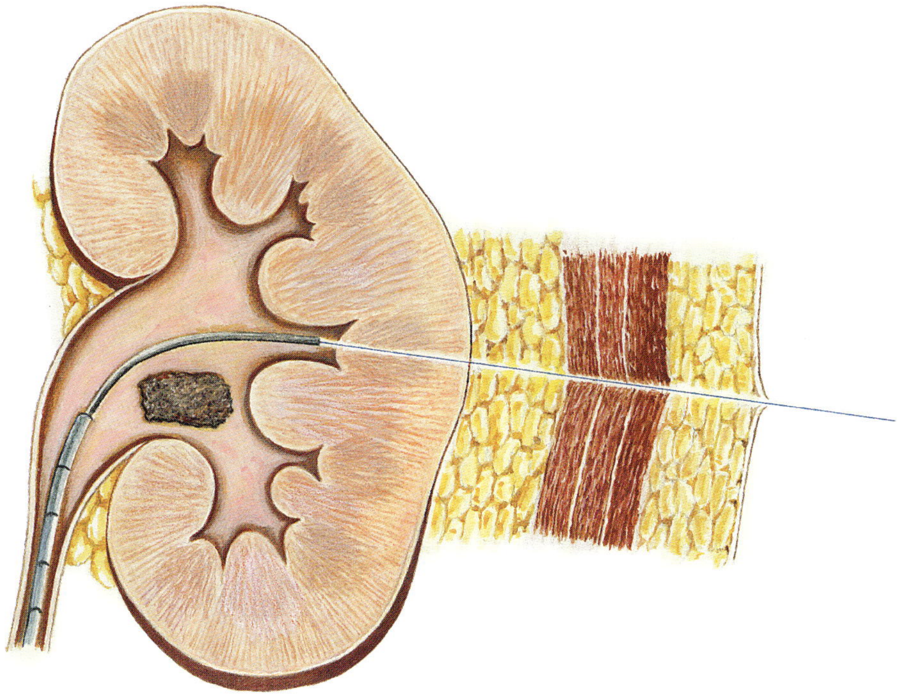

124-2

Procedure

Equipment to be checked and available after sterilization

a. 1 to 80 cm 9 Fr Teflon catheters
b. 2 to 90 cm 5 Fr Teflon catheters
c. 145 cm, 0.35 J-tip torque wire
d. assembled catheters and wire, 9 Fr in size
e. 20 and 21 gauge needles
f. A 260 cm 0.021 inch rocket wire stylet

124-1. One 5 Fr catheter is loaded inside the 9 Fr catheter to help position it in the appropriate calyx selected for nephrostomy. The second 5 Fr catheter serves as a sheath for the nephrostomy needle to prevent a needle from straying, as the nephrostomy needle is advanced through the curved areas of the 9 Fr catheter.

At times the rocket wire may be used inside the needle to provide added stiffness when previous renal surgery has led to cutaneous scarring.

124-2. After the needle exits the flank, the rocket wire is passed through the needle to provide extra length at the flank. This wire guide now allows Amplatz dilators (small to large in series) to be used over the wire needle combination. A small incision into the fascial areas may be needed. Local anesthesia is helpful. The tract is dilated from a 24 to 30 Fr size using the Teflon dilators.

After dilation and with a guide wire in place, the stone is removed or fragmented with the appropriate instrument.[3] After stone removal, a nephrostomy tube is left in place for 2 to 3 days.

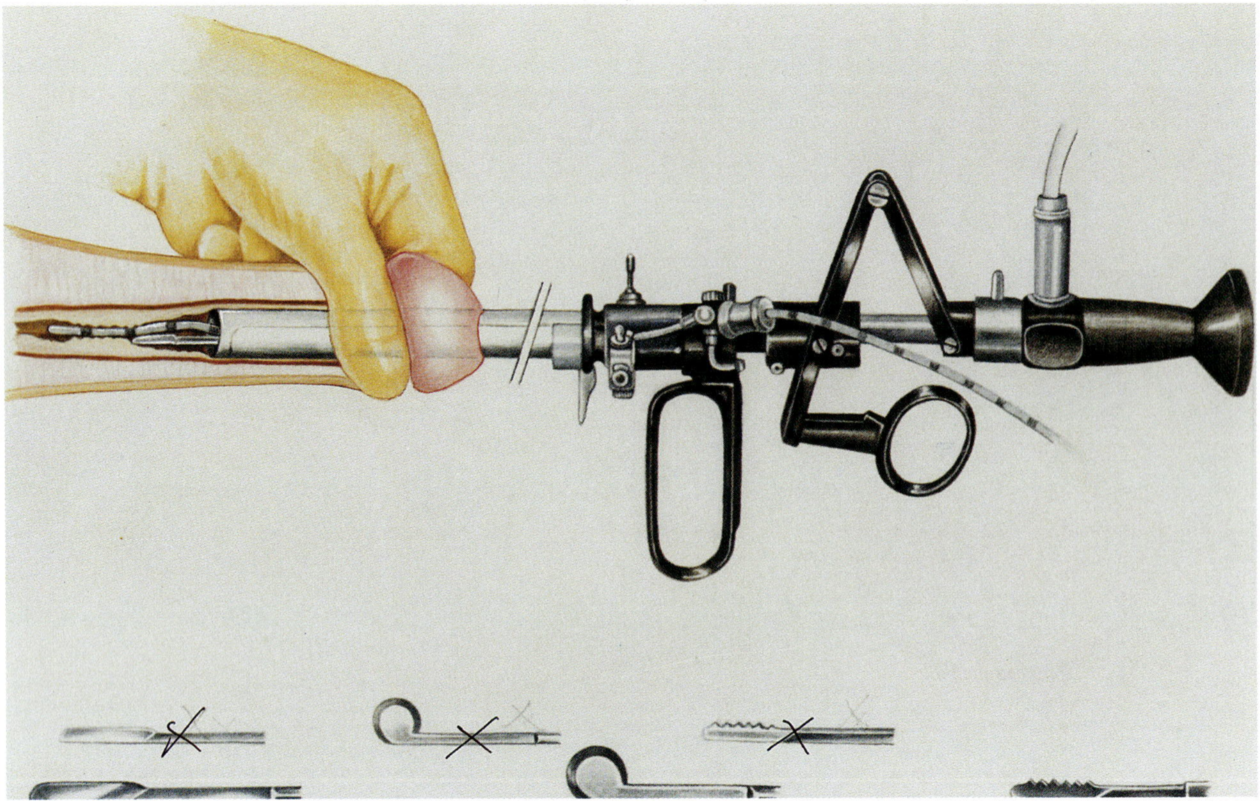

125-1

During establishment of the nephrostomy, manipulation, and positioning of the patient, it is important for the patient to be well hydrated. If the nephrostomy stone extraction is not successful, another attempt at stone manipulation is carried out 2 to 3 days later when the outer tract is mature.

Transurethral Endosurgery

125. Internal Urethrotomy with Storz Instrument

125-1. Karl Storz devised an instrument for internal urethrotomy. The tip of the cutting instrument has several different shapes of knife-like tips. For example, one of the tips can be fitted in the instrument and the tip has an edge like a saw. Another has a round tip with a cutting edge on the rounded portion. The instrument is well designed, and instead of the resectoscope, one places this extended tip into the working element of the instrument. In some instances, by replacing the knife, one can insert a cutting current onto the appropriate tip to perform a urethrotomy.

After instrumentation it is important to insert an indwelling catheter for 24 to 48 hours. Antibiotics are given at the onset.

The use of periodic urethral dilatation (7 to 10 days) may be necessary until full healing has occurred.

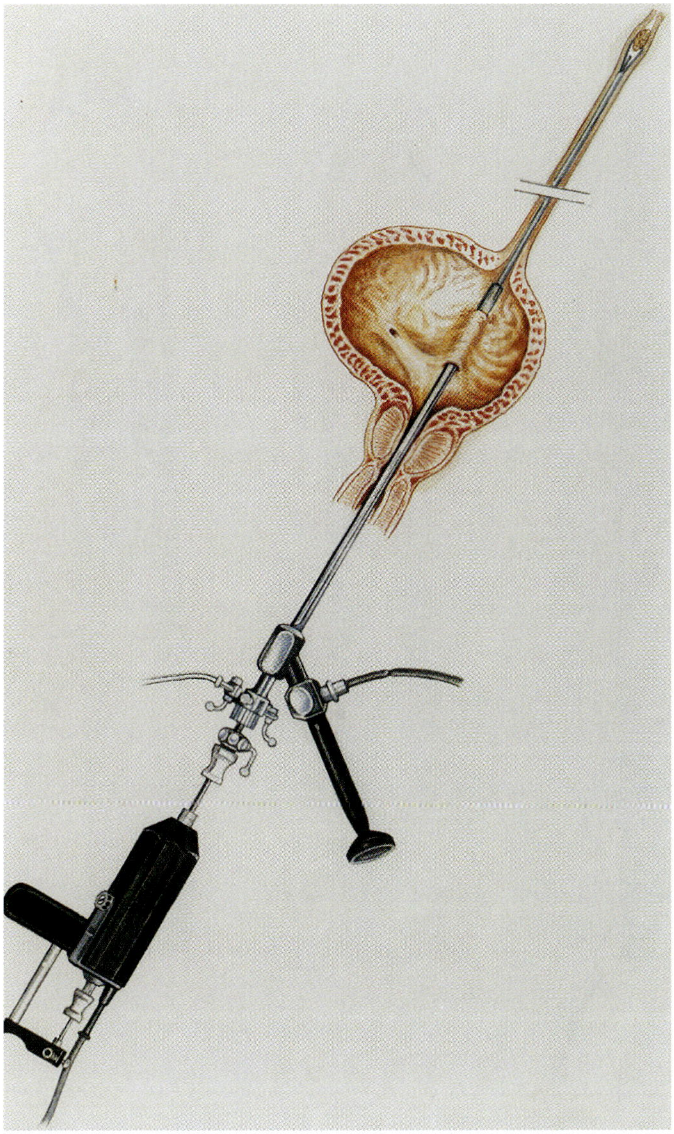

126-1

126. Transurethral Ureterolithotomy (TUL)

This is a special instrument. There are many sizes (5 to 8 Fr) which can be accommodated by the lumen of the left or right ureter.

126-1. The appropriate angulation is important so that the nonflexible ureteroscope can be placed up into the lower half or appropriate part of the ureter, in this case the left ureter. A larger instrument, 8 Fr, is then passed and when the stone is seen, then a grasping forceps can be placed around the stone to hold it.

126-2A-E. From within is a special attachment, the lithotrite that can proceed either with a mechanical force or the stone can be grasped as shown. The stone is thus removed. There is an attachment so that a balloon deflated can be placed beyond or superior to the stone. Then by inflating the balloon the stone can be captured and held. In this instance by immobilizing the stone then the appropriate lithotrite can be brought to the stone to initiate fragmentation or lithotripsy.

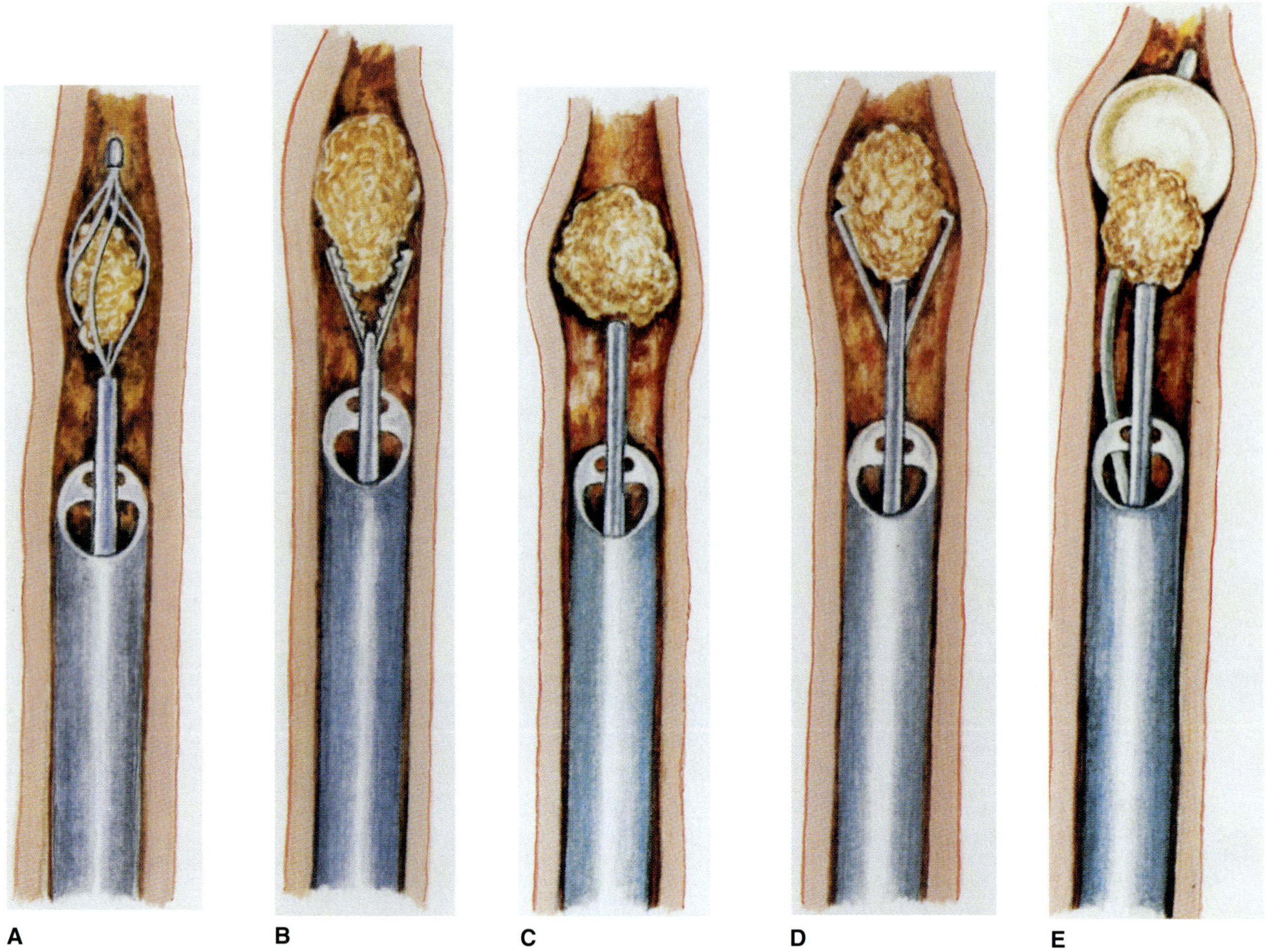

126-2

Laparoscopic Surgery

Recent urologic advances have included the development of specific laparoscopic instruments. These instruments and supporting equipment have led to the expansion of laparoscopic examination and treatment into the peritoneal cavity.

The technique of laparoscopic surgery is, however, still one of the most difficult of all endoscopic operations to master. This difficulty results from several factors. First, laparoscopic surgery does not afford the surgeon a three-dimensional view. The result is a marked reduction in depth perception. A major challenge for the surgeon is the magnified video image but with the visual field limited to a small area. In the beginning, one has difficulty assessing the anatomic relationships and the small working area. Finally, instrument movement is limited by fixation at the trocar entry site. Tactile sensation is diminished because the instrumentation through the trocar and its valve is magnified on the video image even with the slightest movement.

In our view, the younger generation of urologists are more enthusiastic about laparoscopic procedures than are their elders. We believe, however, the instruments and technique will continue to improve and will make this procedure less challenging and less tedious from a technical standpoint.

In the very beginning, laparoscopy was used in the main for inspection and diagnosis within the peritoneal cavity. Now, the skilled laparoscopic urologist can effectively replace the open incisional procedures with his/her endoscopic approach and perform surgery. The procedures include unilateral or bilateral varicocelectomy, treatment of an undescended testicle, bilateral pelvic lymph node dissection, nephrectomy, nephroureterectomy, ureterolysis, and even adrenalectomy. The technique of varicocelectomy is already an established laparoscopic procedure and can be substituted as a treatment of choice instead of the high spermatic vein ligation performed by open surgery.

In this chapter, a basic laparoscopic technique and a standard technique of laparoscopic ligation of the spermatic varicocele are included. The illustrations and technical steps for diagnosis and treatment of nonpalpable testes or intersex, pelvic lymphadenectomy and nephrectomy are also described.

PATIENT SELECTION AND CONTRAINDICATIONS

A careful history and physical examination are essential before patient selection for a laparoscopic procedure. Most of the contraindications will be identified after obtaining a history and performing an initial physical examination. Preexisting conditions that place the patient at risk for anesthesia-related complications, such as severe cardiac or pulmonary disorders, must be considered and may preempt further workup and consideration for intervention.

ABSOLUTE CONTRAINDICATIONS

1. Abdominal wall infection. The danger of dissemination is real.
2. Generalized peritonitis or localized peritonitis.
3. Partial bowel obstruction due to adhesions from previous surgery.
   Associated bowel distension increases the risk of bowel injury during needle insertion and prior to establishing a pneumoperitoneum and proper trocar placement.
4. Uncorrected coagulopathy.
   Any laparoscopic intervention is fraught with hazards when a bleeding tendency is encountered.
5. Large hiatal hernia.
   The diaphragmatic defect associated with a hiatal hernia may allow CO_2 gas to dis sect into the mediastinum, resulting in a pneumomediastinum.
6. Previous medical problems including pulmonary or cardiac insufficiency represent risks.

RELATIVE CONTRAINDICATIONS

1. *Obesity.* With obesity, the increased thickness of the anterior abdominal wall can make the introduction of a trocar and the establishment of a pneumoperitoneum more difficult. Also, in certain patients, a thick and muscular anterior abdominal wall may necessitate the maintenance of a higher insufflation pressure to obtain an adequate working space in the peritoneal cavity. A diminished ability to transilluminate the abdominal wall in order to avoid injury to the inferior epigastric vessels when introducing additional trocars can increase the risk. Also, the large amount of intraperitoneal adipose tissue reduces visibility in the operative field.

2. *Prior abdominal or pelvic surgery.* This can become the most commonly encountered relative contraindication to the laparoscopic procedure. The location of the previous incision and the site of the planned laparoscopic Veress needle insertion must be integrated into the risk/benefit analysis. It may be possible to insert the needle, but

the primary working port trocar must be at a site away from possible abdominal wall adhesions. In such a case, the Hasson cannula, which has a blunt-tipped obturator, can be employed through a minilaparotomy incision.

3. *Intraperitoneal fibrosis.* Patients with a previous history of peritonitis are poor candidates for a laparoscopic procedure. The history of a ruptured appendix or a partially inflamed colonic diverticulum may result in a significant amount of adhesions in the peritoneal cavity. A significant part of the procedure may be involved with adhesiolysis.

4. *Umbilical abnormalities.* The presence of an umbilical hernia or a urachal cyst or sinus is a contraindication to using the umbilicus and requires the lower midline as the primary site for insertion of the Veress needle. The problem can be overcome by choosing a lateral site on the abdomen for instrument insertion in some instances.

5. *Unreducible abdominal or inguinal hernia.* In case of an irreducible abdominal or inguinal hernia, the pneumoperitoneum may result in vascular compromise of the herniated abdominal contents.

6. *Aneurysm of the abdominal aorta and iliac artery.* Patients with an aneurysm of a major abdominal or pelvic artery are obviously at increased risk for vascular injury during needle and trocar introduction. In these patients, an upper quadrant alternative site for insertion of the Veress needle should be considered.

PATIENT PREPARATION

Routine preoperative studies must be done before laparoscopy. Special attention is paid to bleeding time and other coagulopathies. If it is elongated or abnormal, further studies such as prothrombin time and partial thromboplastin time must be determined. Coagulopathies can cause bleeding and need to be evaluated. Anticoagulants, aspirin, and other medications causing platelet disorders should be discontinued at least 5 to 12 days (aspirin) before laparoscopic intervention.

A chest film and electrocardiogram are essential. Besides an informed consent, one must include an explanation of the risk, benefits, alternatives, and potential complications of laparoscopic procedures. It is essential that prior to laparoscopic intervention he/she understands the risks of the procedure.

In laparoscopic varicocelectomy, preoperative patient preparation is rather simple after the infertility workup suggests the need for laparoscopic treatment of the varicoceles on the left and often on the right side.

1. We allow the patient to have a regular diet for supper on the day before the operation. He is asked to refrain from drinking fluids after midnight.
2. An enema before he goes to bed may be part of the preoperative preparation.
3. IVs are started on the morning of the surgery.

In the case of a more complicated procedure such as laparoscopic nephrectomy, regular bowel preparation and cleansing are ordered.

1. A low residue diet is begun 2 days before the operative day.
2. We prescribe 2 to 4 liters of chilled Colyte (Reed and Carnrick, Jersey City, NJ) in the afternoon or early evening of the day before the procedure.
3. The patient is not allowed any oral fluids (NPO) after midnight if the procedure starts in the morning. IV fluids may be started.
4. On the day of operation he is NPO and we continue IV fluids.

ANESTHESIA

Anesthesia for laparoscopy and associated operative procedures must provide adequate amnesia, analgesia, and muscle relaxation. Besides striving for minimal postoperative pain and a short hospital stay, the anesthetic agent must allow for a rapid recovery.

Laparoscopic surgery may be associated with an increased risk of regurgitation and aspiration of gastric contents. It is recommended that patients fast for at least 8 hours before entering the operating room. Metoclopramide, a dopamine antagonist, can be administered preoperatively to stimulate gastric emptying and increase the tone of the lower esophageal sphincter.

The combination of the H2-receptor antagonist (cimetidine, ranitidine) and metoclopramide can be an effective pharmacologic approach, for reducing the risk factors caused by acid regurgitation.

We recommend administering oral ranitidine, 150 mg, combined with oral metoclopramide, 10 mg, 2 hours before introduction of anesthesia to patients with tendencies that increase the risk for aspiration, such as morbid obesity, hiatal hernia, and diabetes mellitus which can cause hypomobility and distension of the stomach.

The stomach must be emptied with a nasogastric tube before abdominal insufflation to reduce the incidence of organ injury. The bladder must be emptied with a Foley catheter.

Laparoscopy can be performed using any one of three major anesthetic techniques: local, regional, and general anesthesia. For brief diagnostic procedures, monitored anesthetic care by an experienced nurse can be sufficient. However, for operative procedures, general anesthesia is required. The patient may become a candidate for an emergency open surgical procedure should laparoscopy result in an emergency situation, such as profuse hemorrhage or visceral injury.

INSTRUMENTS AND SUPPLIES

All of the necessary equipment must be present and functional before any laparoscopic procedure is started. Following is a list of equipment and supplies for a basic laparoscopic procedure:

Laparoscopic tray

1. Veress needle (disposable or reusable)
2. Trocar sheath units
   5, 10, and 11 mm, 2 each
3. Laparoscope
   10 mm 0° lens
   5 mm 0° lens (mainly for an infant under age 4)
4. Forceps
   straight and curved (Maryland) 5 and 10 mm
   toothed and atraumatic (cautery insulated)
   spoon shaped 10 mm
5. Scissors
   insulated straight
   insulated curved
6. Electrocautery instruments
   cutting spatula blade
7. Hemostatic clips
   multiple clip applicator
   endoligature
   needle driver
8. Suction-irrigation unit
   triple lumen Luer-Lok
9. Cords and tubings
   cautery 2
   fiberoptic light cable

video camera adapted for laparoscopy
irrigation system
suction apparatus
CO_2 with accurate gauges to monitor CO_2

10. Miscellaneous
    syringe 10 cc
    Foley catheter, 14–16 Fr, 5 cc balloon
    Salem sump 16 Fr, and nasogastric tube
    minor surgery set

LAPAROSCOPIC BASIC EQUIPMENT

1. CO_2 insufflator
   adjustable high flow (1–10 L/min)
   intraperitoneal pressure gauge
   total CO_2 insufflated gauge
2. Camera, video monitor, light source
   light source—high intensity (xenon)
   video camera attached to 10 mm laparoscope
   sterile camera wrap in place over camera
   two color TV monitors, high resolution
   video monitor, VHS unit

GENERAL EQUIPMENT

1. Operating table with multidirectional movement
2. Electrosurgical unit
   Settings for coagulation and cutting selected
   Grounding pad is included. The patient is "grounded" to eliminate electrical sparks.
3. Laparotomy set-up (for emergency use)
4. Compression stockings (pneumatic); use for major procedures.

ESTABLISHMENT OF THE PNEUMOPERITONEUM

Establishing a pneumoperitoneum is the initial, basic procedure for any laparoscopic technique. The insufflator and Veress needle are the two essential pieces of equipment.

The sterile insufflation tubing is connected to the insufflator. It is important to be sure that the pressure/flow shut-off mechanism is operational. Then the insufflation tubing is connected to the Veress needle. Either a metal or disposable plastic Veress needle (external diameter 2 mm; length 70 or 120 mm) may be used.

The CO_2 flow is turned to 1 L/min and 6 L/min, and the intra-abdominal pressure reading on the insufflator is noted at each setting; the optimal pressure should be 3 mm Hg. A higher reading indicates that there is some obstruction in the needle.

The blunt tip of the Veress needle should be tested so that the blunt tip retracts easily when it is pushed against solid subcutaneous tissue.

127. Introduction of the Veress Needle

127-1. The patient is placed in the supine, 15° head-down position. The site of entry is usually at the level of the inferior border of the umbilicus in an abdomen that has not been previously operated upon. The insertion of the Veress needle can be easily inserted by first making a stab incision that reaches the fascia with a knife and by picking up or pinching the inferior abdominal wall between the thumb and forefinger of the dominant

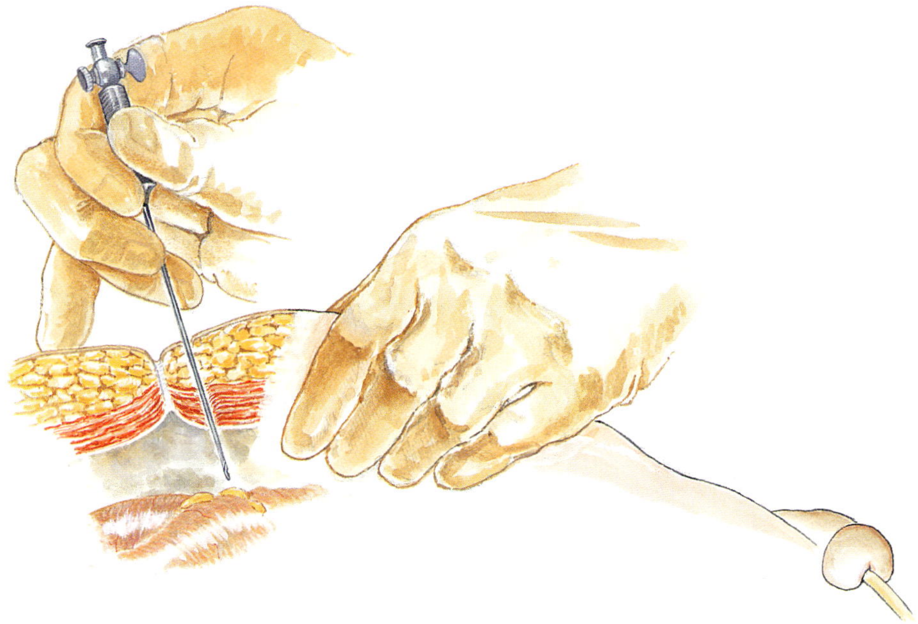

127-1

hand. Then, with the contralateral hand, the shaft of the Veress needle is grasped like a dart and gently introduced into the stab wound perpendicular to the abdominal wall. As the needle touches the peritoneum, a resistance will be felt. When the needle enters the peritoneal cavity, sometimes a distinct click can be heard as the blunt tip of the Veress needle springs forward into the peritoneal cavity.

Then a 10 cc syringe with 5 cc of saline is connected to the Veress needle to assure that the tip of the needle is correctly pointed in the peritoneal cavity. This maneuver is important. The next step is to aspirate and see whether any blood or yellowish fluid (bowel contents) is aspirated into the syringe. If abnormal fluid is seen, remove the needle and re-puncture the abdomen. The second step is to instill 5 cc of saline. It should flow into the peritoneal cavity without any resistance. The third step is to aspirate again. If the location of the tip of the needle is correct, no saline should return. The surgeon will then be able to advance the needle 1 to 2 cm deeper without any resistance.

Now the insufflation line can be connected to the Veress needle to begin CO_2 insufflation. If inflow pressure is less than 10 mm Hg and the CO_2 flow is greater than 1.0 L/min, then the needle is in the correct position. The insufflation should be continued to an abdominal pressure of approximately 10 to 15 mm Hg; this usually requires approximately 4 to 5 liters. Once the 16 mm Hg limit is reached, the flow of CO_2 will cease and actual flow will then fall to 0. A previously unoperated abdomen should expand symmetrically on breathing. When the establishment of the pneumoperitoneum is satisfactory, the Veress needle is removed.

Initial Trocar Insertion: As with the Veress needle, the insertion of the first trocar is a blind procedure with the potential for significant complications.

Trocars are either reusable or disposable. All trocars have two components: a sharp tipped obturator and a sheath through which instruments are introduced. The sheath contains a valve or membrane to avoid loss of CO_2 gas from the abdominal cavity. Some of the disposable trocars are equipped with a self-retaining port sheath which has a ribbed or grooved area on the outside.

In an unoperated abdomen, the initial trocar site is usually at the inferior or supine crease of the umbilicus. The thinnest wall of the abdomen is just on the linea alba and the peritoneum. Also, there are no significant blood vessels in this location.

For insertion of the initial trocar, the patient is placed in a 10 to 30° Trendelenburg position. The skin is incised horizontally until the incision is long enough to accept the 10 to 11 mm diameter sheath. The incision can be spread with a Kelly clamp to provide a more rounded configuration.

Prior to insertion of the trocar through the incision, a technique to elevate and stabilize the abdominal wall with towel clips on each side of the incision is useful. Also, the distance between the abdominal wall and the bowel is maintained.

127-2. The surgeon holds the trocar in the palm of the dominant hand, with the back of the trocar against the thenar eminence. The middle finger should be placed along

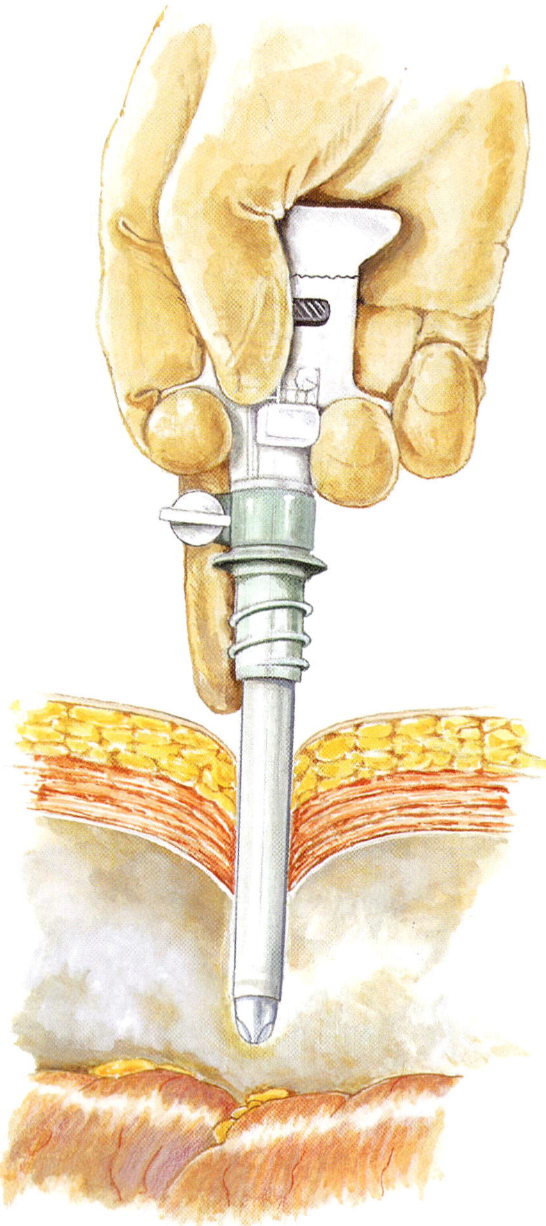

127-2

the trocar shaft. The tip of the finger prevents the trocar from going deeper than necessary and minimizes the risk of visceral trauma.

The angle for insertion of the trocar is initially perpendicular. Once the tip of the obturator is beyond the subcutaneous fat, the trocar handle is tilted cephalad to about a 60° angle; thus, the tip of the trocar is directed inferiorly toward the pelvic cavity. A steady downward twisting force is applied to the trocar unit. After the trocar sheath is positioned, the self-retaining sheath is attached through screws to the abdominal wall.

As the peritoneal cavity is entered, escaping CO_2 gas creates a sound as it rapidly flows out of the opened side port of the trocar. The sidearm is promptly closed and the sheath is advanced deeper into the peritoneal cavity.

INSPECTION OF THE ABDOMEN AND PELVIS

After the initial trocar is properly placed, the obturator is removed. Insert the 10 mm endoscope, attached to the camera and light cord. The tip of the endoscope is treated with an antifogging solution before its insertion into the peritoneal cavity. Allow adequate time for initial inspection of the abdominal cavity and for the cosurgeon to become oriented.

The next step is to observe the underlying loops of intestine. They should be inspected for any sign of injury. Then, a systemic inspection of the peritoneal cavity is performed. The laparoscope is directed caudally into the pelvic cavity. The midline bladder is identified along with the broad-based urachus. The paired prominent medial umbilical ligaments, which course from the lateral aspect of the bladder toward the umbilicus, can be seen.

In the male, the spermatic cord is seen as it enters the internal inguinal ring. In the female, the midline uterus and lateral lying ovaries are seen along with the round ligament. The inferior epigastric vessels are seen on the anterior abdominal wall just medial to the internal inguinal ring and lateral to the medial umbilical ligament. The lateral-lying colon is seen. On the right side, the cecum and appendix are seen.

Caution and care are of utmost importance for this initial inspection. If something appears strange or if the surgeon is unsure of a structure's identity, the surgeon should not proceed with any surgical procedure until he becomes well oriented.

SECONDARY TROCAR INSERTION

Once initial inspection and orientation are accomplished, the surgeon proceeds with the insertion of a second trocar. To perform laparoscopic surgery, two to four trocars must be placed as a conduit for the surgical instruments. These additional trocars are 5 or 10 mm in outer diameter and have a simple membrane to act as a valve. They are inserted under direct vision through the initially placed laparoscope.

The site of placement of additional trocars depends on the type of proposed surgical procedure. Each point of entry should be in proper position to maximally enhance the surgical procedure. To avoid injury to any superficial abdominal wall blood vessels, the room lights are turned off or markedly dimmed, and the proposed trocar sites are transilluminated with the laparoscopic light from inside the abdomen. Larger superficial vessels can often be seen beneath the skin of the abdominal wall; the stab incision for a secondary trocar can be made so as to avoid these vessels. Also, no trocar should traverse the rectus muscle.

When placing the trocars in the lower quadrants of the abdomen, care must be taken to avoid injuring the inferior epigastric vessels. They are seen and identified as a short, bandlike protrusion of the anterior peritoneum.

This area can be located lateral to the medial umbilical ligament and medial to the internal inguinal ring.

Immediately before trocar insertion, the intra-abdominal pressure is allowed to increase to 20 to 25 mm Hg. The stab incision is made transversely, just far enough to accommodate the size of the trocar, usually 5 mm in diameter. A clamp can be used again to spread the incision. The trocar is held with the middle or index finger of the dominant hand and extends down the shaft of the trocar to act as a brake.

Under laparoscopic monitoring, the secondary trocar is inserted into the skin with a slow and twisting motion. The tip of the obturator is seen as it penetrates the peritoneum. Further introduction of the obturator continues until the sheath completely enters the peritoneal cavity.

When all secondary trocars are introduced, the pressure limit is returned to 15 mm Hg.

Operative Techniques

128. Ligation of Spermatic Varicocele

Patient Positioning and Preparation

Under general anesthesia, using an endotracheal tube, the patient is initially positioned in a supine position. The operating table can be rotated in either a side-to side or head-to foot direction. The patient is firmly secured to the operating table with adhesive tapes or restraints across the chest and thighs. Both arms are tucked in at the patient's side to avoid impeding movement of the surgeons.

Initially, the patient is placed in a 15° Trendelenburg position for placement of the laparoscopic ports. Then the ipsilateral side of the table is rotated 30° upward.

A full abdominal skin preparation is performed with an appropriate disinfectant. Scrub from the costal arches to the midthighs and to both midaxillary lines laterally.

A Foley catheter of appropriate size (based on the age of the patient, 16Fr [adult] to 8Fr [infant]) is inserted into the bladder to empty the bladder. The catheter is connected to a drainage bag.

If gastric distension is present after induction of general anesthesia, the insertion of a nasogastric tube is advised to avoid the risk of injury either by a Veress needle or a trocar.

Position of the Surgeon and Placement of Trocars

Usually, the surgeon stands on the side of the operating table opposite the varicocele to be ligated. The assistant stands on the ipsilateral side of the varix for manipulation of the laparoscope and aids in the exchange of instruments. The nurse stands on either side of the table below the surgeon or assistant. In most cases, varicocelectomy is performed on the left side only. When bilateral varicoceles are present, the surgeon and assistant will exchange position after ligation of the first vein or veins.

After establishment of a pneumoperitoneum, the primary 11 mm trocar-sheath for the 10 mm laparoscope is inserted through a skin incision in the inferior crease of the umbilicus.

Then a 5 mm trocar is inserted in the ipsilateral lower abdominal quadrant midway between the umbilicus and anterosuperior iliac spine for access of all 5 mm surgical instruments and irrigation or aspiration instruments.

Lastly, an 11 mm midline port is made midway between the umbilicus and symphysis pubis for the 10 mm clip applicator and an assortment of 5 or 10 mm scissors, dissectors, and graspers.

128-1. While the assistant controls the 10 mm laparoscope that is passed through the

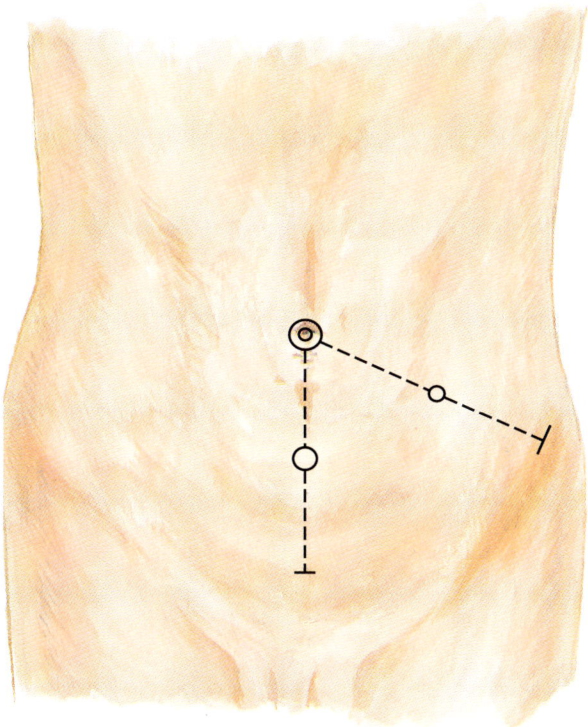

128-1

11 mm sheath just below the umbilicus, the surgeon controls both secondary ports for grasping tissue (mostly through the 5 mm port) and for tissue dissection or application of clips (through the 11 mm lower midline port).

In the case of a small child, when the low midline port is too close to the 5 mm secondary port at the lower abdominal quadrant, one can choose to insert the 11 mm trocar for 10 mm instruments at the contralateral lower abdominal quadrant. When two working trocars are too close to each other, the ability to maneuver instruments within each individual sheath becomes limited as the tops of the sheaths interfere with each other. Moreover, the urinary bladder of a small infant is usually positioned higher above the symphysis than an adults. Therefore, the placement of a secondary trocar midway on the low midline may meet with more risk and can injure the bladder.

Inspection and Peritoneotomy

128-2. On inspection of the pelvic cavity, the internal inguinal ring can be seen and the course of the spermatic cord along the retroperitoneum can be identified. The vas deferens also can be seen emerging from the medial aspect of the internal inguinal ring running towards the bladder under the peritoneum.

It may be necessary to mobilize the sigmoid colon from its lateral abdominal wall attachments to clearly expose the bundle of spermatic vessels. Placement of the patient in a 15° Trendelenburg and 30° upward angle on the ipsilateral side helps to mobilize the sigmoid colon.

128-3. Starting at a point about 5 cm above the internal inguinal ring, a 3 to 4 cm incision is made in the peritoneum towards the internal inguinal ring, just medial to the bundle of spermatic vessels. Usually, the peritoneum is grasped and elevated via the lower quadrant 5 mm port; the scissors are operated through the lower midline 11 mm port. Then a perpendicular incision from the midpoint of the first incision is made and

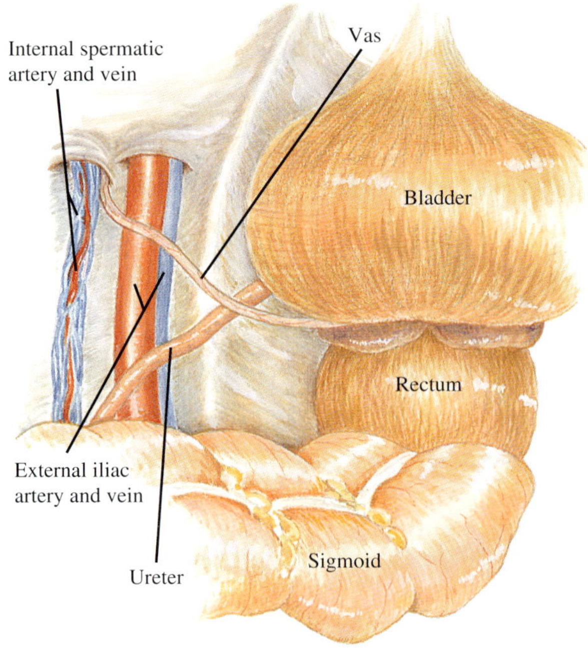

128-2

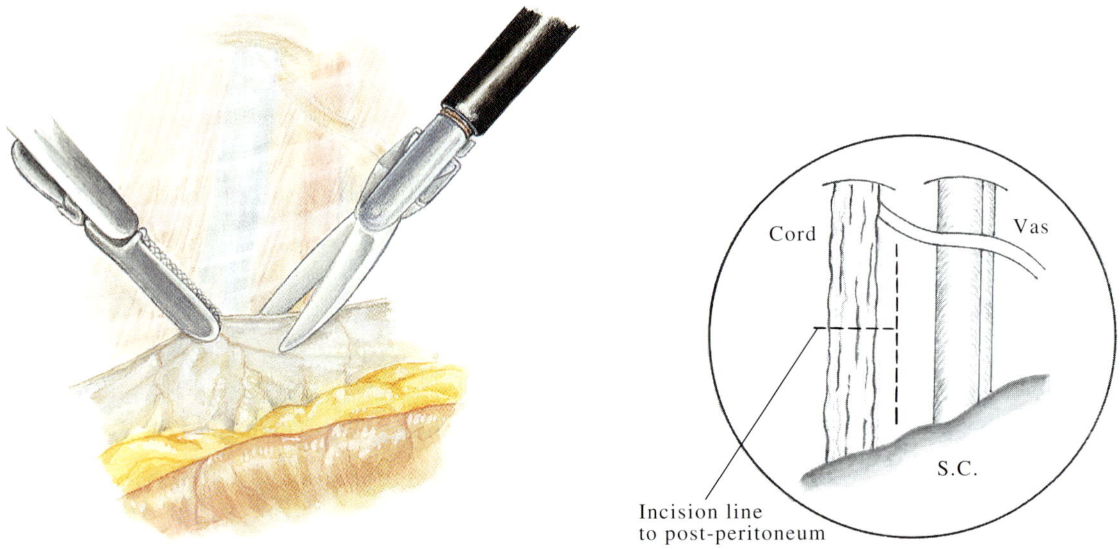

128-3

extended for 3 to 4 cm laterally, crossing the fascial bundle of spermatic vessels.

128-4 and 128-5. Then the spermatic vessels are fully exposed under laparoscopic vision through a window of the peritoneum made by this T incision.

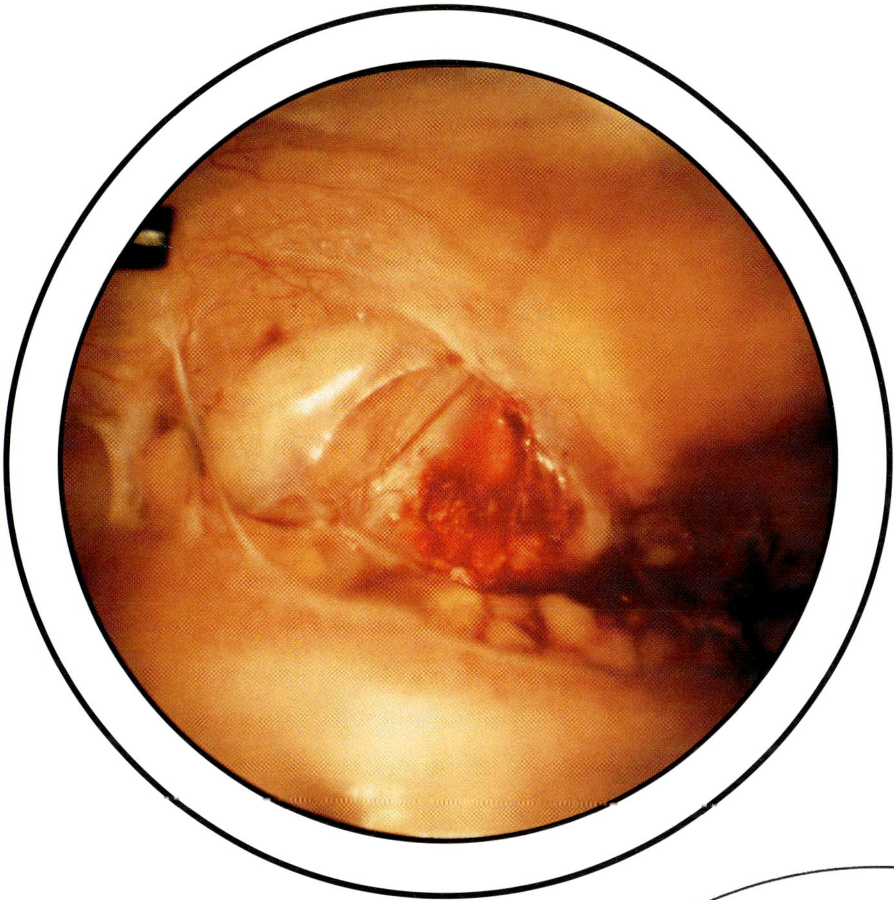

128-4

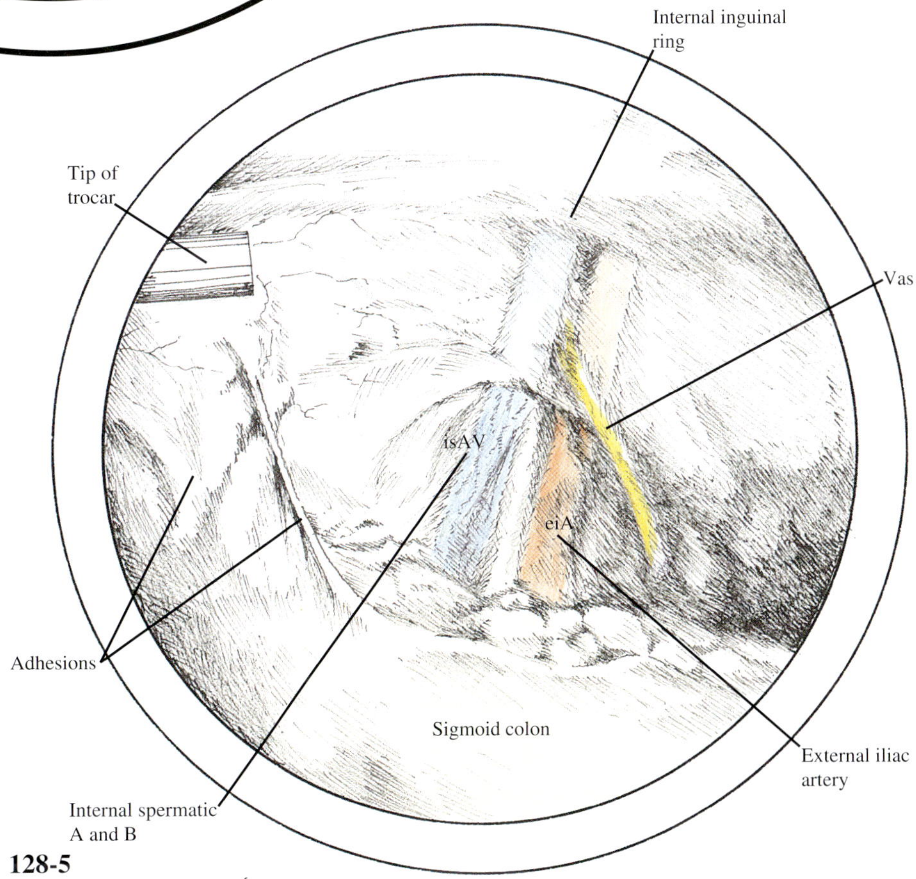
Internal inguinal ring
Tip of trocar
Vas
isAV
eiA
Adhesions
Sigmoid colon
External iliac artery
Internal spermatic A and B

128-5

Isolation of Spermatic Artery and Securing of Spermatic Veins

When the spermatic vascular bundle is still obscure, downward traction of the ipsilateral testis by an assistant's hand will provide tension to the vascular bundle. This helps the surgeon to identify the veins and isolate them from the surrounding tissues.

The entire spermatic vascular bundle is elevated from the retroperitoneum by using blunt and sharp dissection. A curved grasping instrument via the lower quadrant 5 mm port and scissors passed via the low midline 11 mm port are employed.

128-6, 128-7, and 128-8. The major aim of dissecting the vascular bundle is to identify the spermatic artery and to isolate it from the veins surrounding it. The artery can be placed into spasm by the superficial application of papaverine (30 mg/mL) or lidocaine (2%). These solutions applied to the spermatic vessels will relieve the spasm and the pulsation can be observed. Careful and meticulous dissection of the venous bundle is of utmost importance. A clear vision of the operative field must be maintained. Once the spermatic artery is clearly isolated and preserved, the rest of the vascular bundle containing veins can be doubly clip-ligated en bloc proximally and distally with two to three 9 mm titanium clips.

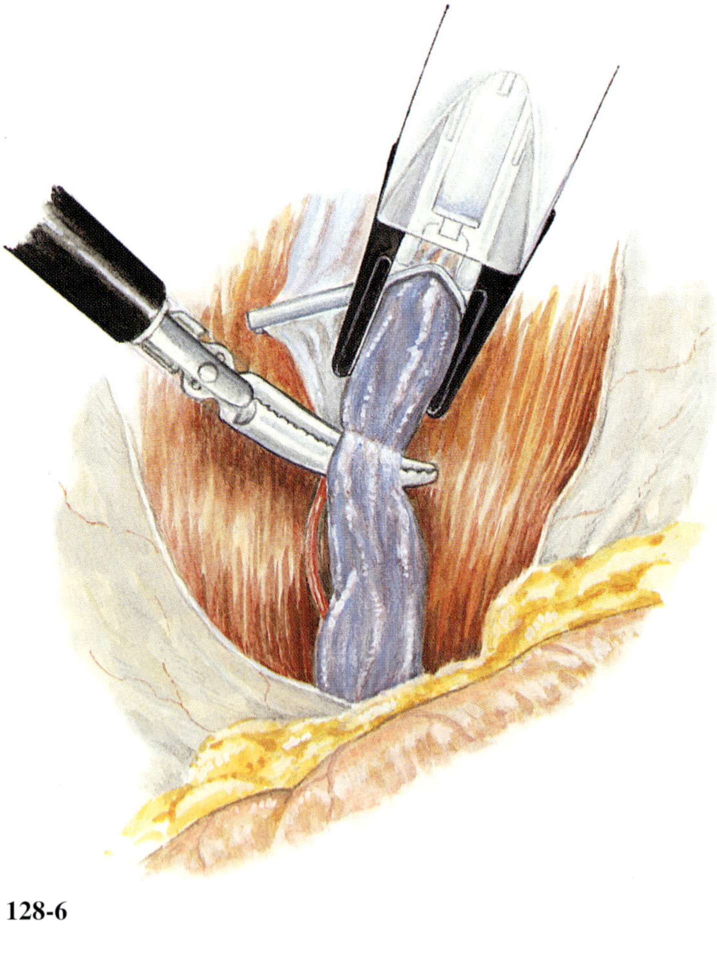

128-6

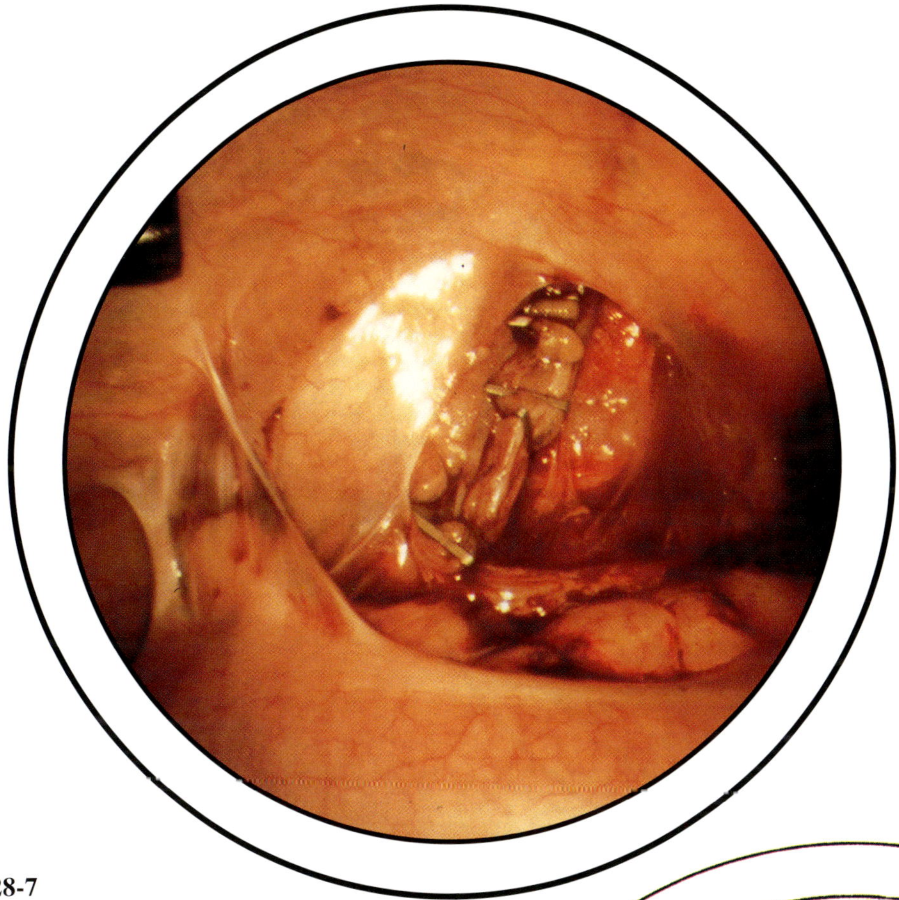

128-7

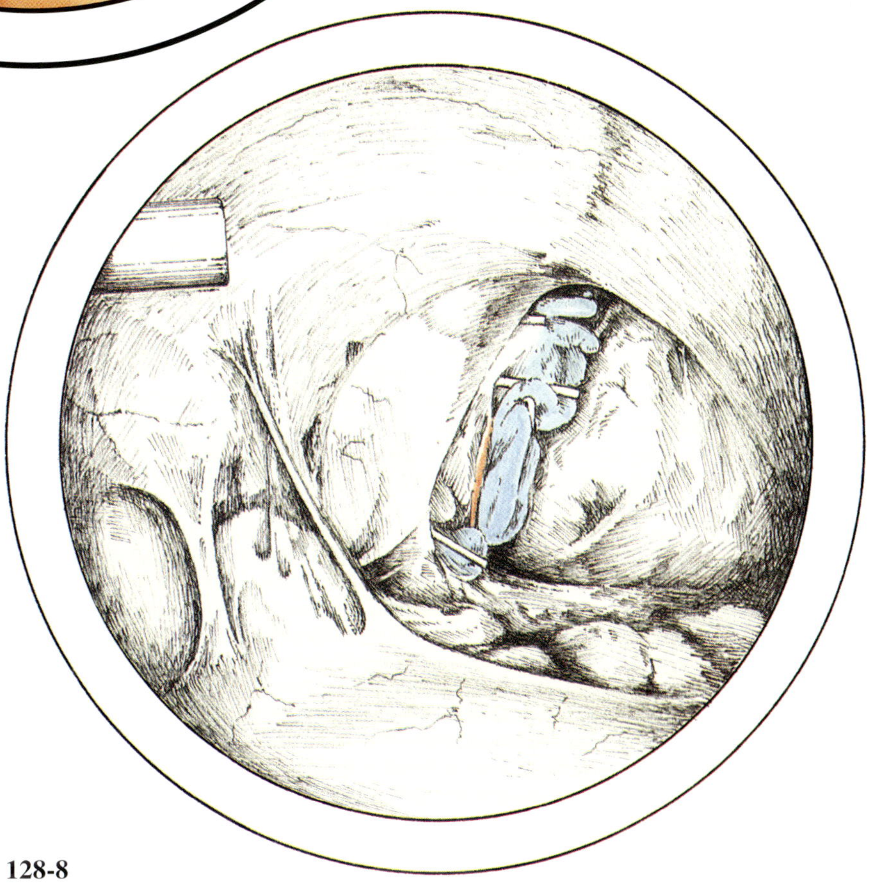

128-8

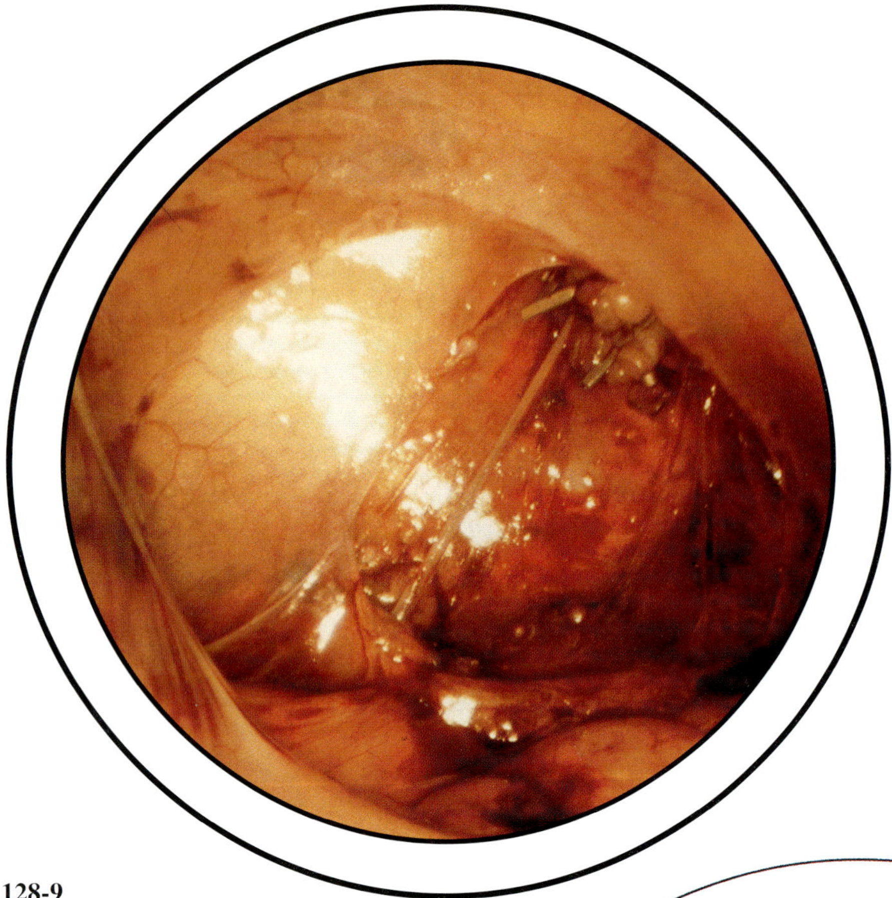

128-9

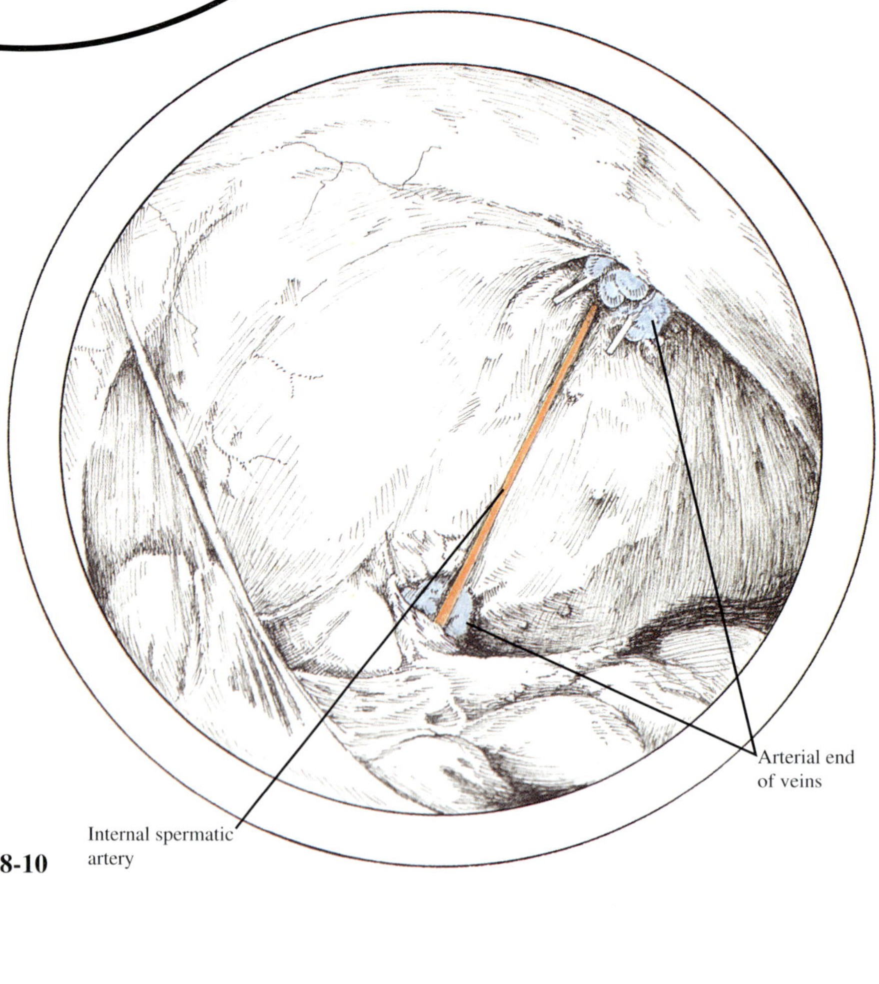

128-10

128-9 and 128-10. The venous bundle is cut in between with cold scissors. Frequently, one or two small veins remain adhering to the spermatic artery. They may grow larger in a relatively short time and can cause recurrence of the varicocele. For occlusion of these small venous channels, a Nd:YAG contact laser beam is useful. Each adherent vein is carefully separated by a curved dissector and retracted at least 1 mm away from the spermatic artery. A fine laser probe with a hemispheric tip is activated at 10 to 15 watts and placed in contact with the retracted vein while irrigating fluid is used to cool the surrounding tissues to avoid injury to the artery.

128-11. Matsuda and associates devised a simple technique for mass clip ligation of the spermatic vessels including the spermatic artery. Two parallel incisions (approximately 1 cm long each) are made along both sides of the bundle of the spermatic vessels. After the bundle is separated from the underlying psoas major with forceps through the incisions, the bundle is clamped with absorbable clips in the mass with overlying peritoneum. Usually two clips are applied. This technique is very simple and can be performed under local anesthesia. There was no notice of testicular atrophy. Also, semen quality was improved in about 60% of the patients. *We believe that the separation of the spermatic artery from the veins is important.* We clip only the veins before dividing the veins between clips.

When artery-preserving varicocelectomy is performed laparoscopically, small veins just beside the spermatic artery may be left intact and may cause recurrence of varicocele frequently. Every effort should be made to tease these veins off the artery. Then clip ligation of the veins can be accomplished.

Termination of the Procedure

On completion of the surgical procedure, careful inspection of the operative field is performed looking for any bleeding. Minor bleeders are usually controlled without difficulty by compressing the area with oxycel for a few minutes.

The intra-abdominal pressure is lowered by 5 mm Hg. This will allow any venous opening tamponaded by the 15 mm Hg CO_2 gas pressure to be recognized. Then the secondary trocars are removed one after another under laparoscopic observation to check for any bleeding or herniation of the abdominal contents into the trocar wound.

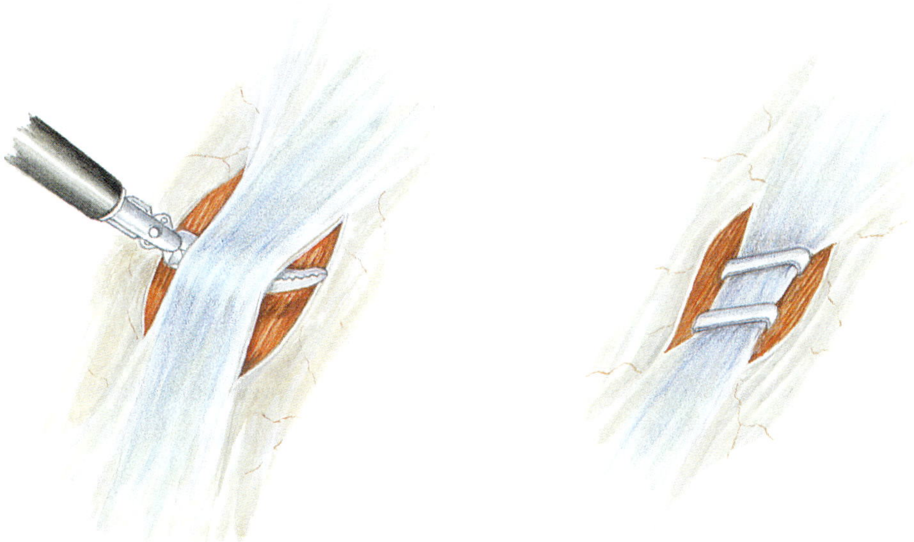

A B

128-11

The initial laparoscopic trocar may now be removed. After satisfactory evacuation of the intra-abdominal CO_2 gas, the 11 mm diameter sheath is removed slowly, checking for any bleeding or herniation of the intestine or omental tissue.

The skin site of the 5 mm port is closed with an adhesive strip. After removal of the 11 mm trocar sheath, it may be advisable to close the fascia with a single figure-of-eight absorbable suture to prevent a herniation. Care must be taken not to entrap bowel or omentum by the fascial suture. The skin at the 11 mm port is also approximated with one or two sutures.

Postoperative Care

The urethral catheter and nasogastric tube are removed in the recovery room. The patient is ambulated 4 to 6 hours after the procedure. Clear liquids can be given when the patient is awake and alert. The diet is advanced as tolerated to a regular diet, usually the evening of the same day or by the next morning.

Postoperative antibiotics are not mandatory. When needed, it is our policy to give one regular dose of broad spectrum antibiotics perioperatively for prophylaxis of infection, especially when the patient returns home on the same day of the operation.

The patient is encouraged to return to full usual activity by the second or third postoperative day.

Postoperative Complications and Management

1. Hemorrhage

Development of abdominal distension; postoperative pain; and a slow, but falling, hematocrit are potential signs of delayed hemorrhage. The anterior abdominal wall at the site of trocar placement is a commonly overlooked cause of delayed hemorrhage, especially at the lateral sites in the region of the inferior epigastric vessels. A computed tomographic (CT) scan of the abdomen is a useful study to locate the site of the hematoma.

In most instances, the symptoms will subside during careful observation. However, if there is significant ongoing bleeding causing a hemodynamic problem, open surgical exploration may be necessary.

2. Incisional Hernia

The incisional hernias may occur at the 11 mm trocar site. The 5 mm trocar sites are at low risk for possible herniation. Development of localized abdominal discomfort or pain several days after the procedure may be a symptom of a bowel herniation or omentum coming through the port sites. It can be reduced without difficulty unless it is caught by a suture. In case of difficulty, it can be reduced and repaired by a secondary laparoscopic procedure or standard open surgical techniques.

3. Peritonitis

The postoperative occurrence of fever and abdominal wall rebound tenderness may be signs of peritonitis. This occurrence can develop due to an intraoperative bowel perforation. A CT scan of the abdomen with oral contrast material will confirm the diagnosis. Surgical exploration, peritoneal lavage, and a diverting enterostomy are the recommended courses of treatment.

4. Bladder Perforation

Gross hematuria associated with pneumaturia in the recovery room is indicative of a urinary bladder perforation. Development of urinary ascites may be secondary to this injury. The onset of azotemia is associated with hyponatremia and hyperkalemia and is indicative of bladder perforation. If the perforation is small, the symptoms will resolve within 2 weeks of continuous bladder catheter drainage. However, if the injury is large, causing considerable intraperitoneal urinary extravasation, insertion of a Jackson Pratt drain or placement of a peritoneal catheter into the pelvic cavity for a several days will enhance closure of the injury.

129. Other Laparoscopic Procedures in Urology

The skilled laparoscopic surgeon can effectively replace open urologic surgical procedures with laparoscopic maneuvers. Some of them can be standard procedures of choice such as varicocelectomy, but others are still challenging procedures with limited indications.

Diagnosis and Treatment of Nonpalpable Testicle or Intersex

Laparoscopic examination in patients with a nonpalpable testicle or an intersex condition has a direct impact on any subsequent surgical procedure. An open exploration can be avoided if a testicle is not found by laparoscopy. If a testicle is present, its precise location determines the incisional site of a subsequent operative procedure. If the testicle is dysplastic, it can be removed. Finally, when a two-step orchiopexy is considered, the first stage of the Fowler-Stephens technique can be performed laparoscopically. Also, this technique is useful for diagnostic evaluation of intersex conditions.

The majority of the patients are in the pediatric age group, including babies. All laparoscopic problems that are seen in adult laparoscopy can also occur in children. The shorter pediatric instruments are rather easy to use. The trocars range from 3 to 6 mm in diameter and their length varies from 15 to 20 cm. A 5 mm telescope with a 6 Fr working channel is used, though the optical resolution is not as good as that of a 10 mm telescope.

Laparoscopic orchiectomy for an intra-abdominal testis was first introduced by Castilho et al. The technique of laparoscopic ligation of the internal spermatic artery as a first stage Fowler-Stephens orchiopexy was reported by Bloom. After 6 months or more, when collaterals are established by the cremasteric and vasal arteries, the second stage procedure can be undertaken.

Pelvic Lymphadenectomy

For cancer of the prostate, pelvic lymph node dissection is an important diagnostic procedure for clinical staging of the localized tumor. It may be performed either as a limited obturator node dissection or as an extended iliopsoas node dissection.

In patients with carcinoma of the penis, a laparoscopic lymph node dissection of the iliac nodes may also be helpful for staging of the disease.

For cancer of the bladder, a laparoscopic pelvic lymph node dissection should be performed only for the purpose of precluding an indication for radical cystectomy.

Fundamental operative techniques are similar to those of laparoscopic varicocelectomy. For the node dissection, the procedure can be performed more easily by placing the patient into a 30° head down position. The side on which the dissection is being done is elevated 30° upward.

For trocar placement, we usually prefer a diamond-shaped pattern: one 11 mm port at the umbilicus, one 11 mm port in the midline between the umbilicus and symphysis, and two 5 mm ports on each side midway between the umbilicus and the anterosuperior iliac spine. This is similar to the way bilateral varicocelectomy is performed. The node dissection is begun on the side that is more likely to have positive nodes. If the positive biopsies are from the midline, usually the right side is chosen initially, because it is easier for a right-handed surgeon. Moreover, the left side usually has adhesions between the pelvic side wall and the sigmoid colon. The adhesions must be divided to provide access to the iliac vessels and obturator nodes.

Incision of the posterior peritoneum is made along a line medial to the external iliac artery, using the electrosurgical probe. The vas deferens may be identified and incised. The lateral umbilical ligament can also be incised to provide a better view. The retroperitoneal adipose tissue is dissected from the medial aspect of the external iliac artery and the external iliac vein is identified. Care must be taken not to injure the external iliac vein, because it is frequently collapsed and appears as a flat blue ribbon due to the pressure of the pneumoperitoneum.

As one continues the dissection caudally, the obturator nerve is seen passing behind the internal iliac vein. The pubic bone is seen just lateral to the symphysis pubis, and it is cleared of overlying tissue. The gleaming white periosteum is seen. This area is the medial caudal corner of the node dissection.

Then the dissection is continued cephalad along the medial aspect of the external iliac artery and vein until one reaches the bifurcation of the common iliac artery and vein. Now the dissection is continued along the medial surface of the internal iliac artery until one meets the medial umbilical ligament (obliterated umbilical artery). Then the entire nodal tissue or packet is freed.

For the dissection of this portion, a 5 mm hook electrode is very helpful. Clips may also be used to secure the cephalad pedicle of the nodal packet.

The nodal packet can be delivered out of the abdomen via the low midline 11 mm trocar. It can be fragmented into smaller pieces with scissors and can be delivered with the 10 mm forceps.

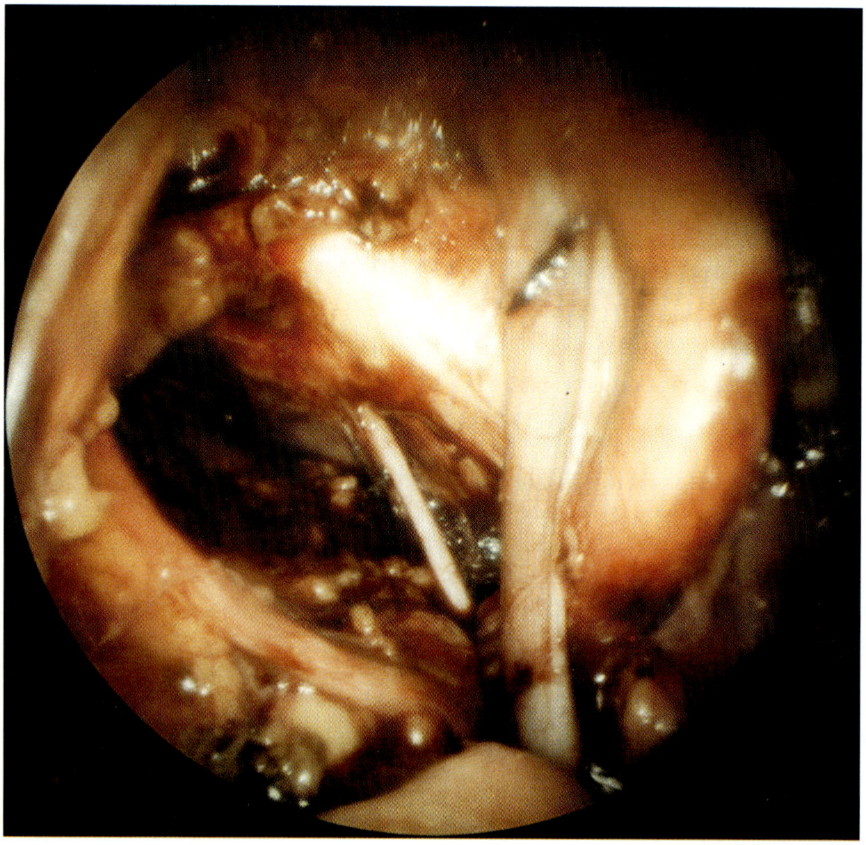

129-1

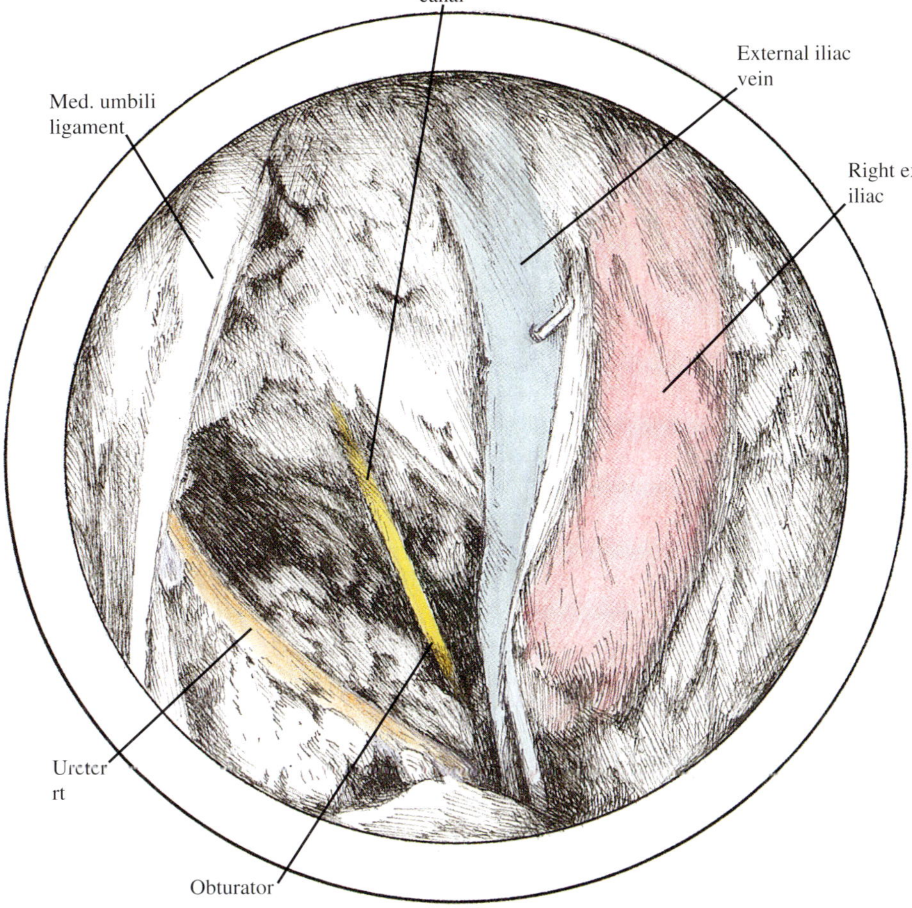

129-2

129-1 and 129-2. The peritoneal incision is approximated and clipped to prevent adhesions to the intestine. If the frozen section results on the first side are negative or if a bilateral dissection is planned from the beginning, the contralateral side is similarly approached.

Nephrectomy

Laparoscopic nephrectomy is indicated for cases in which the kidney must be removed for benign diseases. The indications are a symptomatic, poorly functioning kidney due to chronic obstruction and/or infection; renovascular hypertension; hypoplastic kidney associated with ectopic ureteral orifice causing urinary incontinence; and, occasionally, a multicystic dysplastic kidney. Partial nephrectomy can also be performed in selected cases even in an infant as young as 4 months. The application of laparoscopic nephrectomy on patients with early stage renal cell cancer or transitional cell cancer is still under clinical investigation and is controversial.

Immediately before laparoscopic nephrectomy, renal arteriography should be performed to visualize the location and distribution of the renal artery. Also, the main renal artery or segmental renal artery can be embolized after arteriography. Placement of a ureteroscope up the ureter of the operative side helps identification of the ureter. The illuminating light at its tip can be visualized by laparoscopy.

In all cases of laparoscopic renal surgery, general anesthesia with an endotracheal tube is employed. A nasogastric tube is passed to deflate the stomach. Positive compression stockings of the pneumatic type are placed on both lower extremities.

The initial patient position is supine. The abdomen is insufflated and the initial three ports are placed: one just below the umbilicus (12 mm), one at the upper midclavicular line immediately subcostal (12 mm), and another one at the lower midclavicular line about 3 to 4 cm below the level of the umbilicus. The patient is then rolled into a lateral decubitus position. The contralateral arm is tucked close to the body and wrapped in protective foam padding. The ipsilateral arm is brought over the body and secured to the other screen. A pillow is placed between the legs and the lower leg is flexed to about 30° at the level of the knees. Then the table is flexed to place the patient in a secure lateral decubitus position. Sand bags can be used to further support the patient in this position.

Next, two 5 mm ports are placed in the ipsilateral anterior axillary line, one at the tip of the 12th rib and one at the level of the umbilicus. Five trocars are now in place; the surgeon functionally works with the two midclavicular line trocars; the first assistant operates the two anterior axillary line trocars and the second assistant operates the camera via the trocar at the umbilicus. All trocars are directed towards the renal pelvis.

The incision is made on the white line of Toldt and is continued caudally until the common iliac artery is seen pulsating. The incision is then extended cephalad along the hepatic or splenic flexure, depending on the appropriate kidney. The dissection now proceeds medially until the colon can be completely freed and swung medially away from Gerota's fascia. On the right side, the duodenum is reflected medially to reveal the anterior surface of the inferior vena cava. On the left side, care must be taken in dissecting the colon in the area of the spleen.

Identification of the ureter may be easily made by illuminating the fiberoptic ureteroscope placed up the ureter on the operating side. The ureter is carefully freed from the retroperitoneum and umbilical tape is wrapped around the ureter for retraction. Then it can be dissected rapidly from the rest of the retroperitoneal tissues.

The gonadal vein is visualized; the right side is crossing the ureter and the left side is running along side the ureter. The vein is carefully dissected from surrounding tissue, occluded by two 9 mm clips and transected in between. The left gonadal vein will lead the surgeon to the left main renal vein superiorly.

After the ureter is dissected superiorly to the ureteropelvic junction, the lower pole of the kidney is cleared of surrounding tissue. Since a renal cancer is not present, Gerota's fascia is purposely incised. The renal capsule is then identified and dissected superiorly to the upper portion of the kidney. The surrounding retroperitoneal tissue at the upper pole of the kidney, including the adrenal gland, is pushed in a cephalad direction off the renal surface. This dissection is continued medially until the entire medial surface of the upper pole is exposed. The dissection of the upper pole of the kidney will not be easy on the right side because of the overlying liver. On the left side, care must be taken to avoid lacerating the spleen.

Now the surgeon continues the procedure to secure the hilar vessels. The upper pole of the kidney is retracted laterally and upward by an atraumatic forceps and the umbilical tape wrapped to the ureter is also pulled laterally and upward by the assistant by stretching the renal hilum to provide a better view to the surgeon. Then the surgeon dissects the hilar vessels using electrosurgical scissors through the upper midclavicular line port. An atraumatic forceps through the upper anterior axillary line port is helpful. The renal vein is usually identified first. It is carefully dissected from the surrounding tissue. Then the renal artery is identified and dissected. On the right side, there is usually a single renal vein and single renal artery. On the left side, however, the surgeon should carefully dissect out the branches of the renal vein: the adrenal, ascending lumbar, and gonadal. They can be separately identified. A window is made around each vessel, doubly clipped with 9 mm clips on each side and transected. It is helpful to pass a curved dissector through the 12 mm midclavicular line port to help develop separate windows. For the renal artery, three titanium 9 mm clips are placed on the median portion of the renal artery, two clips are placed on the lateral portion, and the area in between is transected. Following this, the renal vein is similarly clipped and transected.

After securing the hilar vessels, the procedure is continued, and the ureter is incised. After removal of the previously placed fiber ureteroscope or ureteral occlusion balloon catheter, two pairs of 9 mm titanium clips are placed on the ureter, and the ureter is incised in between. The umbilical tape around the ureter is removed. Then, the kidney is freed from all other attachments.

Removal of the kidney from the abdominal cavity is a major challenge. The technique of using an entrapment sack is described in detail by Clayman and McDougall. The 5 × 8 inch entrapment sack is carefully rolled onto its introducer and passed into the abdominal cavity via the upper 12 mm midclavicular line port. The sack is pulled out of the introducer using two atraumatic 5 mm graspers. The laparoscope is then moved to the upper midclavicular line port from the umbilical port to allow three locking/grasping forceps to manipulate and open the entrapment sack. Then, the laparoscope is passed into the sack to open the bag. Use of CO_2 gas insufflation will also help to expand the sack. The freed kidney is pulled toward the open sack by the grasper on the ureter and placed deep within the sack. Then the drawstrings of the sack are grasped with the 5 mm locking forceps that have passed through the umbilical port and are drawn into the sheath; this allows the neck of the sack also to be drawn into the tip of the 12 mm umbilical sheath. At this time, the intra-abdominal pressure is decreased to 5 mm Hg to check for hemorrhage and hemostasis of the operative site. Hemostasis must be complete.

Delivery of the kidney is begun after the patient is returned to a supine position. The laparoscope is maintained in the 12 mm midclavicular line port. When the neck of the sack is secured into the tip of the sheath, the draw strings are released from the forceps, and the forceps and the sheath are completely removed from the abdomen. The surgeon then grasps the drawstrings with his hand and pulls them up until the neck of the sack is delivered onto the abdominal wall. If the removed kidney is atrophied and small, the surgeon can deliver it by enlarging the port site using retractors or extending the incision a little longer with a knife. In most instances, however, the tissue morcellator is used to fragment the organ through the opening of the sack. When the renal tissue is fragmented and the pieces are aspirated into the handle of the morcellator, the sack is withdrawn from the abdominal cavity.

The abdominal cavity can be irrigated with approximately 300 to 500 cc of saline irrigant containing broad spectrum antibiotics and the fluid is aspirated as completely as possible.

When exiting the abdomen, a 5 mm laparoscope is placed in the lower anterior axillary port. Then the 12 mm ports are removed and closed with 0 absorbable figure-of-eight fascial sutures placed under endoscopic monitoring. The subcutaneous tissue is closed with a 3–0 absorbable suture. The 5 mm ports are removed under endoscopic control. The laparoscopic site is removed last, carefully inspecting the path of the port. All skin port sites are approximated with approximating adhesive strips.

References

1. Clayman RV. Techniques in percutaneous removal of renal calculi. Mechanical extraction and electrohydraulic lithotripsy. Urology 23:11–19, 1984.
2. Hunter PT, Finlayson B, Drylie DM, Leal J, Hawkins IF. Retrograde nephrostomy and percutaneous calculus removal in 30 patients. J Urol 133:369–374, 1985.
3. Clayman RV, Surya V, Miller RP, Castaneda-Zuniga WR, Smith AD, Hunter DH, Amplatz K, Lange PH. Percutaneous nephrolithotomy: extraction of renal and ureteral calculi from 100 patients. J Urol 131:868–871, 1984.

Suggested Readings

Ao T, Endo T, Suyama I, Harano Y, Utsunomiya T, Uchida T, Yokoyama E, Koshiba K. Four cases of laparoscopic nephrectomy. Jpn J Clin Urol 47:833, 1993.

Bloom DA. Two step orchiopexy with pelviscopic clip ligation of the spermatic vessels. J Urol 145:1030, 1991.

Castilho LN, Ferreira U, Esteves SC, Valim LA, Netto NR. Laparoscopic Orchiectomy. J Endourol 5:S163, 1991.

Clayman RV, McDougall EM. Laparoscopic Urology. St. Louis: Quality Medical Publishing, 1993:290–301.

Ehrlich RM, Gershman A, Fuchs G. Laparoscopic renal surgery in children. J Urol 151:735, 1994.

Fishburne JI, Keith L. Anesthesia. In: Phillips JM, ed. Laparoscopy. Baltimore: Williams & Wilkins, 1977:69–95.

Griffith DP, Schuessler WW, Vancaillie TH. Laparoscopic lymphadenectomy: a low morbidity alternative for staging pelvic malignancies. J Endourol 4(suppl 1):S84, 1990.

Hodson J. The lobar structure of the kidney. Brit J Urol 44:246–261, 1972.

Matsuda T, Horii Y, Higashi S, Oishi K, Takeuchi H, Yoshida O. Laparoscopic varicocelectomy: a simple technique for clip ligation of the spermatic vessels. J Urol 147:636–638, 1992.

O'Sullivan G, Sear JW, Bullingham RES, Carrie LES. The effect of magnesium trisilicate mixture, metoclopramide, and ranitidine on gastric pH, volume and serum gastrin. Anesthesia 40: 246–253, 1985.

Stoelting RK, Miller RD. Monitoring. In: Basics of Anesthesia. New York: Churchill Livingstone, 1989:211–227.

Winfield HN, See WA, Donovan JF, Godet A, Farage YM, Loening SA, Williams RD. Comparative effectiveness and safety of laparoscopic vs open pelvic lymph node dissection for cancer of the prostate. J Urol 147:244A, 1992.

Transurethral Resection of Prostate (TURP)

10

Transurethral prostatic resection of the enlarged prostate (BPH) is an integral and extremely important part of prostatic surgery. Today, the majority of obstructive prostatic lesions are operated on using this approach.

Although there are two types of transurethral prostatic resection (TURP), cold punch resection and electroresection, the latter is the method employed almost universally and is the procedure usually referred to in relation to TURP.

Modern instruments providing excellent visualization permit the rapid resection of tissue and instant coagulation of bleeding vessels by powerful high-frequency currents. The technique of transurethral resection is, however, still one of the most difficult of all urologic operations to master. Moreover, it requires different abilities plus intensive and prolonged training. The procedure is not simple. The potential exists for many operative hazards and complications when the operation is performed inaccurately and inefficiently by the inexperienced endoscopic surgeon. On the other hand, if carried out skillfully and adequately by a well-trained resectionist, the procedure is better tolerated than an open procedure, especially when the patient is a poor surgical risk. One can expect accurate and more efficient removal of tissue by transurethral resection: the resectionist can remove the surgical capsule or compressed peripheral zone of the prostate. These vestiges always remain when the adenomatous hypertrophied prostate is enucleated by open prostatectomy.

In our view, the younger generation of urologists is more enthusiastic about transurethral resection than are their elders. We believe the instruments and the operative technique will continue to improve and will make this procedure more accurate and less difficult technically. A recent advancement is the small video camera plus videotape apparatus. By attaching the video camera, which then connects to the resectoscope, a novice can observe transurethral surgery being performed by a more experienced urologist. The observer can watch the TV monitor. The surgeon can replay the tape later and learn from his/her experience.

INDICATIONS AND CONTRAINDICATIONS

Any type of prostatic obstruction, whether large or small, benign or malignant, can be treated by transurethral resection. Basically, the indications and contraindications for TURP are the same as those for suprapubic or open prostatectomy.

Obstructive carcinoma of the prostate for which total prostatectomy is not suitable is an important indication for TURP. Many patients with advanced carcinoma, however, are relieved of obstruction by conservative endoscopic means.

One of the contraindications for TURP is stricture of the urethra, but the prostate can be successfully resected transurethrally through a perineal urethrotomy because most urethral strictures are located distally in the bulbous urethra. Another contraindication is a deformity of the pelvis or fixation of the hip joint, prohibiting the introduction of the instrument or the operative movement of the resectoscope to permit adequate visualization of the entire prostate.

Normal bladder function is essential in carrying out a TURP. A patient with an atonic or hypotonic bladder due to neurogenic causes cannot expect to regain normal detrusor action following TURP. The obstruction at the bladder neck and the original neurogenic cause must be treated. On the other hand, a hypertonic or contracted bladder with a very low capacity also presents a serious problem during endoscopy because the period before irrigating fluid fills the bladder is short and the operative time is significantly reduced.

The size of the hypertrophied glands to be removed is an important criterion in deciding whether the transurethral or open surgical approach should be employed. As a rule, glands less than 50 g are generally suited to transurethral operation, allowing completion of the procedure within 60 minutes. This interval will generally prevent unfavorable complications, such as excess absorption of irrigating fluid.

Recent advances in the operative and postoperative management of the patient, including the use of a nonhemolytic isotonic irrigating fluid coupled with the intravenous administration of mannitol containing appropriate amounts of electrolytes, has enabled the extension of the operative time to 2 hours. The size of the glands suited to a one-stage procedure approaches 100 g even for the resectionist who has average endoscopic skills.

PATIENT PREPARATION

Most patients who require transurethral prostatic surgery are in the older age group; therefore, their general condition requires careful evaluation and examination prior to the operation. Proper attention must be paid to the patient's cardiovascular, respiratory, hepatic, and neurologic systems before transurethral surgery is undertaken.

Prolonged urinary-tract obstruction will produce renal insufficiency. Although repeated catheterization frequently causes urinary tract infection, preoperative catheter drainage is indicated in the presence of a large amount (over 200 mL) of residual urine to improve renal function prior to operation. The drainage system should be closed and aseptic. Irrigation of the drainage system is not necessary unless infection with exudate or calculus formation is found.

Diabetes mellitus must be brought under control before surgery. Particular care is required to stabilize the blood glucose by calculating the amount of insulin required. Precise regulation of the diet must be continued. An overdose of insulin is the principal danger to the diabetic patient undergoing surgery. Insulin shock may be difficult to distinguish from shock due to blood loss or to excessive dilution of serum electrolytes during or immediately following transurethral surgery. This is especially pertinent while the patient is under general anesthesia. One may allow some glycosuria the day of operation.

When Kimmelstiel-Wilson's disease with renal insufficiency is documented, transurethral resection may be undertaken if the blood urea nitrogen (BUN) and serum creatinine levels are stabilized at the lower levels (BUN, 35 mg/dL; creatinine, approximately 2.5 mg/dL).

If the patient is receiving anticoagulant therapy for the treatment of cardiovascular disease or an old cerebrovascular accident, the medication should be discontinued for at least 5 days before surgery. Hypoprothrombinemia caused by bishydroxycoumarin (Dicumarol) and its derivatives should be corrected by the use of vitamin K.

If the patient has a history of an abnormal bleeding diathesis or if there is a family history of a bleeding tendency suggesting hemophilia, a complete hematologic workup should be carried out. Transurethral resection is not recommended in the patient with bleeding tendencies of any type.

A concomitant bilateral partial vasectomy is not a guarantee against postoperative epididymitis. Statistics show that the incidence of the complication is significantly lowered when vasectomy is carried out before TURP. If a patient needs prolonged preoperative catheter drainage to improve his renal function, it is recommended that bilateral partial vasectomy be performed at the time an indwelling catheter is introduced.

When the necessary preoperative examinations have been completed and the therapeutic measures for preoperative care have been carried out so that his general condition has reached a satisfactory level, the patient is ready for TURP.

A gentle sedative is administered the night before and an enema is given the morning of operation. For elderly patients, barbiturates should be avoided. If necessary, the enema should be repeated to empty the rectum completely before the patient is taken to the operating room.

ANESTHESIA

Low spinal or epidural anesthesia is satisfactory for patients undergoing TURP. The patient is kept awake during the operative procedure so that he can alert the doctor to abdominal pain if irrigating fluid extravasates outside the prostatic capsule. He may also complain of nausea and restlessness when large quantities of irrigating fluid are absorbed into the circulatory system.

Spinal anesthesia affords complete bladder and muscle relaxation and causes little postoperative discomfort, nausea, or vomiting. Its main disadvantage is that it may lead to a sudden fall in blood pressure unless pressor substances are administered at appropriate intervals. Sudden changes in blood pressure are hazardous to the patient with cardiovascular disease. Prolonged hypotension may cause renal, myocardial, and cerebral damage.

Epidural anesthesia is probably even safer in the poor-risk patient because it has little effect on the cardiovascular system. One of the disadvantages of epidural anesthesia is that 20 minutes are required after administration for the anesthesia to have a satisfactory analgesic effect. Therefore, a significant time loss occurs before the operative procedure is begun. However, this time loss will be minimized by an anesthetist introducing the epidural canula prior to the scheduled time of operation, in the early morning or on the day before. Another disadvantage of epidural anesthesia is that it sometimes causes a mild but bothersome penile erection, which elongates the urethra. The tip of a resectoscope may not easily reach the bladder neck in a tall patient. However, intracavernous injection of 2 mg of etilefrine hydrochloride will promptly reduce the penis to its flaccid state. Once anesthesia has been properly induced, satisfactory analgesia and muscle relaxation are achieved.

Disadvantages to the use of general anesthesia are that 1) it does not provide sufficient relaxation without administration of muscle relaxants and 2) there is an increased risk of respiratory complications. Explosive inhalant gases should not be used in transurethral resection in which high frequency electrical currents are employed. However, for the extremely apprehensive patient, in whom general anesthesia is desired, supplementary general anesthesia with nitrous oxide and oxygen is recommended and complements epidural or low spinal anesthesia.

INSTRUMENTS AND SUPPLIES

Before the operation, instruments and supplies should be carefully checked. The operating table should have a large drainage tray and should be rapidly adjustable to allow elevation or lowering of the patient by a hydraulic or electrical mechanism. The operative chair should also be mobile to allow changes in the position and height of the surgeon.

Two resectoscopes should be prepared in every setup for TURP. A second light source and electrosurgical unit should also be available for rapid substitution in the operating room in the event of malfunction in any one instrument.

In addition to two resectoscopes and loops, the following accessories and instruments are required for transurethral resection:

1. Drapes and a plastic rectal shield, gloves.
2. Male urethral sounds No. 20 through 30 French, lubricating jelly in a medicine glass, and a urethral syringe.
3. Light cord, power cord, and irrigating-fluid conduit with stopcock.
4. Minor surgery tray for vasectomy, meatotomy, and suprapubic drainage; gauze sponges.
5. Two Ellik evacuators and Toomey syringes; a basin for filling evacuators with irrigating fluid.
6. Indwelling Foley catheters, No. 20 through 24 Fr, with a 30-mL inflatable bag; a curved stylet and a glass stopper; and a 50-mL syringe with adapter for inflating the indwelling urethral catheter.

The irrigating system should supply fluid on demand and continuously during the resecting procedure. Two plastic fluid-containing bags (each with a 3 liter capacity) suspended from a stand provide a convenient and easily sterilizable irrigating system that is still popular. The use of a factory-bottled nonhemolytic isotonic solution with disposable tubing units is more convenient if an abundant supply is available.

During the resecting procedure, the level of the irrigating fluid is maintained from 50 to 80 cm above the patient's bladder. The pressure should be maintained at the low level because this keeps the operative field clear of blood and because the lower the pressure, the less danger of bladder overdistension. Less absorption of irrigating fluid occurs at lower pressures.

The use of a nonhemolytic isotonic irrigating fluid, such as glycine or a mixture of mannitol and sorbitol (Cytal) is recommended. We prefer the latter fluid. Mannitol is a potent osmotic diuretic and has a protective effect, discouraging acute renal failure when large amounts of irrigating fluid are absorbed. The irrigating fluid should be delivered at body temperature.

The bladder and prostatic fossa are washed with tremendous quantities of irrigating fluid during the endoscopic procedure. If the fluid is cold, the pelvic area and body temperature are lowered, and the patient may be chilled.

POSTOPERATIVE MANAGEMENT

We usually move the patient to the ward within 1 hour after TURP. Careful observation is done at the ward for the first few hours. It is important to recognize such possible complications as excessive bleeding, low-sodium syndrome, hypotension, renal insufficiency, and respiratory distress. Blood counts, serum electrolytes, and arterial blood gas levels should be monitored in the poor-risk patient as soon as the endoscopic procedure is completed. The data should be compared with preoperative levels and appropriate therapy should be started.

In the immediate postoperative period, the patient should be free of pain except for mild discomfort in the urethra, occasionally accompanied by a desire to void. Ordinarily, a new severe pain is a sign of a complication that must be treated immediately. In most cases, it is a symptom of bladder distension due to catheter obstruction with blood clots; it may also signal a perforation of the prostatic capsule or bladder wall. Prompt action should be taken to treat the appropriate problem. If untreated, it may progress to a significant degree. Excessive blood loss should be replaced with blood transfusions. Appropriate amounts of 5 to 10% sodium chloride should be added to the intravenous fluids to correct hyponatremia.

The necessity for using a urethral catheter means postoperative urinary infection will develop almost inevitably. Now we are seeing a number of patients without postoperative infection by using a closed drainage system. Therefore, frequent bacteriologic culture of the urine is required. Postoperative infection of the bladder, prostatic fossa, and urethra is usually mild and can be controlled by use of appropriate antimicrobial drugs. Maintenance of a high fluid intake and removal of the indwelling catheter at the earliest opportunity help minimize infection.

When urinary infection exists prior to operation, culture and sensitivity tests are performed to identify the invading organism. Appropriate antibiotics to treat the existing infection should be started before and continued during the transurethral procedure.

Catheter care to keep the lumen open and draining is an important principle of postoperative care. When the patient is well hydrated, there may be a steady drip of clear or blood-tinged urine from the catheter. This indicates that there is no undue hemorrhage and that hand irrigation is unnecessary. We prefer to use the regular straight-drainage closed system in such cases. If, on the other hand, there is either intermittent flow from the catheter or a flow of bloody urine, irrigation of the catheter and evacuation of blood clots in the drainage system and bladder are necessary.

Frequently, postoperative hemorrhage may be controlled adequately by evacuating blood clots from the bladder and prostatic fossa; this allows contraction of the prostatic capsule and bladder neck which, in turn, discourages further bleeding. Use of a continuous irrigation system with a three-way catheter, 22 to 24 Fr, is sometimes quite useful.

The traction of an indwelling catheter (50- or 60-mL bag) against the bladder neck is also helpful in controlling undue bleeding from the bladder neck and prostatic fossa. Care must be taken not to inflate the hemostatic bag excessively. If it is inflated with more than 70 mL of water, the tip of the catheter may be elevated at the dome of the bladder, which disturbs the smooth return of irrigating fluid.

As a rule, patients are permitted out of bed the day after transurethral resection unless there is a danger of excessive bleeding. It is advisable to have the patient out of bed, sitting quietly in a chair. The patient is permitted to walk as soon as the danger of hemorrhage has passed.

The indwelling catheter is removed in 3 or 4 days when macroscopic hematuria has disappeared. Too early removal of the catheter sometimes encourages significant hemorrhage.

The patient is ready to be discharged from the hospital on the day following removal of the catheter. He should be afebrile and voiding clear or slightly blood-tinged urine without difficulty. Periodic examination of the urine should be continued at the outpatient clinic or office as long as the urine is infected. Appropriate antimicrobial drugs are administered as needed.

ORIENTATION WITH THE RESECTOSCOPE LENS

Complete observation of the bladder neck and prostatic urethra should be accomplished and all landmarks, including ureteral orifices, should be well visualized before resection is started. The safety of this operation depends upon constant identification of all important landmarks in the operative field. Only pathologic tissue is resected; other structures are spared. Routine use of an oblique lens in the visual telescope system (foroblique) is very helpful for a beginner. Experience will facilitate rapid and accurate identification of all landmarks in the bladder and urethra.

The important landmarks (Fig. 1) seen with the foroblique telescope lens in patients with prostatic hypertrophy are:

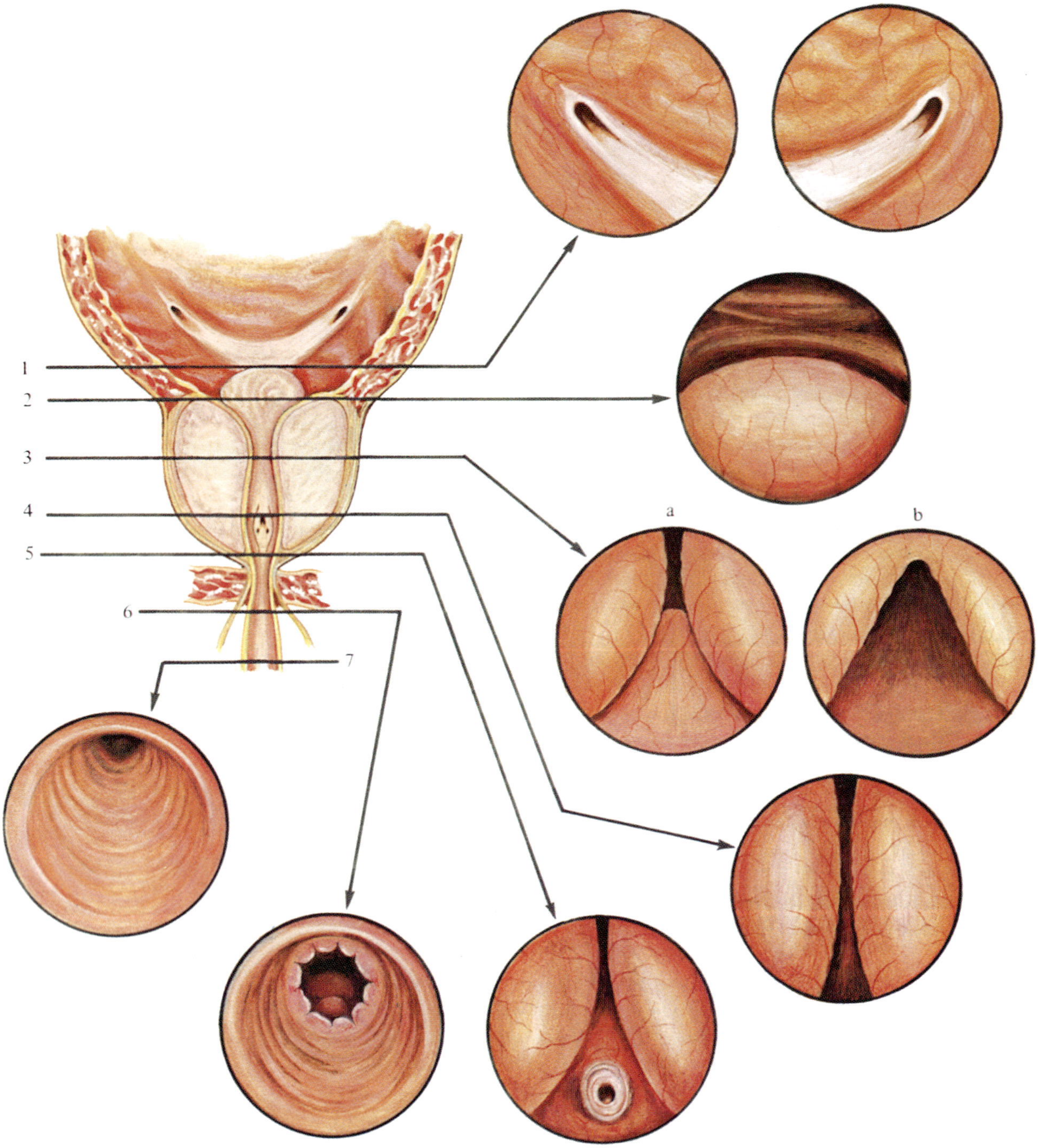

FIG. 1.
Landmarks in patients with prostatic hypertrophy, as seen with the telescope lens.

1. Vesical trigone, right and left ureteral orifices.
2. Intravesical median lobe.
3. a. Both lateral lobes and median lobe at the prostatovesical junction.
   b. Junction of lateral lobes in the 12 o'clock position.
4. Hypertrophied lateral lobes as seen between the bladder neck and verumontanum.
5. Verumontanum and intruding lateral lobes at the lower posterior surface of the prostatic urethra.
6. External sphincter at the membranous urethra.
7. Bulbous urethra.

When significant prostatic hypertrophy with marked intravesical protrusion exists, there will be a considerable blind area. The ureteral orifices may not be identified with the foroblique telescope lens.

The verumontanum is the most important landmark by which the surgeon can be assured that resection is close to the external sphincter. It is found by withdrawing the telescope until the rounded prominence is seen on the posterior floor of the prostatic urethra.

The external sphincter is just distal to the verumontanum. It is a pleated circular band that wrinkles when the telescope and sheath tip are pushed forward and backward. Accurate identification of this point is very important to ensure that resection does not damage the external sphincter when resection is concentrated close to apical tissue at the verumontanum.

POSITION OF THE PATIENT AND PREPARATION OF THE OPERATIVE FIELD

After the patient is properly anesthetized, the patient is placed in a lithotomy position on the operating table. An indifferent electrode is placed beneath the buttocks. The patient's knees should be widely spread to allow adequate space between them for manipulation of the resectoscope. The thighs should be at a gentle angle with the body to avoid elevating the pelvis. If the thighs are flexed at an acute angle, then the prostate is displaced downward into the perineum; during surgery the resectoscope is then tilted upward in an awkward position, and this location prevents smooth manipulation of the resectoscope along the horizontal plane.

The lower abdomen, penis, scrotum, and perineal area are well cleansed with soap and antiseptic solution.

The plastic rectal shield is applied over the perineum with its finger cup well lubricated with a sterile surgical lubricant. The finger cup is inserted into the rectum.

The operative field is draped; the power and light cord are connected to their source. All other instruments are checked and placed in working order before the operation is started.

Preliminary Accessory Urologic Procedures. After bilateral partial vasectomy, or immediately after the patient is draped if vasectomy is omitted, the urethra is well lubricated with a water-soluble jelly. Urethral calibration and dilatation are performed with curved urethral sounds (24 to 30 Fr). If a 30 Fr sound can be passed easily, the surgeon may choose a 28 Fr resectoscope sheath for resection of significant prostatic hypertrophy. When urethral calibration is snug to a 28 Fr sound, a smaller sized sheath, 26 or 24 Fr, is selected according to urethral size.

Urethral dilatation by means of a curved metal sound is helpful when mild urethral stenosis disturbs the free passage of a resectoscope sheath. After the urethra is dilated to the size of a 26 Fr sound, there will be no difficulty in performing transurethral resection with a 24 Fr resectoscope sheath.

Frequently, a narrow external urethral meatus causes difficulty in introducing the resectoscope sheath. External meatotomy is performed by cutting the ventral aspect of the urethral meatus in such cases. It is important to suture the divided urethral mucosa to the adjacent mucosa of the glans penis. If the incision is left open, a more severe stenosis will recur when healing takes place.

When a long urethral stricture or unusual narrowing of the entire anterior urethra is encountered, transurethral resection can be performed through a perineal urethrotomy. It is performed by cutting down vertically on a urethral sound at the perineum. A filiform and follower can be used to identify the bulbous urethra. When the incision is extended into the urethral lumen, anchor sutures are placed through the bulbocavernosus muscle and wall of the urethra on each side. Through this opening the resectoscope sheath can be introduced without difficulty into the prostatic urethra and bladder.

Operative Techniques

The surgeon will have decided upon a well-organized plan prior to starting the resection. Proper strategy will allow a satisfactory operative result in the allotted time. Resection of a piece of tissue from one lobe and then the opposite lateral lobe of the prostate is not an efficient method of performing transurethral resection. Although several efficient operative strategies have been described by excellent resectionists, our favorite plan is introduced herein.

130. Transurethral Resection for Prostatic Hypertrophy

130-1. After *the resectoscope sheath is* introduced through the external meatus or perineal urethrotomy, the Timberlake obturator is removed and the inflow line is connected to the one-way stopcock on the metal rim of the sheath. Then the working element equipped with a cutting loop and the oblique telescope is introduced and locked into the sheath. A light and a power cord are connected to the resectoscope.

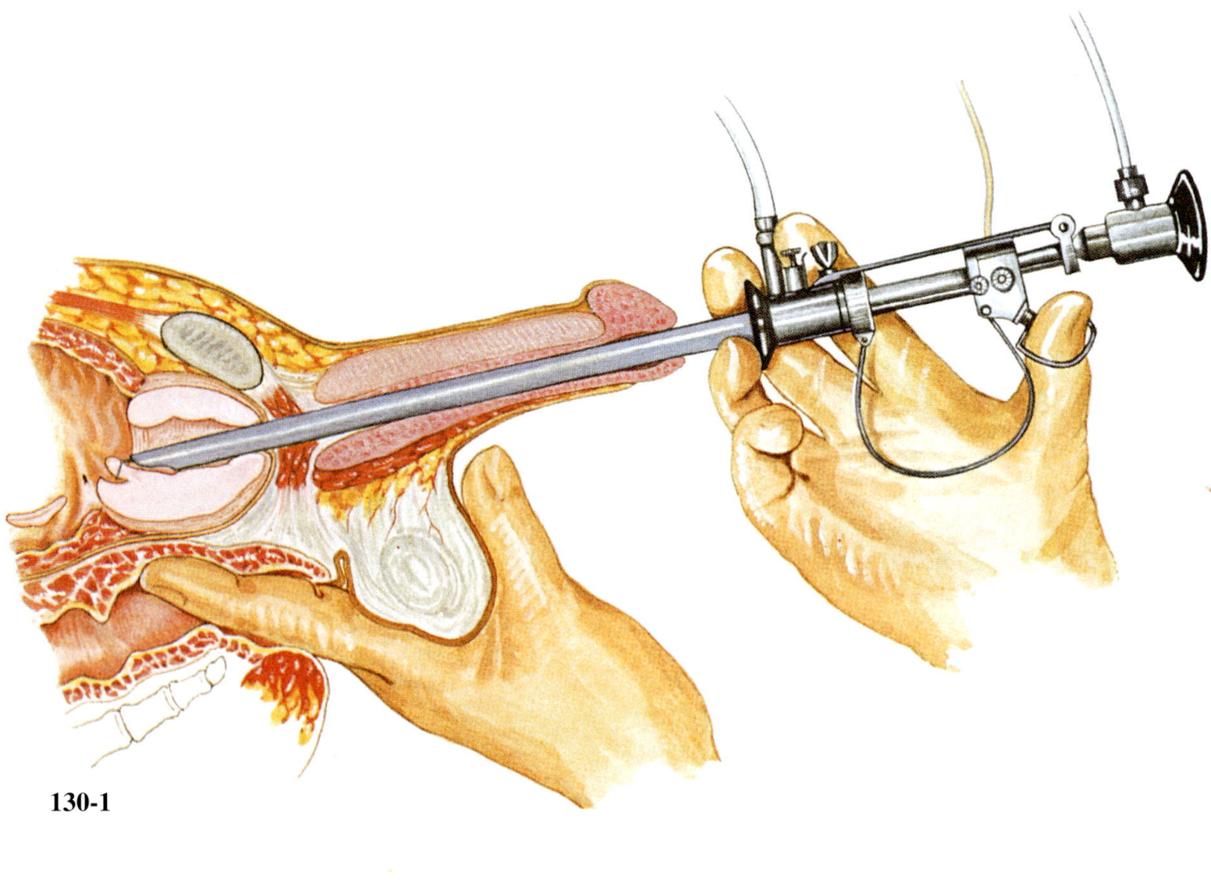

130-1

130-2. *The "landmarks" are now identified.*

130-3. The surgeon starts to *resect at the posterior bladder neck between the 4 and 8 o'clock positions.* The median lobe is removed down to the mid-prostatic zone and the elevated bladder neck is resected close to the circular fibers of the internal sphincter. But never resect too deep into the circular fibers. If the circular fibers are fully exposed by excessive resection, it may cause postoperative bladder neck contracture.

This initial maneuver cuts off some of the main blood supply to the median and lateral lobes at about the 4 and 8 o'clock positions. Careful coagulation of these bleeding points makes further resection of these lobes easier and bloodless.

After this area is flattened, irrigation of tissue fragments into the bladder cavity during the resecting procedure allows the surgeon to maintain a good endoscopic view.

Another advantage of beginning the resection at the posterior portion of the bladder neck rather than at its anterior portion is the greater number of important landmarks existing in this area. Finishing the resection of this area with a clear view in the very beginning of the operation is a great advantage; it helps the surgeon to avoid injuring the trigone and ureteral orifices and cutting too deeply into the circular internal sphincter fibers.

After this initial step is completed, the surgeon returns to this area only for coagulation of bleeding points, not for cutting.

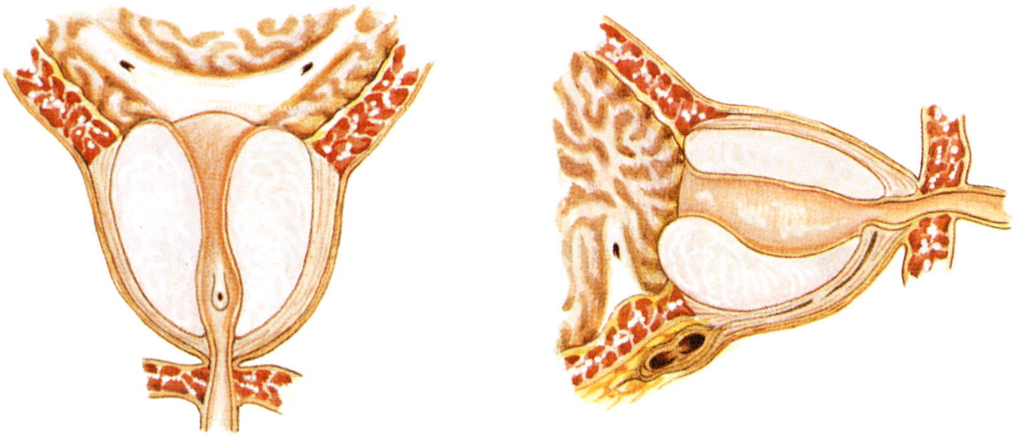

130-2

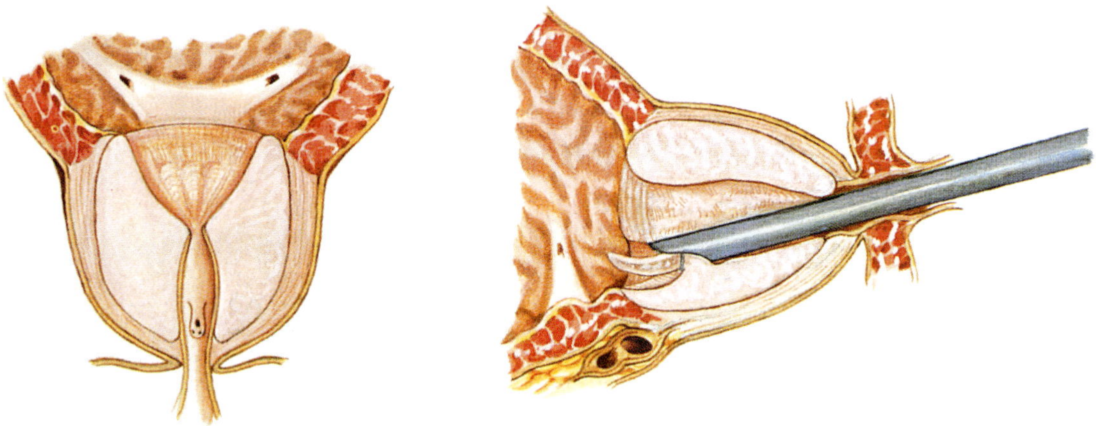

130-3

130-4. *The anterior commissure is resected.* After the first few pieces of tissue are resected, the anterior commissure will widen laterally as the tops of the lateral lobes drop down to either side. After this step, resection of the lateral lobes is initiated, with each lobe being resected separately.

Making the furrow at this point usually produces little anterior adenomatous tissue and with one or two sweeps of the loop, the circular fibers of the bladder neck are exposed. It is helpful to establish this valuable landmark at the early stage.

130-5A and B. *The main part of each lateral lobe is resected from the bladder neck to the level of the verumontanum.* Each side of the lateral lobe is thoroughly resected and the bleeders are coagulated. The surgeon does not move to the opposite lobe until all the active bleeders are stopped and the return of irrigation fluid becomes almost bloodless. This precaution obviates a search of the entire operative field when active bleeding occurs during resection of the opposite lobe.

When resection is completed to this stage, the widely opened prostatic fossa comes into view in front of the verumontanum.

If the patient is a poor risk or in the older age group, the surgeon may stop the operation. Satisfactory clinical results usually can be expected when the resection is carried out to this point.

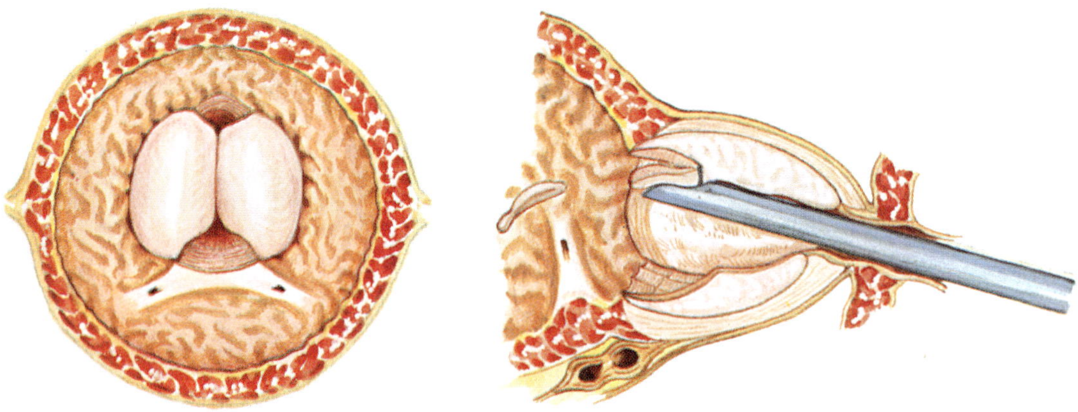

130-4

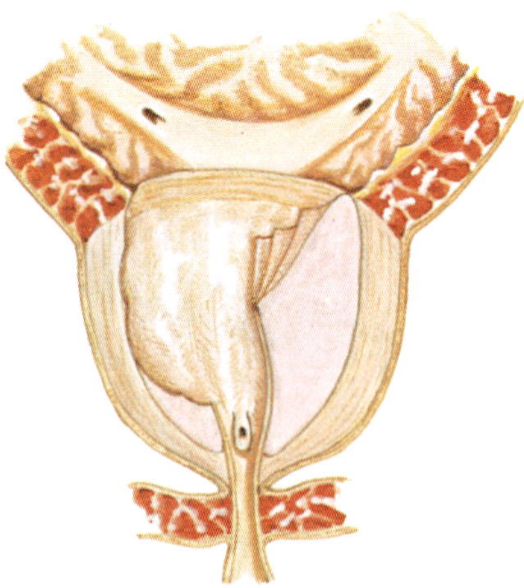

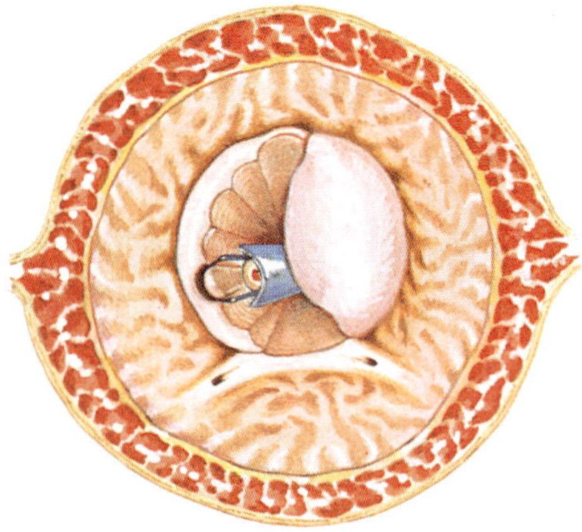

130-5A

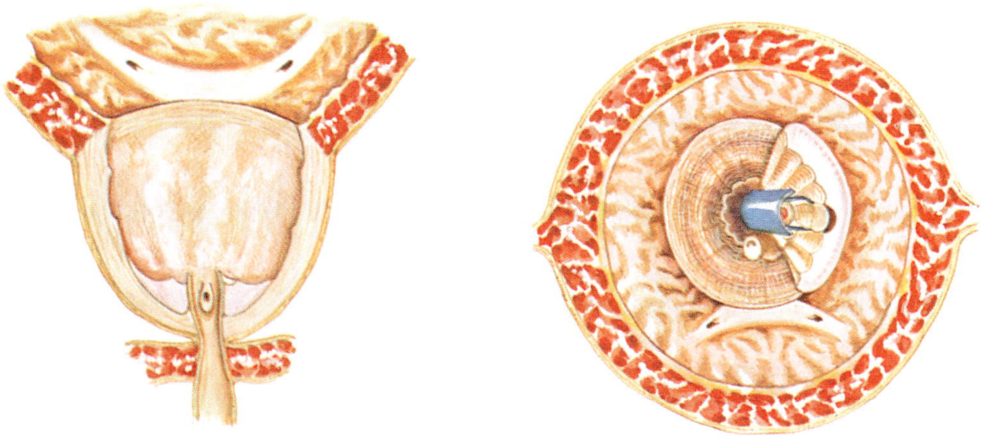

130-5B

130-6. *The resection is completed by removing the remaining tissue around the verumontanum and prostatic apex.* This is the most critical step of the whole procedure and great care is taken to judge the correct amount of tissue to remove. The adenomatous tissue may extend beyond the verumontanum both anteriorly and laterally; therefore, the correct identification of the external sphincter is of utmost importance. The surgeon frequently draws the resectoscope sheath back toward the membranous urethra to identify the external sphincter before resecting the apical tissue.

The membranous urethra is a fixed structure situated at the urogenital diaphragm, whereas the prostate gland, which abuts on this diaphragm, is slightly movable. When the prostate gland is moved by manipulating the resectoscope sheath back and forth, the mucosa bridging the junction is plainly visible as it is thrown into a fold, like an accordion. This wrinkle should never be resected or coagulated. It overlies the external sphincter.

A useful hint in resecting apical tissue is to cover a finger with a plastic shield for protection and insert it into the rectum; the finger can displace tissue medially or upward. The surgeon is able to palpate the resectoscope sheath through the rectum and can be assured that the cutting tip is in the safety zone and not at or in the membranous urethra.

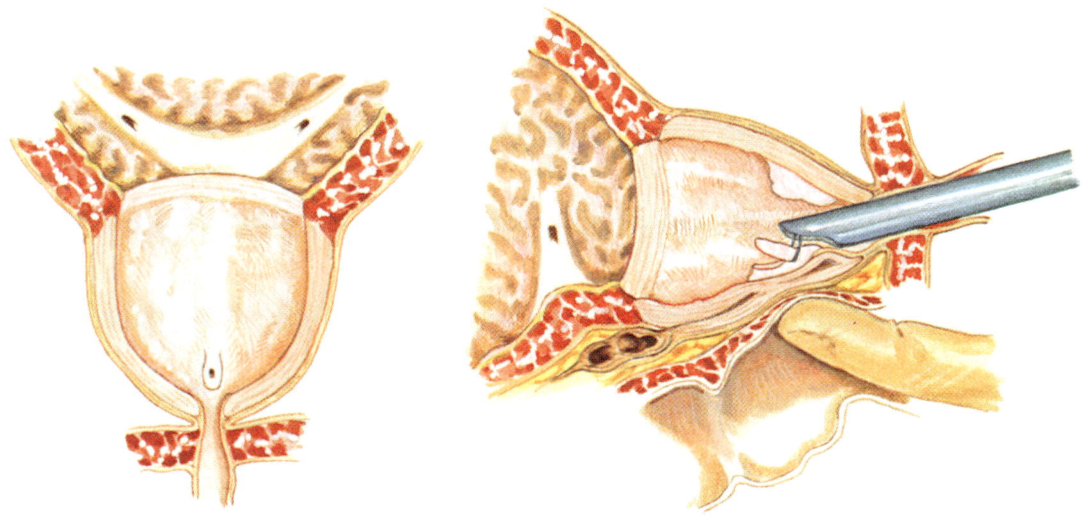

130-6

When the resection progresses to the true glandular or posterior lobe, the fuzzy or cotton-like appearance of the adenoma gives way to the smoother and patterned structure of true prostatic tissue, which does not bulge into the operative field. However, the change is not distinct and, usually, it is difficult to differentiate true prostatic tissue from adenomatous tissue unless the resection continues close to true capsule.

In some cases a layer of prostatic calculi helps to identify the plane between adenoma and true prostatic tissue. The calculi usually lie either between the adenoma and true prostatic tissue or in the superficial layer of the latter. All tissue containing calculi should be removed; care is needed not to resect too deeply to reach the true capsule.

It is wise to stop resecting when true prostatic tissue is identified. Troublesome, multiple fresh bleeders from capsular vessels and venous bleeders are frequently encountered close to true capsule. Unroofing of the capsule is not an indication to stop the resection but is a warning to proceed no deeper in that particular area. It is also a guide to the depth of the capsule in the adjacent areas.

When the resection is completed, no fuzzy-looking adenomatous tissue remains in the prostatic fossa and the important landmarks, such as the ureteral orifices, verumontanum, and external sphincter, should be visible and intact.

131. Cancer of the Prostate

A patient with curable cancer of the prostate without demonstrable metastases or fixation of the gland should not undergo transurethral surgery as a rule. However, a small nodule in the prostate, palpable by rectal examination, can be resected.

131-1. *A small nodule in the prostate is resected by the transurethral approach* and can serve as a biopsy specimen.

131-2. Prostatic cancer is somewhat yellowish on gross examination and appears coarsely granular and friable. When a small cancerous nodule is successfully resected along with the surrounding normal tissue, *true capsular fibers are exposed;* total prostatectomy can be postponed until recurrence or another nodule is detected.

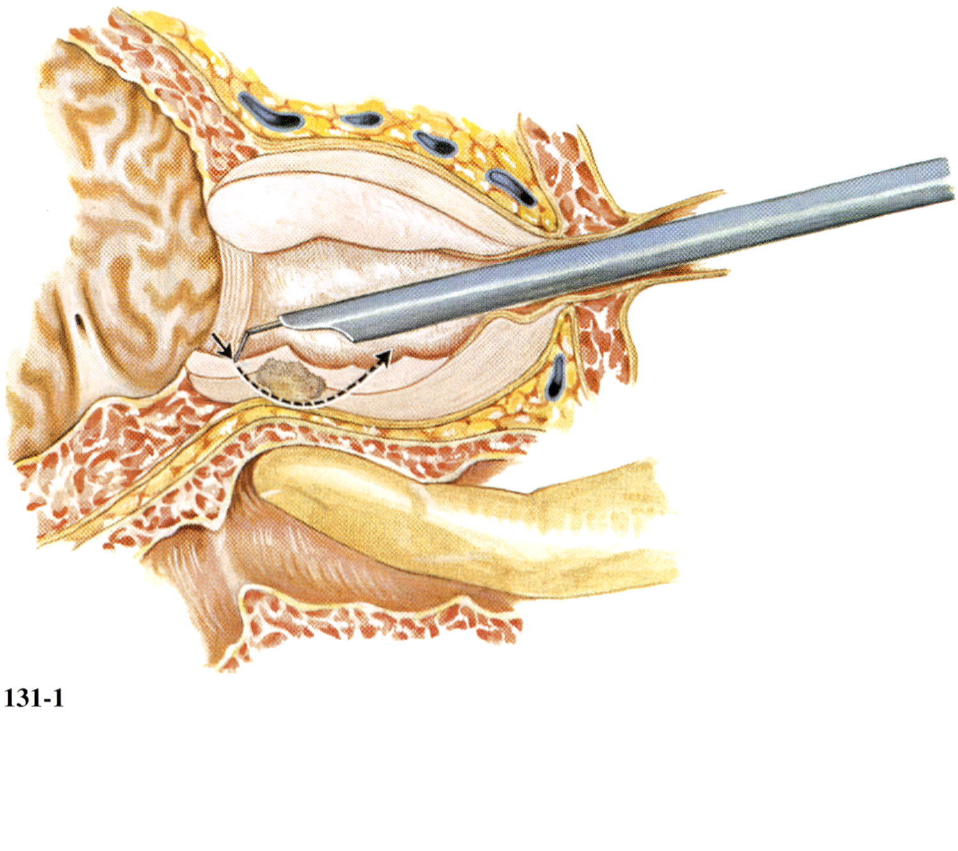

131-1

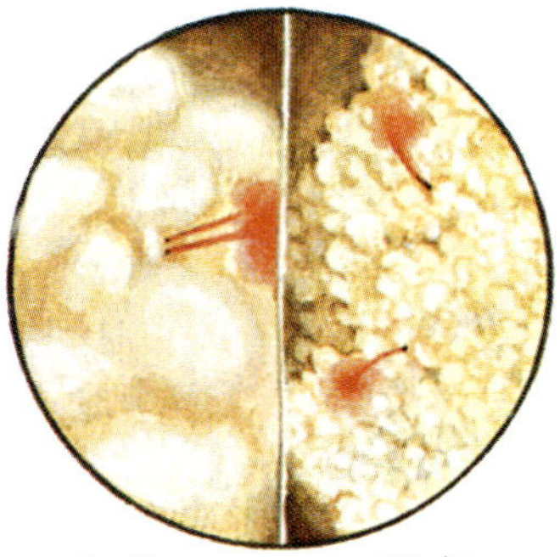

131-2

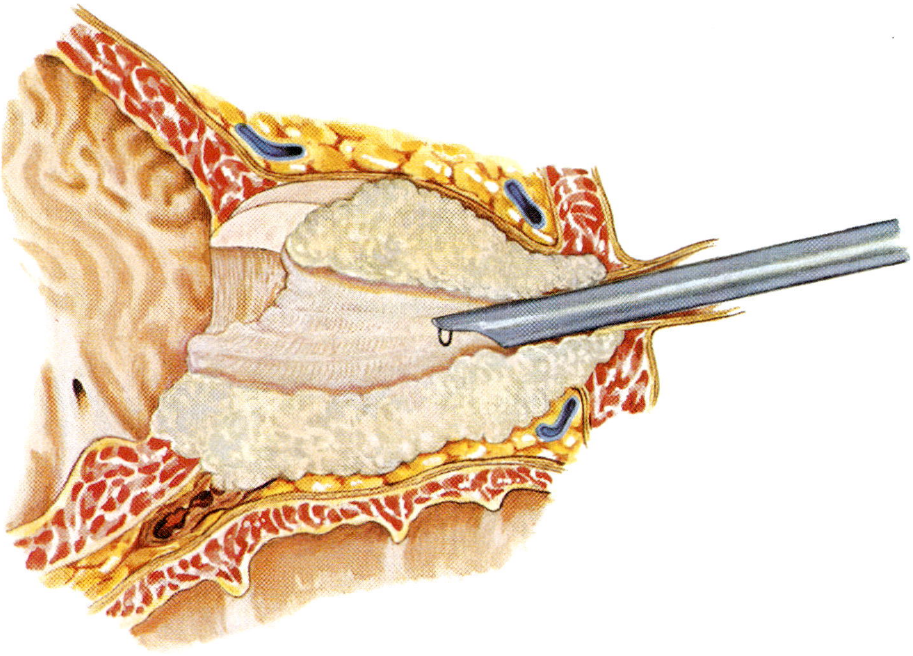

131-3

The main purpose of transurethral resection of prostatic cancer is to provide a channel for urination through the prostatic urethra by resecting obstructive cancer tissue. When the lesion is beyond the borders removable by total prostatectomy, with local invasion and metastases, transurethral resection is the treatment of choice. Hormone trials are always warranted to relieve obstruction.

Obstructive cancer tissue is more difficult to resect than benign adenoma. First, the hard and nonelastic cancer tissue disturbs the smooth cutting movement of a resectoscope. Sometimes the sheath is tightly fixed in the prostatic urethra and only a thin superficial layer is resected by the cutting loop. Second, the true capsule of the prostate is frequently involved with cancer; therefore, a very important landmark is missing, and further resection is hazardous. Third, the verumontanum and external sphincter are frequently involved with cancer. Resection of tumor tissue in this area will cause postoperative urinary incontinence.

131-3. *Resection of obstructive prostatic cancer should cease when a satisfactory channel is made* in the prostatic urethra. Recurrence of obstructive symptoms is rather rare if estrogen or antiandrogenic therapy is continued after the operation.

132. Hemostasis

The most troublesome problem during transurethral resection is bleeding. As large areas of prostatic tissue are resected, the visual field of the telescope is frequently obliterated by arterial bleeders. This is very stressful to a neophyte resectionist and will be discouraging in the early years. However, no arterial bleeder exists that cannot be controlled by fulguration in the operative field.

The protruding stumps of the arterioles usually contract with their thick muscular wall and can be coagulated without difficulty if the loop is pointed correctly over them. Extensive electrocoagulation over a large area, however, is damaging to normal tissue and is usually ineffective in controlling hemorrhage.

A surgeon who becomes flustered may become disoriented and may not see the bleeding sources. However, once the surgeon gains self-confidence in the proper hemostatic technique, resecting ability will improve. The following hints can be of great assistance in learning proper hemostatic techniques.

132-1. *Stop the main bleeders at the vesical neck first.* The most important vessels to the prostate enter the lower quadrants of the vesical neck at about the 4 and 8 o'clock positions. If they are coagulated at the early stage of the operation, large areas will be devascularized. This will minimize the bleeding thereafter, and will provide a better view to the surgeon.

On the contrary, when a large arteriole is encountered during the resecting procedure, the surgeon is advised to return to the freshly resected area to search for arteriolar bleeders.

132-2. Search for bleeding points along the resected surface.

132-3. *Arterial bleeding cannot be localized when an artery is spurting directly at the lens, but is easily seen in profile.* One must advance the lens of the resectoscope very close to the resected surface of the tissue until the spurting vessel is seen in profile. Cessation of bleeding is immediate when the coagulating current is applied to the loop placed exactly on the arterial stump.

132-4. *Beware of the opposite side.* Occasionally blood from an artery spurts across the prostatic fossa, rebounding at the opposite side, making it appear that the source of bleeding is from the area of rebound. The surgeon should direct attention to the opposite side when a vague, nonlocalizable wall of blood appears without any obvious source.

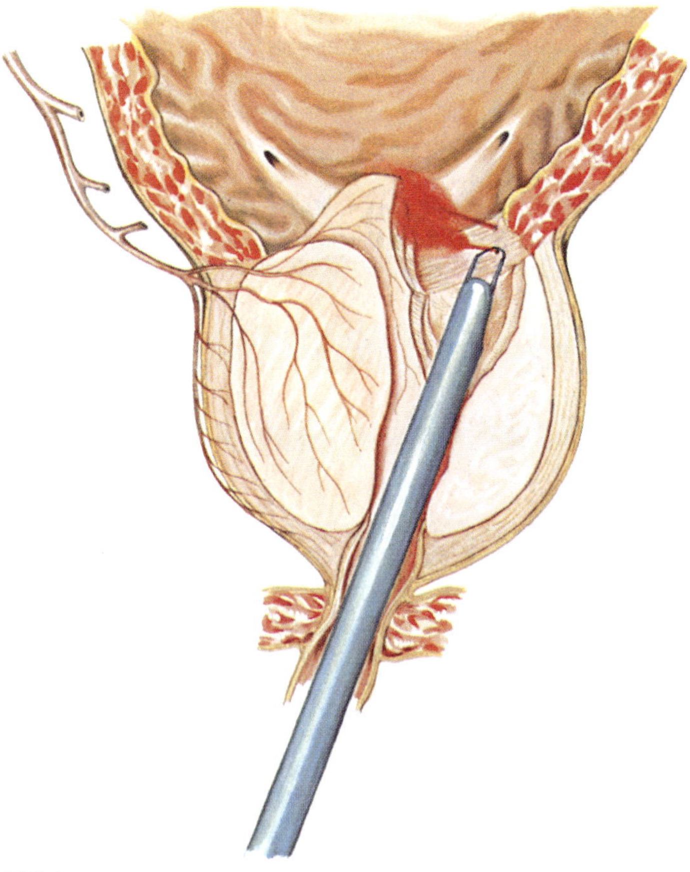

132-1

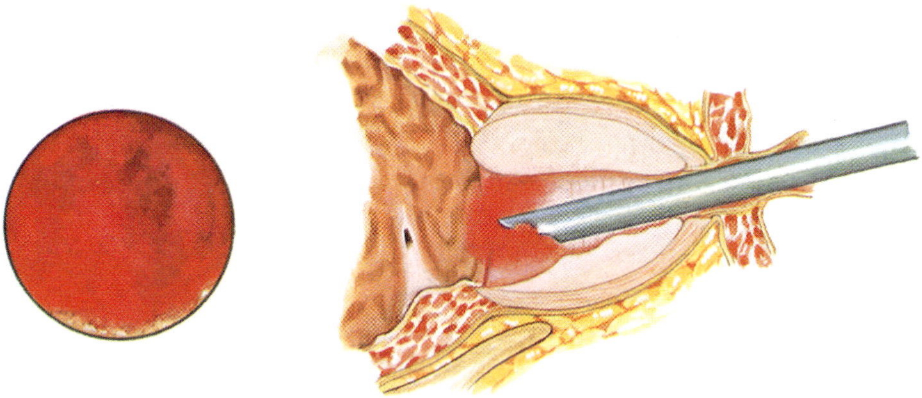

132-2

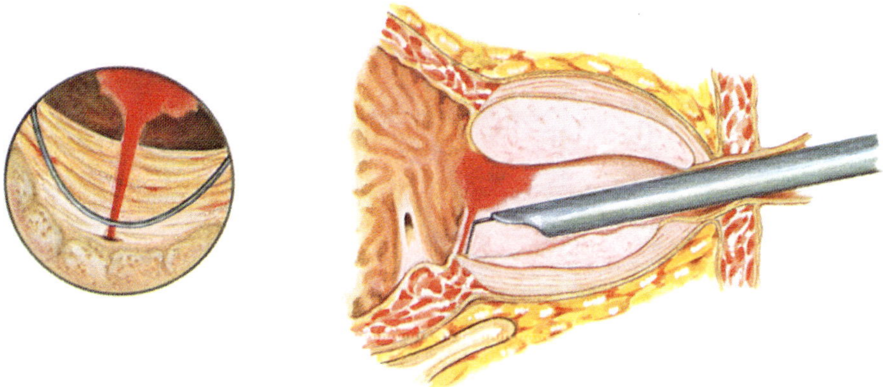

132-3

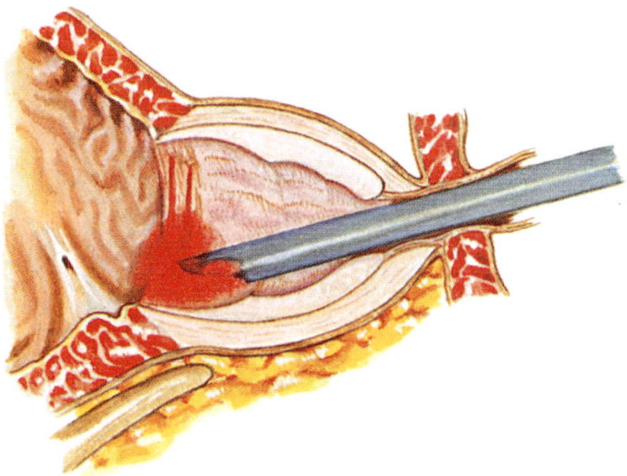

132-4

132-5. Arterial bleeding behind the vesical neck, spurting toward the bladder cavity, cannot be detected with the oblique telescope. It is seen as a vague nonlocalizable show of blood behind vesical neck. *Careful coagulation of the suspected area behind the vesical neck will be successful.*

Localizing a Direct Bleeding Point. The best time to control a bleeding artery is immediately after the cut that started it. However, if the surgeon is working rapidly to remove a large adenoma, bleeding will be more difficult to localize later.

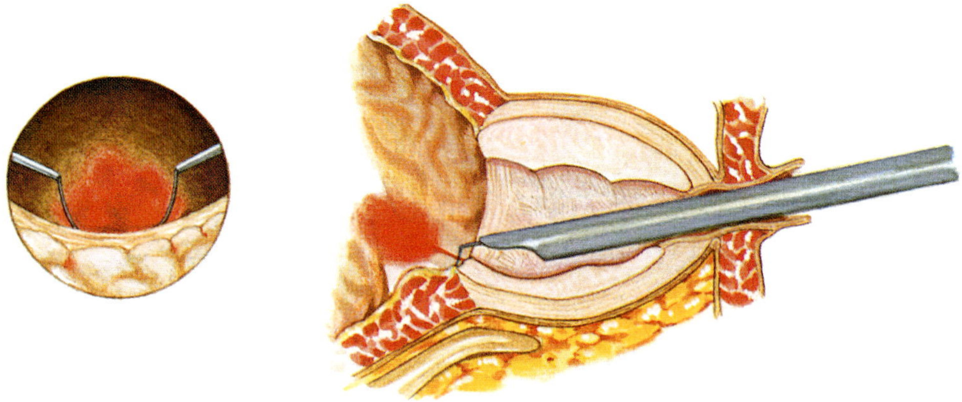

132-5

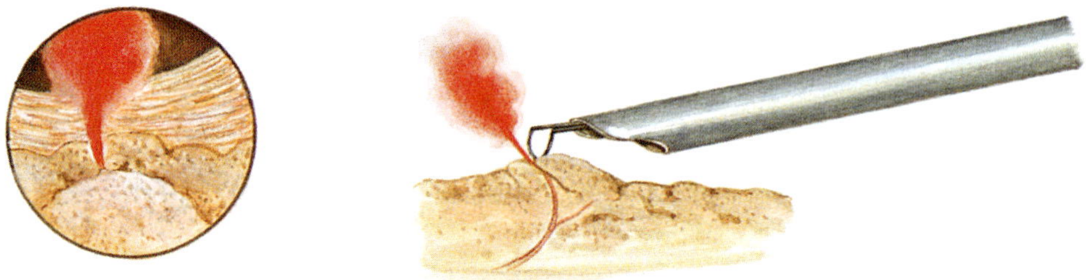

132-6

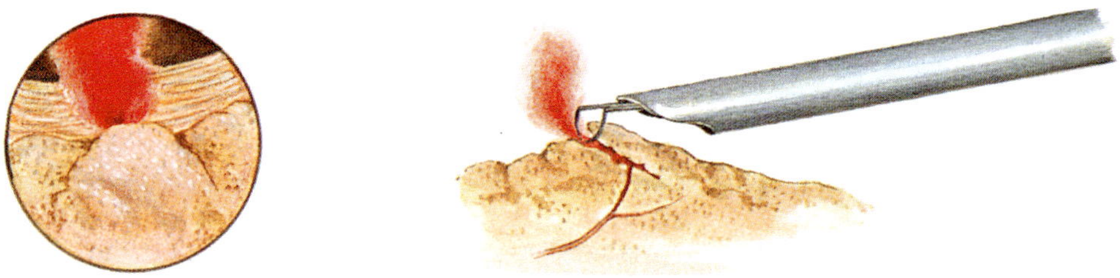

132-7

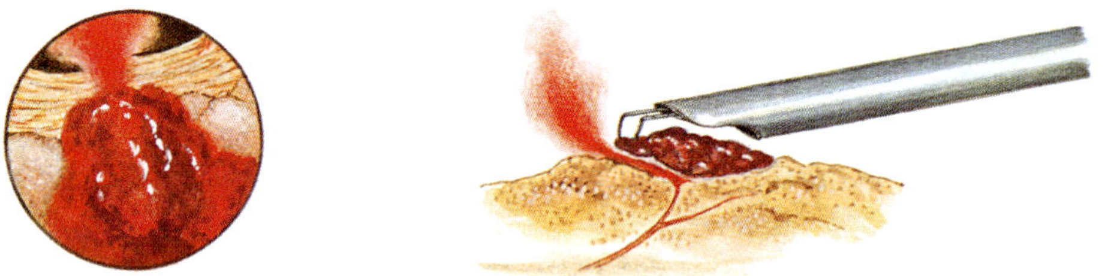

132-8

132-6 and 132-7. Sometimes *tags of tissue or blood coagula* that project in front of the resectoscope lens *obscure the bleeding point.*

132-8. At times, *the cut end of a spurting artery is located in a split tissue cleft.*

132-9. *When a shallow resection is made in this area, the bleeding point is easily seen* on a clean, shining, cut surface and can be readily coagulated.

132-10. *Use the other hand as an aid in the operation.* Rectal elevation of the prostatic fossa with the index finger of the left hand is sometimes helpful in localizing bleeding points after removal of a large adenoma. When the gloved finger is pressed firmly against the bleeding point, the spurting stops; when it is released, it spurts again.

132-11. *Compression of the suprapubic area is also a helpful technique* in coagulating bleeding points at the anterior bladder wall near the neck. Use of the one-hand resectoscope is recommended for these techniques.

132-12. *Do not resect too deeply into the true capsule.* The best result of transurethral resection of the hypertrophied prostate is obtained when the adenoma is completely removed. Most of the surgical capsule should remain untouched. When resection proceeds beyond adenoma, numerous small bleeders from the surgical capsular group of arteries may occur, an indication that the resection has been carried far enough. If one extends to the true prostatic capsule, there will be more troublesome minor bleeders and a greater chance of unroofing venous sinuses.

In addition, the cut ends of arterioles at the true capsule are frequently buried between capsule fibers, making the bleeding points difficult to identify. Intense coagulation of the true capsule may lead to perforation of the capsule and subsequent leakage of irrigating fluid into the surrounding tissue.

Do not attempt to coagulate venous bleeders. Bleeding from veins is easily identified since they do not spurt like arterial bleeders. It ceases with a slight rise of intravesical pressure. It is not necessary to coagulate minor venous bleeders, since they usually stop spontaneously after completion of transurethral resection.

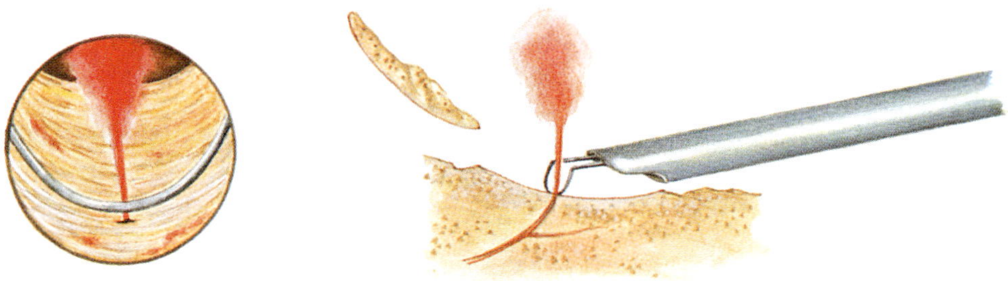

132-9

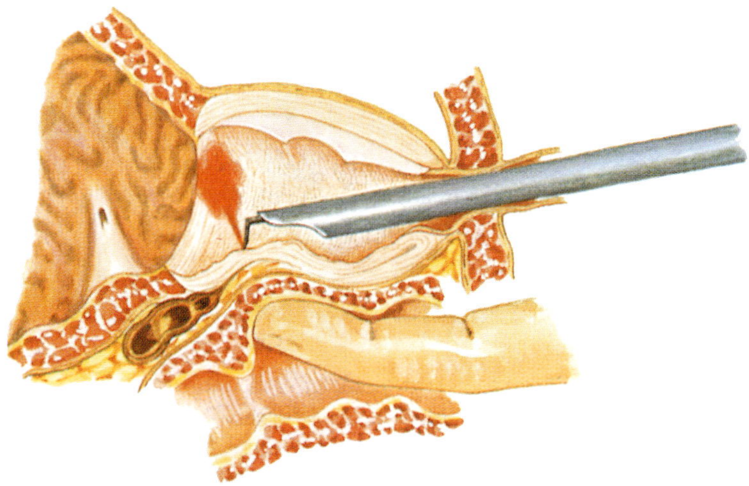

132-10

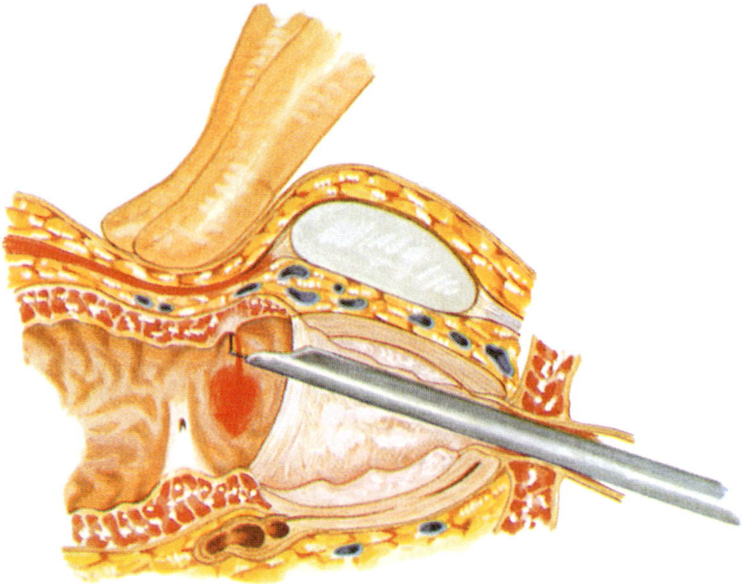

132-11

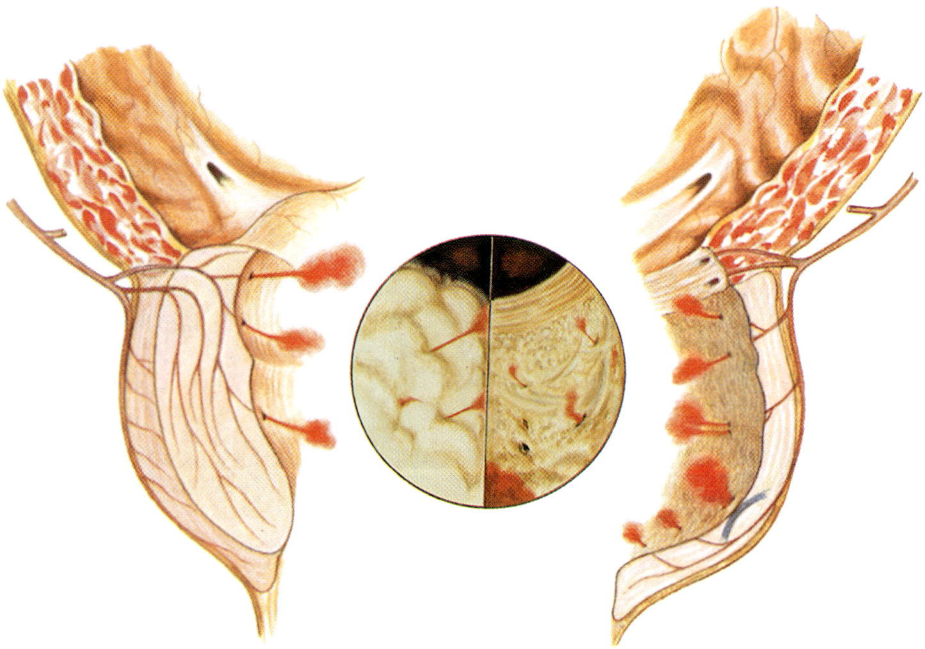

132-12

Bleeding from venous sinuses cannot be controlled by electrocoagulation. It persists in spite of extensive coagulation directly on the venous sinus walls. Continued coagulation may enlarge the opening and produce more profuse hemorrhage with further extravasation of irrigating fluid into the bloodstream.

If blood pours out of the working sheath when the resectoscope is removed, yet bleeding ceases when the bladder is distended with irrigating fluid, the source of bleeding is usually the unroofing of a venous sinus. Bleeding from venous sinuses, however, is easily controlled by slight tension on a Foley catheter with the bag inflated. The catheter is inserted after coagulation of spurting arterial bleeders.

Check the blood pressure level. Hypotension must be evaluated and treated appropriately. In the control of bleeding at the termination of transurethral resection, the surgeon should be aware of any change in the patient's blood pressure. When the blood pressure is maintained at a lower level because of excessive blood loss or spinal anesthesia, bleeding from the operative field is much less and the surgeon may be deceived into thinking hemostasis is satisfactory. However, if the patient's blood pressure rises after completion of the operative procedure, bleeding will increase and bleeders that previously stopped may start again. Therefore, it is recommended that the anesthetist raise the patient's blood pressure to the preoperative level. This maneuver allows inspection of the entire operative field again before the endoscopic procedure is terminated.

133. Prostatic Capsular Perforation

A small perforation of the prostatic capsule or vesical neck may occur when an adequate transurethral resection is under way. This window will permit small amounts of irrigating fluid to enter the periprostatic tissues and venous channels. However, this complication will rarely give rise to difficulty if care is taken to avoid enlarging the perforation by continuing the resection nearby or by overdistending the bladder with irrigating fluid. If there is no clinical evidence of suprapubic pain and muscle rigidity, the operation can continue.

A capsular perforation in the early stage of the operation can occur at the vesical neck or trigone where a depth of one or two bites with the cutting loop may penetrate the wall. Perforations in the late stage of the operation usually occur when the resection has advanced close to the true capsule of the prostate. This may occur in a large adenoma when the capsule is very thin.

133-1. The capsule consists of a meshwork of interlacing fibers and can be easily recognized by its characteristic appearance. *When the capsule is scraped, the fibers separate widely and the interstices are more marked.*

133-2. *If a perforation is deeper, a dark cavity comes into view between the coarse fibers. Pericapsular fat may be seen through the opening of the perforation* or may even protrude slightly into the prostatic fossa. When a perforation occurs, large amounts of irrigating fluid containing blood and tiny tissue fragments may be extravasated into the surrounding tissues. This complication is characterized by gross interference with the free exchange of irrigating fluid through the sheath when the working element is removed.

A patient with a spinal or epidural anesthesia will complain of pain in the suprapubic region that does not disappear on emptying the bladder. If a patient is under general anesthesia, there will be no complaints of pain. However, rigidity of the lower abdominal muscles and distention of the lower abdomen are confirming signs of definite extravasation. If one is uncertain about the occurrence of perforation, a cystogram using an innocuous radiopaque medium and an emptying film are of great value. When a deep perforation accompanied by clinical signs occurs, immediate suprapubic drainage is indicated. Spurting arterial bleeders are then coagulated and a hemostatic Foley catheter with bag is inserted. Mild traction is applied to control other bleeders.

A delay in these emergency measures will lead to extravasation of a large volume of irrigating fluid, and the patient may develop shock and acute signs of distress.

133-3. *Suprapubic drainage is usually performed through a small incision in the midline just above the symphysis pubis.*

133-4. The fascia is incised; the rectus muscles are slightly separated and *the perivesical space down to the region of the prostate is opened by blunt dissection with a finger.*

133-5. *A soft rubber multiperforated, flat tubular Jackson Pratt drain is inserted.* This may be done on the operating table or in the recovery room as soon as the diagnosis is confirmed and while the anesthesia is still effective.

Unless there is profuse bleeding, which requires open hemostasis or packing of the prostatic fossa through a cystotomy, suprapubic drainage is adequate. However, if there is suspicion of intraperitoneal extravasation due to perforation of the bladder wall, the peritoneum should be opened for inspection in the operating room. The peritoneal cavity is emptied by suction and the perforated wound is closed with a running 2–0 chromic catgut suture.

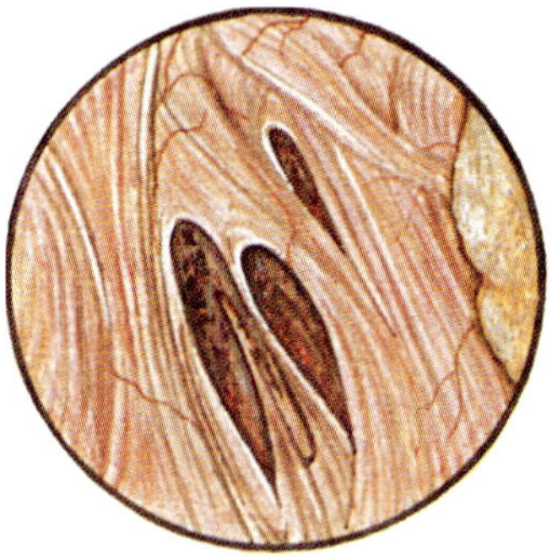

133-1

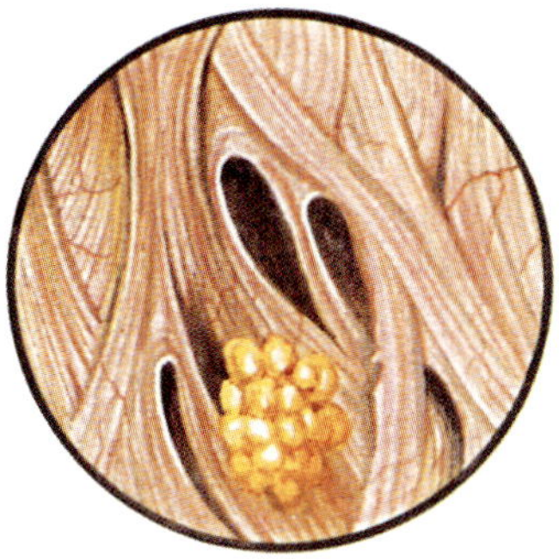

133-2

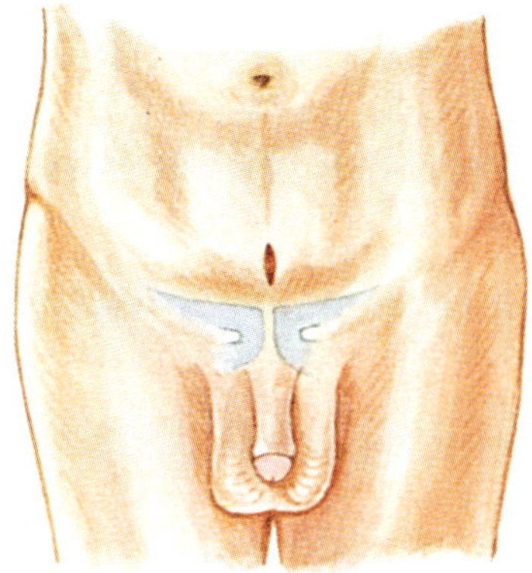

133-3

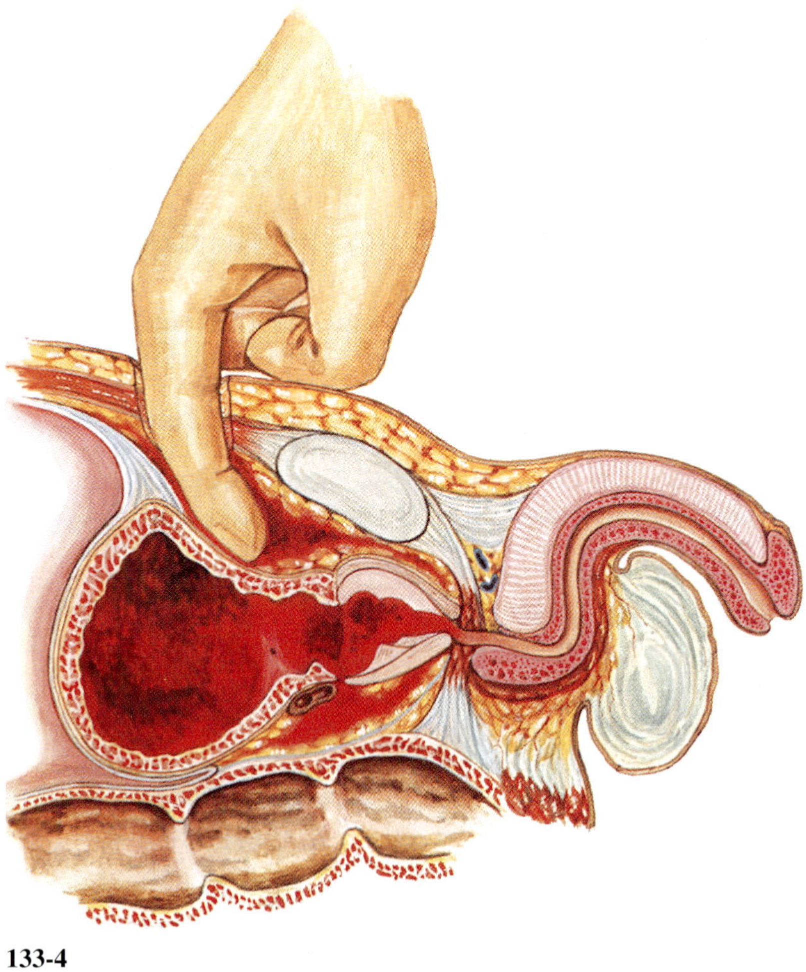

133-4

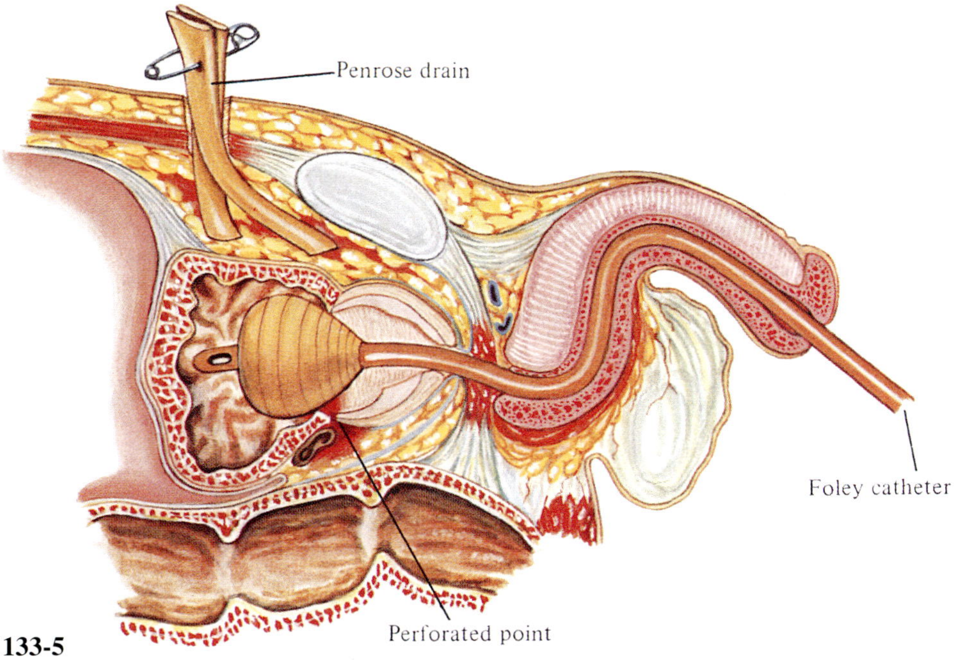

133-5

134. Systemic Complications due to Absorption of Irrigating Fluid

The nonelectrolytic isotonic solutions, such as glycine or a mixture of mannitol and sorbitol, are routinely used now as irrigating fluid for transurethral resection. These are safe fluids and do not cause hemolysis. However, their use may give the surgeon a false sense of security.

134-1. *The rapid transfer of large amounts of irrigating fluid to the bloodstream* during transurethral resection *will produce systemic complications* such as hypervolemia and hyponatremia, as well as diluting the electrolytes in other body fluids. Hypervolemia probably causes a preliminary rise in blood pressure before the patient manifests a symptom complex due to hyponatremia, consisting of restlessness, nausea, vomiting, bradycardia, and agitation. Some of these symptoms are possibly due to cerebral edema. Generalized muscle weakness then appears, but in some instances, muscle cramps may occur, probably as a result of hypocalcemia.

If the operation is prolonged and there are additional complications, such as excessive hemorrhage and prolonged anesthesia, the patient will develop circulatory failure. A serum sodium of 120 mEq/L is conducive to shock. Hyponatremic shock is not easily reversible and may result in acute renal failure.

It is wise, therefore, if the operation is prolonged, to determine serum sodium and hematocrit levels during the operation in a high risk patient.

Central venous pressure monitoring is also a helpful method of assessing hemodynamic changes during the operation in a high risk patient. The severity of the hypervolemia and its associated hyponatremia are directly related to the amount of irrigating fluid entering the venous system through the open venous sinuses.

The intravesical pressure depends on the height of the irrigating fluid. Irrigating fluid with a hydrostatic pressure of 60 cm can easily be forced into a venous system registering 15 cm of water pressure. Therefore, a lower irrigating fluid height and frequent emptying of the bladder are recommended. Using the Iglesias continuous flow resectoscope may help to avoid bladder overdistension. It allows continuous resection under clear vision without the need for periodic evacuation of bloody irrigating fluid.

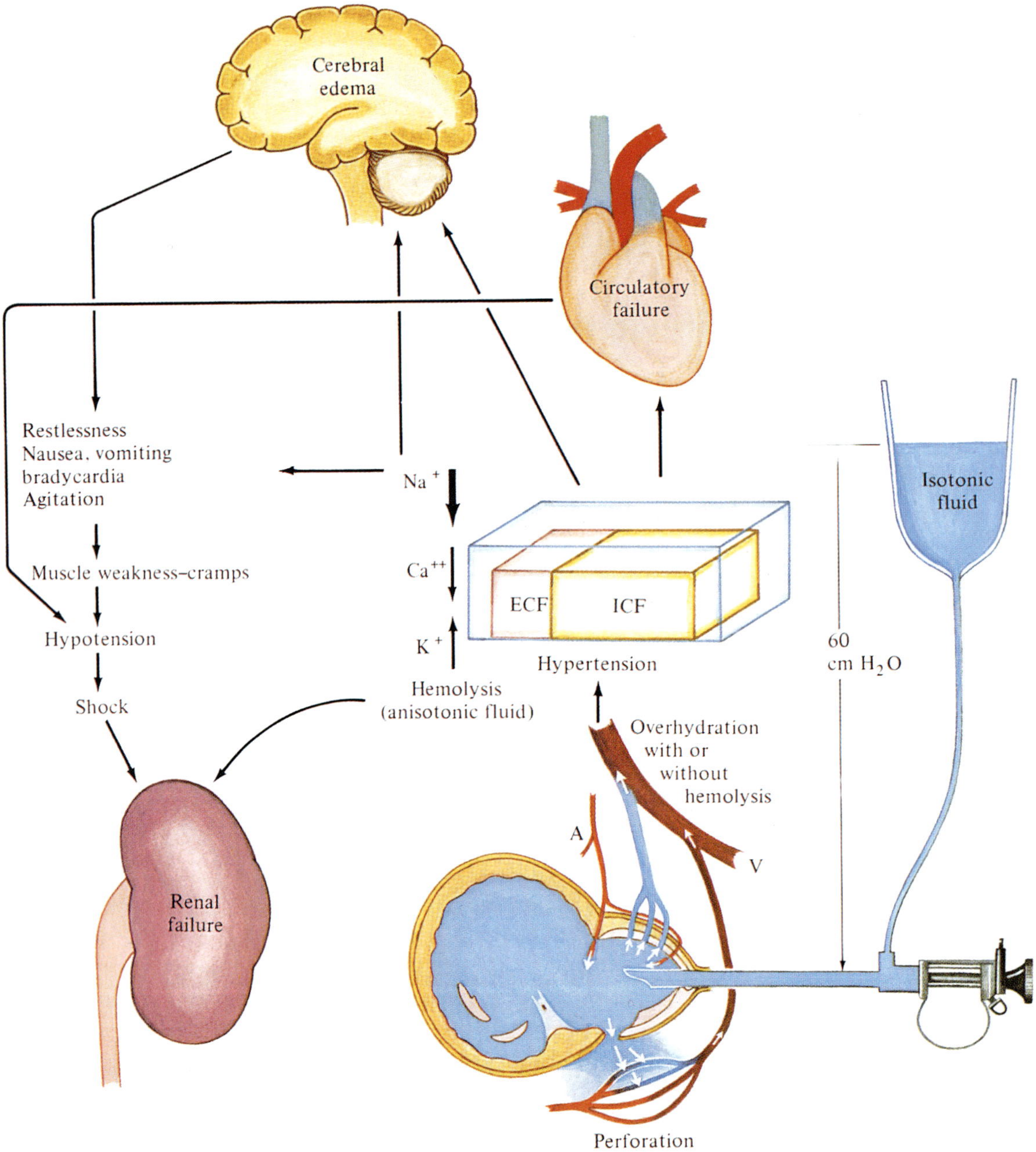

134-1

The intravenous administration of appropriate amounts of 5% sodium chloride is recommended to prevent the hyponatremic syndrome if the operation is a long and bloody one.

Intravenous mannitol will definitely serve to prevent the development of this syndrome. Mannitol is an excellent osmotic diuretic and has a potent diuretic effect when injected into the circulation in high, appropriate concentrations. It can mobilize irrigating fluid that is absorbed during transurethral resection. When using mannitol, however, it is necessary to supplement the electrolytes, particularly sodium, since its use is accompanied by considerable loss of sodium.

In 1964 Bodner reported that mannitol was a useful agent for intravenous use in transurethral resection of the prostate. We have used mannitol successfully. There are two types of mannitol solutions for operative and postoperative use. We have the solutions prepared and use them routinely.

Solution 1 (for operative use) contains 15% mannitol, 5% glucose, 0.85% sodium chloride, and 0.05% calcium chloride. During a transurethral resection lasting approximately 60 min, 500 mL of this solution is administered intravenously.

Solution 2 (for postoperative use) contains 5% mannitol, 5% glucose, 0.25% sodium chloride, and 0.02% calcium chloride. This solution is administered continuously until the next morning at the rate of 200 mL/hour to mobilize substances absorbed during the operation. It corrects abnormal shifts of body fluid electrolytes; it also increases urinary output and obviates the need for frequent catheter irrigation. It diminishes the occurrence of postoperative urinary infection. If the patient has cardiovascular problems, then the rate of infusion is reduced to 100 mL/hour.

Using New Laser Energy Sources

There are a number of new devices and techniques being introduced as alternatives for the surgical treatment of benign prostatic hyperplasia (BPH). Among them are laser devices that offer an efficient and effective means of applying a large amount of energy precisely to a target. Today, laser therapy can be proposed as a treatment modality for bladder outlet obstruction due to BPH.[1–7] There are three major laser devices now being used to treat BPH. They are as follows:

1. A right angle, noncontact laser beam under endoscopic control (VLAP);
2. Angling the noncontact laser beam through a balloon under ultrasound guidance (TULIP);
3. Inserting the laser fiber interstitially into the prostate and cutting or reducing tissue volume by a contact laser beam (ILC).

135. Visual Laser Ablation of the Prostate (VLAP)

In our opinion, VLAP can be easily performed even for high risk patients. Today, many hospital operating rooms are equipped with standard neodymium aluminum garnet (Nd:YAG) laser sources. The only instrument that must be purchased for this procedure is a right angle laser-beam fiber. This laser fiber can be introduced through an ordinary cystoscope attached to a camera for TV monitoring.

The Nd:YAG laser, emitting light at 1064 nanometers, will produce relatively deep tissue penetration resulting in coagulation necrosis. At an energy source up to 60 watts, coagulation and necrosis occur. Tissue sloughing occurs much later. At a power of 100 watts, tissue vaporization occurs. Potential advantages of laser ablation, compared to TURP, have been mentioned by McCullough[8] and are as follows: 1) a short hospital stay, 2) minimal bleeding, 3) no fluid absorption, 4) rapidity of treatment, 5) a simplified procedure, and 6) prevention of antegrade ejaculation.

Initially, laser energy produces considerable tissue edema resulting in potential urinary retention for unpredictable intervals. The procedure requires a catheter for a much longer interval than a TURP.[9,10]

Patient preparation is the same as that for TURP. Low spinal or epidural anesthesia is usually employed. The procedure can also be performed under local anesthesia for patients with smaller glands of 15 to 25 g.[11]

With the patient in a lithotomy position, a 21 Fr cystoscopy equipped with a working port is introduced into the urethra. After careful inspection of the prostatic urethra and urinary bladder, a 7.5 Fr gold-tipped laser fiber is passed through the working port of the cystoscope. This is similar to any other catheter or endoscopic instrument. A plas-

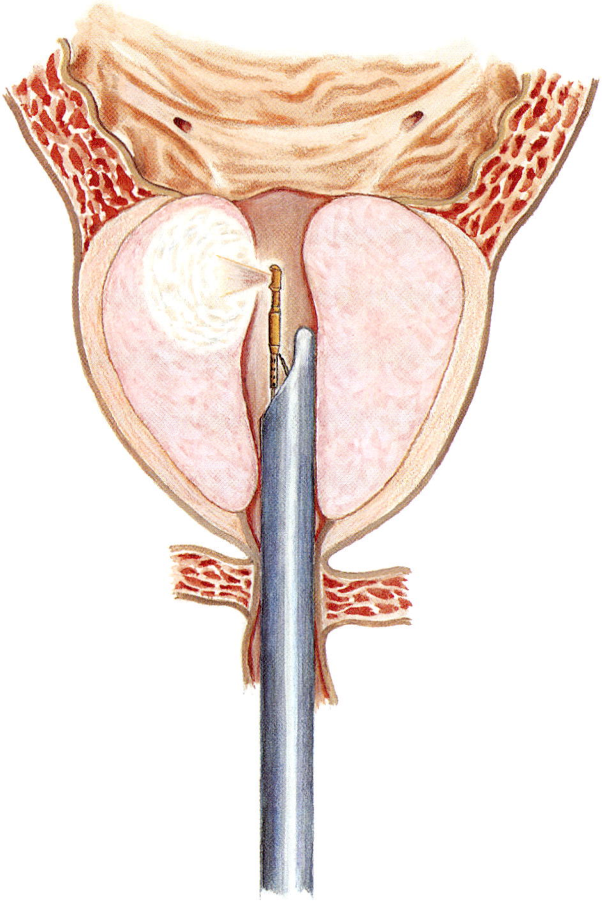

135-1

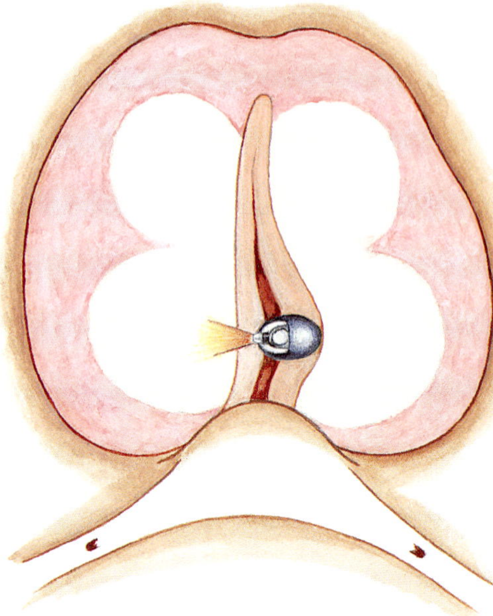

135-2

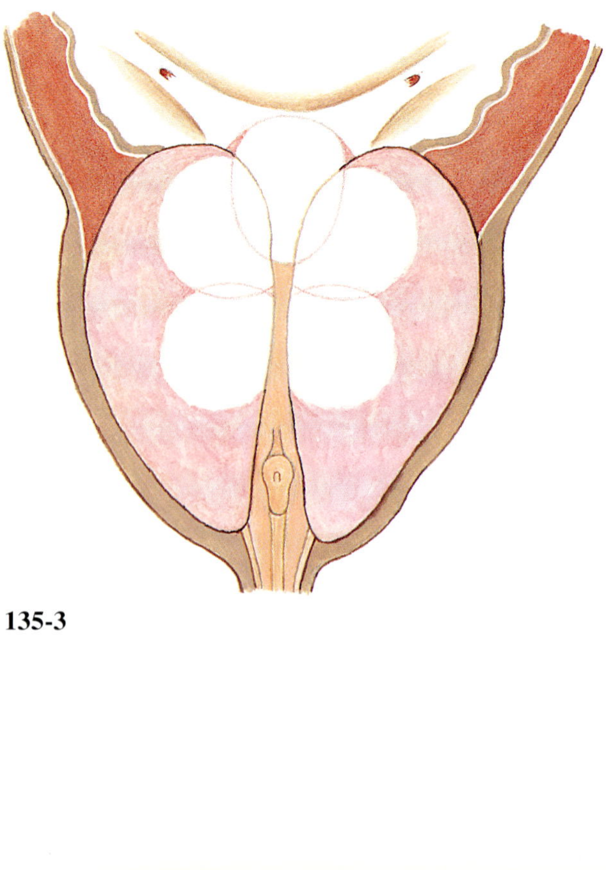

135-3

tic torque handle is attached to the quartz fiber that can be adjusted in a convenient position and tightened to allow the surgeon to have a secure grasp and control of the fiber during operative manipulations.

Because the Nd:YAG laser is invisible to the human eye, the laser sources are routinely equipped with a low-energy helium beam. A visible neon red aiming beam assists in directing application of the laser beam during prostatic surgery.

Sterile water at room temperature is used as the irrigant. The irrigation serves to cool the gold alloy tip of the laser fiber and, thus, assures a constant flow. Before each laser application, the bladder should be emptied.

To produce the desired effect of maximal tissue ablation, each laser application should be continued at a single location for 60 seconds. With a Urolase right angle laser fiber, the laser power usually employed is 40 to 60 watts. This laser energy usually destroys prostatic tissue to a depth and width of 10 to 15 mm, respectively, at each spot. Discontinuous laser firing along the prostatic urethra (painting) will produce less tissue ablation.

135-1. The Urolase, manufactured by the Bard Company, is a right angle laser fiber. The tip of the laser fiber should be held just off the mucosal surface to ensure a clear plane of water between the metal and the prostatic tissue.

135-2. A view from inside the bladder. The technique we employ in Japan for the majority of our patients is to coagulate at the 2, 4, 8, and 10 o'clock positions of the prostatic urethra about 1 cm distal to the vesicle neck.

135-3. VLAP for large BPH with median lobe hyperplasia. For the larger glands, a second set of four-quadrant laser coagulations are performed roughly 2 cm distal to the first sites, staying at least 1.5 cm proximal to the verumontanum. For a large median lobe hypertrophy, additional spot beams can be applied to the tissue.

At the conclusion of laser prostatectomy, a 16 Fr 5 cc balloon Foley catheter is inserted.

The application of laser energy to the prostate produces considerable tissue edema frequently causing urinary retention and requiring catheter drainage—usually for a week or longer. The patient can be discharged from the hospital on the following day and the catheter can be removed at his initial postoperative visit to the office. For the patient who requires the indwelling catheter for a longer duration, placement of a suprapubic cystostomy tube by the trocar technique is recommended.

Use of prophylactic antibiotics is also recommended. For patients with a positive urine culture, antibiotic treatment is appropriately chosen and adjusted in accord with the bacterial antibiotic sensitivities.

Postoperatively, the urine appears whitish and cloudy. This is caused by dissolving prostate tissue and lasts for several weeks. Larger pieces of necrotic tissue are rarely seen. The patient will have an improved urinary stream usually 4 weeks after laser ablation.

References

1. Costello AJ, Bowsher WG, Bolton DM, Braslis KG, Burt J. Laser ablation of the prostate in patients with benign prostatic hypertrophy. Br J Urol 69:603–608, 1992.
2. Johnson DE, Price RE, Cromeens DM. Pathologic changes occurring in the prostate following transurethral laser prostatectomy. Laser Surg Med 12:254–263, 1992.
3. Dixon CM, Lepor H. Laser ablation of the prostate. Semin Urol 10:273–277, 1992.
4. Costello AJ, Johnson DE, Bolton DM. Nd:YAG laser ablation of the prostate as a treatment for benign prostatic hypertrophy. Laser Surg Med 12:121–124, 1992.

5. Kabalin JN. Urolase laser prostatectomy. 1993 monographs in urology 14:23–36, 1993.
6. Marks LS. Serial endoscopy following visual laser ablation of prostate (VLAP). Urology 42: 66–71, 1993.
7. Norris JP, Norris DM, Lee RD, Rueenstein MA. Visual laser ablation of the prostate: clinical experience in 108 patients. J Urol 155:1612–1614, 1993.
8. McCullough DL. This month in investigative urology: transurethral laser treatment of benign prostatic hyperplasia. J Urol 146;1126–1127, 1991.
9. Gibbons RP, McNicholas TA, Koshiba K, Flam T, Jewett MAS, Stein BS, Steg A. Surgical and laser treatment. Proceedings, the 2nd International Consultation on Benign Prostatic Hyperplasia (BPH) 1993:363–374.
10. Uchida T, Koshiba K. Visual laser ablation of the prostate (VLAP) as treatment for benign prostatic hyperplasia. Jpn J Endourol and ESWL 8:10–13, 1995.
11. Leach GE, Sirls L, Ganabathi K, Roskamp D, Dmochowski R. Outpatient visual laser-assisted prostatectomy under local anesthesia. Urology 42:149–153, 1994.

Suggested Readings

Baumrucker GO. Transurethral Prostatectomy. Baltimore: Williams & Wilkins, 1968.

Bodner H, Howard AH, Ross SC. Use of mannitol in transurethral prostatectomy. J Urol 91:287, 1964.

Conger KB. Transurethral Prostatic Surgery. Baltimore: Williams & Wilkins, 1963.

Creevy CD. Hemolysis and transurethral resection. Surgery 39:180, 1956.

Flocks RH, Culp DA. Surgical Urology. Chicago: Year Book Medical Publishers, 1967.

Goodwin WE, Cason JF, Scott WW. Hemoglobinemia and lower nephron nephrosis following transurethral prostatic surgery. J Urol 65:1075, 1951.

Griffin M, Dobson L, Weaver JC. Volume of irrigating fluid transfer during transurethral prostatectomy studied with radioisotopes. J Urol 74:646, 1955.

Hagstrom RS. Studies on fluid absorption during transurethral prostatic resection. J Urol 73:852, 1955.

Iglesias JJ, Sporer A, Gellman AC. New Iglesias resectoscope with continuous irrigation, simultaneous suction and low intravesical pressure. J Urol 114:929, 1975.

Koshiba K. Intravenous infusion of mannitol in transurethral prostatic resection. XIV Kongress der Internationalen Gesellschaft für Urologie 424: Band 2, 1967.

Mebust WK, Brady TW, Valk WL. Observations on cardiac output, central venous pressure, fluid and electrolyte changes in patients undergoing transurethral prostatectomy. J Urol 103:632, 1970.

Melchior J, Valk WL, Foret JD. Transurethral prostatectomy and epididymitis. J Urol 112:647, 1974.

Nesbit RM. Urology, 3rd ed. Philadelphia: WB Saunders, 1970.

Parry WL. Prostate malignancies. In: Glenn JF, ed. Urologic Surgery. Hagerstown: Harper & Row, 1975.

Silber SJ. Transurethral Resection. New York: Appleton-Century-Crofts, 1977.

Schmidt SS, Hinman F. The effect of vasectomy upon the incidence of epididymitis after prostatectomy: an analysis of 810 operations. J Urol 63:872, 1950.

Schulte TL, Hammer HJ, Reynolds LR. Clinical use of Cytal in urology. J Urol 71:656, 1954.

Transurethral Resection of Bladder Tumor

11

Many patients who develop bladder tumors have a history of working in an environment where exposure to chemicals or certain organic products are present. He/she may also be a chronic cigarette smoker in many instances.

In our opinion, a history of gross, painless, total hematuria and the presence of blood and/or red blood cells in both routine examination and collections of urine during an office visit should prompt the urologist to consider the possibility of a bladder growth. Cystoscopy and a bladder wash of the transitional cells lining the bladder surface—a cytology specimen—is often useful. Dr. Leon Wheeless has recently suggested that chromosome 9, present in some of the transitional cells lining the bladder floor, is also an early indicator of bladder cancer. A more serious clinical outcome is probable in many of these patients.

Middle aged men have a higher incidence of bladder cancer than women. In the U.S., however, many women (aged 20–40 years) have a significant history of cigarette smoking and we have seen a rise in early bladder cancer among some women.

Most bladder tumors are papillary initially. They may be multifocal particularly on the trigone or floor of the bladder.

For definitive staging of the cancer, biopsies of the bladder should be obtained under anesthesia. Before the biopsy a bimanual examination is important and useful. Palpating the mass on the bladder floor suggests muscular infiltration by tumor. Fixation of one portion of the bladder denotes a higher stage of cancer.

One of our colleagues—Leon Wheeless—has excellent research experience in the early detection of bladder cancers. DNA slit-scan flow cytometry of cells retrieved after washing the bladder epithelial surface with saline has been useful in detecting early bladder cancer.

Diagnosis of bladder tumors can be easily made by cystoscopy and biopsies under local anesthesia. We believe that staging of the tumor can be accomplished by a computed tomographic (CT) scan using a dilute contrast media. The radiographic media should be introduced by an indwelling catheter.

It is generally agreed that most bladder tumors of low grade and low stage are best managed by transurethral resection and fulguration. The skilled endoscopic surgeon can safely and adequately remove tumors of any size as long as the neoplasms are accessible with the resectoscope and do not deeply invade bladder wall. Bladder tumors that extend deeply through bladder musculature cannot be removed by transurethral resection.

However, the tumors can be managed by transurethral resection for palliation. The tissue obtained may be used in grading and staging the tumor.

PATHOLOGY

Most primary bladder tumors are transitional cell (urothelial) tumors, either of the papillary or sessile (broad-based) variety.

Epidermoid or squamous-cell carcinoma may arise directly from the bladder mucosa from leukoplakia, or from papillary transitional cell tumors. In an early stage, epidermoid or squamous-cell carcinoma may be difficult to recognize. It may not project into the bladder cavity but can infiltrate into deep muscle wall. Poorly differentiated squamous-cell cancers frequently display a highly malignant pattern of invasion even in early stages. These tumors in the early stages are associated with lymphatic permeation far beyond the main tumor.

Adenocarcinoma is rare. It was reported in only 17 of 1400 bladder tumor cases at the Bladder Tumor Registry, Armed Forces Institute of Pathology.

Nonepithelial tumors are extremely rare. They are divided into benign connective-tissue tumors and sarcomas; the latter constitute more than half the neoplasms in this category. All sarcomas invade rapidly, extend extravesically, and metastasize.

In the majority of cases, staging and grading of tumors, as described by Jewett and Strong and modified by Marshall, are probably the most important factors in arriving at a reasonable prognostic evaluation.

We believe the years ahead may provide new diagnostic tools for the staging of infiltrative bladder cancer. CT bladder scans can demonstrate density changes in the bladder wall between tumor and normal wall. The intact perivesical fat line often seen around the bladder wall is a helpful diagnostic sign. Comparisons between fat density, water, muscle density, and neoplasia can be made by properly focusing on the various tissue densities. Bladder cancer has a higher arbitrary tissue density. Careful infusion of a dilute contrast medium into the bladder lumen enhances the bladder mucosa and muscular layers. The other imaging modalities, such as magnetic resonance imaging (MRI) and transurethral ultrasonography are also very useful in the clinical staging of bladder cancer. These new modalities can help the urologist in the proper selection of patients for appropriate therapy—surgery, irradiation, chemotherapy, and/or immunotherapy.

Metastases are rare in most men developing superficial tumors. Satisfactory results can be expected by simple transurethral resection of the primary tumor. It must be emphasized, however, that 65% of stage $T_{3A}(B_2)$ tumors have metastasized by the time of initial cytoscopy (Fig. 1).

According to Jewett et al., the usual O, A, B_1, B_2, C, D_1, and D_2 staging categories are useful. The TNM (tumor, node, metastases) system, as proposed by the International Union Against Cancer is now used around the world. The equivalent stages in both systems are as follows: stage A is T_1, stage B_1 is T_2, stage B_2 and C are T_3, and extension outside the bladder with fixation, stage D is T_4.

PATIENT EVALUATION BEFORE SURGERY

Preoperative evaluation of the patient's general condition is similar to that required for transurethral resection of the prostate. Urethral stricture or a large prostate may hinder use of the resectoscope. The surgeon should rule out these possible problems before scheduling the patient for transurethral resection of the bladder tumor. A urethral stricture should be dilated to allow passage of a 24 French resectoscope sheath without difficulty. An alternative is a perineal urethrostomy. When the patient has a large prostate, it may be necessary to resect it before adequate access to the bladder tumor can be gained. If tumor is located near the hypertrophied vesical neck, it may be necessary to resect the vesical neck before access to the tumor is possible.

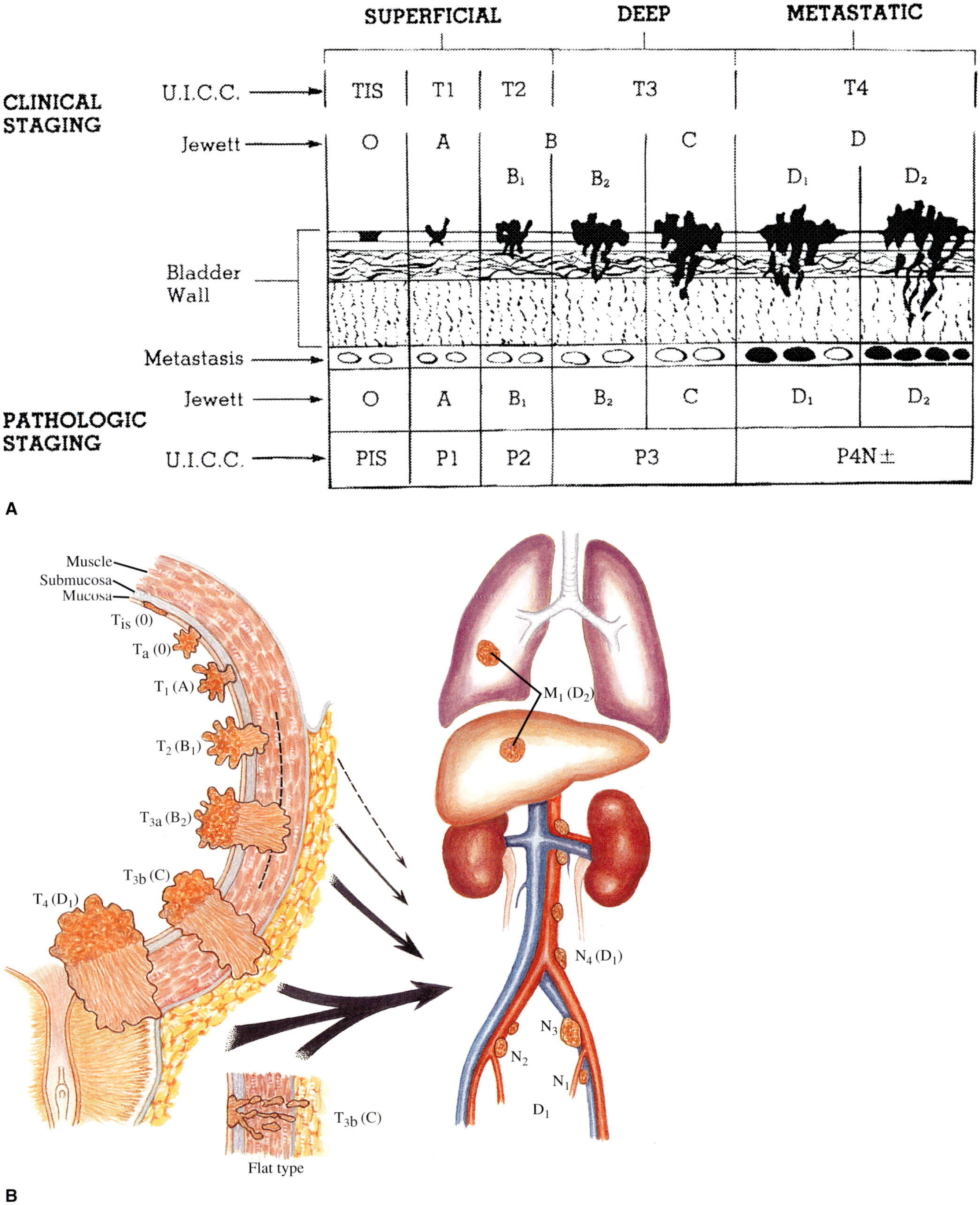

FIG. 1.
A. Staging of bladder tumor. B. Pathologic staging of bladder tumor.

Intravenous pyelography should be performed in every patient. Obstruction of one or both ureters usually means that tumor has infiltrated deeply into muscle to the extent that the tumor may not be managed completely by transurethral resection. On occasion we have found that superficial papillary tumors located near or just at the ureteral orifice may cause urinary obstruction.

CLINICAL STAGING OF BLADDER TUMOR

Figure 1A points out the various stages of bladder cancer—stages O, A, B_1, B_2, C, and D. The second portion of the diagram, with both kidneys and the large vessels, demonstrates sites of lymph node extension (Fig. 1B). It is obvious that if the lymph nodes are infiltrated by cancer in the bony pelvis, then the bladder cancer is probably incurable. This is stage D_1. If the tumor is beyond the pelvic nodes, then this is stage D_2. It is well known that bladder cancer can metastasize to the lung and also to the bones. Again this is stage D_2.

Reference is also made to the same figure that clearly describes the stages using the international and Union Internationale Contre le Cancer (UICC) staging system for bladder cancer.

When using imaging techniques—transvesical ultrasound scan (US) or CT scan—the difference between stage O and A is not clear; however, US, CT, and MRI can differentiate between the types of superficial invasion (B_1 or T_2).

For deeper tumor invasion, CT, MRI, and angiography are useful. Technetium scans are also useful in determining regional metastases, e.g., lymph node or bony invasion. In our experience, Technetium scans can also detect distant metastases, i.e., lung, liver, and brain.

After biopsy, a distinct pathologic diagnosis can be made between stages O, A, and B_1 (T_a, T_1, and T_2, respectively).

After anesthesia, the pelvic bimanual examination can detect advanced bladder cancer with some fixation. There is a zone where the exact tumor stage is unclear after bimanual examination.

The clinical staging of bladder tumor is useful and important (Fig. 2). The illustration describes the imaging techniques which can be used for the different grades and stages of tumor, shown on the left-hand side. On the right-hand side, transurethral resection is proposed where the tumor is still resectable down to stage T_{3a} (stage B_2 in the older American Classification).

It should be kept in mind that there is a border on which further infiltration or progression can lead to an unresectable tumor. A CT scan, MRI study, or angiography is useful in our opinion; however, the bimanual pelvic examination under anesthesia may reveal a mass that is only slightly movable or fixed, particularly in stage C cancers. In stage D cancer there is obvious fixation on bimanual examination. It is probably true that in stage D cancers there will be metastatic spread to other body sites—for example, the lungs and skeletal bones. The tumor is probably unresectable by standard means in this higher stage. Chemotherapy, immunotherapy, and/or irradiation are the only alternatives.

In bladder tumors, accurate preoperative evaluation of depth of infiltration is not always possible. Large tumors with wide and fixed bases, which are palpable by bimanual pelvic examination, are nearly always deeply invasive. The extent of their invasion can often be demonstrated by pelvic angiography. However, these cases preclude any type of radical surgical treatment. They should be considered as candidates for immunotherapy, chemotherapy, and/or megavoltage irradiation.

It is generally agreed that superficial tumors (up to stage $T_2[B_1]$) are best treated by transurethral resection. The deeply invasive tumors beyond the halfway level in the muscle layer (stage $T_{3A}[B_2]$) frequently cannot be removed completely by transurethral resection without perforating the bladder wall. In these cases, more extensive surgical

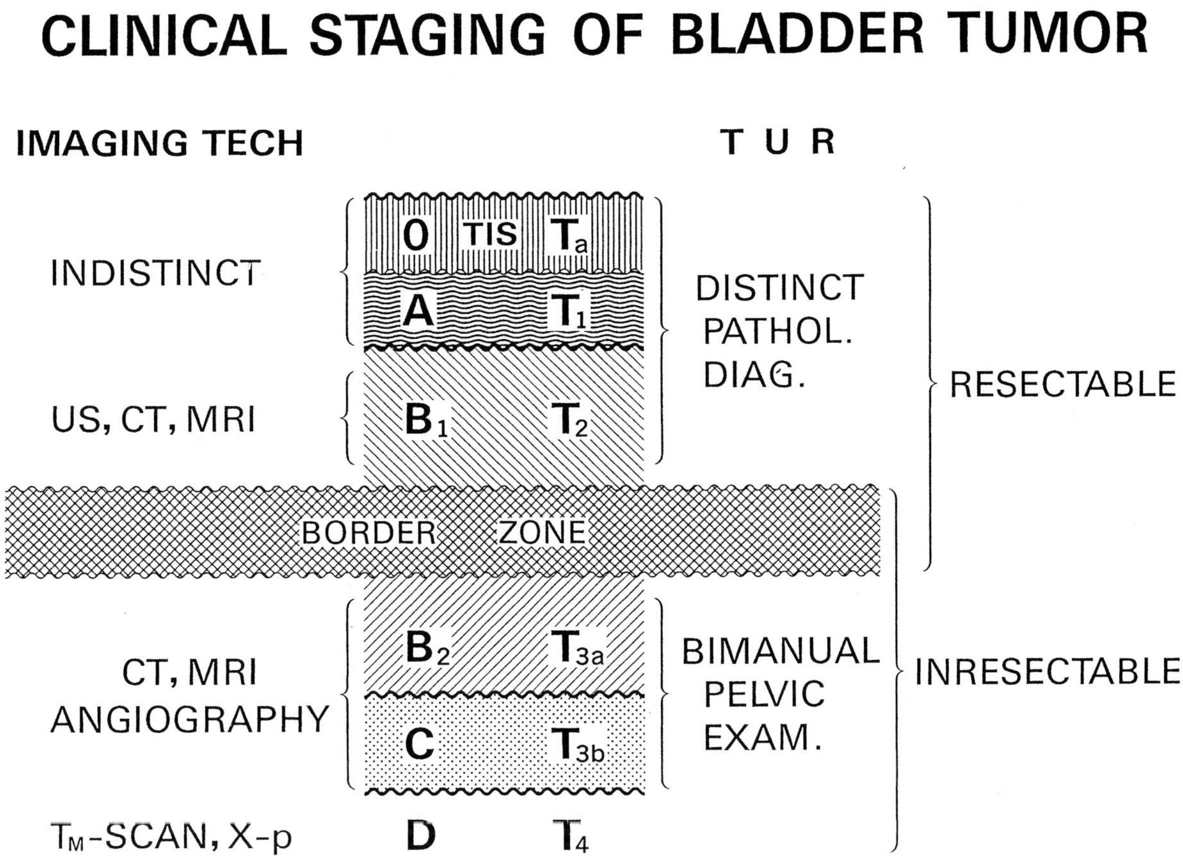

FIG. 2.
Clinical staging of bladder tumor.

measures such as total or radical cystectomy should be considered.

Staging should be precise when it is based on the microscopic study of the removed tumor and muscle at the site of deepest infiltration. Clinical staging before removal or partial, segmental resection of the whole layer of bladder wall is also helpful, although it will be less precise than pathologic staging.

In our experience in Japan, a remarkably high degree of accuracy can be achieved by using imaging modalities such as CT, ultrasound, MRI, and by careful bimanual pelvic examination under anesthesia. Transurethral bladder biopsies and resection of the involved bladder areas are performed. Palpable tumor within the bladder wall, with rare exception, represents deep infiltration of tumor. Therefore, the major clinical challenge is the accurate staging of tumors that cannot be felt by bimanual pelvic examination (Fig. 3).

Clinical staging of nonpalpable tumors depends principally on tissue removed by transurethral resection. In our experience, the majority of early nonpalpable tumors can be completely removed by a wider, transurethral excisional biopsy using the resectoscope.

The steps for removal consist of the following: 1) resecting all the tumor mass that projects into the bladder lumen down to the level of surrounding mucosa and placing the tumor in specimen bottle one; 2) resecting the bladder muscle beneath and at the periphery of the tumor, usually to the depth of one loop and placing the tumor fragments in specimen bottle two; and 3) resecting a thin layer of deeper wall, if it is possible, when tumor tissue is demonstrated on frozen section in tissue fragments at the convex border of the tumor.

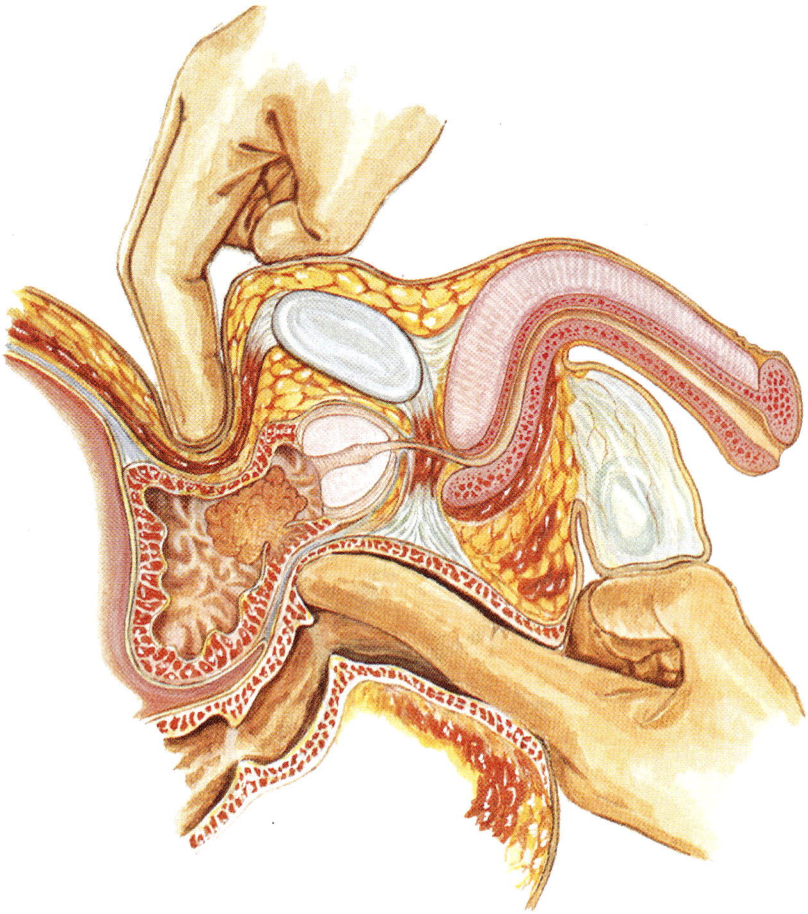

FIG. 3.
Bimanual pelvic examination in tumor staging.

Microscopic invasion into deep muscle should be suspected when tumor cells are detected on the convex side of the semicircular area resected, and narrow slivers of muscle are obtained. These tumors should be diagnosed as stage T_2 or higher. Tumors that have invaded only the concave or flat side and have not reached the convex side are nearly all in stage $T_2(B_1)$. The tumors that have invaded the submucosa but have not reached the muscle layer are usually in stage $T_1(A)$. According to Jewett, staging by multiple biopsies carefully performed by transurethral resection is very reliable.

However, significant staging inaccuracies may occur if we draw a midpoint or halfway line with this technique. The only clinically reliable information is whether the depth of the tumor infiltration was shallow enough to be removed or too deep to be removed by transurethral resection.

The resectable cancers may contain some tumor at the borderline $T_{3a}(B_2)$. On the other hand, unresectable tumor may also contain some borderline $T_2(B_1)$ growth. The long-term results between these two groups are quite different, and we can draw clear cut survival patterns from the group.

It is our present policy, when we have a borderline case, to subject the patient to a transurethral resection initially and remove the tumor as completely as possible. When we find that the transurethral resection was inadequate and we did not remove all the local tumor, or, when the tumor is unresectable, we consider further treatment such as radical cystectomy, irradiation, chemotherapy, or immunotherapy. On the other hand, when we find the tumor is resectable, transurethral resection of the tumor—monotherapy—

will be the treatment of choice, unless the pathological grade of the tumor is grade 3 or higher.

Regardless of location in the bladder, nearly every tumor can be removed by transurethral resection; success depends largely upon the training and skill of the surgeon. A tumor located in a vesical diverticulum is one of the most difficult to remove endoscopically. In our experience, nearly 99% of primary bladder tumors are accessible with the resectoscope.

For those inaccessible tumors that deeply invade muscle, partial cystectomy, total cystectomy, or radical cystectomy should be considered, depending on the grade and depth of tumor infiltration.

Tumors that have spread to the perivesical tissue and beyond as metastases are usually not amenable to complete surgical removal. They are best treated by immunotherapy, chemotherapy, and/or radiotherapy. Palliative operative procedures, such as urinary diversion and ligation of the internal iliac artery for bleeding, are performed if indicated.

STAGING BY TRANSVESICAL ULTRASOUND AND CT FOR BLADDER CANCER

Ultrasonic scans are depicted in Figure 4A–D. Subtle differences in the scans are due to a different response between the normal bladder wall and a pathologic bladder containing tumor. The examples are clearly shown in each of the four tumor samples. The tumor can be seen in varying sizes.

The patient has a tumor on the floor of the bladder and different ultrasonic views from the same tumor are demonstrated. In Figures 4A and B, the tumor is superficial. In Figures 4C and D, the tumor size and depth is increased, showing greater tumor depth.

COMPUTED TOMOGRAPHY OF BLADDER

A second patient has undergone a CT scan of the bladder (Fig. 5). Air occupies the lumen. A urine level on the floor is noted. The CT imaging clearly demonstrates the tumor area on the upper surface of the bladder.

We have had some experience with staging of bladder cancer by CT. In an early paper by our group,[1] we showed that one can clinically stage bladder cancer quite accurately by putting in a very low contrast urographic medium that will outline the lumen of the bladder. One is then able to see the differences in staining of the tumor itself using CT scanning. This staining, down to the mucosal lining, is absorbed by the tumor and one can actually see contrast differences. Intramuscular invasion superficially or in a deeper muscle layer can be ascertained with CT scans.

CYSTOSCOPIC FINDINGS OF BLADDER TUMOR

In this series of illustrations, Professor Koshiba has carefully drawn different configurations of bladder tumor. The very low stage O, or the early papillary tumor, has finger-like projections as shown. A higher stage has a broader base and the elevation from the base to the lumen of the bladder does show some growth in a vertical fashion.

Neovascularization can be seen and described (Fig. 6). In the earliest stages, only a few vascular markings may be seen next to the very small papilloma. As the tumor progresses, even though the actual volume may not increase, many more neovascular vessels can be seen as shown. This is classified as a high grade early tumor. When the tumor becomes invasive, such as we see in carcinoma in situ (CIS), the tumor borders are less well defined and the actual neovascularity takes on a much more impressive pattern, becoming more intense.

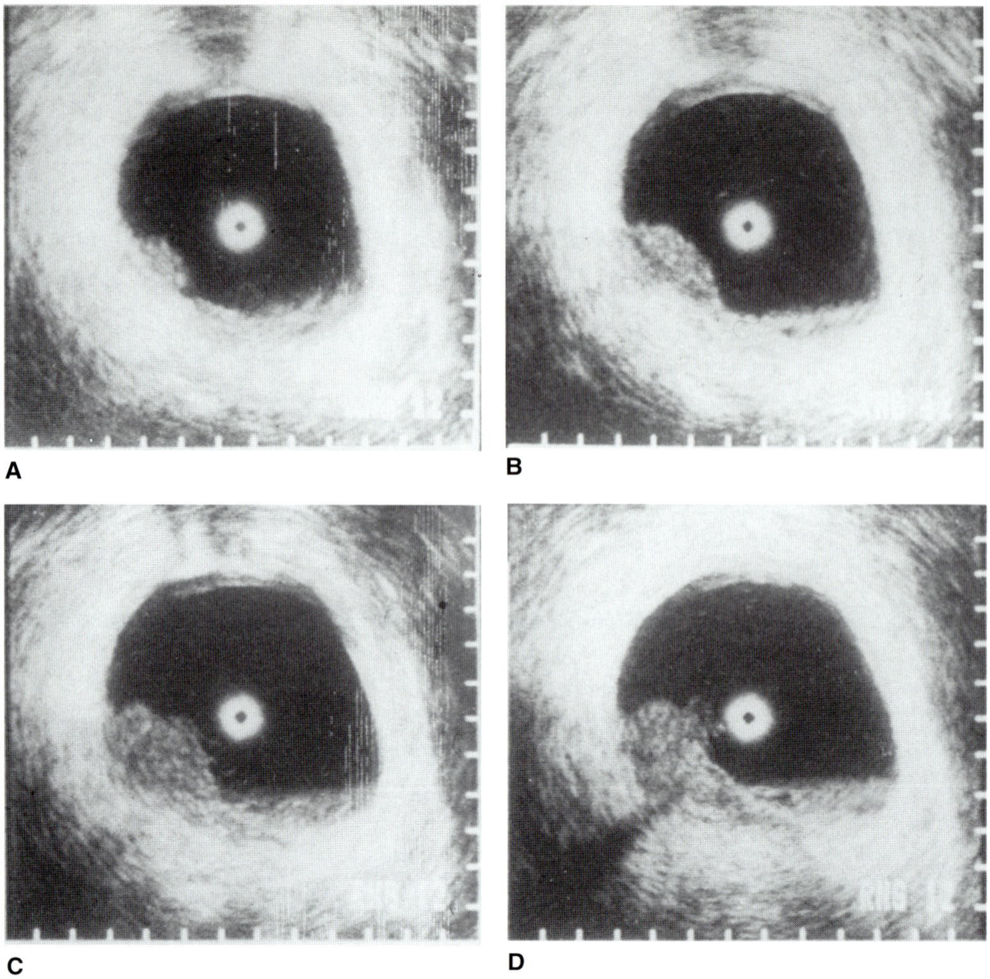

FIG. 4.
A–D. Different ultrasonic views of the same tumor on the floor of the bladder.

Preparation of the Patient and Anesthesia

The preoperative preparation is similar to that used in transurethral prostatic resection (TURP). A mild sedative is administered the night before. An enema is given the night before or the morning of the operation. Preoperative infection is treated by appropriate antibiotic therapy before the transurethral procedure.

Low spinal anesthesia is usually sufficient for the majority of cases. Epidural anesthesia is not adequate. The obturator muscular reflex that is caused by stimulation of the obturator nerve cannot be avoided with epidural anesthesia. Straining and sudden movement of the patient's leg during electroresection is seen when the high frequency current is used. Complete perforation of the bladder wall may occur in this instance. General anesthesia with an endotracheal tube and adequate use of muscle relaxants is recommended when deep resection is attempted at the lateral wall near the ureteral orifice, a site near the obturator nerve. However, local obturator nerve blockade,[2] unilateral or bilateral, will successfully prevent occurrence of violent jerking of the leg during resection of the tumor at the inferior, lateral bladder wall.

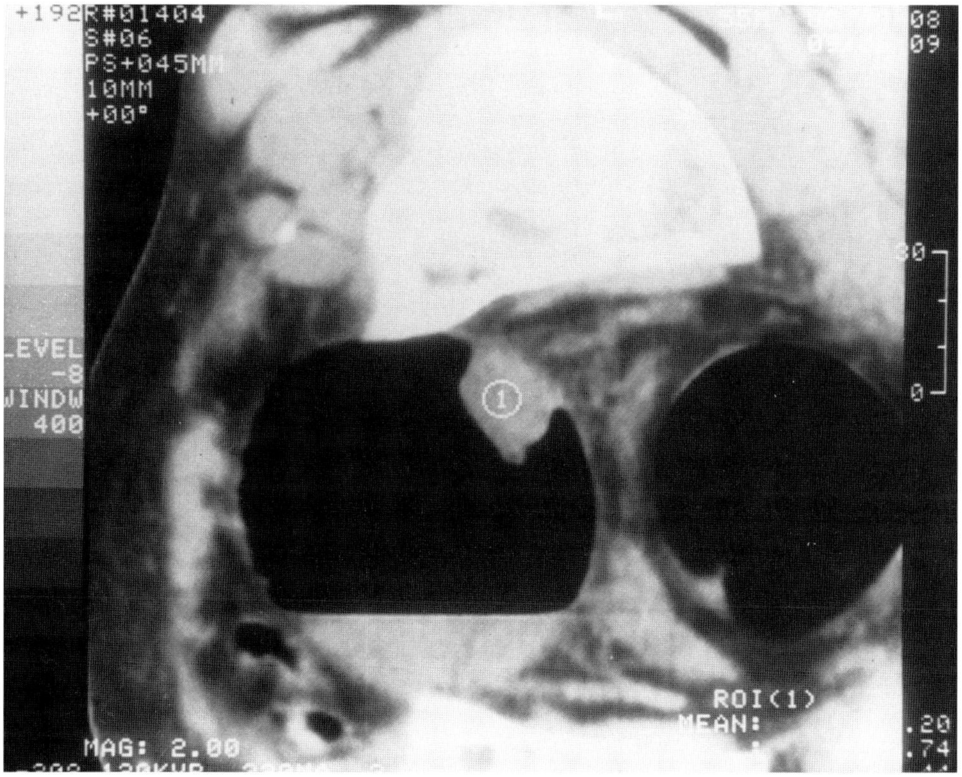

FIG. 5.
Computed tomography scan of the bladder.

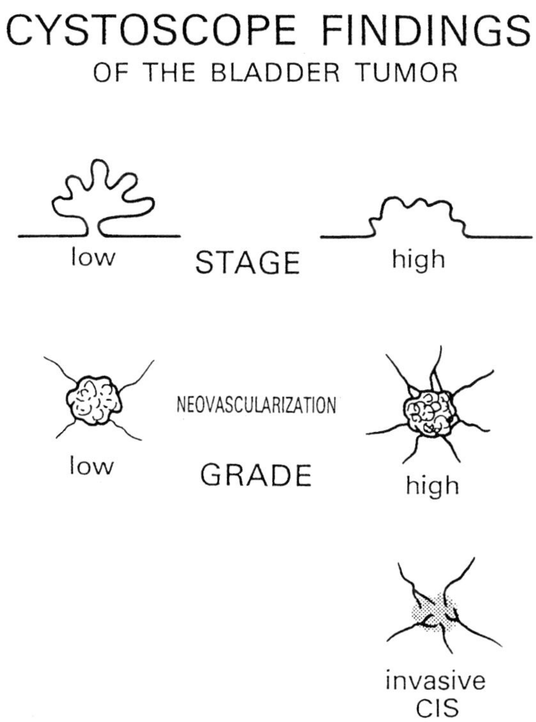

FIG. 6.
Cystoscopic findings of the bladder tumor.

Postoperative Management

A 22 French Foley catheter is used for postoperative urinary drainage and is maintained as long as hematuria is evident. If the tumor is small, the catheter is left indwelling for only a few days.

The use of appropriate antibiotics is recommended for treatment of existing infections and to prevent septicemia. Maintenance of a high fluid intake, and the intravenous use of mannitol solutions will increase urinary output and obviate the need for catheter irrigation. The increased urinary output will also diminish the occurrence of postoperative urinary infection.

FOLLOW-UP

Cystoscopic examination of the patient for possible recurrence is carried out at 3-month intervals for high-grade tumors and at 4-month intervals for low-grade tumors during the first 2 years. Cystoscopy procedures are increased to 6-month intervals during the second and third years; then they are performed at yearly intervals.

In most instances, the resected bladder wall will show complete healing in 3 or 4 months after transurethral resection; however, extensive fulguration or previous high-dose megavoltage irradiation may retard healing.

Recurrence of a tumor of equal or higher grade malignancy at the original site on the bladder wall is a grave clinical sign. In most instances this means either that the previous transurethral resection was inadequate, or that infiltration was of a higher stage. Tumors could not be completely removed even by a skilled surgeon. If there is a raised edge at the periphery of the resected area, it signifies unresected tumor; the patient should be readmitted for transurethral resection.

If there is a recurrent wide-based tumor at the bottom of the previously resected scar, it usually signifies that the tumor has invaded far more deeply and cannot be removed by transurethral resection. The patient should be readmitted for partial or total cystectomy and lymph node dissection. Preoperative megavoltage irradiation should also be administered (2000 rad) prior to surgery.

Complete healing of the resected bladder wall, covered by urothelium, signifies complete transurethral resection of bladder tumor in that area, even though there might be multiple recurrences in other areas of bladder mucosa. Transurethral resection should be repeated to remove these new tumors regardless of the number of recurrences, as long as they are accessible with the resectoscope.

Operative Techniques

136. Routine Strategy

The position of the patient on the operating table and the preparation of the operative field are the same as those employed in transurethral resection of the prostate. After satisfactory anesthesia is induced, bimanual pelvic examination is performed. A plastic anal-rectal shield for the gloved index finger is useful for this purpose.

The number and size of each lesion and the degree of infiltration must first be estimated. The resection is then begun on the surface of the lesion. The loop is always placed at the posterior and superior borders of the lesion to begin the resection. Bleeders must be controlled individually as they occur in order to maintain good visualization throughout the procedure. The steps of resection are as follows:

136-1A. *The tumor mass that projects into the bladder cavity is resected down to the level of the bladder mucosa.* Fragments are placed in specimen bottle one.

136-1B. *Bladder muscle beneath and at the periphery of the tumor is resected to the depth of one loop.* Sections of this tissue are placed in specimen bottle two.

136-1C. The pathologist should be oriented regarding the significance of different tumor samples; he/she must be informed of the fact that the *deep side of each tissue fragment will have a convex contour* corresponding to the shape of the loop. The insertion of a pin through selected tissue fragments for frozen section, from superficial to deep sites, is of great assistance to the pathologist; this helps to orient him/her in preparing the vertical tissue sections and in properly staging the tumor. Gross invasion deep in the muscle layer can be recognized by the granular appearance of the resected surface, with a lack of normal pattern in the muscle fibers.

136-2A. When the tumor has been proven by frozen section to invade tissue fragment obtained at the contex border of the muscle layer, the tumor possibly invaded deeper. Gross invasion deep in the muscle layer can be recognized by the granular appearance of the resected surface, with a lack of normal pattern in the muscle fiber.

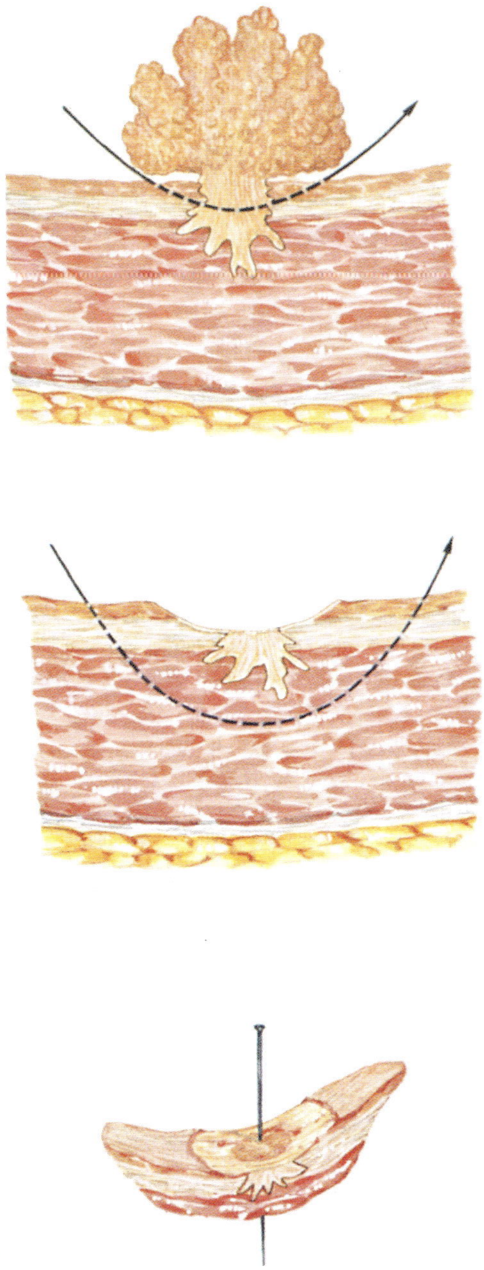

A

B

C

136-1

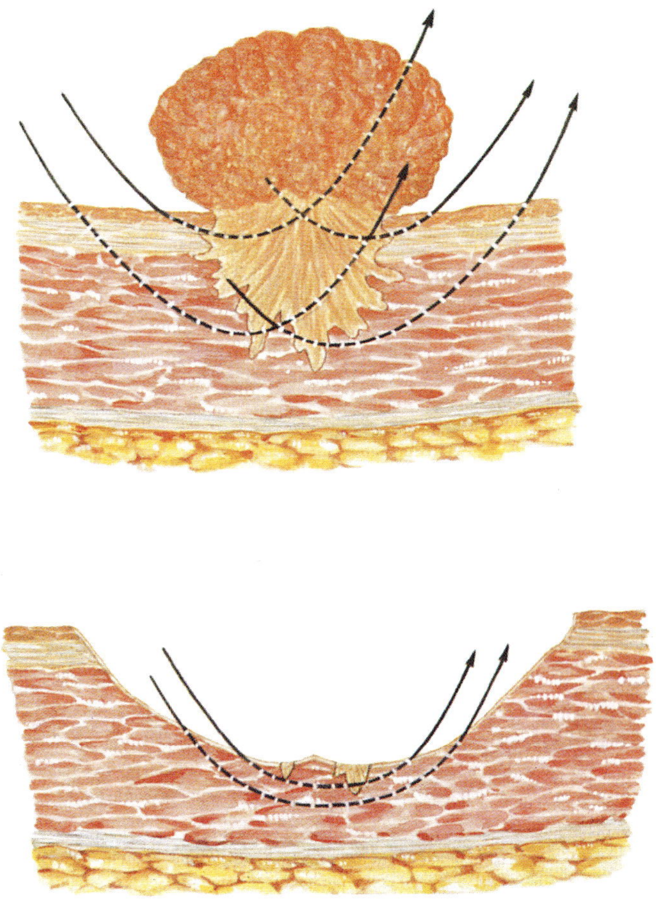

A

B

136-2

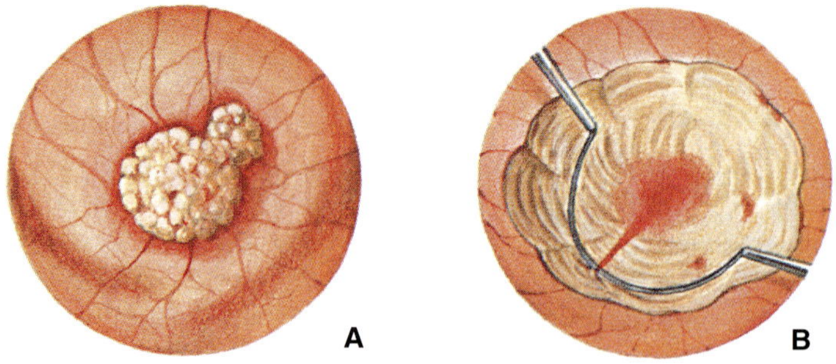

136-3

136-2B. *A thin layer of tissue from deeper muscle is resected,* if possible. This thin section is also placed in bottle two.

It is inadvisable to proceed deeper; but an experienced surgeon can proceed deeper into the muscle layer, even at the upper portion of the bladder.

136-3A. Endoscopic appearance of a sessile papillary tumor of the bladder.

136-3B. A spurtin arterial bleeder is secured after complete resection of the tumor intohe muscle layer.

137. Specific Operative Hints

The bladder should not be overdistended with fluid. When the bladder is overdistended with irrigating fluid, the wall becomes thin and may be easily perforated, even with a "shallow scoop" by the resectoscope loop. In addition, the lesion fades away from the tip of the resectoscope as the bladder becomes distended and the procedure becomes more difficult and troublesome.

137-1. *A lesion near the anterior or lateral vesical neck may fall away from the visual field* of the resectoscope as the bladder becomes distended; this also makes the tumor inaccessible.

137-2. On the other hand, *when the bladder is not distended, the lesion is more easily visualized and may be trapped by the loop.* The bladder wall is also thicker in its empty state and will not be easily penetrated even by a deep resection.

Once a deep resection is made in the bladder wall, overdistension of the bladder is avoided to prevent secondary rupture of the bladder wall. Therefore, the surgeon frequently empties the bladder and never overdistends the bladder with irrigating fluid throughout the operative procedure.

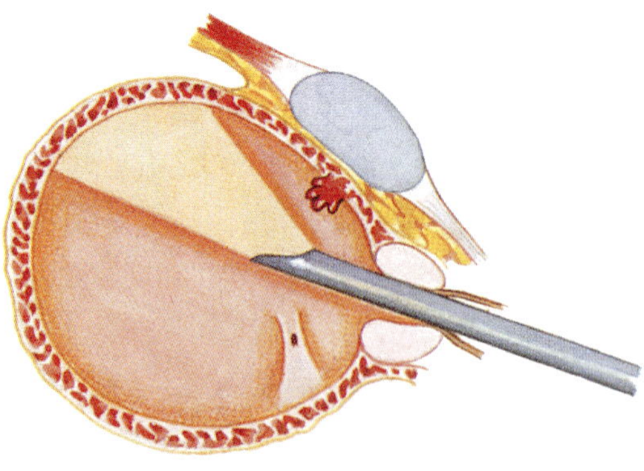

137-1

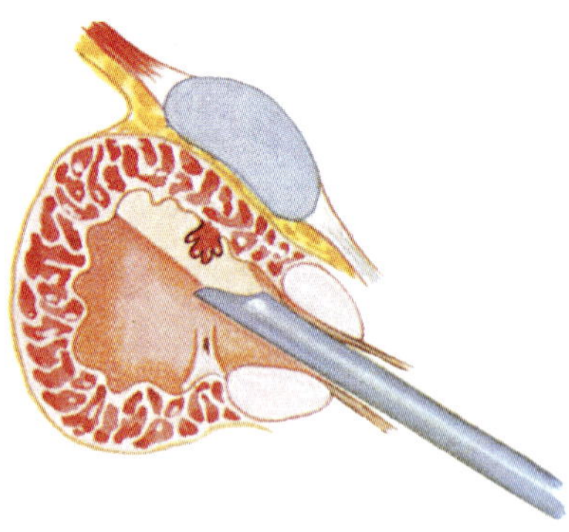

137-2

Use the Other Hand as an Aid During Resection

137-3. *Elevation of the bladder wall,* with the index finger of the opposite free hand in the rectum or vagina, *is very helpful in gaining access to the lesion* with the resectoscope loop.

137-4. *Compression of the suprapubic abdomen is also a helpful technique* in gaining access to a lesion at the dome or anterior wall of the bladder. Use of the one-hand resectoscope is recommended for these procedures.

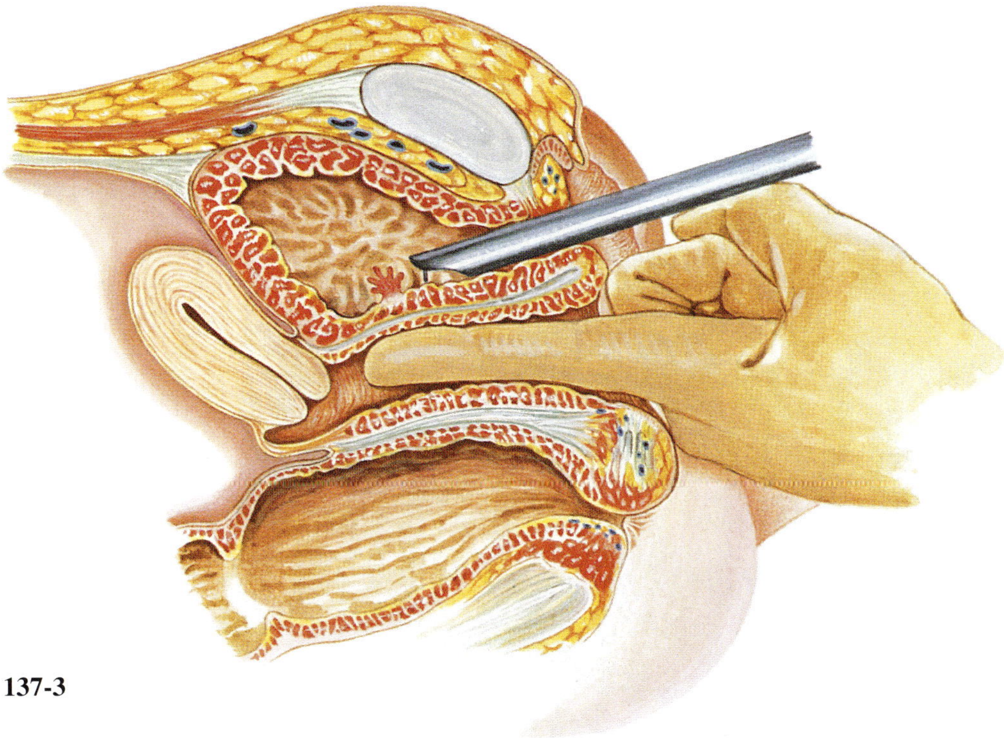

137-3

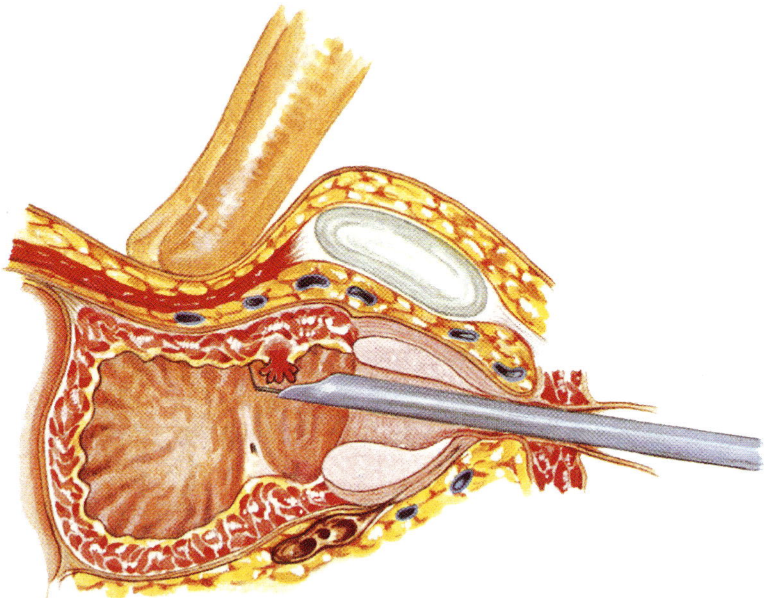

137-4

138. Patient Positioning

The position of the patient is the same as that used for routine cystoscopy. The knees should be widely spread to allow adequate space between them for manipulation of the resectoscope, especially in resecting a lesion at the lateral wall of the bladder.

When a lesion is observed at the anterior wall of the bladder, the thighs should be at a less acute angle with the body. Sharply abducted thighs displace the posterior urethra downward into the perineum, limiting accessibility of the resectoscope to the lesion at the anterior wall and dome of the bladder.

138-1. *The operating table is lowered and the surgeon's chair is elevated for resecting a lesion in the recess behind the trigone or posterior wall.* This position places the instrument in a more direct line to the lesion.

138-2. This advantage becomes more evident when *the operating table is shifted to the head-up and hip-down position.*

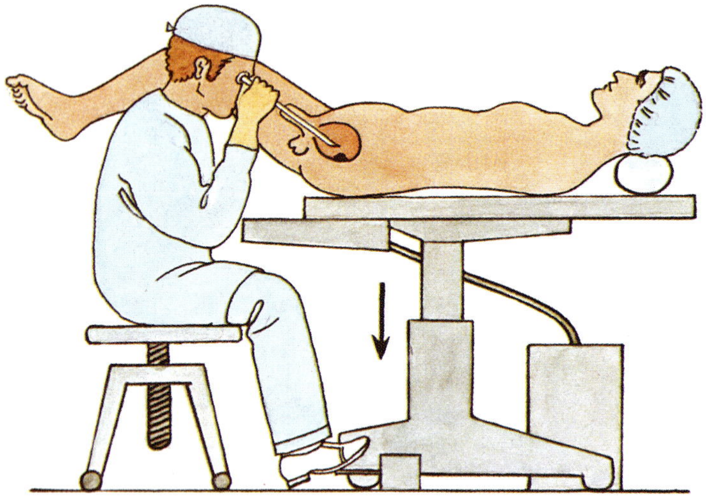

138-1

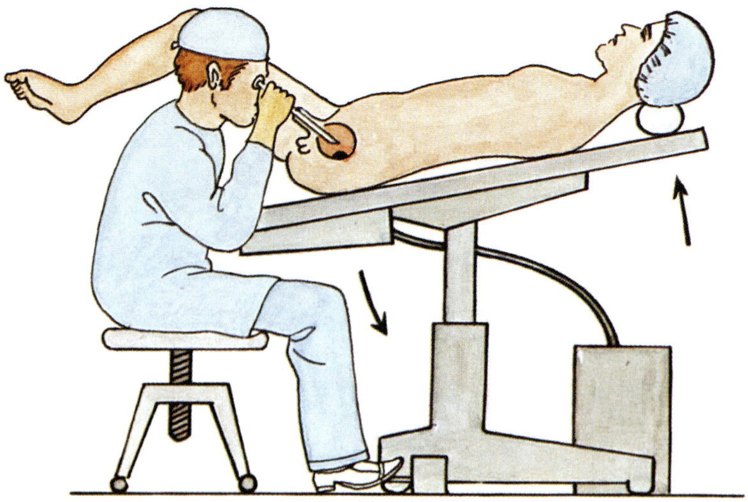

138-2

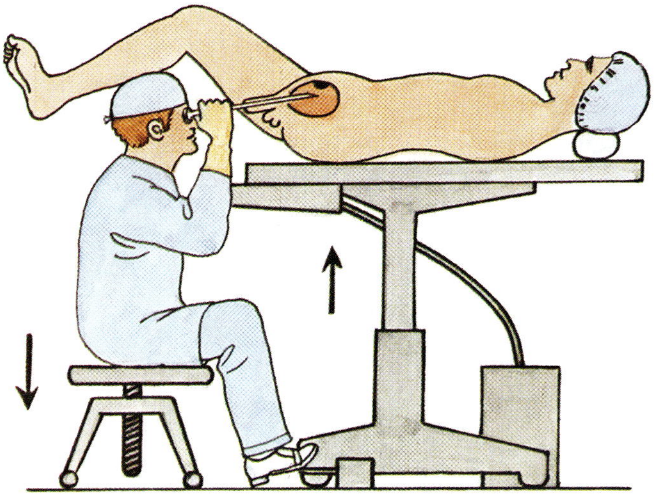

138-3

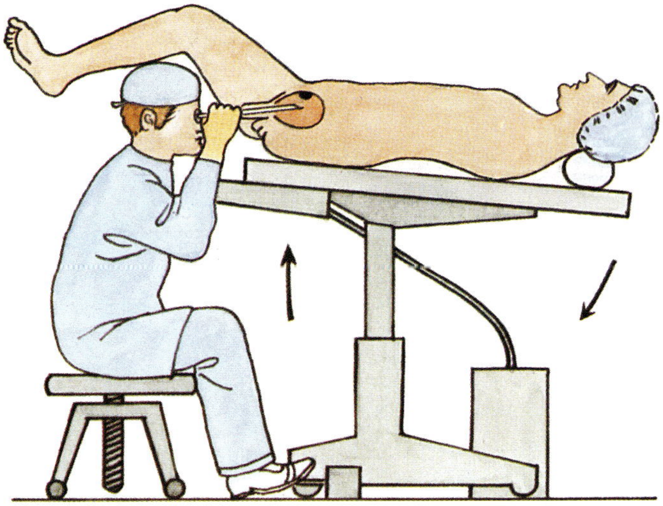

138-4

138-3. *Raising the operating table and lowering the surgeon's chair when a lesion is located on the anterior bladder wall helps the surgeon gain access to the lesion.*

138-4. This advantage also becomes more evident if *the operating table is shifted to the head-down and hip-up position.*

An effective combination of these three techniques increases the surgeon's access to the bladder lesions. In our experience, about 99% of early stage tumors are accessible with the resectoscope.

Management of Complications

OPERATIVE AND POSTOPERATIVE BLEEDING

Bleeding should be controlled as it occurs during the procedure. All arterial bleeders should be completely controlled before the transurethral resection is terminated. Sudden elevation in blood pressure or any straining, retching, or abrupt movement of the patient, after the patient has been moved from the operating table, may result in profuse bleeding. Vigorous bleeding, not controlled by continuous irrigation, is usually from one of the bladder arterioles in the resected area. It is recommended that the patient be immediately returned to the operating room so that the bleeding points may be fulgurated. It is unwise to procrastinate and hope for spontaneous cessation of arterial bleeding. Blood loss can be quite significant and must be replaced.

The quantity of blood lost cannot be accurately measured; gross estimations can be made by hemoglobin determinations during and after the operative procedure. It is advisable to start blood replacement before signs of shock appear.

Secondary hemorrhage is not frequent but may be anticipated 1 or 2 weeks after transurethral resection. It usually results from separation of the eschar from the resected bladder wall; delayed bleeding occurs if there is retained, devitalized tissue and infection. Bleeding usually is managed by bladder irrigation with removal of all clots and indwelling catheter drainage for 1 or 2 days.

PERFORATION OF THE BLADDER

Perforation of the bladder into the perivesical space is of no serious consequence if extravasation is recognized early and is limited to a small area. If any tumor is left at the time this occurs, care should be taken not to overdistend the bladder. The resection should be completed and hemostasis obtained while the bladder is only partially filled with irrigating fluid.

Foley catheter drainage should be maintained for at least 4 to 5 days. Irrigation of the bladder with an antitumor solution at the termination of the operation may be an effective measure in preventing tumor dissemination to the perivesical tissue. For example, thiotepa in the United States, triethylene glycol diglyceridyl ether (Epodyl) in Great Britain, and mitomycin-C (MMC) in Japan have been used for this purpose.

If extensive extravasation through a perforation of the bladder wall is suspected and if pain and swelling are predominantly suprapubic, surgical drainage should be instituted immediately. The technique is similar to that used for perforation of the prostatic capsule (see section 133–5). A small incision is made in the midline just above the symphysis pubis and extends through the fascia. The rectus abdominis muscles of the abdomen are separated; the prevesical space down to the region of the prostate is opened by blunt finger dissection; and one or two flat tubular drains are inserted into the inferior bladder surface, depending on the size of perforation.

INTRAPERITONEAL PERFORATION

This complication should be infrequent. The patient under spinal anesthesia will almost immediately complain of pain under the left diaphragm. Treatment is an immediate laparotomy to drain the intraperitoneal fluid and close the perforated wound in the bladder. If any tumor remains, a partial cystectomy may be performed at this time.

DAMAGE TO THE URETERAL ORIFICE AND SUBSEQUENT OBSTRUCTION

Damage to the ureteral orifice can occur during resection of a tumor near or at the orifice. The main problem to be avoided during resection of the tumor is destruction of a ureteral orifice. This complication may lead to ureteral stricture and partial or complete obstruction. It is important, therefore, to recognize the orifices. Indigo carmine given intravenously (5 mL) can help in locating the orifice. When ureteral damage occurs, the patient must be observed after the operation; every attempt must be made to preserve kidney function.

The ureter does not usually become obstructed if a pure cutting current and a fine gauge loop are used. The use of a blended or coagulating current is harmful to the ureteral orifice. When an active bleeder is observed near the ureteral orifice, careful "spot coagulation" should be done just on the bleeding point. Multiple coagulations of a large area should be avoided.

When damage to a ureteral orifice is observed, no special measures are required at the time of operation. The danger lies in fibrosis and stricture formation. Stricture of both ureters may lead to loss of kidney function. The patient should be under careful observation. A ureteral stent (JJ) may be used if dilitation of the appropriate orifice is deemed necessary. Creatinine determinations should be obtained at intervals. Necessary measures to relieve obstruction, such as ureteroneocystostomy, should be accomplished before the kidney loses significant function.

PROPHYLAXIS OF TUMOR RECURRENCE

A major problem is the high incidence of bladder tumor recurrence after transurethral resection.

Irrigation of the bladder with an antitumor solution at the termination of the operation is an effective measure in preventing tumor dissemination to the bladder wall or to the perivesical tissue.

Today, intravesical use of antitumor solutions either for treatment or prophylaxis of recurrence (or regrowth) have been employed worldwide. Adriamycin (ADM), MMC, Bleomycin (BLM), and Bacilllus Calmette-Guérin (BCG) are the popular antitumor drugs used for this purpose. However, the therapeutic dose of these antitumor solutions are often too irritative to the bladder mucosa. BCG cannot be used in the immediate postoperative period. We wait at least 8 weeks before instilling BCG into the bladder lumen.

Our present policy is to do a continuous instillation of more diluted and less irritative antitumor solutions for 3 consecutive days following transurethral resection of the bladder tumor while the patient is in the hospital. The antitumor drugs are diluted with saline solution 10× their intravesical treatment dose. A three-way Foley catheter, 22 Fr, is employed for this purpose and a slow drip of one of the antitumor solutions is continued at the rate of 2000 mL in 24 hours. Either ADM, MMC, or BLM are equally effective in reducing the recurrence rate by about 50%.[3]

References

1. Hamlin DJ, Cockett ATK, Burgener FA. Computed tomography of the pelvis: sagittal and coronal image reconstruction in the evaluation of infiltrative bladder carcinoma. J Comput Assist Tomogr 5:27–33, 1981.
2. Augspurger RR, Donohue RR. Prevention of obturator nerve stimulation during transurethral surgery. J Urol 123:170–172, 1980.
3. Koshiba K. TUR and implantation. In: Prout GR, Tanaki H, eds. New Concept of Bladder Cancer. Medical Research Center Co Ltd. 243–248, 1983.

Suggested Readings

Dean AL, Mostofi FK, Thompson RV. A restudy of the first fourteen hundred tumors in the Bladder Tumor Registry, AFIP. J Urol 71:571, 1954.

Hamlin DJ, Cockett ATK. Computed tomography of bladder. Staging of bladder cancer using low density opacification technique. Urology 13:331, 1979.

Hata T, Sano Y, Sugawara R, Matsumae A. Mitomycin, a new antibiotic from Streptomyces. J Antibiot Ser A 9(4):141, 1959.

Jewett HJ. Carcinoma of the bladder: influence of depth of infiltration on the 5-year results following complete extirpation of the primary growth. J Urol 67:672, 1952.

Jewett HJ, King LR, Shelley WM. A study of 365 cases of infiltrating bladder cancer: relation of certain pathological characteristics to prognosis after extirpation. J Urol 92:668, 1964.

Jewett HJ, Strong GH. Infiltrating carcinoma of bladder: relation of depth of penetration of bladder wall to incidence of local extension and metastases. J Urol 55:366, 1946.
Jones HC, Swinney J. Thiotepa in the treatment of tumors of the bladder. Lancet 2:615, 1961.
Kano M, Ito S. The effect of intracavitary chemotherapy after transurethral resection on the recurrence rate of superficial bladder cancers. Jpn J Clin Urol 27:403, 1973.
Koshiba K. Urinary bladder biopsy by means of transurethral resection. Jpn J Clin Urol 28:31, 1974.
Marshall VF. The relation of the preoperative estimate to the pathologic demonstration of the extent of vesical neoplasms. J Urol 68:714, 1952.
Milner WA. Urologic Surgery, 2nd ed. Hagerstown: Harper & Row, 1975.
Mishina T, Oda K, Murata S. Mitomycin C bladder instillation therapy for bladder tumors. J Urol 114:217, 1975.
Ogawa H. Intracavitary treatment of tumors of the bladder with cytotoxic agent (mitomycin C) and radioactive phosphorus. Jap J Urol 60:746, 1969.
Veenema RJ, Dean AL Jr, Uson AC, Roberts M, Longo F. Thiotepa bladder instillations: therapy and prophylaxis for superficial bladder tumors. J Urol 101:711, 1969.

Index

C

L

M

R

V

W